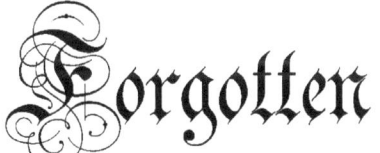 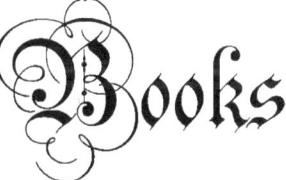

ISBN 978-0-260-23784-2
PIBN 11012729

1 MONTH OF
FREE
READING

at
www.ForgottenBooks.com

By purchasing this book you are eligible for one month membership to ForgottenBooks.com, giving you unlimited access to our entire collection of over 1,000,000 titles via our web site and mobile apps.

To claim your free month visit:
www.forgottenbooks.com/free1012729

English
Français
Deutsche
Italiano
Español
Português

www.forgottenbooks.com

Mythology Photography **Fiction**
Fishing Christianity **Art** Cooking
Essays Buddhism Freemasonry
Medicine **Biology** Music **Ancient
Egypt** Evolution Carpentry Physics
Dance Geology **Mathematics** Fitness
Shakespeare **Folklore** Yoga Marketing
Confidence Immortality Biographies
Poetry **Psychology** Witchcraft
Electronics Chemistry History **Law**
Accounting **Philosophy** Anthropology
Alchemy Drama Quantum Mechanics
Atheism Sexual Health **Ancient History**
Entrepreneurship Languages Sport
Paleontology Needlework Islam
Metaphysics Investment Archaeology
Parenting Statistics Criminology
Motivational

MEDICAL DIAGNOSIS

WITH

SPECIAL REFERENCE TO PRACTICAL MEDICINE.

A

GUIDE TO THE KNOWLEDGE AND DISCRIMINATION OF DISEASES.

BY

J. M. DA COSTA, M.D.,

LECTURER ON CLINICAL MEDICINE, AND PHYSICIAN TO THE PENNSYLVANIA HOSPITAL; FELLOW OF THE
COLLEGE OF PHYSICIANS OF PHILADELPHIA; MEMBER OF THE AMERICAN PHILOSOPHICAL SOCIETY;
OF THE PATHOLOGICAL SOCIETY OF PHILADELPHIA; FORMERLY PHYSICIAN TO THE PHILA-
DELPHIA HOSPITAL; CORRESPONDING MEMBER OF THE NEW YORK PATHOLOGICAL
SOCIETY, ETC. ETC.

Illustrated with Engravings on Wood.

THIRD EDITION, REVISED.

PHILADELPHIA:

J. B. LIPPINCOTT & CO.

1870.

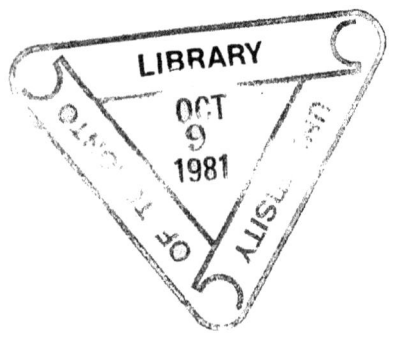

PREFACE TO THE THIRD EDITION.

ANOTHER edition of this work having been called for, I have revised it, and in some parts extended it; I trust, in all, improved it. In submitting it again to the profession, I indulge the hope that this edition may meet with the same favor as its predecessors.

1609 WALNUT STREET,
  PHILADELPHIA, July, 1870.

(iii)

PREFACE TO THE FIRST EDITION.

My chief aim in writing this work has been to furnish advanced students and young graduates of medicine with a guide that might be of service to them in their endeavors to discriminate disease. I have sought to offer to those members of the profession who are about to enter on its practical duties a book on Diagnosis of an essentially practical character,—one neither so meagre in detail as to be next to useless when they encounter the manifold and varying features of disease, nor so overladen with unnecessary detail as to be unwieldy and lacking in precise and readily-applicable knowledge.

In executing my undertaking, two plans offered themselves: either to describe morbid states in compliance with the usual pathological classification followed in treatises on the Practice of Medicine, or to group them according to their marked symptoms. The former plan would have been far the easier, but the latter seemed to me the more suitable for a volume of this kind; and although it has involved much labor, and has rendered the task much more difficult of accomplishment, its advantages appeared to me so great that I have adopted it throughout. That this attempt at a purely clinical classification is not perfect, I am fully aware. But with all its shortcomings, I venture to hope that it will not be devoid of value as an aid in their studies to those for whom it is intended.

Some of the statements made may appear too absolute, and as not taking sufficient notice of the many exceptions which may arise; but it was impossible to avoid this without very lengthy discussion: and even in the lengthiest discussion all exceptions and all possible points of fallacy would not have been mentioned: for Nature does not limit herself in her irregularities any more than in her rules. The text must, therefore, be looked upon as treating only of general laws and of their most notable infractions ; in fact, but as a series of etchings, with here and there a prominent figure shaded, but not as an attempt to reproduce the colors of an original whose varied hues could not be closely copied, even by the hand of a master.

The main object of this work is, what its title implies, the consideration of Medical Diagnosis.   In connection with this, however, I have endeavored to take cognizance of the prognosis of individual affections, and, where it could be done without interfering with the plan of the book, to give a summary of the indications for their treatment.   Occasionally the record of cases has been introduced by way of elucidation.   To have done this to a much greater extent, though in some respects desirable, would have swelled the work to an inordinate size.

The wood-cuts employed as illustrations are all original.   Many are from sketches, or at least are based on sketches, taken directly from cases of interest, and improved either by the skilful hand of Dr. Packard, or by Mr. Wilhelm, the artist who has so faithfully engraved them.   While acknowledging my obligations to them, I must also express my indebtedness to Dr. Richard J. Dunglison for his valuable assistance in making the index to this volume.

PHILADELPHIA, *April*, 1864.

CONTENTS.

INTRODUCTION.

CHAPTER I.

EXAMINATION OF PATIENTS, AND SOME SYMPTOMS OF GENERAL IMPORT

CHAPTER II.

DISEASES OF THE BRAIN, SPINAL CORD, AND THEIR NERVES.

CHAPTER III.

DISEASES OF THE UPPER AIR-PASSAGES.

CHAPTER IV.

DISEASES OF THE CHEST.

SECTION I.

DISEASES OF THE LUNGS.

CONTENTS.

CHAPTER V.

DISEASES OF THE MOUTH, PHARYNX, AND ŒSOPHAGUS.

CHAPTER VI.

DISEASES OF THE ABDOMEN.

SECTION I.

DISEASES OF THE STOMACH.

SECTION II.

DISEASES OF THE INTESTINES AND PERITONEUM.

SECTION III.

DISEASES OF THE LIVER.

CHAPTER VII.

ON THE URINE, AND ON DISEASES OF THE URINARY ORGANS.

CHAPTER VIII.

DROPSY.

CHAPTER IX.

DISEASES OF THE BLOOD.

CHAPTER X.

RHEUMATISM AND GOUT.

CHAPTER XI.

FEVERS.

CHAPTER XII.

DISEASES OF THE SKIN.

CHAPTER XIII.

POISONS AND PARASITES.

LIST OF ILLUSTRATIONS.

MEDICAL DIAGNOSIS.

INTRODUCTION.

GENERAL CONSIDERATIONS.

THE study of any complicated subject leads of necessity to its arrangement into branches. Closely connected as these are, and forming always parts of a whole, they are not only capable of distinct treatment, but frequently become more intelligible as they are so treated. This is made very manifest in investigating disease. The extent of ground the inquiry covers has rendered it imperative to map it out into various provinces, which, however intimately united, may be with convenience separately surveyed. One comprises the laws and facts common to individual affections; in another are gathered together all relating to their causes; another embraces the consideration of their detection and the full recognition of their nature. It is the purpose of these pages to examine this department somewhat minutely, and especially that portion of it coming within the range of the practitioner of medicine. In so doing it will become apparent how *diagnosis*, for such the distinction of disease is technically called, is partly a science, partly an art: a science, because it comprehensively takes account of general facts, and of principles based on those facts; an art, because it demands a cognizance of the means, and their application to arrive at the desired result.

To consider, then, medical diagnosis in all its bearings, it will be necessary not only to hold up to view the morbid states met with in the examination of the sick, but to inquire

2 (17)

in what manner they may be most readily recognized and explored, and how their differences may be made available in the discrimination of one ailment from another. In a study of this kind, an investigation of symptoms plays unavoidably a prominent part. In truth, the detection of disease is the product of close observation of symptoms, and of correct deduction from these symptoms.

The first requirement therefore for an accurate diagnosis is to learn to recognize morbid signs. But the art of observation this implies is not easy, and cannot be thoroughly acquired except by practice. No one aspiring to become a skilful observer can trust exclusively to the light reflected from the writings of others; he must carry the torch in his own hands, and himself look into every recess. The knowledge obtained from reading is, however, serviceable in this way. It aids in overcoming one of the main difficulties at first experienced,—to know where to look and what to look for. There are in almost every affection some symptoms which can hardly escape the merest beginner; but also some which do not appear on the surface, and which to find tax the skill of the experienced physician. And it is especially in this search after hidden signs that medical information as well as cultivated tact is demanded.

Now, to recognize the manifestations of disease, whether they are or are not readily perceptible, we have to employ our eyes and ears, our sense of touch and of smell. Formerly we could go no further than these senses unassisted would carry us. But science has lent its aid, and furnished means by the help of which we can detect clearly what before we could not detect at all, or of what at best we only caught a glimpse. We now possess instruments by which we ascertain with accuracy the size of organs and their play. With thermometers we tell the heat of various parts of the body to a fraction of a degree. Specific-gravity bottles, and other measures devised for the purpose, inform us of the relative gravity of fluids. The microscope gives at a glance insight into matters which the naked eye fails even to perceive. And chemistry, with its marvellous teachings, is rendering our knowledge of many morbid states admirably and amazingly complete. Then the sagacity of modern times has taught us to enlist the sense of hearing, and demonstrated how a disciplined ear may detect the workings of disease in cavities into which the eye cannot penetrate. The effect of all these improved methods of study has been to give an immense impetus to clinical research, and in this manner to lead to the construction of a solid groundwork of experience in striking contrast with the looseness and wild vagaries of former times. The advance in diagnosis thus attained forms indeed one of the most pleasing portions of medical history.

When, by means of the aided or unaided senses, the symptoms of the malady have been discovered, the next step toward a diagnosis is a proper appreciation of their significance and of their relation toward each other. Knowledge, and, above all, the exercise of the reasoning faculties, are now indispensable. The daily habit of investigating disease; a scrutinizing study of the anatomical lesions; chemistry, with its most searching analyses; the microscope, with the wonders it reveals,—are all of little use, unless we have been taught the necessity of placing the morbid signs they lay bare in connection with each other, and of considering in individual cases their respective value. Were it otherwise, the science of diagnosis would be simply a matter of memory. It is, however, this very analysis of symptoms, and the lengthy process of induction attending it, which make medical diagnosis so difficult and so unattractive to the beginner. He sees that by reflection and reasoning on what are frequently but indirect manifestations, he must find the seat and nature of disorders hidden from his view. Nor is it reasoning on the ascertained facts alone that is required: the premises may be but probabilities; for, in truth, diagnosis deals at times with the logic of probabilities as much as with the logic of patent facts.

Now we are greatly aided in appreciating the import of morbid signs, and in interpreting them correctly, by already existing knowledge. We look to landmarks which our predecessors have erected, and the gradually accumulated science of semeiology, rightly employed, furnishes the clue to the

discovery of the disease. Thus the stores which medicine
has laboriously collected during centuries can be used with
advantage by all, and exist for the good of all.

But an acquaintance with semeiology is far from being the
sole guide to diagnosis, nor does it at once help to a recognition of the malady. There are few symptoms in themselves distinctive; and often a symptom may be due to one
of several causes. Semeiology informs us of these different
causes; but to find out the precise meaning of the abnormal
manifestation in an individual case, we have to draw our
inference from all the signs encountered—to compare them
with each other; to seek out those that are in the background.
We are thus arriving, step by step, at the explanation of the
morbid appearances, the starting-point in deduction always
being what is known of the affection whose presence is suspected, and whose symptoms we are contrasting with those
before us. For the conclusion to be valid and exact, it is of
course requisite that each part of the testimony have the
proper position assigned to it. In reasoning correctly on
symptoms, the same laws apply as in reasoning correctly on
any other class of phenomena : the mental process is the
same; the facts have to be sifted and weighed, not merely
indiscriminately collected. And while the intellectual act is
being performed, much collateral evidence is to be sought
for before a final judgment is given; especially is it necessary
to view the symptoms with constant reference to the age, sex,
and habits of the patient, and to the circumstances amid which
the disorder develops itself.

To accomplish all this effectually, the physician has need
of much and varied knowledge. He must be master of
something more than of that information supplied to him by
semeiology. He must be an anatomist to pronounce with
certainty on the seat of the malady; a physiologist to appreciate the aberration of functions. Above all, he must be a
pathologist in the full sense of the term: he must understand
the antagonism between diseases; the frequency with which
they coexist; the influence of remedial agents on them; and
be cognizant of their natural history and of the general laws
governing them,—for how else can he form an estimate of

morbid action while it is in progress? Then it is desirable that he should be aware of what are their current divisions and classifications. From what has already been represented, it is evident that he must also be a correct reasoner; for even a good observer will, by bad reasoning, arrive at a faulty diagnosis, just as sometimes a bad observer may, by the same process, blunder into the truth. There is, indeed, no end to the extent of knowledge which may be brought to bear in working out a conclusion regarding the character and seat of a malady. The habit of observation once acquired, information of the most varied kind will, by an accurate reasoner, be made tributary to the completeness of the diagnosis. Every fresh acquirement tends to enlarge our powers of insight. Just as in nature, the higher we ascend, the more fully lies the view before us.

Having thus indicated the elements of an accurate and thorough diagnosis, we may next inquire in what way it is most speedily and conveniently arrived at when at the bedside. The main facts of the case on which the deductions are to be based are of course first elicited; and we shall presently see how this may be most effectually done. We lay hold of the main facts, and especially of those which are the most direct signs of the morbid action. They are coupled together, and the inquiry started as to what organ they point as the seat of the malady. This often has been already determined by the very method of the examination, and we therefore proceed at once to investigate the precise nature of the disorder by analyzing the symptoms and the previous history. Sometimes, however, the site of the disease does not admit of being definitely fixed upon, or we can only in a general manner decide upon the function impaired. Again, as in idiopathic fevers, we may find no signs of local disease, —merely those of a general disturbance. In any of these instances clinical experience steps in to explain the phenomena as far as possible, and to inform us in what affections they occur. It may be only in one, then the desired goal is at once attained. But, as above stated, there are few signs in themselves pathognomonic. It is therefore to be ascertained which one of the disorders is before us that special pathology

teaches may yield the symptoms encountered.   One of these
is taken up.   Its symptoms are placed side by side with
those present.   They accord in some respects, but not in all.
Moreover, in searching for some of the phenomena which
the supposed malady gives rise to, these are not found.   The
view is abandoned, and another taken up.   It agrees in all
particulars.   The diagnosis is made.   Yet when the diagnosis
is thus arrived at, we have, before it can be considered as
complete and be acted upon, still to determine whether or
not any other morbid state exists, and to take into account
the patient's general condition and his individuality.

To cite a case in illustration.   A person consults us for a
cough brought on by exposure.   He has been sick for four
or five days, having been previously in good health.   We
notice, on examining him, that his breathing is hurried, and
that he has fever; the lower portion of one side of the chest
is dull on percussion, and the respiration there is wanting;
the action and sounds of the heart are normal.   The facts
point to the lung or its covering as the seat of the disorder.
We know, furthermore, from the history and the febrile
symptoms, that we have to deal with an acute affection.
What are the acute pulmonary affections? Acute bronchitis;
acute phthisis; acute pleurisy; acute pneumonia.   In all
occur fever, cough, and impaired breathing.   Is it acute
pneumonia? No; for, notwithstanding there is in this complaint, in addition to the general symptoms mentioned, dulness on percussion, such as we have here, the dulness is
associated with a blowing respiration; whereas in the case
before us no respiration is heard.   Let us look at the sputum,
and see if it is tenacious and rusty colored.   It is not; it
is thin and frothy.   Moreover, the breathing, although hurried, is less hurried than it is apt to be in inflammation of
the lung.   But acute pleurisy may explain all the signs.   The
patient, too, when questioned, states that he had at the onset
a sharp pain in his side; and this, we are aware, takes place
in pleurisy.   The vocal vibrations, likewise, are noticed to
be absent on one side of the chest, which, when measured, is
found to be enlarged.   This corresponds in all points with
what happens in pleurisy in the stage of effusion.   The disease

is, therefore, acute pleurisy in the stage of effusion. We finish the diagnosis by ascertaining the existence or non-existence of other maladies, and by taking note of the severity of the complaint; that it has occurred in a young and robust person of good habits; and that the symptomatic fever is very active.

This process of arriving at an opinion is the simplest. It is one in which the investigation of the case is to some extent carried on while the deductions are being made. And by habit it is astonishing how rapidly it may be performed. The mind works unconsciously, and a decision is, to all appearance, formed intuitively, which surprises the inexperienced by its readiness and precision. This method aims, so far as the symptoms permit, at a direct diagnosis. But, in truth, it is often what is called *differential*: that is, it takes cognizance of and dwells on the essential signs by which one disease can be discriminated from another which it resembles.

Sometimes, instead of attaining the desired result in the manner proposed, we are obliged to judge of the nature of the malady entirely by finding out what it is not. The various diseases capable of producing all, or even some, of the striking symptoms observed, are enumerated. They are one by one considered and set aside, until by this process of pure *exclusion* the mischief is brought to light. Thus, to use again the example just given, we should have to assign reasons why the disease is neither acute pneumonia, nor bronchitis, nor acute phthisis, and in this way determine it to be acute pleurisy. But to prove what a thing is, by proving all that it is not, is a very tedious process; and we must be quite certain that really *all* morbid states which may give rise to the symptoms encountered are thought of and inquired into, otherwise our conclusion may be fallacious, though reasoned out in the most logical manner. Moreover, our knowledge of many pathological conditions is so imperfect that we are not fully cognizant of, or able at once to discern the more characteristic signs; nor can the symptoms be taken hold of and arranged in such a way as shall permit us to make nice distinctions without a lengthy and laborious plan of procedure. Owing to these drawbacks, diagnosis by exclusion is not, on ordinary occasions, much employed, nor, indeed, is it to be recommended. Yet in difficult and obscure cases, where the accustomed pathway is blocked up, it may enable us to pass by obstacles otherwise insurmountable.

But can we by this, or by any other road, always reach a certain diagnosis? We cannot, and for several reasons: The patient may deceive us, wilfully or unintentionally. It may be necessary, for the confirmation of the opinion formed, to obtain an accurate history of the case, and circumstances may render this impossible. The disorder may be so rare that its symptoms are not understood. There may be several lesions present, the signs of one masking or neutralizing the signs of the other.

The first of the causes mentioned is a source of error difficult to guard against. To escape punishment, to avoid disagreeable duty, to excite compassion, to obtain a compliance with unreasonable wishes, or sometimes from the mere love of deception, symptoms may be stated to exist which do not exist, or may be imitated and artificially produced. Persons who thus feign disease are numerous. They are found in all occupations and all classes of society. They abound in the army and navy. Hysterical women and hypochondriacs go to swell the list. These, indeed, suffer mostly some inconvenience, but exaggerate it immensely, and, by deceiving themselves, end by deceiving, unless he be on his guard, their physician. On the other hand, disease actually in progress may be carefully concealed from motives of delicacy or from fear of the consequences.

An incorrect diagnosis from want of a proper history does not, on the whole, often occur. Patients are generally very willing to give a full account of themselves and of their distresses. Sometimes, however, the reverse happens. Mental anxiety or sorrow may be wearing the body out while the sufferer obstinately persists in hiding the cause of his waning health. We meet also with individuals so stupid that the most elaborate cross-examination fails to elicit anything like a connected history. Again, we may be unable to do so from the patient having lost the power of speech. A man is brought into a hospital unconscious. It is of the utmost importance to know how long he has been in this state, and what were his prior symptoms; unless some friend can supply the information, the most valuable diagnostic data are wanting.

In the rarity of a disease we have a serious drawback to its recognition. This may occasion an error of diagnosis in a twofold manner. The more distinctive symptoms may be so little understood, and the prominent features so nearly identical with those of a malady with the manifestations of which we are well acquainted, that a conclusion of the presence of the latter forces itself almost immediately on the mind. Or, the disorder may give rise to phenomena wholly unknown, nothing but the autopsy revealing their true meaning. Every physician encounters such cases. It is true that the progress of science and the aggregation of clinical facts are from year to year bringing them into a narrower circle. But is, for instance, our knowledge of affections of the nervous centres anything like complete? Are there not still diseases, nay, groups of diseases, that have eluded discovery to the manifold means of research of the present day, as they have to the accumulated experience of the past?

But the most serious obstacle to a precise diagnosis lies in the fact that frequently several lesions coexist. Disease is a very complex state, and when one portion of the economy gets out of order, another is apt to follow. How close, for example, the connection between affections of the heart and of the kidney! Here it is easy to arrive at a conclusion, since we have the means of judging accurately of the condition of both organs. But there are instances in which it is very difficult, especially when a part contiguous to one chronically affected is attacked with acute disease. A person applies for relief, presenting all the symptoms of a severe local peritonitis. The inflammation spreads; death results. The exciting cause of the inflammation is discovered to be a structural alteration of one of the abdominal viscera, the signs of which were completely merged in the more marked signs of the recent inflammation. And this disguisement is effected not only by the supervention of another and more acute complaint, but also sometimes by the prominence of those remote sympathetic derangements which an affection of any viscus may produce. Thus, the disturbed action of the heart in dyspeptic persons throws at times the symptoms of the gastric malady into the shade. Yet it must be admitted that errors of diagnosis from this source are not apt to occur to the careful practitioner. A thorough examination of the case is a safeguard against them.

These, then, are the various causes rendering a diagnosis uncertain, or wholly unattainable. Let us add to them one that does so temporarily. There are disorders the early manifestations of which are so much alike, that it is next to impossible to tell with which of several we have to deal. In fevers this often happens. Here, however, a few days, or even less, will almost always solve the difficulty. But not so in other diseases. It is only after a much longer time, and by careful watching of the patient, that the appearance or disappearance of a striking symptom, or the greater prominence a hitherto indistinct sign assumes, inclines the scales toward one or the other of the affections between which judgment has been kept in suspense.

In some such instances, the treatment becomes the touch-stone of the diagnosis. Now it may be asked, Does this demonstrate that the diagnosis of a case is not necessary for its treatment? Not at all. It simply proves that we are sometimes obliged to aim at removing symptoms without understanding their source. But it does not prove that if we understood their source, we should not be better able to remove the symptoms. The practitioner who undertakes to relieve disease simply by attempting to allay its symptoms, regardless of their cause, and without understanding their true relation and significance, is groping in the dark. His treatment is vacillating; drug replaces drug; alleviation is taken for a cure; and the experience obtained is utterly untrustworthy. One great advantage, indeed, of attending carefully to diagnosis is, that it enables us to use remedies knowingly, and with decision; to appreciate what they are effecting; to abstain from such as must be injurious. There is less needless meddling, more calmness; the treatment rises above the consideration of the moment, and takes into account what is for the patient's ultimate good. It is sometimes urged that the accurate detection of disease makes timid practitioners, and deprives them of confidence in medicines. More just is it to say, that it shows how wide is the chasm between our acquaintance with morbid conditions and with remedies; how far, unfortunately, our skill to detect disease outruns our power to cure it.

There is undoubtedly, however, a danger which may arise from paying very minute attention to diagnosis. The study of it is so interesting, and capable of being conducted so entirely without reference to other points, and especially to the treatment of the complaint, that some minds are carried away, and, lost in the pursuit of diagnostic knowledge, forget for what purposes chiefly that knowledge is profitable. Its main use is to enable us to foretell the course and probable issue of a malady, and to frame, with understanding, plans to relieve the sufferings and disorders of those who have entrusted their health and their lives into our hands. Nor ought we ever to be unmindful how important it is, in basing the management of a disease on its diagnosis, to found that diagnosis on a general survey of all the circumstances; how necessary not to assign prominence to minor points; and how the extent of the disorder, the circumstances under which it has occurred, the sympathetic disturbances produced, and the vital state of the patient, belong, rightly considered, quite as much to the diagnosis as the recognition of the precise seat and exact anatomical character of the malady, and are, in truth, frequently its more important part.

CHAPTER I.

To elicit the facts of a case by a careful examination is, as has been stated, the first requisite for diagnosis. To con-duct, however, a clinical inquiry with precision and facility, requires continual practice, and is rendered easier by following some well-digested plan. The advantage of adopting a method is clearly seen, if the attempts of a beginner be watched. He wanders in his search from one part of the body to another, attracted by different symptoms in turn; pointless question succeeds to pointless question; and a conclusion, almost cer-tainly erroneous, is finally jumped at, or an acknowledgment made of inability to arrive at any.

Now there are several ways which have been proposed to overcome this embarrassment. One of the principal consists in first questioning the patient with regard to his history. His age; his occupation; the diseases from his childhood up; his habits; his constitution; the affections hereditary in his family,—are all minutely inquired into. After this are traced the origin and progress of the existing disorder, and the remedies ascertained that have been used against it. The present condition is then explored; each organ or each sys-tem being in turn interrogated. The investigation is now regarded as complete; the facts are considered, and the diag-nosis, prognosis, and treatment determined. This method of examining is termed the *synthetical* or historical; another, the *analytical*, reverses the order. The present condition is first ascertained, and subsequently the patient's history or *anam-nesis*. Both of these courses have something to recommend them, and some strong objections. The synthetical method is the more purely scientific; but it is too full, and calls for too

(28)

much labor, to meet the requirements of ordinary professional life. It is much better adapted for recording cases in the pursuit simply of pathological knowledge, and decidedly the best where the history is obscure and the symptoms ill-defined. The plan which I habitually prefer is to take a general survey of the history and of the prominent symptoms, and having thus obtained some clue to the part most likely to be affected, to explore that with care. For instance: we are brought to the bedside of a patient for the first time; we inquire how long he has been sick; how that sickness began; in what way he is now troubled,—whether he has pain, or what is the main source of his annoyance. While questioning him, we are scanning his appearance, the position of the body, his movements, his manner of breathing. The hand is applied to the skin; the pulse is felt. Partly from this examination and partly from the history, some organ is fixed upon to be specially investigated: say pain in the epigastrie region and vomiting are complained of—our attention is directed to the stomach. We explore this organ, its physical state and its functions. Then we look to the parts that are anatomically or physiologically nearest related to it, which are, in the case cited, the intestines and liver. The examination is completed by taking heed of the condition of other portions of the body; by reviewing the history of the case; and by endeavoring to elicit fully such points as bear upon the diagnosis, which the mind, consciously or unconsciously, has already commenced to frame. Then the balance between the symptoms is struck, the diagnosis recast, modified, or extended, and the treatment decided upon.

There is some repetition in this plan, but it is the one which appears practically the most suitable. It has the advantage of bringing together the marked features of a case, and especially those most clearly indicative of the general or vital condition. But whatever scheme be chosen, it should, for us to become proficient in it, be as constantly and closely adhered to as the varying circumstances of disease will permit. Yet thoroughly to acquire the habit of examining with accuracy and care, and also to obtain the full fruits of experience, it is indispensable to keep written records. This, too, should, so far as possible, be done according to a uniform design, since it both prevents us from overlooking important symptoms, and enables cases to be more readily compared. I subjoin a schedule which I have used for some time, and which is based, as closely as practicable, on the plan of examination just mentioned.

Date of Examination; Name; Age; Color; Place of Birth; Present abode; Occupation or social state; In females, whether married or not, number of children and date of last confinement.

HISTORY.

1. *History antecedent to present disease:* Constitution and General Health — Hereditary predisposition — Previous Diseases or Injuries—Habits and mode of life; hygienic influences to which exposed, etc.

2. *History of present disease:* Its supposed exciting cause—Date of seizure—Mode of invasion; subsequent symptoms in order of succession—Previons treatment.

PRESENT CONDITION OF PATIENT.

1. *General Symptoms:*

Position $\begin{cases} \text{in bed—mode of lying;} \\ \text{out of bed—movements;} \end{cases}$

Aspect $\begin{cases} \text{of body;} \\ \text{of countenance;} \end{cases}$

Skin;

Pulse;

Respiration—as to frequency, etc.;

Tongue;

General state of Digestion $\begin{cases} \text{appetite;} \\ \text{thirst;} \\ \text{condition of bowels;} \end{cases}$

General state of Urinary Secretion;

Sensations of patient: pain, etc.

2. *Examination of special regions or functions,* commencing with the one presumably the most affected.

DIAGNOSIS.

TREATMENT.

REMARKS.

The history is here placed first; then the symptoms of general import, such as those furnished by the pulse and tongue, are made to precede the examination of special regions. These general symptoms are of great value in the recognition of disease, and of yet greater value in determining its treatment. They are something more than the mere physical signs of textural affections; they indicate vital conditions, and partly from their value, and partly from their not being linked to a disease of any organ in particular, they demand a separate and detailed consideration.

Position of the Body.—By noting whether the patient is in bed or out of bed—how he lies, or how he walks—a general idea may be formed as to the acuteness of an attack, the impairment of strength it has produced, and sometimes even as to its nature. Let a person who has been actively attending to his usual occupation be suddenly confined to his bed, and the inference that the disease, if not dangerous, is at all events a severe and acute one, will be commonly correct; certainly so, if no mishap to the organs of locomotion has necessitated a resort to the recumbent position. When the patient lies for a long time on his back, it is generally from exhaustion, or from paralysis, or it is owing to the pain which pressure or motion of any kind occasions. Such is the cause of the dorsal decubitus in peritonitis, and in rheumatism. Lying fixedly upon one side may be looked upon as an indication that the action of the lung of this side is impeded, and that the respiration has to be carried on with the other. There are exceptions to this rule, but not enough to destroy its value. The patient may be confined to bed, and yet unable to lie down in it, on account of the distress in breathing to which the recumbent posture gives rise: he leans forward, or sits erect. This necessity of breathing in the upright position, or " orthopnœa," is a form of dyspnœa encountered especially in diseases of the heart, or where fluid is effused into the air-cells or into both pleural cavities.

If a person is able to be about, his posture and movements become important manifestations of his condition. The young and the strong walk erectly, quickly, and firmly; the aged and weak, stoopingly, slowly, and with difficulty. In diseases of the spine the body is bent: so, too, in affections of the larger joints of the lower extremities.

When, after a fever, or any other prostrating malady, the patient leaves his bed, he totters, moves slowly, and is soon obliged to rest: returning strength brings with it a quicker and steadier gait. In some diseases of the brain the movements are staggering; in one-sided palsy they are uncertain, and the affected side lags, or its motions, if it can be moved at all, are laborious. Excessive and uncontrollable movements are observed in mania and in chorea; trembling motions in states of extreme debility, in shaking palsies, and in the delirium of drunkards.

General Aspect—Expression of Countenance.—The eye of an experienced observer notices rapidly whether the body is bulky or wasted, and whether the surface is discolored or otherwise changed. The indications afforded by the latter appearances will be more conveniently spoken of in connection with the morbid states of the skin; but to those furnished by the former a few lines may be here devoted. A bulky aspect of the whole body is the result of corpulency, or arises from universal anasarca. In some acute diseases, too, a general tumefaction may take place—for example, in the exanthemata. A partial increase, or a swelling, arises from the local extravasation of fluid or air into the cellular tissues. If air, the tissues crepitate under the finger; if fluid, the skin pits. A swelling may, further, proceed from an inflammatory thickening, or from a tumor or any morbid growth.

A diminution in bulk is a more frequent and a more striking symptom than an augmentation. It may take place very rapidly, as witnessed in Asiatic cholera. More generally the wasting is gradual, and is a sure indication of the nutrition of the body not being properly carried on. It occurs in the course of protracted fevers, and in most chronic diseases. In dangerous and slowly fatal maladies, and in those attended with constant discharges—for instance, in chronic diarrhœa —the loss of flesh reaches its highest point.

Emaciation is most readily recognized in the face. It gives rise to that significant change in the features which at once reveals the existence of disease. Not that emaciation is the only striking alteration observable in the countenance when health has failed. There may be pallor, sallowness, a livid hue of the lips, a puffy appearance of the eyelids, a flush on the cheeks. Now these changes in the features, added to the expression which pain or special trains of thought produce, make up that peculiar physiognomy of disease so pregnant with meaning. But I shall not attempt to describe in detail the cast or the play of features in the sick. The shades of expression are so numerous that they baffle description, and are only to be learned by continuous bedside experience. I will merely set down a few broad facts which this experience teaches.

Among the countenances most frequently met with, is that of apathy and stupor. The eye is dull and listless; the face pale, or flushed with fever. This look is very common in fevers of a low type, and is often combined with blackish accumulations on the lips, gums, and teeth.

Unnatural fulness and congestion of the features are sometimes observed in hypertrophy of the heart, and oftener still in habitual drunkards. The same aspect is seen in apoplexy and in typhus fever.

A pinched expression is found when there is intense anxiety or pain, or a wasting malady attended with constant suffering. It is specially observed in acute peritoneal inflammation. When very marked, and accompanied by change of hue, it is the face which Hippocrates has so graphically described. In the great master's own words, "a sharp nose, hollow eyes, collapsed temples; the ears cold, contracted, and their lobes turned out; the skin about the forehead rough, distended, and parched; the color of the whole face green, black, livid, or lead colored." This is the physiognomy of approaching death, and generally its speedy forerunner, excepting in those cases in which it proceeds from want of food, from protracted vigils, or from excessive discharge from the bowels.

The face of shock, with its great pallor, its anxious or frightened look, and its fixed or oscillating eye, often with a contracting pupil, is a face seen after severe injuries, and as such familiar to the surgeon. But in many of its main traits it may be also met with in diseases that make a sudden and overwhelming impression on the nervous system; for instance, it is at times encountered in cerebro-spinal fever and in cholera.

An aspect serious and dull on one side, while the other side is in full play, is witnessed in hemiplegia, or in paralysis of the facial branch of the seventh nerve. The difference in the cast of the features may escape observation when the face is in repose, but as soon as an attempt is made to laugh, it shows itself plainly.

Independently of these lineaments which may be said to be common to several diseases, we read frequently in the countenance the signs of special disorders. A dusky flush on the face, if associated with rapid breathing, is almost a certain indication of inflammation of the lung. Puffiness of the eyelids in a pallid person is very apt to be expressive of Bright's disease. A bluish color of the lips shows plainly that the venous circulation is interfered with, or that the blood is but imperfectly aerated. Then there is the straw-colored, anemic hue of malignant disease; the jaundiced, melancholy look of a hepatic affection; the downcast expression and mobility of the features in hysteria; the thickened upper lip, delicate skin, and fair complexion of scrofula, and the various traits which tend to mark not only the special diathesis, but also the peculiar temperament with the morbid tendencies that belong to it. But this is not a subject to be pursued here any further; it was merely touched upon to exhibit the diagnostic importance of a study of the countenance.*

Skin.—By the state of the skin we can, to a great extent, judge of the activity of the circulation and of the character

---

* For fuller information on the Physiognomy of Disease, and especially on the physiognomical value in diagnosis of special features, as the jaws, palate, teeth, ears, hair, the reader is referred to Laycock's Lectures, Med. Times and Gazette, vol. i. 1862; also to a paper, *ib.* Sept. 1867. The individual muscles concerned in physiognomical expression have been made the subject of careful study by Duchenne: Proceedings of French Academy, Arch. Géner. de Méd., 1862, *et seq.;* also in Physiologie des Mouvements, Paris, 1867.

of the blood. Moreover, it is a fair index of the secretions, and of the condition of the system at large. In fevers, along with the quickened circulation, the temperature of the skin is increased; the attending dryness is produced by defective perspiration. Coldness of the surface indicates a weakened capillary circulation, and is met with at the invasion of acute diseases, and when the nervous power is under the sway of some highly deleterious influence. If heat of surface succeed a cold skin, we know that reaction has taken place, that the circulation has again become active. Protracted coldness, whether attended with dryness or with clamminess, is of evil augury; it implies a seriously diminished vital force.

The cutaneous covering is pale whenever the blood is poor and watery. If it be seriously vitiated and deprived of its fibrin, as in putrid fevers, black spots are seen, due to extravasation. Ofttimes the surface is overspread with eruptions, some of which bear a close relation to disorders of internal organs, while others are connected with febrile or general maladies; and others, again, are owing to a disease of the texture itself.

Tension of the skin is met with in acute affections accompanied by active excitement. In wasting and prostrating ailments, on the other hand, the skin feels very relaxed and soft; and in those producing rapid emaciation, it is inelastic and lies in folds.

Pulse.—The study of the pulse, elevated into a science by Galen and his disciples, has come down to us with the sanction of centuries; and to feel the beat at the wrist is still, in the opinion of many, as indispensable to the understanding of a case as it was thought to be by the Arabs, and in the Middle Ages. Yet the advance of science has shaken the belief in the paramount importance of the pulse. It has shown that, although a most valuable means of information, it is not exclusively to be relied upon, and has proved the many divisions and refinements of the physicians of by-gone days—who endeavored by the pulse to judge of every conceivable morbid condition—to be practically useless. Indeed, were even all their distinctions founded in fact, we have now better ways of judging of lesions than by feeling the radial artery. The same may be said of the prognostic indications drawn from the pulse. It affords us in this respect much instruction ; but any attempt to revive the various critical pulses, as taught by Solano or Borden, would be received with the same derision as we do the pretensions of our Chinese brethren to distinguish diseases by feeling the pulse of the right or the left side, or to determine, by its aid, the sex of the child in a pregnant woman.

The pulse enlightens us on the action of the heart, and on something more—on the state of the artery itself and of the blood. In a healthy adult a beat of some resistance is felt, recurring from sixty-five to seventy-five times in a minute. It becomes slower with advancing years, though it may rise in the very aged. The pulse of infancy is one hundred and ten to one hundred and twenty; and of a child three years old, from ninety to ninety-five. Warmth quickens the pulse, so do rapid breathing, forced expiration, and the process of digestion. In the recumbent position and during sleep it falls.

At the bedside we study in the pulse its frequency, its rhythm, its volume and strength, and its resistance.

Increased *frequency* of the beat denotes increased frequency of the heart's action, and arises from any cause which excites the heart. Hence exercise, rapid breathing, mental emotion, or restlessness, will occasion the number of beats to exceed the average of health as readily as fevers or acute inflammatory diseases. In great debility, too, the pulse rises; and the more depressed the vital condition, the higher the pulse becomes. The heart may thus quicken from so many and such varied causes acting temporarily or permanently, that increased frequency of pulse, taken by itself, has no significant diagnostic meaning.

A *slow* pulse, too, happens in many different states—from cold, exposure to wet, in icterus. It is also produced by an intense and prostrating shock, or is found coexisting with pressure on the brain. In some persons the pulse is naturally very slow.

The *rhythm* of the pulse is often perverted. Instead of the beats following each other in regular succession, they are unequal, or one or two intermit. An irregular pulse occurs from digestive troubles or from debility; but it is more frequently the indication of a cerebral or cardiac lesion. It is sometimes a difficult beat to count; and we must be careful not to regard at once a pulse as irregular because it appears to intermit. The seeming irregularity may be caused by a slipping of the fingers from the artery, which they are very apt to do after they have been on the vessel for some time.

The *volume* and *strength* of the pulse are of much more importance than either its rhythm or its frequency. Volume and strength are often associated, and are much alike; but they are not identical. When the beat of the artery is large, we call it a *full* pulse. This is owing to the distention of the vessel with blood—its complete expansion with every beat of the heart. A full pulse is, therefore, the pulse of plethora; the pulse of the young and robust in health, or in inflammatory diseases; the pulse in the early stages of fevers, or in obstruction of the capillaries. It is usually a pulse of power, just as its opposite, a *small* pulse, is usually the pulse of debility. Yet a full pulse may be produced by the distention of an artery which has lost its tone, and which the finger easily compresses. Such a pulse, the " gaseous pulse," denotes exhaustion, and proves that a full pulse and a strong pulse are not always synonymous. Indeed, into the idea of *strength* enters something more than mere fulness. A strong pulse is a natural pulse heightened in all its characters. It has more fulness, but, in addition, more impulse, and less compressibility than an ordinary pulse. A strong pulse, therefore, indicates activity of the contraction of the heart, and a normal, perhaps increased tonicity of the arterial coats. It is found in active inflammations; also in hypertrophy of the heart. Its opposite, a weak pulse, betokens want of force, often want of healthy blood. It is generally small as well as weak. But as little as the full pulse is always strong, is the small pulse always weak. The small, choked pulse of peritoneal inflammation may be fine and wiry; but who would call it a weak pulse?

The *resistance* or tension of the pulse is another valuable guide in the appreciation of morbid action. Is the pulse hard and resisting? is it soft and compressible? are questions on the solution of which the application of remedies may hang. A *hard*, tense pulse denotes increased contractility of the arteries, and high-wrought power. Be the beat full or small, slow or frequent, it tells us that the blood is being driven with force along the arterial system. But it also tells us that the irritation has implicated the coats of the arteries themselves, as their extreme resistance to the finger plainly shows. A tense pulse is met with in active, violent inflammations, or sometimes, though not often, in states of extreme and continued excitement without inflammation. It is almost needless to add that changes in the coats of the arteries may also be a cause of a hard and resistant beat. Where no local alterations are present, and where no acute symptoms explain the sympathetic disturbance of the heart and arterial system, a tense pulse will be commonly found to be associated with hypertrophy of the left ventricle.

The opposite of the hard pulse is the *soft* or compressible pulse. This implies deficient impulsion, loss of tone in the vessel, and is the pulse of low fevers and of debility. But it is also, when following a tense state of the artery, the pulse which denotes returning health, and imminent danger passed.

Such are the meanings attached to the various characters of the pulse. Yet they do not often present themselves thus isolated. The following are usually combined, and bear this explanation:

A hard, full, frequent pulse occurs in active inflammations, and in most of the acute diseases of robust persons.

A hard pulse, full or small, bounding or not, if unconnected with acute symptoms, leads to the suspicion of cardiac disease, or of an affection of the artery itself.

A tense, contracted, and frequent pulse is met with in a large group of inflammations below the diaphragm, as in enteritis, peritonitis, gastritis.

A frequent pulse, full or small, but rarely tense, is the pulse of most idiopathic fevers.

A very frequent pulse, but very feeble and compressible, is the pulse of marked debility, of prostration, of collapse.

A pulse frequent, and changeable in its rhythm, is produced, for the most part, either by disease of the heart or of the brain.

The appreciation of these different kinds of pulses requires considerable practice. But even this scarcely teaches us to estimate the exact degree of the alteration of the beat, certainly not with sufficient distinctness to convey to others an accurate idea, or even to be able ourselves to compare one observation with another. To attain these desirable results, physiologists have sought for instruments by means of which the pulse might be examined with precision, its finer shades of difference recognized, and its movements recorded. The best instrument as yet invented is the *sphygmograph* of Marey,* which registers with correctness not only the frequeney and regularity, but also the form of pulsation, and may be applied almost as readily to the study of the cardiac impulse and of pulsatile tumors as toward gaining a knowledge of the pulse wave. Slight irregularities which wholly escape the finger may be, through its aid, discerned with facility, and we can tell at once in how far these irregularities belong to one or to a succession of beats. Double beats, too, not appreciable

FIG. 1.

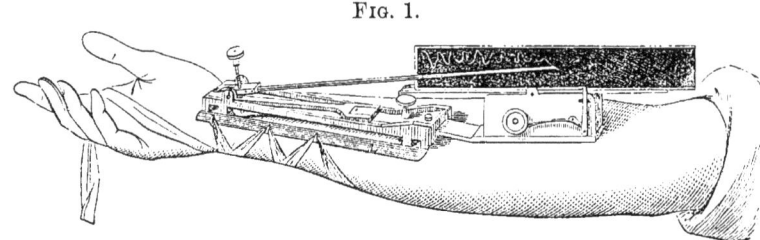

The sphygmograph attached to the wrist. Its tracings are seen by the white lines on the black background.

to the hand, are easily detected. Indeed, one of the most valuable results arrived at by the sphygmograph concerns the type of pulse in which a double beat is perceived to each contraction of the heart. This, the "dicrotic" pulse, or the *pulsus biferiens* of the older authors, is most commonly met with in fevers of a typhoid form, and preceding or during the

---

* Physiologic Médicale de la Circulation du Sang. Paris, 1863.

continuance of hemorrhages. Yet the phenomenon of di-
erotism may be stated to be really a physiological one, since
the sphygmograph proves it to exist in almost every person.
The rebound is chiefly due to the oscillation of the column
of blood in the arteries, and is very much influenced by their
elasticity. It is rarely sufficient to be determined by the
touch, except when the arterial tension or contractility is
lessened and the elasticity of the tubes increased, as happens
in the disorders in which the dicrotic pulse is encountered.
In old persons, in whom the coats of the arteries are inelastic, dicrotism is but feebly marked. A rapid circulation
renders the pulse more obviously dicrotic. The rebound
may occur during the systole or diastole of the vessel; and
instead of one, there may be four or five of the secondary
pulsations.

When we apply the sphygmograph for clinical purposes,
we study chiefly in its tracings, the line of ascent, the summit,
and the line of descent. Each pulsation is composed of these
three parts. The line of ascent tells us the manner in which
the blood enters the vessels. The more rapid the flow, and
the more quickly the artery distends, the more vertical the
line. The force, too, is indicated by this line, or rather by
its height; though here we find that the strength of the ventricular contraction is far from being the only cause influ-
cueing the amplitude of the tracing. Indeed, as we may
note in old persons, a large volume of the artery gives very
considerable height to the lines of ascent, so does a long interval between the pulsation, or the obstruction of the vessel
below the point where the observation is made. A state of
feeble tension in the capillary system, further, has the same
effect, whereas when the passage in the ultimate ramification
of the vesicular system is difficult, the lever descends slowly
by a line convex upward, and is soon again raised by the
next pulsation. The line joining the summit of a series of
pulsations, or the maxima of tension, is generally a straight
line; a similar imaginary line connecting the bases, or the
minima, is apt to run parallel to it; but irregularity of pulsation leads to irregular lines, and the lower line may be irregular while the upper is straight.

The *summit* of the pulsation informs us of the time during which the entrance of blood balances the onward flow. This summit may be a horizontal line of some length, and an extended plateau of the kind is very apt to happen in induration or ossification of the arteries. In some instances we find a little hooked point preceding the usually transverse mark of the summit. This occurs by the rapid movement of the lever, and is a valuable sign of regurgitation through the aortic valves.

The *line of descent* follows the closure of the semilunar valves. It is sometimes purely oblique, and the more rapidly the pressure is lessened in the arterial system, the more oblique is the line. It often shows a series of undulations, giving rise to the dicrotism in the pulse which has been above mentioned.

These points must all be attended to in examining sphygmographic tracings; but, unfortunately, the mode of adjusting the instrument, and of proportioning the pressure of the spring, has something to do with the kind of delineation obtained. To secure greater accuracy, Anstie* and Sanderson have made improvements in the instrument. Sanderson, especially, has fixed the centre button at a definite pressure, thus insuring an arrangement very useful for purposes of comparison. Still, with all its perfection, the precise value of the instrument for clinical research is yet to be fixed. After using it considerably, I think it much more likely to be of avail in investigations on the exact action of medicines than in aiding us very materially either in questions of diagnosis or in decisions on treatment. At all events, I do not think it has been shown that it supersedes the older and more usual means of research.

Tongue.—When a patient is told to put out his tongue, it is not because the physician thinks it obligatory to see whether or not this organ is the seat of a disease, but because experience has taught him that the tongue is a mirror, more or less perfect, of the condition of the digestive functions, and that it reflects the complexion of the nervous

---

* Lancet, No. 35, 1868.

power and of the blood, and the state of the secretions. To judge of these varied circumstances, we have to examine the tongue in regard to its movements, its volume, its dryness or its humidity, its color, and its coating.

The *movements* of the tongue are impeded and tremulous in all conditions of the system attended with exhaustion. It is protruded slowly and with difficulty in fevers of a low type, and in nervous disorders which are accompanied by marked debility. The action of the muscles is seriously impaired in paralysis. In hemiplegia one side is crippled, and the tongue turns toward one of the corners of the mouth. When imperfect articulation is associated with difficulty in moving the organ, it commonly announces a serious cerebral lesion.

The *volume* of the tongue is changed by its own diseases; more rarely by the condition of the system at large, or by disturbances of the abdominal viscera. Yet a swollen or a broad and flabby tongue, on the sides of which the teeth leave their marks, is sometimes found in chronic ailments of the digestive organs, and as the result of the action of mercury, and of certain poisons. It is further observed in some affections of the brain, or as a consequence of the disturbed circulation attending diseases of the heart, and in distempers, like the plague, typhus, or scurvy, in which the blood is much altered.

Dryness of the tongue indicates deficient secretion. In acute visceral inflammations, and still more frequently in the exanthemata and in typhoid fever, the tongue is dry; it may be so dry as to cause the papillæ to become prominent and the whole organ to appear roughened. This condition is one which, in acute diseases, is always to be dreaded, especially if the tongue be, in addition, of a dark color, or furred or fissured; for it is then a proof not only of arrested secretions, but of depraved blood and of ebbing life force. Yet a fissured tongue is not, by itself, indicative of great and imminent danger; it may occur in chronic affections of the liver, or in chronic inflammation of the intestines; and in some persons it is congenital. The opposite of dryness, *humidity*, is, unless excessive, a favorable sign. It is extremely so, if it succeed to dryness, because it is a proof that the secretions are being re-established.

The *color* of the tongue is subject to many variations. It is remarkably pale whenever the blood is watery and deficient in red globules. It is exceedingly red and shining in the exanthemata, especially in scarlet fever. The tongue is also very red, if inflammation have attacked its substance, or the fauces, or the pharynx. It is bluish and livid when there is an obstruction to the flow of the venous blood or deficient aeration, as in some structural diseases of the heart and in dangerous cases of pneumonia or bronchitis.

Equally as important as the color of the organ are the color and form of its *coating*. In health the tongue has hardly a discernible lining; disease quickly gives it one. In inflammation of the respiratory textures, at the commencement of fevers, in disorders of large portions of the abdominal mucous tract, the epithelium accumulates, and the tongue has a loaded, whitish appearance. The coat is apt to be yellowish in disturbances of the liver, and of a brown or very dark hue when the blood is contaminated. But we must be sure, in drawing our inferences, that the abnormal aspect be not due to the food partaken of or to medicine. Its color is also modified by the character of the occupation. Thus, as Chambers tell us, there is a curious, smooth, orange-tinted coating on the tongues of tea-tasters. A local cause sometimes gives rise to a thick, opaque coat. For instance, decayed teeth may produce a yellow sheathing on one side. Affections of the fauces also occasion a deep-yellow hue. Again, some persons, even in health, wake up every morning with their tongues covered at the back with a heavy coating which wears off during the day.

In some diseases the epithelium, which is either formed in excessive quantities or not thrown off, collects between the papillæ, leaving these uncovered and prominent. This is especially noticed in scrofulous children. When the epithelium is sticky and adherent, it winds itself chiefly around the filiform papillæ, giving to the surface of the organ a *furred* appearance. Although this kind of tongue, as almost every other variety, is met with now and then in persons who are not sick, yet it may generally be looked upon as denoting serious trouble. It occurs sometimes in chronic diseases of the abdominal viscera, but much oftener in grave acute maladies.

To sum up, before leaving the subject, the manifestations afforded by the tongue which are indicative of danger. They are, tremulous action; dryness; a livid color; a very red, shining, or raw aspect; a marked fur, or a heavy coating of a dark or black hue. Any change from these to a more natural look bears a favorable interpretation; so, too, when the red, glazed tongue becomes covered with a distinct coat.

The state of the *digestion* and the character of the discharges have so close a connection with the nutrition of the body, that they become important general symptoms. But for sake of convenience, their value will be inquired into while discussing the diseases in the recognition of which they occupy the foremost place. A few words here, however, on the sensations of patients.

Sensations of Patients.—Sick persons are subject to many disagreeable feelings. They complain of chills, of heat, of languor, of restlessness, and of uneasiness; but their most constant complaint is of pain. Now *pain* may be of various kinds: it may be dull or gnawing; it may be acute and lancinating. In its duration it may be permanent or remittent. A *dull* pain is generally persistent. It is most often present in congestions, in subacute and chronic inflammations, and where gradual changes of tissue are taking place. It is the pain of chronic rheumatism, and shades off into the innumerable aches of this malady. The only acute affections in which it is apt to exist are inflammations of the parenchymatous viscera and of mucous membranes.

Acute pain is in every respect the reverse of dull pain. It is usually remittent, and not so fixed to one spot. It is met with in spasmodic affections, in neuralgia, and, with extremely sharp and lancinating pangs, in malignant disease.

Pain varies much in intensity; it is sometimes so extreme as to cause death. We have to judge of its severity partly on the testimony of the sufferer, partly by the countenance, and partly by the attending functional disturbances. The latter are not to be overlooked, for they enable us, to some extent, to appreciate whether the torments are as great as they are represented to be.

The seat to which the pain is referred is far from being always the seat of the disease. A calculus in the bladder may produce dragging sensations extending down the thighs; inflammation of the hip-joint gives rise to pain in the knee; disorders of the liver occasion pain in the right shoulder. Pain felt at some part remote from that affected, is either transmitted in the course of a nerve involved, or is sympathetic.

The same abnormal action does not always create the same kind of pain. Inflammation, for instance, causes different pain as it involves different structures; the pain from an inflamed pleura is not the same as that from an inflamed muscle. Speaking generally, the tissues themselves seem to determine the form of pain more certainly than the precise character of the morbid process does. Thus, pain in diseases of the periosteum and bones, no matter what may be the exact nature of the malady, is mostly boring and constant; in the serous membranes, sharp; in the mucous membranes, dull; and in the skin, burning or itching.

Pain produced by pressure is called *tenderness*. It indicates increased sensibility, and is most constantly associated with inflammation. Yet tenderness may be present without inflammation; the tenderness, for example, of the skin in hysteria. Commonly it is combined with pain occurring independently of pressure; but a part may be tender and not painful.

Temperature of the Body.—There is one more symptom having a general significance which must be mentioned, namely, that connected with the function of calorification, and based on the determination of the heat of the body. To measure this a thermometer is necessary; and the thermometry

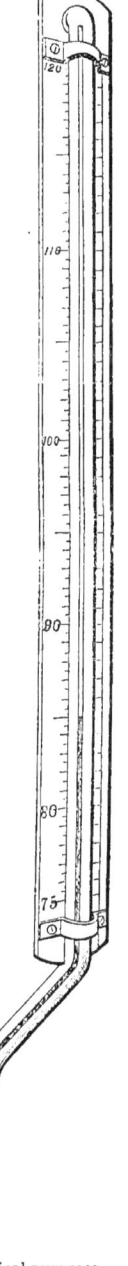

Fig. 2.

Thermometer for clinical purposes.
Nearly natural size.

of disease has been of late very carefully studied, and has been found to afford much aid in the recognition of morbid states, particularly of febrile conditions, and of affections attended with marked tissue changes.

The thermometer used for clinical purposes should be very sensitive. A convenient form is to have it curved, and with an elongated bulb. The scale, extending from about 75° Fahr. to 115°, ought to be very correctly and uniformly graduated. For minute investigations it should be divided so as to exhibit fifths or tenths of a degree; but for ordinary purposes one registering half of a degree is sufficiently accurate.

It is a matter of some dispute as to which is the most appropriate part to place the thermometer. To put it under the tongue or in the rectum has been strongly recommended. But the most suitable site seems to be the axilla. The bulb is pressed into the armpit and kept in close contact with the skin for from three to five minutes,* and the degrees marked are read off while the thermometer is still in position. The instrument may be conveniently introduced just below the skin covering the edge of the pectoralis major muscle; and to insure exactness, the patient should be kept in bed for at least one hour before the examination, and the axilla be well covered. The best posture is found to be neither completely on the back nor side, but diagonally on the right or left side.†

In all cases of any importance, not less than two observations should be made daily, and every day at the same hour. Between seven and nine o'clock in the morning, and about seven o'clock, or somewhat earlier, in the evening, are regarded as the most appropriate periods. If only a single observation be taken, it is best done in the afternoon or evening. Before fitting the thermometer into the armpit, it should be warmed in the hand or slightly heated in water; and in every record of the temperature, the pulse and the respirations must be also noted.

---

* Yet, even after this, the thermometer may go on rising. Indeed, the variations may extend over an hour. (See the observations of Goodhart in Guy's Hospital Reports, vol. xv.) I think, however, that for practical purposes the statement in the text is correct.

† Ringer on the Temperature of the Body. London, 1865.

The average heat of the body in temperate climes is estimated by Wunderlich as 37° centigrade in the axilla; that of freshly voided urine is about the same.* Expressed in the scale used in this country and in England, it may be stated that the average heat of sheltered and internal parts of the body is 98·6° Fahr.† It rises with the temperature of the air, and fluctuates during the day, being in temperate climates greatest early in the morning. It is heightened by exercise, and reduced by sustained mental exertion, and changes even when we are at rest.‡ But no cause, as a rule, except disease induces a variation of much more than 1°; and even in the extreme heat of tropical climates, the animal heat does not surpass 99·5°. Thus a temperature above this, or more than a degree below the average stated, when persistent, indicates some morbid action in the economy. At all events, it does so in adults; in very aged persons, a temperature of 97° may still be normal; and we must bear in mind that in children the daily range is much greater than in adults. There may be a fall in the evening amounting to between 2° and 3° Fahr.§ A further point, too, to be taken into account in those of all ages is, that the temperature is influenced by food and stimulants. And these are elements apt to be overlooked, and which make deductions from single observations or comparatively slight changes untrustworthy.

In ordinary cases the pulse and temperature rise synchronously, and every degree above 98° Fahr. corresponds with an increase of ten beats of the pulse. The fever temperature ranges from 100° to 106°. When it exceeds this, the

---

* Die Eigenwärme in Krankheiten.   1868.

† It may be useful, for the sake of comparing the results of observers in different countries, to recall the fact that one degree of Fahrenheit is equal to ⅝th of a degree of the centigrade thermometer, and ⅘th of a degree of Reaumur; and also that the freezing point of the first is placed at 32°; that of the others at zero. To convert centigrade into Fahrenheit, we multiply by 9 and divide by 5; to convert Reaumur, we multiply by 9 and divide by 4, and when above zero, in either case, add 32.

‡ See an instructive paper by Garrod, on the Minor Fluctuations of the Temperature of the Human Body, Proceedings of Royal Society, May, 1869.

§ Finlayson, Glasgow Med. Journal, Feb. 1869.

patient may be looked upon as in danger, except the rise be due to malarial fever. Under these circumstances it is rapid, occurring in a person who but yesterday was healthy. In typhoid fever, the thermometer during the earlier stages does not rise to more than 103·5° Fahr. in the evening, and is lower in the morning; at any period of its course, a temperature of 105° is a proof of a grave disease. A temperature of 101° to 103° shows a mild attack. In severe cases of yellow fever, the heat in the armpit has been noted as 108°.* In pneumonia, a temperature above 104° Fahr. is stated to be a symptom of a very serious seizure; so, too, is it in acute rheumatism a symptom either of danger or of some complication. "Stability of temperature," says Aitken,† "from morning to evening, is a good sign; on the other hand, if the temperature remains stable from evening till the morning, it is a sign that the patient is getting or will get worse." In convalescence the temperature declines until it attains its norm, or even falls somewhat below this. If the thermometer again indicate a decided rise, it shows a return of the malady, or the supervention of some complication or new disorder; and the persistence of even a slight degree of abnormal heat after apparent convalescence, is a sign of imperfect recovery, or of the existence of some lingering secondary complaint. Further, in cases of low fevers, the skin, particularly of the hands and feet, may feel cool, while the instrument in the axilla marks 104°.

Specific forms of febrile diseases have their characteristic variations of temperature. In measles, for instance, the temperature rises toward the breaking out of the rash, reaches its height with the period of eruption, and in the twenty-four hours succeeding it falls rapidly. If it remain elevated, 104° to 105°, particularly after the rash has faded, it is due to the presence of some complication. In scarlet fever the thermometer marks 105° or 106°, or upwards, until about the third day. From the third to the ninth day it ranges from a fraction below 104° to somewhat under 103°, and then gradually subsides.

---

* Wragg, Charl. Med. Journ., vol. x.
† Science and Practice of Medicine.

In other than febrile states, too, the thermometer may assist materially in diagnosis and prognosis. Thus it enables us to judge between increased frequency of pulse due to fever and to debility; it indicates that sweating which is not preceded by a previous elevation of temperature, and caused by it, is the result and not the source of exhaustion; and according to recent observations, there is probably a continuous rise of the heat of the body in all cases in which a deposition of tubercle is taking place in any of its organs, and more especially in the lungs; while, on the other hand, I have noticed that in cancerous affections the heat of the body is but little influenced, and is sometimes even below the normal standard.

Such are some of the main facts connected with the thermometry of disease, and in the course of this volume there will often be occasion to refer to others. But even those here mentioned are sufficient to show that the accurate study of the temperature may be of much service in the recognition of a malady and in foretelling its issue. But to make it so we must look to connected observations, and particularly must we avoid laying too much stress on fluctuations comparatively slight, and which may be due to other causes than to disease.

4

CHAPTER II.

THE study of the disorders of the brain, and, in truth, of those of the entire nervous system, is very difficult. Nor, owing to our deficient knowledge of the physiology of these vital parts, and to our inability to appreciate the minute structural changes of nerve tissue, does it yield as precise and accurate results as the importance of the subject renders desirable, and as our improved means of research have attained in affections of most other portions of the economy. Yet considerable advance has been made of late years in untangling many knotty problems; and at least the more tangible evidences of nervous disease are much more clearly recognized. It is these with which this sketch is intended to deal.

But first, of a few symptoms and morbid states having a general significance rather than a specific connection with any malady.

DERANGED INTELLECTION.

The great instrument of the intelligence, the brain, manifests its ailings, whether primary or merely sympathetic, by derangement of thought of every conceivable degree and kind—from dulness and confusion of the intellect to its utter perversion and absolute prostration. When one intellectual function is disturbed, generally all are, or soon become so; yet we may find impairment of judgment and of imagination without deterioration of memory or of the powers of attention. One of the most marked signs of mental infirmity is a disordered memory. This is especially encountered in chronic cerebral diseases, or in such nervous affections of uncertain seat as epilepsy. Another signal of mental de-

(50)

rangement is loss of judgment, or rather loss of power to appreciate the logical sequence of ideas; yet another is depression of mind, or its opposite, exaltation. All these abnormal conditions may happen in acute as well as in chronic maladies, but they are more striking and become of more aid in the diagnosis of the latter than of the former; and they may or may not be joined to appreciable textural changes. To the psychologist their significance is very great, as they are often the only premonitory symptoms of that departure from mental health which terminates in confirmed insanity.

In acute disturbances of the brain, whether functional or organic, we meet with these striking phenomena connected with disordered intellection: delirium, stupor, coma, insomnia.

Delirium.—This is a wandering of the mind, manifesting itself by the expression of ill-associated thoughts, of the incongruity of which the patient is not conscious. It most frequently occurs in those of susceptible nervous system, and is, in consequence, more common in the young than in the old. It is almost invariably united with restlessness, and rises as night approaches.

The character of the delirium is very various. There is first the *quiet* delirium, of a low or passive type. The patient mutters incoherent words, moans without any assignable reason, or lies silent, with his eyes open, his thoughts preoccupied with his vague illusions. If strongly aroused, he gives a rational answer, but not a long or a connected one, for he soon returns to his dreams and his ever-changing hallucinations. He picks at his bedclothes, moves in bed, and may even occasionally try to leave it, although he is very easily prevented from so doing.

Then there is a delirium of somewhat more active type, but still, on the whole, quiet; the patient wanders, yet not boisterously. He is irritable, and often does not show that his mind is disturbed, excepting in some one particular: in irascibility about trifles, or in expressions and modes of thought quite foreign to his nature.

An active, *fierce* delirium presents different characteristics.

The patient is wild, noisy; he sings, screams, gets out of bed; his face during the excitement becomes congested; the eye is bright, often fiery.

Now all these forms of delirium occur in many different maladies, and are very far from being of necessity linked to an organic cerebral affection. Nay, not even the most violent kind of mental wandering is positively indicative of a lesion of the brain; at least, not of such a lesion as can be determined by the aid of the scalpel, or indeed by any of our present means of investigation. As a rule, we find the low, quiet delirium in conditions of vital exhaustion, partienlarly in those depressed states of the nervous system which are connected with quickened vascular action, and with a deterioration of the blood, as, for instance, in the low fevers. The fierce delirium may, however, be associated with prostration or depraved blood. Thus the delirium of pneumonia is sometimes of a violent kind, owing to the maddening effect of the ill-oxygenated vital fluid on the brain. In most of the ordinary fevers the delirium is of a moderate type; in inflammatory diseases of the brain and in acute mania it is fierce.

Delirium is not difficult of recognition: yet we must be very careful not to confound with it the troubled dreams to which ailing children are so liable, and which occasion confusion of thought on first awaking and until consciousness is fully aroused. Delirium is most likely to be mistaken for insanity. There is, however, this palpable difference: an insane person is commonly in good health in all save his intellect; a delirious person is sick, and exhibits other evidences of his sickness in much besides his delirium. It is true that, when the patient is first seen, doubt may arise; but it is not generally of long duration. The most perplexing cases are those in which insanity follows or attends inordinate drinking. But this is a subject we shall discuss in reviewing the clinical phenomena of mania a potu.

Another perplexing group of cases is furnished by the occurrence of that singular form of delirium which is met with at times in acute diseases, especially in fevers, and which, as it is apt to be associated with insufficient nutrition, has been called the *delirium of inanition*, or of collapse.* Its outbreak is sudden, like an attack of mania, but it is found to be combined with a feeble pulse, a skin bathed in perspiration, cold hands and feet,—in one word, with the signs of great prostration or of collapse. The seizure happens usually early in the morning, and is quite unexpected, for it occurs very commonly at the end of the febrile state, and when the condition of the skin and pulse bespeaks convalescence. The exhausted nervous centre betrays itself in the sudden mental wandering, which has generally this characteristic, that there is but one fixed delusion, and this ordinarily one connected with the subjects which have most engrossed the mind before the illness. The seizure lasts from six to forty-eight hours, and at its termination the patient is apt to awake out of a sleep with a calm mind, remembering, perhaps, his hallucination as a vivid dream. There may be more than one attack, but this is not common; and the duration is materially abridged by opium and the employment of stimulants and nourishment. The form of delirium under consideration has been spoken of as linked to, or rather as a sequel of, febrile conditions. But it may also succeed exhausting discharges and drains from the system, or inability to obtain the proper amount of food or to digest it. Thus it may happen in malignant diseases of the stomach; also in mere gastric irritability and persistent vomiting. The most marked instance of this kind of mental wandering I have encountered was associated with functional gastric disorder, which prevented enough food from being retained. In this patient the hallucination was on one subject—a business matter which had been annoying him greatly just before his illness assumed a decided character.

Delirium is sometimes simulated. I saw not very long since an instance of the kind. It differed from real delirium by the absence of all other signs of sickness, and by the *sameness* of the mental wandering. The man whined when spoken to, and pretended to rave; but his ideas always ran

---

* See Weber, Medico-Chirurg. Transact., 1865; Becquet, Archiv. Génér. de Médecine, 1866; also the Clinical Lectures of Chomel and of Trousseau.

on the same subject, and he was very solicitous about his food, and about other matters of which a delirious person takes no notice, and for which he cares nothing. Delirium is more or less continuous; once delirious, a patient remains so for some time, and until the exciting cause subsides. In this respect hysterical delirium is exceptional; it does not last long, or it intermits and then reappears.

Stupor.—A blunted state of mind, a partial drowsy unconsciousness, constitutes the phenomenon called stupor. The patient lies in a deep slumber, from which he cannot be roused save with great difficulty, and when roused he answers reluctantly and briefly, and soon resumes his heavy sleep. The expression of his face is dull, yet now and then a ray of intelligence, excited by some object which attracts his attention or by some pleasant reverie, flits across his features.

Stupor is met with in several cerebral affections, and seems to be chiefly owing to a congestion of the brain. It is frequently seen in typhoid fever, immediately after an epileptic fit, or as the result of narcotic poisons; and is, in these states, also probably due to cerebral congestion. But there is nothing pathognomonic about it in these various conditions, nothing by which we can judge positively of its origin.

Coma.—Coma is complete loss of consciousness: perception and volition are alike suspended, and there is an appearance of the profoundest sleep. The face wears a confused look; the pupils are sluggish, often dilated. Sensation may be blunted, but is not destroyed; neither is motion, for the patient moves when his skin is pinched or tickled. Coma is always of grave augury: it betokens a very serious disturbance of the functions of the brain.

The most thorough coma is seen in apoplexy; it comes on very quickly, and is attended with a noisy respiration and a slow pulse. Another form of coma, scarcely less complete, is caused by narcotic poisoning; it, however, does not appear suddenly, and when from opium is associated with contraction of the pupils. The coma of fevers and of acute diseases, whether cerebral or not, is also gradually produced, but, unlike that due to the toxical effect of opium, is ordinarily preceded for days by insomnia, by delirium, and by other signs of cerebral disturbance. The coma of epilepsy is recognized by its following epileptic seizures. In Bright's disease, among the nervous phenomena of which coma as well as stupor and delirium may happen, the loss of consciousness is apt to occur subsequently to either of the two other morbid phenomena, and its cause is made evident, as is further on more particularly explained, by the coexistence of albumen and tube-casts in the urine.

Sometimes a person may appear to be comatose when his intellect is really but little disordered. He may be paralyzed, and not have the power to communicate his ideas. This state is distinguished from coma by noting that the patient's attention is always directed to the questions asked him, nay, that he strives to answer them, but cannot; and that he has lost all control over the muscular movements of one or of both sides of the body.

Insomnia.—The deprivation of sleep is a frequent concomitant of cerebral congestion and of the earlier stages of cerebral inflammation. But a person may be sleepless from excessive pain, from exhaustion, from grief, or from mental excitement or fatigue; and sometimes insomnia is engendered by habitual working late at night. However, in several of these states congestion, though of a passive character, is, in all likelihood, the immediate cause of the wakefulness.

Insomnia often precedes or attends delirium, as appears in typhoid fever. Among purely nervous affections it is most marked in delirium tremens. It is a very troublesome symptom; but, occurring in so many abnormal conditions, it cannot be looked upon as having a distinct and specific diagnostic value.

DERANGED SENSATION.

The signs of perverted or impaired sensation are very numerous. They may be either those due to an alteration of the general sensibility, or be the signals of a derangement of a nerve of special sense. Let us look at a few in detail.

Hyperæsthesia.—An exalted irritability of the sensitive surface nerves—of those of the skin, the mucous membranes, or even of those of deeper seated structures—in other words, a hyperæsthesia of these parts, is a symptom of much diagnostic importance; not so much, perhaps, on account of the light thrown on any particular disease by the increased sensibility, as because its presence makes it requisite to determine its origin and to separate its phenomena from those of inflammation. And in truth the distinct acknowledgment that acute sensibility is not of necessity inflammatory, is one of the triumphs of modern pathology. How many cases, for example, of abdominal tenderness, which would formerly have been supposed to be indicative of peritoneal inflammation, are now known to be merely instances of hyperæsthesia! We may, as a rule, distinguish the peripheral sensibility from the tenderness of subjacent inflammation, by its extension over a larger surface; by deep pressure producing no more pain than a very light touch; by the absence of signs of functional disturbance of the part apparently involved in inflammatory disease; by the uniformity of the symptoms, no matter how long the duration of the disorder; and by the sensitiveness exhibiting distinct intermissions and exacerbations.

But in what affections do we encounter hyperæsthesia? Is it only in those of the brain or spinal cord? By no means; indeed we may say that, in organic diseases of these structures, such at least as we can detect, it is not common, and rarely reaches a high degree of development, with the exception of tumors pressing upon the pons varolii and corpora quadrigemina, and of alteration of the posterior columns of the cord, or in some cases of meningitis, or in injuries dividing transversely and completely a lateral half of the spinal cord. By far the most usual causes of hyperæsthesia are impoverished blood and that mysterious malady called hysteria. Sometimes it is produced by rheumatism or gout, or by disturbance of the function of the kidney. It is further met with in hydrophobia; in inflammations in internal cavities involving the ganglia of the great sympathetic; after the use of ergot and of opium; and in some of the diseases of the skin. It also attends paroxysms of neuralgia, as witnessed in the exquisite sensitiveness of the skin during an attack of *tic douloureux;* the painful spots, too, in the course of local neuralgias, are thought to be hyperæsthetical.

The exaltation of sensation may disclose itself in other signs besides pain and tenderness; in a general irritability of the surface, in itching, and in unnatural feelings of various kinds. Its seat is ordinarily the skin, and commonly the cutaneous nerves near the point of irritation which causes the heightened sensibility.

Hyperæsthesia may affect the nerves of the special senses, manifesting itself, for instance, by intolerance of light, or of sound. But this variety of hyperæsthesia need here be but alluded to, as we shall presently look more fully at the signs of disturbance of these nerves.

Of the minute anatomical changes in hyperæsthesia we know nothing; our present means of research are insufficient for investigations of this character. Physiologically speaking, the phenomenon belongs, for the most part, to the reflex order—a term under which we conveniently hide much ignorance.

Anæsthesia.—Loss of sensation, or anæsthesia, is of various degrees. It may be complete or partial: a perfect absence of sensibility or its mere benumbing. Not to speak of its meaning when displaying itself only in the organs of the special senses, we find it in diseases of the brain; in several of the neuroses; after the use of large doses of Indian hemp, of lead, of arsenic: we see it accompanying or preceding cutaneous eruptions, such as elephantiasis or pemphigus; and as the result of abnormal conditions of the blood. In the mucous membranes, too, it may exist, either in consequence of the general causes just mentioned, or of some purely local irritation. But it does not attack these structures nearly as often as it does the skin; indeed this is so well understood that, when we speak of anæsthesia without qualifying it, we mean that of the cutaneous nerves. In the parts affected with anæsthesia the nutrition is less active, and there is a feeling of numbness. The temperature is diminished, and, if the impaired sensibility be at all general, the patient is not susceptible to alternations of heat and cold. Frequently the circulation in the skin is retarded, occasioning a perceptible lividity and discoloration of the surface.

Loss of sensation has a much more constant connection with organic affections of the nervous centres than increased sensibility. It may precede acute attacks of cerebral disease, and indeed sometimes exists for years before any marked cerebral symptoms are perceived. Thus, a case of apoplexy was observed by Andral* in which deficient sensation was noticed at various portions of the thorax for a long time previous to the loss of consciousness; another in which the tips of the fingers were benumbed, and felt continually as if they had been subjected to intense cold. Forbes Winslow† mentions instances in which circumscribed conditions of impaired sensation were the premonitory symptoms of softening of the brain; the defective feeling being manifested in some cases in the skin, in others in the tongue and fauces. In the insane, especially in monomaniacs, anæsthesia is very common, and ordinarily very extended; so, too, in general paralysis. Indeed, with few exceptions, an *extended* anæsthesia points to an affection of the nervous centres. Loss of sensation from this source has, moreover, the significant feature of being associated with motor disturbances.

If the defective sensibility be owing to a spinal malady, it is generally found in the lower extremities, and coexists with paralysis; for anæsthesia without paralysis of motion is not met with in the ordinary diseases of the spinal cord. Impaired sensibility of spinal origin is usually indicative of the gray matter of the cord having been disturbed or altered; in the affection known as sclerosis of the cord the sensation is retarded rather than lost.‡

Anæsthesia is sometimes the result of reflex action. It may thus arise in disorders of any of the viscera, and from an irritation of any sensitive nerve. It has, for instance, been observed in both lower limbs in sciatica.§

---

* Clinique Médicale, tome v.   † Obscure Diseases of the Brain, page 549.
‡ Vulpian, Arch. de Phys., i. No. 3.
§ For some striking observations on this subject, the reader is referred to the tenth lecture of Brown-Séquard's work on the Central Nervous System.

A *localized* and curious form of anæsthesia happens now and then in consequence of an affection of the fifth nerve. The extent of loss of sensation depends very much upon the part of the nerve at which the cause of disturbance is seated. The skin of the nose and cheek may become devoid of sensation; the reflex movements of the muscles of the face may cease; the conjunctiva, or the whole surface of the eye, or one-half of the tongue be deprived of sensibility. Only one, or all of these phenomena may be conjointly encountered, according as part of one, or one, or all of the branches of the fifth nerve are affected. Sometimes, as Romberg proves, *trigeminal anæsthesia* is of rheumatic origin. When it is complicated with disturbed functions of adjoining cerebral nerves, it may be assumed, says the same distinguished observer, that the cause is seated at the base of the brain.

In endeavoring to form a correct opinion of the complete-

Fig. 3.

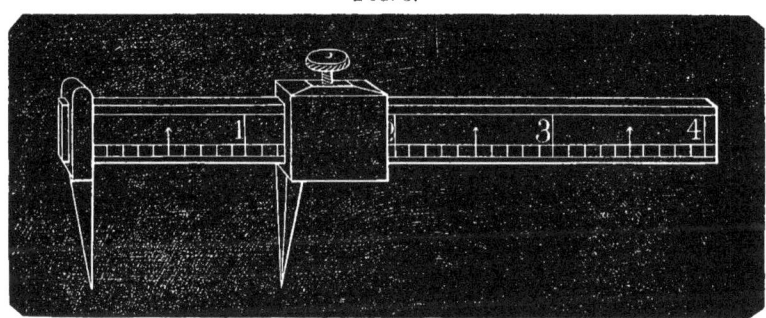

The æsthesiometer.

ness of anæsthesia, it will not do to trust entirely to the patient's statements. We must resort to means by which we can make accurate comparisons; and one of the best is to pursue the method used by Weber in his researches on the tactile properties of the skin. It consists in determining how closely the points of a pair of compasses sheathed with cork may be approximated on the skin, and yet be felt as two distinct points. An instrument for the same purpose, called the "æsthesiometer," was invented by Dr. Sieveking, and can be applied in paralysis to ascertain the amount and extent of sensational impairment, as a means of diagnosis between actual paralysis of sensation and mere subjective anæsthesia in which the tactile powers are unaltered, and as affording us assistance in determining the progress of a case of palsy for better or for worse. A similar instrument, though differing in having a larger handle, is used by Brown-Séquard;[*] and yet another, combining the principle of the beam compass with that of the mathematical one, has been contrived by Dr. Ogle.[†]

To understand, however, any results obtained regarding the tactile sense, it is absolutely necessary that we should be aware how this differs in some parts of the body. Most works on physiology contain an account of the researches of Weber and of those who have prosecuted the inquiry he started.[‡] It would therefore be useless to quote them here at any length, yet a few of the conclusions arrived at may be advantageously mentioned. At the tip of the tongue two points can be readily distinguished when only separate from each other about the $\frac{1}{22}$ of an inch, or half a Paris line; at the palmar surface of the third phalanx the limit is one line; on the palm of the hand, the check, and extremity of great toe, five lines; on the back of the hand, fourteen lines; on the skin over the patella and dorsum of the foot, eighteen lines; over the middle of the arm, thigh, and over the spine, thirty lines. But these observations are found to vary somewhat even in perfectly healthy persons, some being able to distinguish at a much shorter distance than others.

Besides the impairment or loss of tactile discrimination, the altered sensibility may show itself in the loss of the faculty of feeling pinching, pricking, and other acts which excite pain; or in insensibility to tickling; or in the want of appreciation of heat and cold; or of the sensation which attends muscular contraction, whether produced by the will or by a galvanic current. Now, it is of interest in individual cases to note which particular kind of sensibility is affected, though, as yet, we are not in possession of sufficient facts to draw, from the

---

[*] Journal de Physiologie, tome i., 1858.

[†] Beale's Archives of Medicine, vol. i.

[‡] See especially Carpenter's article, "Touch," in Cyclopædia of Anatomy and Physiology; also Valentin's "Lehrbuch der Physiologie."

absence of one form of sensibility or the other, any positive conclusions as to the seat or character of the disease.

In affections of the base of the brain, we have been recently told there is this peculiar modification of tactile impression, that the patient feels three points instead of the two of the æsthesiometer.*

Anæsthesia may be limited to one-half of the body. In diseases of the spinal cord this is a symptom of the gray matter in the opposite half of the cord being altered.

Anæsthesia and hyperæsthesia follow, or, to speak more accurately, manifest themselves only in connection with external impressions. Let us now look at some abnormal sensations which are not objective, but subjective,—arising, so far as we can judge, independently of external impressions. Headache and vertigo are of this character.

Headache.—In every case of headache we must first ascertain that the pain really originates within the cranium, and that it is not owing to supra-orbital neuralgia; to rheumatism of the scalp; to disease of the bones; to periostitis, syphilitic or otherwise; to affections of the ear; in fact, to those numerous causes which occasion cephalic pain. To accomplish this is generally not difficult. An inquiry into the history of the case, the particular locality of the pain, and its augmentation on pressure in most of the disorders named, furnish evidence which, rightly used, decides the source of the cephalalgia to be external to the cranium.

Having settled this point, we have next to determine the probable cause of the headache—a question the solution of which depends frequently more upon the symptoms attending the pain than upon its character. But let us glance at some of the more common causes and characteristics of intra-cranial headache.

Headache is an important, and, on the whole, rarely absent symptom of *diseases of the brain*. In inflammation of that organ it is generally agonizing, and, although subject to exacerbations, continuous; it is associated with fever, with vomiting, and with delirium. In abscesses of the brain, in

---

* Brown-Séquard, Archive de Physiologie, i. No. 3.

tumors, softening, and similar affections which run a chronic course, the headache is also persistent, but less violent, and only occasionally paroxysmal; it is usually accompanied by signs of disturbed intellection and of deranged motion. In congestion of the brain the pain is dull, increased by stooping or lying down, by long sleep, and by bodily or mental fatigue; its concomitants are a flushed face, throbbing of the arteries of the neck, and a heated head. In diseases of the meninges, especially those of a chronic character, the pain is constant and fixed, and sometimes very sharp. The latter kind of pain when persistent is very significant either of disease of the membranes, or, at least, of parts of the superficial structure in contact with them, and is usually felt at the place on the head which corresponds to the lesion within the skull. There is generally in meningeal affections coexisting heat of forehead, with signs of local vascular excitement.

Nervous or neuralgic headache is most common in women, especially in anemic women. It is unremitting and very severe, yet of short duration; but after it is over there is a great lassitude, and even some local soreness. It is not attended with fever, nor with any signs of disturbance of the brain, excepting at times with a confusion of vision and an inability to carry on a connected train of thought. Anything that agitates the nervous system produces an attack; stimulants and food often relieve it.

Sympathetic headache is of kindred nature. It is found mainly in connection with disorders of the alimentary tube and of the uterus, and is often worse in the morning, before food has been taken.

Headache may be dependent upon various *poisons*, whether generated in the system or introduced from without; for instance, in organic diseases of the kidney the retention of a large quantity of urea in the blood becomes the source of constant pain in the head. In lead poisoning, in opium eaters, in drunkards, and after the use of strychnia or of large quantities of quinia, headache is a common phenomenon.

In studying headache as a symptom, we must always note what influence position and movements of the head have on the pain: whether, for instance, stooping, swinging the head from side to side, or rising rapidly from the horizontal to the erect posture affect it, and cause it to be combined with vertiginous or other abnormal sensations.

Vertigo.—This is a transitory feeling of swimming of the head, a sense of falling, or illusory movements of external objects. The curious sensation is apt to occur whenever the circulation within the cranium is disturbed, and is often symptomatic of a disease of the heart, liver, kidneys, stomach, or blood, or it follows long-continued and exhausting discharges. Vertigo may attend any disorder of the brain. The cerebral form is recognized, in part, by the absence of those affections of other organs which would induce the dizziness; in part, by its being joined to headache, and to further signs of an encephalic malady. Moreover, it is most usually objective in character: surrounding objects appear to the patient to move, not he himself; and unlike the subjective vertigo, so common in mere sympathetic disturbance of the brain, closing the eyes relieves it.

There is a kind of vertigo to which Trousseau especially has called attention. The abnormal sensation is very short in its duration, but severe; the patient momentarily loses all consciousness. The vertigo recurs at uncertain times: while actively engaged, sometimes while in bed and half asleep. The head feels heavy after an attack, and the mind is temporarily stupefied; otherwise the health is good. This type of vertigo is dangerous. It is often the precursor of epilepsy, and after a time becomes associated with convulsions.

Another kind of vertigo is that which arises from overwork of the brain, and which, when at all persistent, must make us fear that the organ has begun to soften. Yet another is found to be associated with partial deafness, or with irritation of the auditory nerve. In some instances the giddiness is the only symptom of disorder, and is present for many years, the patient enjoying otherwise excellent health. I have known a number of such instances in which this tendency appeared to have been inherited.

Besides headache and vertigo, there are various unnatural sensations, such as a feeling of momentary unconsciousness without giddiness; a feeling within the cranium of weight, of constriction; the feeling described as a rush of blood to the head; ocular spectra, and other false perceptions of many kinds and of every gradation. But I shall do no more than advert to this subject, and will merely, in concluding the examination of the evidences of deranged sensation, consider some of the morbid phenomena of the special senses, and particularly of the sense of sight and of hearing.

Derangement of Special Senses.—The sense of *vision* may be exalted, impaired, or perverted, in disorders of the brain, whether organic or functional. It is exalted in inflammation; impaired, even totally lost, in softening, in tumors, in apoplexy, and during violent hysterical attacks simulating apoplexy. Perversions of the sense of vision are more frequent than its abolition, and probably more peculiar to cerebral affections. They are of all kinds—some of great consequence, others of but little. *Muscæ volitantes*, or the delusion of spots and various small objects floating before the eye, have the latter significance; for they may happen in almost any form of cerebral disturbance, also in anæmia, in cardiac maladies, in the neuroses, and in states of nervous exhaustion. Some persons see but *half* an objcet. This may be dependent upon an injury to the brain, or be owing to some purely local affection of the eye. In the former case there is coexisting headache, and the mind generally shows signs of disorder. *Double* vision, unless connected with strabismus, is almost always the result of cerebral disease. Of other manifestations of deranged sight, such as illusions, ocular spectra, and phantasms, I cannot here take cognizance: I shall only state that they are more common in derangement of the mind, temporary or permanent, than in recognizable organic disease of the brain.

The *appearance* of the eye is often of as much significance as the derangement of sight. There, for instance, is strabismus, which is of very usual occurrence in cerebral ailments. We find it during an attack of convulsions; in meningitis; in tumors of the base of the brain; in effusion into the ventricles; and previous to an attack of apoplexy. In some cerebral maladies the eye has a fixed stare; in others the eyelids are constantly moving: but the latter is a sign more frequent in chorea or hysteria. Great brilliancy of the eye is often noticed in meningitis and in insanity.

The *pupils* are very variously affected by cerebral disorders. We find them dilated or contracted, sluggish or rapidly altering, on the admission or exclusion of light. We observe a difference in the size of the two pupils, and in their relative irritability. A dilatation of both pupils is found in compression of the brain, whatever its immediate cause, but especially in compression from a collection of fluid in the ventricles and in the subarachnoid spaces; the pupils likewise react very sluggishly, sometimes hardly at all, under the stimulus of light, and the retina appears insensible. A similar state, although not carried to the same degree, is met with in the congestion of the brain accompanying low fevers. We also find dilatation of both pupils in chlorosis, and when the system is under the influence of belladonna.

Contraction of the pupils exists in the earlier stages of cerebral inflammation. It is then associated with intolerance of light, which does not occur if the contraction be produced by narcotism or by coma. Contraction of the pupils happens also in spinal diseases.* One-sided contraction, like one-sided dilatation of the pupil, is ordinarily the result of a one-sided lesion of the brain ; yet it may also be owing to tumors at the root of the neck.

But in estimating the value of any morbid evidences furnished by the state of vision or the appearance of the eye, we must make allowance for the purely local diseases of the organ, and exclude them from consideration before we draw conclusions as to the condition of the brain. We are greatly aided in this by the use of the ophthalmoscope, which gives not only information as to many of the mere visual disturbances, but as to the changes brought about in the eye by cerebral affections.

The fundus oculi, as revealed by the *ophthalmoscope*, presents various lesions, which, although not pathognomonic of any one condition, furnish additional information of value in locating more definitely the particular disease. These lesions

---

* See Cases, Edinb. Med. Journal, Dec. 1869.

depend either on an extension of inflammation of the brain to the internal structures of the eye, or on the amount of resistance offered to the circulation within the cranium. This resistance may arise either from a marked " coarse" lesion, or it may be exerted through the sympathetic nervous system.

We should invariably examine with the ophthalmoscope the eyes of patients suspected of having disease of any part of the cerebro-spinal nervous system, and not wait for the development of symptoms which belong to a later stage to elucidate the diagnosis. Changes in the eye, indeed, often occur early enough to be the first certain sign of the disease, and this, too, without any impairment of sight; on the other hand, lesions indicating cerebral or other organic trouble have been found in cases in which failure of sight only was complained of, the ultimate cause being unsuspected by the patient. But particularly is the ophthalmoscope valuable in enabling us to diagnosticate, oftentimes at once and with certainty, organic from functional disorder.

The changes in connection with organic disease have been observed chiefly in the retina, the optic disk, and the choroid, and for the most part indifferently in both eyes, even when the causative disease is limited to one hemisphere.

Retinitis occurs most frequently in connection with intra-cranial lesions, constitutional syphilis, and Bright's disease. It is characterized by a reddish-gray, opaque, swollen, and somewhat hyperemic optic disk, with an irregular and indistinct outline, which passes into the retina without any clear line of demarcation. The retina presents a hazy appearance, particularly marked in the vicinity of the optic papilla and macula lutea; its arteries are but slightly changed in appearance, but the veins are enlarged, dark in color, and very tortuous. Hemorrhagic extravasations are common.

In *syphilitic retinitis* the disk and retina are veiled by a faint, bluish-gray film, due to serous transudation, most marked along the course of the vessels, and which shades off imperceptibly into the healthy retina. Minute punctiform opacities are strewn irregularly over the retina, and they undergo rapid changes, appearing and disappearing in the course of a few days. Galezowski has found syphilitic retinitis and neuritis to be always accompanied by color-blindness. In patients who were the victims of hereditary syphilis, Mr. Hutchinson has frequently observed pigmentary retinitis.

The syphilitic form of retinitis should not be confounded with that which accompanies *disease of the kidney*, and which is characterized by the formation on the retina of brilliant white stellated spots in the region of the macula lutea, and of a broad, glistening, white mound encircling the optic disk. ·These spots are constant, and are due to a fatty degeneration of the connective tissue element and sclerosis of the optic nerve fibres. Retinal hemorrhage is also of frequent occurrence.

A peculiar form of retinitis has been observed, in some rare cases, to accompany diabetes.*

Optic neuritis always results directly — so, at least, we are told by Dr. Allbutt — from meningitis or cerebritic softening, whatever may be the indirect cause. Yet it has been observed in cases of phlebitis of the sinuses, acute and chronic meningitis, chronic encephalitis, cerebral hemorrhage, tumors of the brain, particularly when situated near the optic tract or chiasm, cerebral compression, chronic hydrocephalus, abscess of the brain, syphilitic deposit, hydatid cyst, acute myelitis, locomotor ataxia, certain forms of epilepsy, paralysis or neurosis connected with organic disease of the nervous system, and in diphtheria, rheumatic fever, etc. Being found in so many states, its exact value in each is still to be settled. In cases of hemiplegia, Dr. Hughlings Jackson has noted its greater frequency in connection with left-sided paralysis. In lesions of the encephalon or meninges, Bouchut thinks it is in general more marked in the eye corresponding to the hemisphere which is more seriously affected; Hughlings Jackson, however, denies the existence of any relation between the side of the brain diseased and the eye affected.

The essential ophthalmoscopic sign of optic neuritis is serous infiltration and prominence of the papilla, aecom-

---

* Vide Compte Rendu du Congrès Ophth. de Paris, 1862, p. 110.

panied by vascular turgescence. The disk, owing to its infiltration, presents a woolly appearance. As the walls of the vessels are mostly healthy, the extravasations which are seen in the retinitis of albuminuria do not frequently occur in optic neuritis.

Perineuritis is the name given by Galezowski to inflammation which seems chiefly to affect the outer neurilemma. The papilla is enlarged and prominent, but the exudation appears to be confined to the margin of the papilla, the outlines of which are veiled, while the centre is transparent, and resembles the normal state. This condition is very suggestive of meningitis.

Simple hyperæmia of the disk may be due to encephalic disease, to meningitis, or to Bright's disease. A transient form of hyperæmia may be seen in the changes of cerebral vasenlarity attended with convulsions, in affections of the heart, such as aortic regurgitation, and in Graves' disease.

Diseases of the spinal cord, as acute myelitis, spinal sclerosis, locomotor ataxia, frequently induce a congestive lesion of the optic papilla, which, at a later period, becomes atrophic. These changes do not become established in cases of spinal disease which run a short course, but they slowly supervene in more chronic cases.

Dr. Hughlings Jackson has described[*] a peculiar condition of the retina, which he observed in a patient with epileptiform convulsions, and which he calls *epilepsy of the retina*. The retina is entirely anemic, a condition dependent in all probability upon a contraction of the retinal vessels similar to that which occurs in the vessels of the brain during an epileptic fit.

Atrophy of the optic nerve is met with in cases of cerebral tumor, in meningitis, hydrocephalus, constitutional syphilis, sun-stroke, after typhoid fever, and in paralysis and symptomatic epilepsy. Allbutt has found[†] that atrophy of the optic disk happens in nearly every case of general paralysis of the insane, beginning as a pink suffusion of the nerve, without much stasis or exudation, and ending as simple

[*] Royal Ophthal. Hosp. Rep., vol. iv. p. 14.
[†] Brit. Med. Jour., March 14, 1868.

white atrophy—a process which he likens to "red and white softening" of the brain. Atrophy frequently occurs in loco-motor ataxia, and has been observed in some cases of chronic myelitis, etc. It may occur as a secondary effect of cerebral hemorrhage. According to Bouchut,* it is never seen in cases of meningitis, except when this is a complication of chronic meningitis, an old encephalitis, or an old tumor of the brain. It is never found as a result of spinal injuries; and repeated scrutiny has convinced Bouchut that the fundus is entirely unaffected in rachitis.

The causes of *choroiditis*, with the exception of the syphi-litic form, are very obscure. It appears most frequently as circumscribed white patches in the choroid, over which the retinal vessels may be seen coursing. It, however, occa-sionally assumes most varying appearances. The syphilitic form is by far the most common, and is distinguished by the presence of patches of many colors at the back of the eye, some being of a brilliant white, others of darker tints, such as red or brown.

Tubercles of the choroid are a manifestation of the tuber-cular diathesis, and one, too, which is probably of more frequent occurrence in miliary tuberculosis than is generally supposed. In eighteen cases of miliary tuberculosis which were examined in the Berlin Pathological Institution, Cohn-heim found tubercles in the choroid of one or both eyes in every instance. They appear, ophthalmoscopically, in the form of small circumscribed spots, of a pale rose-red color, or grayish-white tint, and vary in size, according to Wells, from one-third to two and five-tenths of a millimetre. They are chiefly situated in the vicinity of the optic disk. The sight may remain unimpaired. In the retina and choroid, the existence of tubercles indicates either tubercular meningitis or general tuberculosis. If, with tubercular granulations of the choroid, fever and disturbances of intellect, of movement and sensation be present, the existence of tubercular menin-gitis may be determined.

As regards the *sense of hearing*, the same may be said as

---

* Diagnostic des Maladies Nerveux par l'Ophthalmoscopie.

of vision. It, too, is perverted and impaired in various cerebral affections; yet to be certain that the cause of the trouble is cerebral, the ear must first be carefully examined with reference to any physical imperfection.

Great acuteness of hearing and intolerance of sound are generally symptoms of extreme nervous irritability, or of commencing cerebral inflammation. Deafness may be owing to softening of portions of the brain; but it is also found as a temporary, and by no means unfavorable symptom in the continued fevers. Imaginary sounds and ringing noises in the ear, or *tinnitus aurium*, are frequent accompaniments of cerebral disorders. But the latter is encountered in so many different conditions—in diseases of the cerebral vessels, in congestion of the brain, in affections of the heart, in anæmia —that it is a sign of but little moment; and, in truth, its most usual cause is local, namely, an accumulation of wax in the meatus.

DERANGED MOTION.

The chief manifestations of deranged motion resolve themselves into the phenomena called paralysis, tremor, ataxia, spasms, and convulsions.

Paralysis.—When we speak of paralysis, we mean a loss of muscular contractility, and, as a consequence, of the power of motion. It is true, there is also a paralysis of sensation, which may be conjoined with the paralysis of motion; but the latter often happens alone, and is the morbid state alluded to when we use the term paralysis without qualifying whether of sensation or of motion.

Paralysis may be general, or it may be partial. It may affect the majority of the muscles of the frame, or be limited to one muscle. It may be strictly confined to one side, or exist solely in the lower half of the body. It may come on rapidly, or appear slowly. But under any circumstance it is not a disease, but a symptom. We must, in individual cases, therefore, aim at determining, so far as possible, its cause, before we attempt to remedy the palsy. The causes which give rise to paralysis may be thus summed up:

Paralysis due to a lesion, or any morbid condition of the nervous centres.—Softening of the central nervous textures, or any process which materially alters them, occasions loss of power in the part over which their influence in health extends. The complete paralysis attending most of the diseases of the brain or of the spinal cord belongs, therefore, to this category.

But besides these palsies of organic origin, there are palsies dependent upon what, so far as we are aware, is simply a functional derangement of the great centres of innervation. How else explain a hysterical paralysis, or the transitory palsy sometimes seen to follow low fevers, or that occurring after overwork or excesses, and so evidently from nervous exhaustion ?

Paralysis due to a lesion in the course of a nerve.—The nervous force may be properly generated, but the nerve fibres may be incapable of conducting it. For instance, if a nerve be wounded, or lacerated, or compressed, paralysis of the muscles which it supplies takes place. Palsy from this cause is local.

Paralysis due to an affection of the nerves at their extremities.— A paralysis originating at the periphery of a nerve is a rare complaint. But we meet every now and then with undoubted illustrations of such a disorder: for example, the palsy resulting from exposure to cold. Peripheral palsies lead quickly to atrophy of the muscles. They are, from their very nature, local, and commonly remain so. But there is a notable exception to this in the so-called creeping palsy; a disease which commences with a feeling of numbness and a slight loss of muscular power in one arm or leg, but which gradually spreads to other portions of the body.

Paralysis due to reflex action.—Here the paralysis is produced through the medium of the great seat of the reflex system, the spinal cord, which reflects the irritation communicated to it to parts healthy in themselves. At all events, cases are from time to time met with which admit of no other explanation. How else can excitation of the dental nerves in teething children, or disorders of the intestines both in adults and children, or disease of the bladder, urethra, uterus, lungs or pleura, or irritation of the nerves of the skin, occasion paralysis ? or how else can a wound of a nerve on one side of the body lead to palsy on the other ?

Paralysis brought on by reflex action is rarely of long duration. It is increased or diminished as the causes which produce it increase or diminish, and, as a rule, soon disappears after the source of irritation is removed. It may affect almost any part of the body, and even assume the paraplegic form.

Paralysis due to serious interference with the circulation.—This kind of palsy is observed if the principal artery of a part be obliterated. But it is not often encountered; and when met with, is not unusually found to be connected with gangrene of the paralyzed part. It is sometimes noticed as a transient phenomenon after the ligature of a large artery; in a more permanent form it is apt to be caused by a plug of fibrin impacted in a vessel.

Paralysis due to a morbid state of the muscles.—Any process which materially impairs the normal structure of muscular tissue will entail loss of muscular power; but in point of fact, the disease which commonly occasions this form of paralysis (if it be correct to call that paralysis in which the nervous system is not to appearance particularly concerned) is muscular atrophy, and especially the progressive muscular atrophy connected with fatty degeneration.

Paralysis due to the presence of poisons in the system.—The toxical effects of lead, arsenic, mercury, of alcohol, and of sulphuret of carbon, may exhibit themselves by producing palsy. Malarial poisons, and poisons formed in the system, such as that of rheumatism or of gout, may act in the same way. The former occasion that singular "intermittent paralysis" which may come on either as one of the phenomena of a fit of ague, or as an apparently independent complaint; which assumes either the quotidian or tertian type, and in which both sensation and motion may be affected. How any of these poisons operate, whether by interfering with the nutrition of the nervous centres and weakening their generating force, or by enfeebling the conducting power of the nerves, is unknown. The palsies coming under this head being, as it were, functional, are not ordinarily intractable. Those due to malaria yield speedily to decided doses of quinine.

In the parts affected with paralysis, the nutrition and secretion are disturbed and the circulation is sluggish. They are frequently swollen and edematous, the pulse is weaker than in the sound members, and the sensation is impaired. The nails grow slowly; the perspiration is defective; the skin feels cold, is prone to break from the effect of pressure, and the ulcers heal but tardily. The condition of the muscles is very various. In some cases they are completely relaxed, in others rigid; at times they become agitated with convulsive movements. These phenomena are apt to be most evident in palsies of organic origin, especially in those dependent upon a brain lesion, and in those due to disease of the spinal cord in which anæsthesia is present. Where hyperæsthesia occurs, the increased sensibility is attended with a larger supply of blood and a higher temperature than normal.

Having thus briefly alluded to some of the general traits and to the causes of paralysis, let us now examine its chief varieties with reference to their clinical significance and their diagnosis. In so doing, it will be convenient to be guided by their marked coarse features rather than by their presumed origin.

Hemiplegia.—And first, of hemiplegia, or one-sided palsy. This state of things may affect all the voluntary muscles on one side of the body; but it generally exists only in those of the limbs and face. Neither the legs nor arms can move, and the muscles of the face on the side corresponding to the paralyzed limbs are motionless. The cheek hangs; the mouth is drawn toward the healthy side, because the muscles on the other are powerless to resist; the tongue, when protruded, is ordinarily slowly pushed out toward the palsied side; the articulation is imperfect.

But the rule with respect to the face being paralyzed on the same side as the rest of the body has its exceptions. Indeed, when we reflect that the nerves which supply the facial muscles are given off above the pyramids, therefore above the point of decussation of the nervous fibres in the cord, it is perplexing that it should be a rule at all. The solution of the question has been attempted by assuming, in accordance with the physiological researches of Stilling and Phillipeaux, a crossing of the facial nerves. Should, then, the lesion be seated in the brain above this crossing, both face and body are paralyzed on the side opposite to the diseased spot. Should, however, the lesion involve the facial nerve fibres at a point below or after the crossing, there will be paralysis of the face on one side, and of the limbs on the other, the facial palsy being direct, and that of the body, crossed.

Now according to Gubler,* who has investigated the intricate subject with much skill, this form of paralysis is always indicative of a lesion of the pons varolii, close to which the facial nerves originate, and through which the nerve fibres for the limbs pass before they decussate lower down. But in adopting this conclusion, we must always remember that there are rare cases of " alternating paralysis" due to a combination of several lesions, one affecting a cerebral lobe on one side and the facial nerve on the other. And even when the lesion is unilateral, we may meet with exceptional cases; so that the whole matter cannot as yet be regarded as fully settled. With reference to the other cerebral nerves, should we find any of them paralyzed on one side and the body on the other, we shall very generally be correct in assuming that the palsy is not due to disease on both sides of the brain, but is rather a disturbance of the affected nerve near its origin or in its course, and on the side on which the brain is injured, while the paralysis of the limbs is on the opposite side.†

Hemiplegia results, in the vast majority of instances, from cerebral disease. Hence we find it commonly associated with disordered mental powers, and other signs of a brain lesion. Hemiplegia caused by an affection of one-half of the

---

* De l'émiplégie alterne envisagée comme signe de lésion de la protubér. ance annulaire. Gaz. Hebdom., 1856, 1859.

† Minute anatomical researches, particularly those of Lockhart Clarke, on the internal structure of the brain, are beginning to remove much of the obscurity in attempting to explain these double palsies, as well as the dissimilar manner in which the facial nerve is affected. Connecting nuclei on the floor of the fourth ventricle and elsewhere are traced. (See Philosophical Transactions, Part I. 1868.

spinal cord, near its commencement, is not combined with a decay of the mental faculties, and the muscles of the chest and abdomen are involved in the paralysis, which they are not in cerebral hemiplegia, unless the lesion be very extensive. Then in spinal hemiplegia there is apt to be coexisting anæsthesia; and the umbilicus is with every act of inspiration drawn toward the sound side; and according to the statement of Romberg, spinal hemiplegia is more persistent in the leg than it is in the arm. We possess a further test in electricity. Marshall Hall long since enunciated the doctrine that the irritability of the muscles, when the influence of the brain is withdrawn, is increased; and that, therefore, in cerebral paralysis the palsied limbs are more excitable by electricity. This statement is qualified by Duchenne, who asserts that in cerebral hemiplegia the electro-muscular contractility remains as in health, while it is diminished or abolished in spinal disease. Unfortunately, this admirable and easy test is liable to certain drawbacks, and its accuracy depends greatly upon the state of resolution or of rigidity of the muscles of the unsound limb. At least such is the conclusion to be drawn from the experiments of Todd;* and the observations of Althaus, also, lead to a similar inference.† The results obtained by him would seem to show that in a certain number of cases of cerebral paralysis, the muscles are flaccid, and the contractility is diminished; while in another class of cases no difference in contractility can be discerned between the healthy and the palsied limb; but in a third class the affected muscles are, by a current of the same intensity, more powerfully convulsed than those of the sound side, and then we may infer that the paralysis is due to brain disease of an irritative character.‡

---

* Clinical Lectures on the Nervous System, page 39; and Med.-Chirurg. Transact., vol. xxxvi.

† On Paralysis, Neuralgia, etc., 3d edition, 1864; also Medical Electricity, 2d edition, 1870. As in the cases of Rosenthal, quoted Retrospect of Sydenham Society, 1868; also cases of Brown-Séquard.

‡ These remarks apply to the effects obtained by the induced current, or to faradisation of the muscles. A continuous current may, however, in cases of palsy, give different results. The muscles of a palsied part may respond actively to galvanisation and not at all to faradisation. How far these dif-

But supposing that we have satisfactorily settled the hemi-plegia to be cerebral, the points next to be investigated are, where is the lesion situated? and what is its probable nature? Now the former question may be answered in a general way by stating that it is on the side opposite to the palsy, if the lesion, which it almost always is, be seated above the point of decussation of the pyramidal columns of the medulla oblongata; for a lesion below the decussation gives rise to palsy on the same side, and a lesion on a level with the decussation, to double-sided palsy. Furthermore, we may reasonably conclude the morbid process to have affected the corpus striatum, if motion be seriously impaired, or to have attacked the optic thalamus, if there be paralysis of sensa-tion; yet in point of fact, so intimate is the union between these two bodies, that one is hardly ever much disorganized without the other being drawn into the disease. The more superficial the lesion, and the nearer therefore to the surface, the more incomplete the palsy, and the more the disease ex-tends toward the corpus striatum, the more thorough does the paralysis of motion become. We may further distinguish the palsy which ensues from that caused by an affection lower down, as of the pons varolii, by observing that, besides the peculiar crossed paralysis of the face and limbs which so often happens in this, and which has been above described, we find extreme coldness of that side of the body which is to become paralyzed after a time; also giddiness and a tend-ency to vomit; jerkings of the muscles of the face, on the side opposite to the injury; sensations of tickling in the face; and one-sided facial anæsthesia, with a loss of sense of taste on the corresponding side, though with unimpaired motion of the tongue. Should we encounter paralysis of sensibility and motion on one side of the body, and both sides of the face be palsied as to motion and sensation, the recti muscles

ferences may be made available for diagnostic purposes is undetermined. In accordance with the recent researches of Erb (Archiv für Klinische Medi-cin, Bd. ii.), the alterations of excitability only affect the muscles, since, when there has been an injury to the motor nerves, there is loss of excitability alike to the induced and continuous current. (See Erb; also Meyer's work on Electricity, translated by Hammond, and Althaus on Medical Electricity.)

of the eye be paralyzed, and taste lost over the anterior part of the tongue, we may infer that the injury is seated rather above the lower portions of the pons, and affects the spot where the facial nerve and part of the trigeminal cross.*

The *nature* of the paralyzing lesion can only be arrived at by a careful scrutiny of all the facts of the case. A sudden paralysis occurring simultaneously with coma almost always has its origin in an apoplectic effusion; a sudden paralysis without coma is generally due to a rapid giving way of a softened brain. A gradual development of palsy indicates some chronic cerebral disorder, such as softening, or a tumor, or any affection compressing the nervous substance. We may also gain much knowledge by carefully exploring the organs of circulation and the kidneys. Thus, a paralysis found to be conjoined to a cardiac malady or to a diseased state of the arteries, is, in all likelihood, owing to softening, to an apoplectic effusion into the brain, or, as happens in rare cases, to a stopping up of one of the cerebral arteries with a mass of coagulated fibrin. When the kidneys are seriously disordered, it is not unreasonable to suppose that the hemiplegia has been caused by some chronic disease of the brain, the result of the altered nutrition produced by the ill-purified blood.

A further clue to the character of the cerebral lesion is obtained by examining the palsied muscles. Todd, who has most clearly and forcibly directed attention to this subject, declares that when the paralyzed limbs exhibit a rigid state of the muscles from the moment of, or soon after the attack, we may assume the lesion to be of an irritative nature, such as an inflammation, or a compression of healthy brain tissue by an apoplectic clot or by an accumulation of puriform fluid in the subarachnoid spaces. When the muscular contraction does not take place until late in the complaint, and becomes associated with wasting of the muscles, it may be presumed to be caused by an irritation from an attempt at cicatrization. When the muscles are flaccid and relaxed, and there is, for instance, no resistance in the flexing of the forearm upon the

---

* Brown-Séquard, Dublin Quart. Journ., May, 1865.

arm, or the leg upon the thigh, we may conclude the lesion to be of a depressing kind, such as white softening of the brain, with or without rupture of the blood-vessels. In paralysis with resolution of the muscles, as before stated, the electric excitability of the unsound limb is far less than that of the sound one, while in early rigidity it is much increased.

A curious phenomenon connected with paralysis is, that reflex actions can be excited in the apparently lifeless limb. The application of a hot iron, or the tickling of the sole of the foot, will often give rise to violent movements.

Paraplegia.—This differs from hemiplegia in the palsy occurring on both sides, yet being limited to the lower extremities. It almost never depends on disease of the brain, its most frequent cause being a lesion of the spinal cord. There are, however, cases in which it results from poisons, from fatigue, from excesses, and in which it exists independently of any recognizable structural change.

The disorder generally comes on slowly. At first the patient only loses the steadiness of his gait; gradually he is deprived of all power of motion, but the intellect and the nerves of special sense remain unaffected. If the lesion be in the lumbar part of the cord, the paralysis is confined to the lower extremities and to the pelvic muscles; if the dorsal portion be attacked, we find, in addition, signs of paralysis of the abdominal walls and of the sphincters, tympanites, and a somewhat impeded breathing. In diseases of the upper section of the cord there is coexisting palsy of the upper extremities, with difficulty in deglutition and in respiration. In the muscles supplied by the nerves which originate in healthy marrow, involuntary retractions or reflex phenomena may be induced, and the striking effects of strychnia, when given in doses sufficient to produce its peculiar muscular spasms, are manifested. To the effects of electricity we have already alluded. The palsied muscles do not respond to the electrical stimulus; at least they do not after their nutrition has become impaired.

Paraplegia is generally more marked on one side than on the other, and the paralysis of motion is apt to be associated with very complete and permanent anæsthesia. When, as sometimes happens, the mischief is limited to a lateral segment of any part of the cord, there is paralysis of motion on the same side of the body, and of sensation on the other.*

Preceding, or even attending many cases of paraplegia, is a very curious symptom which belongs exclusively to affections of the cord: a spasm of the flexor muscles of the lower limbs, so powerful that the anterior parts of the thighs come almost in contact with the abdomen, while the heels are drawn up so as to touch the back of the thighs.†

Let us now take a cursory view of the different forms of spinal paraplegia.

Sometimes the paralysis occurs *suddenly*, and in cousequence of an injury to the spine, of a displacement subsequent to a disease of the bones, of blood extravasated into the canal, or of poisons, as the lathyrus sativus.‡ When either of the former two causes has led to the sudden palsy, the diagnosis is materially aided by the history of the case, and by a close examination of the vertebral column. But if there be no history of an injury, if no signs of a disease of the bones or the intervertebral cartilages can be detected, we may suspect a spinal hemorrhage to have produced the sudden paraplegia; and this suspicion becomes much strengthened if violent pain in the back exist, if the patient be unable to retain his urine or feces, and if the affected limbs become rigid. And we are not kept in doubt long, for spinal apoplexy has generally a speedily fatal termination.

But besides these causes, others lead rapidly to paraplegia. Softening of the cord may have progressed latently until the degeneration destroys the continuity of the conducting tubules, when palsy at once takes place. Then there are cases following sexual excesses, cases for which neither during life nor after death any organic causes can be assigned,§ and which must therefore be viewed as due to enfeeblement

---

* Brown-Séquard's Lectures on the Nervous Centres.

† Ibid., page 114.

‡ Irving, Indian Annals, No. 12, referred to in Brit. and For. Med.-Chirurg. Rev., Oct. 1860.

§ For instance, Case XVIII. in Gull's admirable Series of Cases of Paraplegia, in vol. iv. Guy's Hosp. Rep., 3d series.

of functional power. Similar cases of spinal paralysis, more
or less complete, may occur after fatigue and violent exercise,
and would even seem to have been induced by exposure to
cold and wet. In all instances of spinal palsy due to impaired nerve power, the disorder is much more apt to come
on quickly than gradually, and a tonic treatment is likely to
be followed by decidedly good effects.

Yet another variety of paraplegia which may happen
rapidly, is that form which has been described as *acute ascending paralysis*, and to which evidently many of the cases of
creeping palsy that have been reported belong. It may come
on after fatigue and exposure in persons in perfect health.
Numbness and pain in the lower extremities are soon followed by loss of muscular power, which, in turn, goes on
rapidly to complete paraplegia. The upper extremities now
may become implicated, and sensation, which at first was
normal, is enfeebled. The patient is restless, sleepless, but
his intelligence is unimpaired. The respiration and circulation are then apt to become embarrassed, and sudden death
ensues within a month from the time of the seizure.* But
all cases do not run so rapid a course; and, in truth, we
meet with instances in which the disorder is rather chronic
than acute. The muscles in any case atrophy; and in those
involved, the electro-muscular contractility is diminished or
abolished, and, as Jaccoud† tells us in the cases he observed,
there is anæsthesia localized over the affected parts, and the
reflex movements are abolished. Whether the primary lesion
be in the peripheral nerves or in their spinal centre is as yet
an undecided question.

Gradual paraplegia occurs in congestion, in acute and
chronic inflammation of the meninges, in myelitis, in softening, in atrophy, in compression of the cord, and from
reflex irritation. It is very difficult to determine the features by which these different morbid conditions may be
distinguished from each other; indeed, a distinction is not

---

* As in the case reported by Hayem. Travaux de la Société Médicale
d'Observation, tome ii. 1867.

† Clinique Médicale.

always possible.   These are some of the marks of discrimination:

In *congestion* of the cord there is dull pain, generally confined to the lumbar and sacral regions; the palsy progresses slowly from below upward, is preceded by a feeling of numbness, is almost always incomplete, and rarely combined with paralysis of the sphincters.   Moreover, the difficulty in walking is much greater on arising after a night's rest, or indeed whenever the patient has been for any length of time in the recumbent posture.   We may often, too, trace the congestion to some disturbance of the circulation, especially of the abdominal circulation; or to alterations in the composition of the blood, as in rheumatism, small-pox, or typhus; or we find it as a result of exposure to cold and wet.

In *inflammation* of the meninges we encounter severe pain in the back, but little influenced by pressure upon the spine, yet aggravated by movement, even by the acts of defecation and of urination; sometimes a sensation as if a cord had been drawn around the belly; pains in the limbs similar to those of rheumatism; cutaneous hyperæsthesia; muscular contraetions, more or less permanent and painful; still only very incomplete paralysis, or, indeed, none at all.   When marked paraplegia follows the symptoms mentioned, we may suspect that an effusion has taken place which compresses the spinal cord.   Cases of spinal meningitis are not unusual among soldiers who have slept on damp ground.

Myelitis presents many of the same symptoms.   But they generally come on by slow degrees, and the paraplegia becomes very complete.   Contractions of the muscles are uncommon, and certainly not permanent, the muscles are usually limber; there is comparatively little pain, none on pressure at any part of the spine, or on motion, and anæsthesia is apt, sooner or later, to show itself.   Further, we generally, though not constantly, find the urine alkaline, and, as a rule, a want of control over the bladder and rectum exists. In acute cases there are, as in acute spinal meningitis (with which, indeed, myelitis may be complicated), heat of skin and a frequent pulse.   In many instances we notice erection of the penis.   Reflex movements are gradually abolished in

6

the palsied limbs, and involuntary contractions can no longer be excited in them.*

Softening of the cord cannot, with any certainty, be distinguished from chronic inflammation, often, in truth, a cause of the softening. Nor can the paraplegia consequent upon *atrophy* of the cord be clearly separated. Indeed, although it is stated that we may infer its presence, if the history of the patient prove him to have been subject to tremulous movements, and an unsteady gait; if difficulty in urination, spasmodic muscular contractions, or sudden muscular jerks have preceded, or accompany the failing sensation and the loss of motion; yet of atrophy, excepting when in connection with locomotor ataxia, we have no trustworthy knowledge. In the form of atrophy with hardening, the so-called *sclerosis* of the cord, we find chiefly the symptoms of atrophy just alluded to. But a great deal depends on the seat of the lesion. Thus, when limited to the posterior column, the symptoms are those of locomotor ataxia; when to the anterior lateral, we meet with a paraplegia of slow development and with coexisting derangement of the bladder and rectum; in more general sclerosis, or when diffused and in patches, attacks of severe pain, cramps, or permanent contractions are apt to accompany the gradually extending and very general palsy.† In *tumors* pressing upon the spinal cord or seated in its substance, especially those of a cancerous nature, there is much pain over the seat of the tumor, with very gradual paralysis, which is conjoined to impaired sensation manifest from the very beginning of the disease, and in some instances to priapism; and emaciation and signs of a grave constitutional disease often attend the palsy.

But what of the *reflex* paraplegia, to which Brown-Séquard has of late years so cogently called attention, and which is

---

* An altered sensibility to heat and cold when, for instance, a sponge soaked in warm water or a piece of ice is applied to the spine over the inflamed spot, has been spoken of as a diagnostic test. In either case the sensation, when the diseased part is reached, changes to a burning sensation. This symptom is. however, far from constant, and cannot be accepted as conclusive.

† See, for instance, the cases referred to in Jaccoud's Clinique Médicale; also in an elaborate article by Meredith Clymer, New York Medical Journal, May, 1870.

caused "by the most varied irritations of the skin, the mucous and serous membranes, the abdominal or thoracic viscera, as well as of the genital organs or the trunks of the spinal nerves?" Can we isolate it from the paraplegia of organic spinal origin? Not with any certainty, unless we can discern the source of the irritation, obtain a clear history of the case, and satisfy ourselves of the absence of the special symptoms of an organic disease of the spine or its contents. Some distinctive features are, that the muscles do not become atrophied; that their reflex power is comparatively unimpaired; that anæsthesia is exceptional; that the palsy is seldom complete; that some muscles are much more affected than others; that spasms in the paralyzed muscles are extremely uncommon; that there are very rarely pains in the spine, either spontaneously, or on pressure, or by percussion, or by applying ice, or a hot moist sponge. Then it is stated that "in a short time a much greater probability of the accuracy of the diagnosis will spring from the correspondence between changes in the degree of the paralysis with changes in the visceral disease or external irritation that is supposed to have produced the paraplegia."*

So much for paraplegia. We shall now examine some of the other clinical varieties of paralysis; and first, that connected with hysteria.

In *hysterical paralysis* there is no structural affection of the brain, and yet all looks as if this were the case. What distinguishes this paralysis from that of organic cerebral disease, is its occurrence in markedly hysterical persons; its sudden appearance, and frequently its just as sudden disappearance; its coming on generally under the influence of some powerful emotion; the usual absence of any signs of a lesion of the nervous centres, excepting the paralysis; the incomplete character of the palsy, the patient being sometimes able to move while under strong excitement; the unimpaired motion of the muscles of the face and of the tongue; and the ease with which reflex movements are brought on in the

---

* Brown-Séquard, Lectures on the Diagnosis and Treatment of the Principal Forms of Paralysis of the Lower Extremities. 1861. See also G. Echeverria on Reflex Paralysis. New York, 1866.

helpless limb. Moreover, we have a valuable differential test in electricity. The muscles, except in cases of very long standing, respond perfectly to its stimulus, although, as we are told by Duchenne, the electro-muscular sensibility —the sensation produced by the contractions caused by the current—is either diminished or abolished, while in cerebral paralysis it is intact.

Hysterical paralysis may seize only upon one limb, or part of one limb, or it may, although it rarely does, assume a hemiplegic or paraplegic form. Hysterical hemiplegia presents a peculiarity in the gait, on which Todd* lays great stress. "In walking, when the palsy is pretty complete, the leg is drawn along as if lifeless, sweeping the ground." It is not swung round, describing the arc of a circle, as it is in ordinary hemiplegia. The palsy is almost invariably left-sided. It may be conjoined to very decided anæsthesia, which passes beyond the paralyzed part to the nearest portion of skin and mucous membrane, though, as a rule, still limited to the same side. Thus we find the pituitary membrane of one nostril rendered insensible, if the loss of feeling should affect the face.

Rheumatic paralysis resembles hysterical paralysis in being ordinarily very limited. It may affect any muscle, or any group of muscles in the body; sometimes the rheumatic poison disorders the portio dura, and we observe, in consequence, facial palsy. Rheumatic paralysis is recognized by the history of the case; by the evidences of a rheumatic attack; by the rapid development of the palsy; by the pain that attends it; and by its being unaccompanied by symptoms strictly referable to a disease of the brain. The muscles themselves are readily acted upon by electricity, unless their structure be altered.

Paralysis from lead poisoning occurs primarily, and sometimes only, in the extensor muscles of the arm, occasioning the well-known wrist-drop. Gradually other muscles become involved: there is loss of power in the ball of the

---

* Clinical Lectures on Paralysis and other Affections of the Nervous System. Lecture XIII.

thumb, in the deltoid, and in the triceps; but not in the intercostal muscles, or in those of the lower extremities. The disturbed muscles on both sides of the body waste, and entirely lose their irritability to electricity. The patient is weak, his movements tremulous; he has the peculiar blue line on the gums; is obstinately constipated, and subject to colic. Sometimes the poison seizes upon the brain, and epileptic convulsions and other signs of a serious cerebral trouble appear. From the locality of the palsy, in addition to the accompanying symptoms and the knowledge of the man's employment, the diagnosis is usually arrived at with ease.

Diphtheritic paralysis is a remarkable sequel of diphtheria. It follows an attack of that disease within a fortnight or two months, and, therefore, after the patient is apparently fully convalescent. It may be very localized, merely affecting the palate or the pharynx; or very general, fastening upon both of the lower, and even upon the upper extremities. When extensive, it is always ushered in by a throat palsy. It ensues gradually,—day by day the muscular power is more and more enfeebled. The loss of motion is often preceded by numbness and formication. The palsy mends as slowly as it comes on, yet most cases fully recover. How it is produced is difficult to determine. It may be that the poison acts directly by enfeebling the nervous force, or that the paralysis, like that sometimes attending extreme anæmia, is primarily due to the marked impoverishment of the blood, by which means ultimately the nutrition of the nervous centres is deteriorated. The brain itself shows no signs of disease; at least there were no symptoms of cerebral mischief in the cases which have come under my observation.

Paralysis from syphilis we find in persons presenting signs of constitutional syphilis, and in whom any serious nervous disturbance may be looked upon as pointing to a local manifestation of syphilis in the nervous centres. Not unusually the syphilitic exudation is localized in the course of one or several nerves, and we have, for instance, paralysis of one of the sixth pair, or paralysis of the fifth with or without paralysis of some other cerebral nerve. But as syphilis attacking the nervous system is chiefly characterized by a want of uniformity in the lesions it produces, so we find very dissimilar phenomena preceding or attending the palsies. Thus we may or may not, though, in point of fact, we most usually do, find them associated with pain in the head, with optic neuritis, with vertigo, and sickness at the stomach. Decided vertigo is prone to occur where the syphilitic trouble has led to a disease of the vessels, and is apt to be the forerunner of local softenings, and of a rather extended hemiplegia. When disease of the membranes has happened, headache is generally very severe, and convulsions occur; the same symptoms are encountered when there is a mass in the hemisphere; though here again this form of mischief may be comparatively latent, the patient have only occasionally convulsions, the paralysis be slight or improving, and yet a fatal coma follow a few convulsions. Instances of this kind have lately come under my observation.   ·

But, as a rule, syphilitic paralysis does not terminate fatally. In truth, the ease with which the palsy and its attending phenomena yield to treatment, if we except marked instances of hard nodules, the result of the poison, forms one of the traits of the malady. Other common traits, to speak in general terms, and guarded by what has been said of the dissimilar character of the lesions, are—that it commonly affects persons younger than those in whom we find paralysis dependent upon disease of the nervous centres, and chiefly of the brain; and that its manifestations are very shifting and capricious. These same traits characterize syphilitic diseases of the nervous system in which paralysis is not among the symptoms.

The mischief to the nervous system may not happen for years after the infection. It may be the result of an inherited trait. But such cases cannot be recognized with any certainty unless there are other signs of syphilis than the suspected nervous symptoms; and chief among these signs is that valuable test of congenital syphilis discovered by Mr. Hutchinson—a malformation of the two upper central permanent incisors, which consists in their being narrower at their cutting edges than at their insertions, and often notched.

The forms of paralysis which have just been noticed are mainly such as are designated as partial. When the loss of power is very limited, the palsy is commonly spoken of as *local*. Several of these local paralyses are of very great interest; the one, however—from its comparative frequency, and on account of its being often mistaken for a sign of intra-cranial disease—of particular importance, is the facial, or *Bell's* palsy. The disease consists in an affection of one of those facial nerves the course and functions of which Sir Charles Bell did so much to determine, namely, the portio dura of the seventh pair. In consequence of the derangement of this motor nerve, nearly all the muscles of the face lose their faculty of motion, and as it is their play which gives expression to the countenance, the appearance of the face is extraordinary. The eyelids are open and fixed; the features rigidly composed on one side of the face—for the disease is a one-sided one—and reflecting every change of feeling on the other. In some cases the velum palati is involved in the paralysis. But sensation remains unimpaired so long as the fifth nerve is not disturbed.

The causes of this palsy are such as influence the distressed nerve in its course or at its periphery: a wound; mumps; otitis; exposure to cold. Not being due to a cerebral malady, it is not a sign of serious danger. It is easily discriminated from the facial palsy of disease of the brain by the inability to close the eyelids, owing to the paralysis of the orbicularis palpebrarum; by the absence of impaired sensation, of headache, vertigo, mental confusion, of loss of memory; by the much more complete, though strictly local character of the paralysis, and, ordinarily, by the lost electro-muscular contractility.*

In rare instances the facial palsy is seen on both sides.

---

* But here again we must remember that the continuous current may give different results from faradisation. Meyer, *op. cit.*, tells us that those facial palsies in which, a week after their appearance, faradisation produces no muscular movement, while a feeble, continuous current causes vigorous contractions in the muscles, furnish a much more unfavorable prognosis, and recover slowly and imperfectly. He supposes the lesion to be in the facial nerve while in transit through the petrous portion of the temporal bone.

Now the disorder may be within the cranium or affect the nerves in their course. When dependent simply on a local affection, and therefore limited to the manifestations of paralysis of the portio dura, we find the same causes at work which give rise to the more usual one-sided disease. Exposure to cold and rheumatism are most frequently mentioned in the recorded cases; but syphilis is also cited among the causing elements. In an instance detailed·by Todd, in his clinical lectures, there was disease of the temporal bone, and the portio mollis was also implicated. The face is immovable, or nearly so, and the palsy is generally more complete on the left side than on the right. The muscles do not respond to electricity, or respond but imperfectly, and we notice, as in the one-sided malady, that a continuous current may excite their action, while faradisation does not. Nay, the two sides may give different results in this respect.*

About other local palsies, such as of the pharynx and œsophagus, of the larynx, of the tongue, of the muscles of the eye, of the diaphragm, of isolated muscles of the trunk or of the extremities, it is impossible here to enter into particulars. But there are some forms of local palsy which, from their striking interest, it is necessary to describe. One is the loss of power in the wrists, arising from atrophy of the muscles in the overworked parts of persons whose stomachs do not take in a sufficient supply of nutriment, as in poorly-fed and hard-worked shoemakers;† another, the paralysis of the tongue and parts concerned in deglutition, to which attention has been chiefly called by Trousseau.‡ In this

---

* Case of Baerwinkel, Schmidt's Jahrb., Bd. cxxxvi., No. 1. Baerwinkel suggests that the dissimilar reaction is always owing to different exudation and condition of pressure on the affected nerve. Thus, in any case, whether single or double, where galvanization produces contraction, and the induced current fails to do so, he thinks that a firm and extensive exudation compresses the nerve, whereas in slight or serous exudations, faradisation acts, and a speedy recovery may be anticipated.

For other cases of double facial palsy, see Gairdner, Lancet, May 18, 1861; Pellet, Travaux de la Société Médicale, 1867; Wright, British Medical Journal, Feb. 1869.

† Chambers on the Indigestions, p. 101, Am. edition.

‡ Clinique Médicale.

glossopharyngeal paralysis, the first symptoms which are likely to attract attention are, that the tongue seems less supple and the utterance becomes thick; the food lodges between the teeth and cheek, and the saliva is apt to dribble from the lips and corners of the mouth. As the paralysis progresses, the shape of the tongue is altered—it lies motionless in the mouth; the posterior nares can no longer be closed by the velum and muscles of the posterior palatine arch; deglutition becomes very difficult, and the patient is tormented with hunger. The mucous membrane of the larynx is frequently insensible, the respiratory movements are unusually weak, and fits of suffocation ensue. Thus general debility becomes extreme, and the patient is apt to perish by the sudden stoppage of the heart's action. The disease is an unmistakable one; the only affection at all resembling it is double facial palsy; but here the tongue is not involved, and, on the other hand, in glossopharyngeal paralysis only the lower part of the face is motionless. This curious disease may have an acute beginning.* It is sometimes complicated with weakness of the muscles of one side of the body. Of its morbid anatomy nothing positive is known. In a case described by Trousseau the roots of the vagus, of the right hypoglossal, and several of the anterior spinal roots were atrophied. It may be that the lesion is in the nuclei at the floor of the fourth ventricle, from which, as Lockhart Clarke has shown, the hypoglossal, the spinal accessory, the vagus, and the facial are connected.

Now, before passing on to other matters, we shall here discuss a few points of general clinical interest. We are sometimes much perplexed to know if a palsy is the result of commencing disease of the brain or spinal cord, or if it is purely local. To speak first of the brain: the cerebral symptoms may not be very marked, or they may be so contradictory as to afford no real help in diagnosis. We may have nothing to fall back upon but our knowledge of the anatomy and physiology of the nervous system; and if we discover that the palsy affects muscles that are supplied by

---

* Hérard, l'Union Méd., No. 35, 1868.

differeut nerves, and such as have no communication with
each other, we may set down the complaint as having a central origin.

Another most important question which may arise—and not
only with reference to limited, but also to extended palsies—
is, whether the loss of muscular power be not in reality dependent upon changes in the muscular tissue, and especially
upon that change found in the disorder known as " wasting
palsy," or *progressive muscular atrophy*. Of the nature of this
strange affection we are as yet in doubt. It was once thought
to be owing to a disease of the anterior roots of the spinal
nerves ; but the researches of Aran and of Duchenne have
led to the opinion that it consists in an atrophy connected
with fatty transformation of the muscular fibres, due primarily to changes of these structures. Still, though this
view is perhaps the one most generally adopted, and would
seem to be favored by the cases brought together and analyzed by Dr. Roberts, in his Essay on Wasting Palsy, it is
very possible that, by patient and careful examinations of the
spinal cord, we shall find minute structural changes in its
substance confined to isolated spots, and sufficient to account
for the disease in the muscles.   This was done by Lockhart
· Clarke, in a case recorded in Beale's Archives for 1861. The
sympathetic has been found diseased in its cervical ganglions
by Schneevogt and by Jaccoud ;* and, on the whole, the con
nection with some nervous lesion is too constant for us to look
upon it as a coincidence.

The main, and always the most striking sign of progressive
muscular atrophy is a constantly increasing inability to perform certain movements. When the muscle chiefly concerned
in the attempted motion is examined, it is found to have dwin-
dled.   Soon other muscles follow ; and their wasting, too, is
accompanied by still further impaired motion.   Portions of
the disorganizing muscles sometimes twitch, much to the
annoyance of the patient.   The circulation in the affected
part becomes languid ; it is also very susceptible to cold, and
indeed its temperature is lowered, there is a feeling of numb-

---

* Clinique Médicale; also Simon, Nouveau Diction. de Méd., 1866.

ness in it, but very rarely neuralgic pains; to pressure it is soft and yielding. The muscles most frequently attacked are those of the hand; the flexors and supinators of the forearm; the biceps, the deltoid, and the other muscles of the shoulder; sometimes the disease commences in the trunk and lower extremities. The decrease of the muscular fibres gives rise to strange and palpable deformities, and when the muscles of the trunk are involved, to extraordinary positions of the body, in consequence of all antagonism to the healthy muscles having been removed.

When we contrast this curious malady with the forms of paralysis with which it may be confounded, we find several features at variance. From cerebral hemiplegia it differs by its much more gradual invasion, by the rapidity but want of uniformity with which the muscular atrophy takes place, and by the absence of disordered intellect and of other signs of disease of the brain. From extended general paralysis of cerebral origin it is separated by the non-existence of cerebral phenomena, and by the capricious and unequal manner in which the atrophy seizes upon the muscles. Difficulty in articulation and in deglutition may occur in either; but in the one case they are associated with disturbed mental faculties, in the other they are not. From general spinal paralysis it is mainly diagnosticated by the spinal malady affecting primarily all the muscles of the lower extremities before those of the upper become involved.

Another means of distinguishing the muscular atrophy from the diseases just considered, is by means of instruments by which portions of the affected textures can be removed and subjected to microscopical examination. Duchenne has invented a trocar for the purpose, and so have other pathologists.*

Then we possess a touchstone in the use of electricity. In progressive muscular atrophy the muscles respond feebly, still they respond; and in portions where there are many sound fibres they contract energetically. In general paral-

---

* For an exact description of these different instruments, see Amer. Jour. of Med. Sciences, Oct. 1869, p. 434.

ysis of spinal origin their contractile power is lost; no effort of the patient, no current, whatever its strength, causes them to move. In general cerebral paralysis, on the other hand, their electrical contractility is intact. The difficulty of distinguishing cases of local paralysis from progressive muscular atrophy is at times very great. Yet generally we may separate the latter, say, for instance, from rheumatic paralysis, by noticing that this affects a group of muscles rather than one muscle, or than one muscle here and another there. Further, the atrophied muscle in the rheumatic disorder is the seat of pain intensified by movement, and it contracts well under the electric stimulus,—phenomena the reverse of those presented by fatty transformation of the muscular textures. The same test by the electric current is of service in discriminating the muscular disease from hysterical paralysis, from paralysis consequent upon injuries to nervous trunks, and upon lead poisoning. In the first of these palsies the electrical contractility is intact, in the others it is abolished; while in progressive muscular atrophy it is simply enfeebled.*

Paralyzed muscles atrophy, and, as especially happens in children, may subsequently undergo a fatty change. To distinguish such a condition from progressive muscular atrophy is difficult. We have to lay great stress on the symptoms which ushered in the paralytic state. This is particularly important in attempting to discriminate with reference to the so-called *essential paralysis* from which children suffer; for we attach great weight to the fever and the cerebral symptoms so commonly preceding the palsy, or to its occurring suddenly during teething. Besides, an entire limb,

---

* These remarks are based on the results obtained by Duchenne by means of faradisation (*De l'électrisation localisée*, Paris, 1861); and are, I think, in the main, correct. But, as above mentioned, the condition of the muscles influences somewhat the electro-muscular contractility; some of the statements may be, therefore, too absolute, and cannot be solely relied upon in forming a differential diagnosis. The modifying circumstances alluded to, as I repeatedly have had opportunities of observing, show themselves chiefly in some old-standing cases of cerebral, of rheumatic, and, though this is less certain, of hysterical, paralysis, in all of which the excitability of the muscles may be very much impaired, or even temporarily lost.

or even both legs and arms, may from the onset be affected. The subsequent history, too, is dissimilar. There is often a steadily progressing recovery within six months or sooner; though the disorder may last for three or four years, or even much longer. The affected muscles are apt to begin to atrophy after the paralysis has lasted a month, and when their wasting is marked they no longer respond to the induced electrical current, though they may still react strongly under the constant galvanic current.* In protracted cases, contractions of the joints take place, and atrophy of portions of the osseous system occurs, or rather a want of its development in the blighted parts. Then in forming a diagnosis we may take into account the extreme rarity with which children are attacked with progressive fatty atrophy—a disease of adults, and pre-eminently of those of the male sex who use their muscles continuously and violently.

The same difference in age helps us also to distinguish that curious disorder, chiefly described by Duchenne, and which he names *pseudo-hypertrophic muscular paralysis.* A disease exclusively of childhood, it is characterized by weakness in the lower limbs primarily, the muscles of which, and particularly the gastrocnemii, increase greatly in size. Yet, notwithstanding this apparent hypertrophy, there is debility, with a waddling gait, and as the disease progresses and becomes more general, complete paralysis may ensue, with rapid dwindling of the affected muscles. These, when examined microscopically, show, in the stage of increase, large masses of interstitial fatty matter and an augmentation of the interstitial connective tissue.†

The *prognosis* of paralysis, viewed in a general manner, is unfavorable; but to this general view there are many and palpable exceptions. The cause of the palsy materially influences its probable termination. Palsies produced by poisons usually end in recovery; so do those owing to cachexias, to alterations in the blood, to syphilis, to hysteria, and to wounds of nerves. Rheumatic paralysis is frequently very ob-

---

* Hammond, Journ. of Psychology, vols. i. and ii.
† Archives Gener., tome i., 1868.

stinate, as is also the paralysis which has its origin in nervous exhaustion occasioned by excesses. The palsy resulting from a chronic cerebral or spinal lesion yields a grave prognosis.

In the *treatment* applicable to paralysis two main indications arise. The first is, to treat the palsy as much as possible—and the more recent it is, the more this is possible—according to its cause. The second is, to keep up so far as it can be kept up, the nutrition of the paralyzed parts and to stimulate them to action. The former indication is best fulfilled by constitutional, the second by local means.

Before proceeding, we will examine the main forms of paralysis which we have been studying, arranged in a tabular form, and chiefly with the view of ascertaining its seat, premising that the statements must be received rather as generally true than as statements which are absolutely so.

TABULAR VIEW OF PARALYSIS.

Symptoms.	*Seat of Lesion.*
Inability to move leg and arm of one side. Sensation unimpaired, or slightly impaired. Incomplete paralysis of muscles of face; mouth drawn toward healthy side. Electro-muscular contractility, as a rule, preserved; may be increased.	Corpus striatum chiefly, less markedly optic thalamus, both on side opposite to the palsy.
Same symptoms, but paralysis of face on opposite side to that of arm and leg, and usually marked facial palsy; loss of sensation on one side of face; giddiness; nausea, etc.	Pons Varolii, on side opposite to palsy of limbs. The part affected is below decussation of facial nerve.
Same symptoms, but face paralyzed on both sides.	Pons Varolii, and at level of decussation of facial nerve.
Paralysis of arm and leg on one side; slight paralysis of face; third nerve paralyzed on other side.	Crus cerebri on side corresponding to paralysis of third.
Motion more or less completely affected on both sides of body; sensibility diminished or lost on one side; increased on the other; the same with temperature.	Medulla oblongata on side of increased sensibility and temperature, and at level of decussation of anterior pyramids.

Symptoms.	*Seat of Lesion.*
Both legs paralyzed as to motion and sensation. Paralysis of muscles of respiration; loss of power over bladder and rectum; electro-muscular contractility diminished or lost.	In the cord at upper limit of lumbar region, or higher up.
Both legs paralyzed as to sensation and motion, except muscles supplied by anterior crural and obturator nerves; loss of power over bladder and rectum. .	In the cord at upper limit of sacral region.

Locomotor Ataxia.—In this disorder we have uncertainty of motion and apparent palsy; or, in the words of Duchenne, who gave it the name of progressive disorder of locomotion —*ataxie locomotrice progressive*—it consists in "a progressive abolition of the co-ordination of movement with apparent paralysis contrasting with the integrity of muscular force." The patient is not deprived of the power of motion, but of the power of controlling his motion : hence he staggers in his walk, or cannot walk at all without support; it is evident that the muscles do not obey the will.

"The affected individuals," says Duchenne, in summing up the main signs of the malady, "present a group of identical phenomena: the same commencement, same symptoms, same progress, same termination. Thus, in the majority, paralysis of the sixth pair or of the third pair, a weakening or even a loss of vision, attended with inequality of the pupils, are the phenomena present either at the onset, or are precursory·to the disturbance of the co-ordination of movement. Very characteristic piercing pains, wandering, erratic, of short duration, rapid as lightning, or similar to electric discharges, returning in paroxysms, and attacking all the regions of the body, accompany or follow these local paralyses. These phenomena constitute the first stage. Subsequently, after a time varying from several months to several years, there appear in the second stage: vertigo; difficulty in maintaining the equilibrium of the body and in co-ordinating movements; soon afterward, or sometimes simultaneously, a diminution, or a loss of tactile sensibility or of sensibility to pain (analgesia and anæsthesia), at first in the inferior, more rarely in the superior extremities. Finally, in the third stage the disease becomes general.

" During the course of the malady occur frequently disorders of the functions of the rectum and of the bladder, without sugar or albumen being present in the urine. The intellect remains unimpaired; speech is neither hesitating nor embarrassed; the electro-muscular contractility is intact; and the muscles undergo no alteration of nutrition or of their tissue. Ordinarily, too, the malady is *progressive* in the strained sense which Requin has given to the term, namely, that the disease has not merely a tendency to become general, but it often has also a fatal termination."*

Trousseau, in his Clinical Lectures, points out, as a diagnostic sign, of value even in the early stages of ataxia, the strange effect of closing the eyes: this gives rise to an increase of the uncertainty of the patient's gait to such an extent that he is incapable of taking a single step without falling, or to an utter inability to stand erect with his feet in juxtaposition without instantly losing his balance. But the same sign is occasionally observed in beginning paraplegia and other forms of palsy, and is thus not strictly pathognomonic. And as regards some of the other symptoms, admitting now, as beyond doubt, that the so-called Duchenne's disease is, in its essential features, identical with a form of palsy clearly recognized by Todd, and with the malady described by Romberg and several German pathologists under the name of *tabes dorsalis*, it may well be a question whether we can take as distinctive, that in the affection described by Duchenne the disturbance of the cranial nerves precedes the uncertainty of movement of the muscles of the lower extremities; whether we can consider that the early symptom, accounted by him as the most pathognomonic—the violent pains (and which he declares not to have met with only once in one hundred cases)—is so characteristic that we are justified in regarding as belonging to a separate disease those instances of apparent paralysis, which exhibit, on close examination, an imperfect power of co-ordination of the muscles, and par-

---

* Electrisation Localisée. Paris, 1861.

ticularly of those of the lower limbs, but in which the signs just alluded to are absent. If, then, we admit the identity of tabes dorsalis and of progressive muscular ataxia, and do not even view the latter as a distinct variety of the former, we must also admit, in accordance with other observations than those of Duchenne, that the first symptom of the affection often consists of a sense of weakness and weariness in both legs, or only in one, and that the darting pains in the lower extremities are not constant. The dwindling of the muscles, especially of those of the nates, legs, and back, and their weakened or lost contractility when subjected to a galvanic current, which Romberg[*] notices, may be due to coexisting chronic myelitis. It is indeed undoubted that some of the phenomena which have been ascribed to tabes dorsalis more strictly appertain to concurring complaints, and thus there is some confusion in determining its exact clinical history.

But summing up the truly significant features of locomotor ataxia, we find a peculiar gait, stumbling, staggering, without true paralysis; shooting, neuralgic pains; numbness in the feet and legs, with sensibility defective, excepting to temperature; frequent, but by no means invariable impairment of sight or hearing,—all coexisting with undisordered mental faculties, with well-nourished, vigorously contracting muscles, and with an absence of tremor or spasm. Moreover, though there may be some want of perfect action in the muscles of the upper extremities, the real features of ataxia are met with in the lower.

This curious affection is probably due to a peculiar degeneration and atrophy of the posterior column of the cord, beginning or having its chief seat in the lumbar region. Yet it is not certain that this is the invariable anatomical change, or that the group of symptoms constituting muscular ataxia may not be linked to various diseases of the cord and brain.

But to return to a consideration of the diagnosis of the malady under discussion. Let us first examine how it differs from the *general paralysis* of the insane. Both maladies are

---

[*] Nervous Diseases. Sydenham Soc. Transla., vol. ii.

very chronic in their course, and in both there is loss, or certainly impairment of the faculty by which we co-ordinate the action of the muscles. In the one case, however, it exists with tremors, with thickness of speech, with dementia, and, at least in its earlier stages, with a certain amount of force in the irregular muscular movements; but without strabismus, without amaurosis, and without the sharp, peculiar pains of ataxia. Then, in this malady, the upper extremities share far less frequently in the disorder, and when they do, there is in them rather cutaneous anæsthesia, with some trembling and incomplete paralysis, than an obvious failure of co-ordinating power.

With reference to the distinction of progressive locomotor ataxia from most of the *diseases of the spinal cord*, it is only necessary to remark on the extreme rarity of real muscular spasm in ataxia; from the ordinary spinal paraplegia the result of myelitis, it differs in the fact that the muscles act with strength, the patient can flex and extend his legs and kick vigorously, while in paralysis the affected limbs cannot move.

A diminution or loss of the muscular sense—that guiding sense by which we judge of the position of the limbs, of the degree of resistance opposed to muscular movements, and are conscious of these movements, and which, particularly in hysterical patients, may become very much disturbed—is apt to occasion some difficulty in diagnosis, since in locomotor ataxia the muscular sense may be also deficient, and, on the other hand, in the former morbid state the muscular motions be somewhat impaired, and, as in ataxia, the feet feel numb in standing and in walking, and the patient be unable to walk in the dark. But there is this difference: where merely the muscular sense is affected, he can walk and perform all movements, even those of a complex nature, without vacillation, so long as his eye is fixed on them and superintends and gives them direction; while, in ataxia, the derangement of muscular co-ordination renders, even with the aid of sight, the movements uncertain and irregular. Then cutaneous anæsthesia is apt to coexist with this malady; and the treatment will throw light on a doubtful case,—the local use of electricity will usually cure the loss of muscular sense in hysterical paralysis, but it has no curative effect in ataxia.

Diseases of the cerebellum produce many of the phenomena regarded as peculiar to locomotor ataxia. But the gait of the patient in cerebellar disorders is precisely that of a drunken man: when attempting to walk, he leans to one side, moves in the arcs of a circle, or describes zigzags; and when standing erect, his body swings backward and forward, or from side to side, though his feet remain quietly fixed on the ground. In ataxia, on the other hand, the muscular contractions in the erect position or during attempts at walking are strong and sudden, more like spasms, yet not spasmodic, and have as their object to keep the body in the line of gravity, and the walk, though accomplished with difficulty, is straight, not reeling; the affected person, too, while he is walking. does not take his eyes off the ground or from his feet for fear of falling, but he is not giddy. Moreover, in diseases of the cerebellum we find marked vertiginous sensations, especially during attempts at locomotion; vomiting, particularly at the onset of the complaint, and aggravated or brought on by the erect posture; frontal pain when the head is bent; defective vision, becoming very much so when an object is looked at for any time, or double vision; no diminution either of power of motion or of sensibility;* and in some instances rotary movements.

Chronic alcoholism gives rise to extended hyperæsthesia and neuralgic pains, and motor disturbances which may be like those of ataxia.† But in the history and the other evidences of the ravages of alcohol we find the distinguishing traits. In *chorea* the irregular muscular movements are very dissimilar from those of locomotor ataxia. Moreover, there is an absence of the neuralgic pains, and chorea is a disease of childhood; locomotor ataxia of adults. The closest similarity to locomotor ataxia I have seen has been in several cases of *hysteria*. One in particular, in a very anemic woman, similated it closely; and it may be a question

---

* Duchenne, Gaz. Hebdomad., 1864.

† Leudet, Arch. Génér., Jan. 1867.

whether the nutrition of the parts affected in ataxia were not disordered, and the nervous structures functionally disturbed. I desire particularly to call attention to these cases, which can be distinguished by their history, the usual coexistence of anæmia, and the absence of severe darting pains. Moreover, the apparent want of muscular co-ordination is more irregular in its manifestations; and the cases recover. So I think may other cases of locomotor ataxia due to special causes. For I have seen cases in *syphilitic* patients, typical in everything excepting perhaps the severity of the neuralgic pain, essentially typical in the muscular phenomena, and in the inability to walk with closed eyes, in whom a gradual and nearly complete recovery took place. Here the lesion was probably removed or greatly influenced by the antisyphilitic treatment.

Tremor.—Any involuntary agitation of the body, or of part of it, without marked muscular contraction or impediment to voluntary movement, is called tremor. The trembling depends upon a weakening of the muscular and nervous systems. It is common in old age, in convalescence from debilitating diseases, and during chills. We also find it in workers in mercury and lead, and in those who abuse alcoholic stimulants or coffee, or are addicted to the use of opium. In some cases it seems to be connected with an organic disease of the nervous centres. It constitutes the main symptom of the singular disorder known as shaking palsy, or paralysis agitans; an affection thought to depend upon a lesion of the tubercula quadrigemina, or the upper portion of the spinal cord.

Tremor is easily recognized. Yet it may be confounded with muscular twitchings, which, like it, spring from a deranged innervation rather than from organic disease. But it differs from these spasmodic movements by being more incessant, and unconnected with decided muscular contractions. In nervous susceptible persons laboring under an acute attack of disease, it is at times combined with great restlessness, and is apt to be mistaken for a convulsive state. Again, it may be distinguished by the absence of muscular contractions, and by the unintermitting, irregular motions.

Spasms—Convulsions.—Both these terms are applied to involuntary muscular contractions, with, perhaps, this difference: the word spasm is used when we wish to express the idea of less universal muscular derangement, but especially when the muscles of organic life are believed to be involved; and convulsions, when the disorder affects the muscles of the whole body, or at least many muscles at once, and chiefly those of volition. Yet these are not distinctions that can, or indeed ought to be, very strictly carried out, for the two phenomena often coexist; and being produced by the same causes, and obedient to the same laws, can hardly be separated.

Spasms may be clonic or tonic. In clonic spasms the muscles are agitated by successive contractions and relaxations of their fibres. Clonic spasms are very extensive; in truth, so generally is this is the case, that, if we make any distinction between spasms and convulsions, we are bound to contemplate clonic spasms as convulsions rather than as spasms. In tonic spasms the muscles are rigidly set, and retain for a time their contraction, in spite of every effort on our part, or on the part of the patient, to relax them. The most marked type of this disorder is seen in tetanus; the most perfect illustration of clonic spasms is furnished in hysteria.

Convulsions may be accompanied by a loss of consciousness, and by impaired or abolished sensibility, as in epilepsy, or they may coexist with unclouded thought and unaltered sensibility, as in tetanus. What their immediate cause, is very difficult to determine, for as yet we possess little positive knowledge; and as to the portion of the nervous centres where they arise, or the structural changes that attend an attack, we know next to nothing. The seat of the disturbance is in some cases evidently the cerebro-spinal system, but many convulsions have their origin in a perturbation of the reflex system. Of their exciting cause we may say that, in those of susceptible nervous organizations, any extrinsic irritation, such as teething or disordered digestion, leads to a fit. Further causes are diseases of the brain; sudden interference with the circulation; profuse hemor-

rhages; a contaminated blood. Children, who are partie-
ularly liable to convulsions, often have them as the precursors
of febrile diseases. In point of diagnosis it is of great importance to distinguish whether their inroad is or is not
symptomatic of a cerebral lesion. If there have been a
previous disorder of the intellectual functions, or any other
manifestation of a brain trouble, we may assume the convulsions to be the signal of cerebral mischief. But when
no such phenomena are met with, we are likely to find the
source of irritation in some other portion of the body.
Practically speaking, when convulsions are among the first
signs of a malady, they are not apt to depend upon a disease
of the brain; and even if recognized to form part of the
symptoms of a cerebral lesion, we may conclude that the
lesion has not reached its highest degree of development,
but is still, as it were, irritative, and has not led to cerebral
disorganization.

Besides separating convulsions or spasms in conformity
with their eccentric or their centric origin, we must always
attempt to ascertain the particular nature of the cause. If
centric, is it congestion, or inflammation, a tumor, or cerebral hypertrophy; or is the convulsion essential and idiopathic, due to influences the cognizance of which is not
within our narrowly-bounded horizon? If eccentric, is it
owing to an impure or impoverished blood, to retained poisons, to intestinal or other visceral irritation, and what is the
probable share the reflex system has in the visible disturbance of the muscles? To solve these questions is often a
very difficult matter, and nothing but a careful analysis of
all the phenomena of the case enables us even to approximate the truth.

Closely connected with spasms and convulsions, and indeed, in a certain sense, not separable from them, are other
kinds of irregular muscular movements, such as cramps—
a short contraction of one or several muscles occurring in
paroxysms, and attended with severe pain; rigidity—a permanent tonic contraction of the muscles, often encountered
in diseases of the brain, especially in cerebral softening; and
the jerking movements of chorea.

DERANGED NUTRITION AND SECRETION.

Among the subjects connected with the nervous system which have of late years received most attention, there is none of more interest than the association of its disorders with derangements of nutrition and secretion. Now such are very manifest in paralyzed limbs or after nerve wounds. But these obvious alterations need here but be referred to. It is rather my intention to speak of the less palpable phenomena, and those in which, at first sight, the nervous system is not so distinctly concerned. For instance, the skin may become the seat of diverse eruptions, undergo modifications of color and structure, the secretions may be augmented or diminished, the muscles and joints show textural changes, swellings may happen affecting various portions of the body, either external or internal,—yet all be due to disturbed nervous influence, and the real disorder, therefore, be in parts very different from where it appears.

To particularize with reference to a few of the derangements alluded to. There is the affection known as herpes zoster, of which there can be no longer any doubt that the vesicles encircling half the circumference of the trunk are not a primary skin affection, but the local expression of irritation of a nerve. They closely follow the distribution of some superficial sensory nerve, and this unilateral herpes is really but a sign of localized neuralgia,—from its seat, most generally of a dorso-intercostal neuralgia. Then again we encounter instances of large vesicles or bullæ accompanying other neuralgias, as of the sciatic; and attacks of erysipelas having their origin in facial neuralgia, as has been ably demonstrated by Anstie. Furthermore, the most various kinds of spots and blotches, and thickenings of the skin have been noticed, by different observers, after this and other forms of neuralgia.

Oftentimes, too, these morbid appearances on the skin are combined with evidences of altered secretion. Thus, in a case related by Parrot,* in addition to the neuralgic parox-

---

* Gaz. Hebdom., 1859; quoted in Handfield Jones on Funct. Nervous Disorders.

ysms attended with sanguineous exudations at the painful parts, there occurred, at times, bloody sweating on the knees, thighs, hands, and face. Lachrymation was noticed in nearly half the cases of trigeminal neuralgia analyzed by Notta;* and one-sided furring of the tongue is a not uncommon phenomenon in this complaint. Associated with these evidences of altered secretion may be signs of altered nutrition, such as iritis, corneal clouding, and inflammation of the fascia or of the periosteum in contact with the aching nerve. And let us here add that these evidences of perverted nutrition are not confined to neuralgic disorders. They occur also in diseases of the central nervous system. Thus affections of the joints have been observed to follow cerebral hemorrhages, and various spinal disorders; and a form of joint-mischief, of hydrarthrosis, has been, of late, specially described by Charcot† in locomotor ataxia.

Among the phenomena of altered secretion, connected with nervous affections, one of the most striking is *excessive sweating.* In lesions of the cervical sympathetic on one side, we may have strictly unilateral sweating of the face and neck, the other side remaining perfectly dry;‡ and greater vascularity and increased temperature are concomitants. In lesions of the abdominal ganglia profuse sweating also happens, and is apt to be combined with impeded secretion from the mucous coats of the bowels, as we occasionally find in instances of abdominal aneurism. Not that excessive sweating, whether localized or general, is always linked to an affection of the great sympathetic ganglia. We find, indeed, local sweatings limited to the hands and feet without any signs of other trouble. And general sweatings, irrespective of those of colloquative character attending phthisis, or those of malarial diseases, happen after low fevers, in inactive states of the liver, and in some persons go on for years without any obvious cause. It may be, however, that in most, if not all these cases, the sympathetic system is really at fault, at least in so far that there is a reflex de-

---

* Archiv. Gén., 1854.   † Archives de Physiologie, 1868.
‡ As in the case recorded by W. Ogle, Med.-Ch. Transact., vol. lii.

rangement of the vaso-motor nerves, and of course, then, of the subcutaneous blood-vessels and the glands' they supply.

But these are not questions which we can here consider. Indeed, the *why* and the *how* of all these changes of secretion and nutrition attending nervous affections are very uncertain, and such a consideration touches on the question whether or not there are special trophic nerves, and on other unsettled points of physiology.

To return to the clinical phenomena. Besides the external manifestations of altered secretion and nutrition, there are certain changes in internal organs, the expression of nervous derangements. Modern research has rendered it most probable that the triple lesion known as exophthalmic goitre is of this kind, and due to disease of the sympathetic nerve. And the Medicine of the Future will most likely acquaint us with many more disorders of glands and viscera which originate in altered nerve-structure and perverted power.

So much for the chief manifestations of nervous complaints. From the preceding pages it will have become apparent how many of them are functional, or are at least of necessity so regarded, and how these functional disorders may be attended with the signs of quite as great, or even greater, disturbance than the organic maladies. And nothing is more difficult than to fix their seat; for after death not the slightest structural alteration may be discernible, or it may be of a character insufficient to account for the phenomena during life. In consequence, there is very great confusion, and much doubt is thrown over any anatomical or pathological classification of nervous diseases. I subjoin a table of the main affections, arranged according to their supposed sites. It may not suit a strict critic, since, in several of the disorders regarded as functional, modern research has indicated the probable organic cause. But from the stand-point of the physician it would be as yet premature to recognize a fixed organic nature, and I contend rather for the classification being clinically than pathologically unimpeachable. Nor will it be adhered to in the description of nervous disorders about to follow; which will be traced according to divisions formed by groups of symptoms rather in obedience to a pathological classification.

TABLE OF THE DISORDERS OF THE BRAIN AND SPINAL CORD.

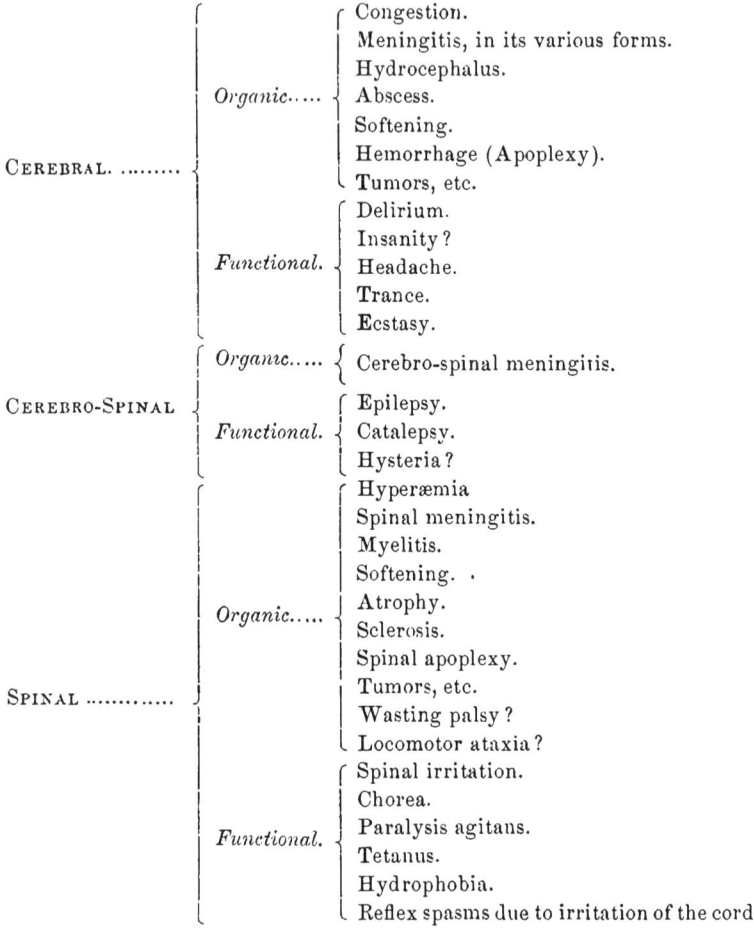

CEREBRAL.

    Organic.....
- Congestion.
- Meningitis, in its various forms.
- Hydrocephalus.
- Abscess.
- Softening.
- Hemorrhage (Apoplexy).
- Tumors, etc.

    Functional.
- Delirium.
- Insanity?
- Headache.
- Trance.
- Ecstasy.

CEREBRO-SPINAL

    Organic.....
- Cerebro-spinal meningitis.

    Functional.
- Epilepsy.
- Catalepsy.
- Hysteria?

SPINAL

    Organic.....
- Hyperæmia
- Spinal meningitis.
- Myelitis.
- Softening. .
- Atrophy.
- Sclerosis.
- Spinal apoplexy.
- Tumors, etc.
- Wasting palsy?
- Locomotor ataxia?

    Functional.
- Spinal irritation.
- Chorea.
- Paralysis agitans.
- Tetanus.
- Hydrophobia.
- Reflex spasms due to irritation of the cord.

Acute Affections of which Delirium is a Prominent Symptom.

This clinical group embraces the different forms of meningeal inflammation, delirium tremens, and acute mania— affections in all of which the brain is the seat of the disturbance.

Acute Meningitis.—By this term is now understood an

inflammation of the membranes of the brain, especially of the arachnoid and pia mater. The dura mater is far less frequently attacked; very rarely, unless the morbid action be of syphilitic origin, or have extended from the bones of the cranium.

The disease generally presents two well-marked stages. The first, or the stage of excitement, is characterized by intense headache, great restlessness, vomiting, a hard, frequent pulse, fever, injected eye, often with a contracted pupil, an increased sensibility to light and sounds, obstinate constipation, irregular respiration, and soon by active delirium, and convulsions; the second stage is marked by an evident ebbing of the life forces: the extremities are cold, the pupils dilated, the pulse is feeble and much slower, and intermitting, or it becomes extremely rapid and threadlike; involuntary passages occur, there is utter loss of mind and of sensibility —in one word, coma or collapse.

Not every case, however, has all these symptoms, or goes at once from the stage of excitement to that of collapse. There may be a well-defined period of transition, during which the heat of skin, excepting of the head, diminishes, drowsiness appears, and the pulse sinks somewhat in frequeney. Again, the disease may be arrested before the signs of prostration are very evident.

The attack may be preceded by sick stomach, buzzing in the ears and vertigo, or set in with severe pain fixed to the forehead, and increased by movements. In some cases it begins with delirium or convulsions.* And among its symptoms, even in the earliest stages, a persistent pain, attacking one or both knees, violent, intensified on motion, unrelieved by local means, and connected neither with swelling nor with any other change in the form or appearance of the joint, has been particularly noticed.†

The malady may pass rapidly through its stages, so rapidly that their distinctive features become confused and

---

* On the other hand, these symptoms may be absent. In a paper by Church, in St. Bartholomew's Hospital Reports, vol. iv., are several cases without delirium.

† Lund, quoted in Amer. Jour. of Med. Sciences, Oct. 1864.

blended.   Generally it does not last less, nor much more, than a week.

Acute meningitis is brought on by exposure, by depressing cares, by intense application to study, by a blow or fall upon the head, by disease of adjacent structures, or by syphilis. It sometimes affects mainly, or wholly, the coverings of the convex portion of the brain; at other times the inflammation is limited to the base. According to Duchatelet,* meningitis of the base may be discriminated by remissions in the delirium, and by the coexistence of spasmodic symptoms with profound and early coma. These signs, at all events, are said to be distinctive in children, who, more than adults, are disposed to this form of the complaint.

Acute meningitis is not always easy of diagnosis. Leaving out for the present the other disorders belonging to the same group, such as acute mania and delirium tremens, it may be confounded with

CEREBRITIS;

ACUTE SOFTENING :

HEAD SYMPTOMS OF CONTINUED FEVERS;

HEAD SYMPTOMS OF ACUTE RHEUMATISM;

HEAD SYMPTOMS OF PNEUMONIA; OF PERICARDITIS.

Cerebritis.—There is very little appreciable difference between inflammation of the brain tissue and inflammation of the meninges. In truth, what we commonly call meningitis (because the evidences of the morbid action are most distinct in the meninges) is often also cerebritis; since the diseased process extends very readily from the tunics of the brain to the adjacent cerebral substance. We may suspect this structure to have become involved, if the sense of vision or of hearing be suddenly perverted; if the convulsions, the agitation of the limbs, and the tremors be very marked; if they occur chiefly upon one side; and if coma succeed rapidly to the period of excitement, and be accompanied or preceded by one-sided palsy.

Acute Softening.—The form of acute softening which simulates meningitis is that associated with delirium. But it

---

* Inflammation de l'Arachnoide, page 230.

occurs only in very old persons, is apt to be preceded by restlessness, some mental confusion, and signs of a general breaking up of nervous force, is soon associated with disturbances of the bladder and rectum, and the patient gradually passes into a comatose state. In the cases which I have seen there was neither much headache nor febrile disorder.

Head Symptoms of Continued Fevers.—In all the varieties of continued fever, but especially in typhoid and typhus, cerebral symptoms at times arise which bear a very strong resemblance to those of idiopathic meningitis; and such symptoms, it has been fully proved, may appear without the examination of the dead body revealing even traces of inflammation. How, then, are we to distinguish these fever cases from meningitis; or how ascertain, if inflammation of the brain be really before us as a complication and product, if thus it may be called, of the fever? Unfortunately, there is no sign absolutely diagnostic. Perhaps future researches may determine that the increase of phosphates in the urine, found by Bence Jones to occur in inflammatory affections of the nervous textures, is a valuable source of distinction. But we know that this increase may also be due to other causes, and as yet we are too little cognizant of the exact chemistry of the secretions in the maladies under discussion to make the urine the differential test. Nor does cerebral auscultation afford us any help; for the few authors, like Fisher,* Whitney,† or Roger,‡ who have at all investigated the subject, are not even agreed whether the *souffle* that is perceived is constantly present in meningitis, whether it may not exist in any cerebral disturbance, nay, whether it may not be heard in health. As matters stand, a diagnosis can only be established by a careful consideration of all the symptoms, and of the history of our patient: by searching for the eruption of typhus or typhoid fever; by taking note of the expression of the countenance; of the character of the delirium, ordinarily so much more active when the brain or its membranes are inflamed, and attended with much more intense head-

---

* Am. Journ. of Med Sciences, Aug 1838
† Ibid., Oct. 1843.   ‡ Ibid., Oct. 1862.

ache, with throbbing of the arteries of the neck and face,*
and not unfrequently with convulsions. But how difficult it
may be to arrive at a correct conclusion, unless we possess a
full knowledge of all the circumstances, is shown by this
case :

A man, about thirty-five years of age, was admitted into
the Philadelphia Hospital on February 8th, 1861, with a cer-
tificate that he was laboring under typhoid fever. No clue
could be obtained to the history of the malady. The man
himself was unable to afford any information, as he was not
in a state to answer any questions. His pulse was excessively feeble, and somewhat irregular; the eye was not injected, but suffused and watery; the pupils sluggish and the
eyeballs in constant motion ; the tongue was dark, dry, and
fissured; the breath offensive. There appeared to be pain
on pressure in the right iliac fossa, but the bowels were
constipated, and no eruption could be detected. The most
striking feature of the case was the delirium, which was
noisy and violent, and accompanied by great restlessness;
the man sang, screamed, was constantly attempting to get
out of bed and to upset his medicine bottle. What was the
nature of the malady? It did not seem to me to be typhoid
fever: the symptoms belonged more to inflammation of the
brain, but, knowing neither how nor when the delirium had
commenced, I could not be positive that such was the lesion.
The bowels were opened by a turpentine injection, and as
the patient was evidently sinking, he was stimulated; but to
no purpose—he died the day after his admission into the
hospital. The autopsy showed the intestines to be sound.
The membranes of the brain, after the dura mater was removed, were found to be opaque, and between the convolutions were shreds of lymph and a puriform liquid. There
were but traces of inflammation at the base, excepting in
the neighborhood of the pons varolii, where some lymphy
effusion was discerned. The ventricles were filled with fluid,
and the nervous structure in the neighborhood of the thalami
and corpora striata was softened.

---

* Still, even this symptom is not certain, for I have repeatedly noticed
throbbing of the vessels of the neck in low fevers.

Subsequently to the man's death it was ascertained that he had been sick for only four days before he entered the ward; which fact, had it been previously known, would have materially assisted the diagnosis. Irrespective of the difficulty of its recognition, this case is of peculiar interest. It illustrates the possibility of the absence of convulsions and of paralysis, notwithstanding the most evident cerebral disorganization.

Head Symptoms of Acute Rheumatism.—In rheumatic fever cerebral symptoms occasionally arise which may be referred to inflammation of the brain, or which, by their prominence, may mislead the practitioner, causing him to regard the signs of the rheumatism as of little importance, if indeed he does not wholly overlook them. And the morbid manifestations are very much like those of acute meningitis: restlessness, headache, and violent delirium, succeeded by coma. The delirium is commonly of gradual approach, but it may come on suddenly. Generally it does not appear until the patient has been suffering for at least a week with acute rheumatism; and the heavy sweats and swollen joints point out the malady with which it is combined.

Formerly the cerebral phenomena were looked upon as due to metastasis of the rheumatic inflammation to the brain. But this view is now abandoned; for examinations of the head, in cases which proved rapidly fatal, have failed to detect, save in rare instances, any evidences of inflammatory action within the cranium. The abnormal signs are, as a rule, much more probably attributable to the altered condition of the blood, and are often found to be connected with the setting in of pneumonia or of inflammation of the membranes of the heart, or to plugs of fibrin in the capillaries of the brain, and are apt to be associated with a very high temperature.

Head Symptoms of Pneumonia; of Pericarditis.—In both these maladies delirium may be met with of a character so violent as to lead to the belief that the brain or its membranes are involved in an inflammatory disease. The diagnosis is cleared up by a careful examination of the chest. Then we may lay stress on the furious delirium, being unattended with spasmodic movements or with paralysis. The form of pneumonia which is mostly associated with delirium, is inflammation of the upper lobes.

Tubercular Meningitis.—This is a rare disease in adults; not a rare disease in children. Its distinct recognition belongs to the present generation of physicians; and nearly all of the cases of so-called acute hydrocephalus, and most of those of meningitis of the base, have now been ascertained to be instances of tubercular meningitis, or, to define the morbid state, of an inflammation of the meninges occurring in tubercular patients, and ordinarily accompanied by the deposition of tubercles at the base of the brain.

The premonitory signs of the malady are of great importance. The child has generally been ailing for some time; is restless, peevish, sleeps ill, complains of headache, and is troubled with a frequent, short cough, and with constipation. To these symptoms are soon superadded thirst, a coated tongue, vomiting, a dry skin, and generally an accelerated pulse and grinding of the teeth, constituting the most prominent features of the first stage of the affection. After four or five days the second stage is reached, and the brain symptoms become much more clearly developed. The child shuns the light, puts its hand frequently to its head, and utters every now and then a peculiar, sharp, distressing cry. At night the headache exacerbates, and is attended with fleeting delirium. A slight strabismus is observable, and the eyeballs oscillate. The pulse is very irregular in its rhythm, sometimes rapid and intermitting, then suddenly falling and becoming quite slow. The vomiting ceases, and there may be a remission in the symptoms with restored intelligence; but the pulse remains irregular, the bowels are even more constipated than before, and the abdomen appears retracted. The third stage is one of complete stupor, accompanied or preceded by convulsions. The expression of the face is idiotic; the pupils are dilated; there is subsultus, and one side of the body is paralyzed. Deglutition is very difficult: the surface is covered with cold sweats. This condition, so painful to behold, may last for days; repeated convulsions hasten its termination.

Can we distinguish this formidable complaint from ordinary meningitis? Seldom from meningitis of the base; generally from meningitis of the convexities. As regards the discrimination from the former malady, we are, it is true, sometimes enabled to pronounce the affection to be tubercular meningitis, if we are familiar with the patient's antecedents, and are cognizant, previous to the seizure, of the presence of tubercle in any of the internal organs, or are able at the time to detect the signs of phthisis. But without knowledge of this kind, a positive diagnosis is impossible; we have nothing to direct us excepting the probability that the case is tubercular, because most instances of meningitis of the base are of that nature. This uncertainty does not exist with reference to the usual form of simple meningeal inflammation. We may generally distinguish the tubercular malady by its occurrence in an unhealthy person; by its insidious approach; by the absence of violent delirium; by the appearance of convulsions, not early, but late in the disease; by the far less violent headache, and less degree of febrile excitement; by the notable remissions in several of the cerebral signs; by the chest symptoms, and the long duration of the affection.

Tubercular meningitis is ordinarily attended with an effusion of serum into the ventricles, and it is very plain that many of the symptoms are attributable to pressure of the fluid on portions of the brain. Now, how can we separate the malady, acute hydrocephalus, as many still call it, from dropsy of the brain, or *chronic hydrocephalus?* Partly by the history of the case, and partly by the normal size of the head; for the water on the brain is not sufficient in amount, nor is it there long enough, to produce an appreciable augmentation of the cranium. Then, in chronic hydrocephalus the symptoms manifest themselves for years, from childhood even to adult life. The signs of a profound cerebral lesion appear gradually, the special senses are by degrees enfeebled, but it is a long time before they are wholly abolished, or before complete loss of consciousness takes place.

As regards the diagnosis between tubercular meningitis and *acute hydrocephalus*, it need only be stated that this

8

affection is in the vast majority of cases à synonyme for the former. Yet we occasionally meet with instances in which acute hydrocephalus occurs unconnected with tubercle. It then runs either a latent course, or appears as an acute malady with symptoms similar to those of acute meningitis, commencing either with fever or with convulsions, and often attended with intense restlessness, succeeded by drowsiness, and having periods of intermission of the symptoms and of apparent improvement. Toward the end convulsions are very common. The complaint, unlike tubercular meningitis, happens in previously healthy children, begins suddenly, and is of shorter duration. But the effusion may remain, and the disorder lead to chronic hydrocephalus.

There is a functional disturbance of the brain which it is of great importance to discriminate from tubercular meningitis—the *hydrocephaloid* disease described by Marshall Hall. It has a stage of irritability, and a stage of torpor: a stage in which the little patient is restless, feverish, irritable; and a stage in which the countenance becomes pale, the breathing irregular, the voice husky, the pupils uninfluenced by light. These symptoms indicate nervous exhaustion. They generally come on after an enfeebling attack of illness, especially subsequent to protracted diarrhœa; sometimes they follow premature weaning. In the history of the case; the less tendency to vomiting; in the regularity of the pulse; in the flaccid and hollow state of the fontanelle, so dissimilar to its prominent and tense condition in inflammation; and in the arrest of the threatening signs by stimulants and by tonics, we find the guides which enable us to decide against the existence of an organic disease of the brain or its membranes.

But other affections besides those of the brain may be confounded with tubercular meningitis, such as typhoid and remittent fevers. From *typhoid fever* tubercular meningitis may be distinguished by the frequent vomiting; by the retracted abdomen, so unlike the swollen, tender belly of enteric fever; by the constipation instead of the diarrhœa; by the absence of an eruption,* and of enlargement of the

---

* Fox, Clinical Observations on Acute Tubercle   St. George Hosp. Rep., 1869.

spleen; by the irregularity of the pulse; by the occurrence of convulsions and anæsthesia, and other signs of profound motor and sensorial disturbance, and by the lower heat, the thermometer seldom rising above 102°.*   The duration of the two complaints affords no help in diagnosis, since the one may last as long as the other.

Tubercular meningitis is very often mistaken for *infantile remittent*, and indeed there are many points of close resemblance between them. Without mooting the question whether the remittent fever of children be really a distinct disease, we may here accept the group of clinical phenomena supposed to be characteristic, and point out the differences between them and those of tubercular or scrofulous inflammation of the brain. In the first place, excepting in those rare cases of coexisting acute tubercularization of the intestines, we do not perceive in the cerebral disorder a tongue red at the edges, diarrhœa, and other manifestations of intestinal irritation; and vomiting and nausea are more prominent and protracted symptoms than in remittent fever. But in this complaint the heat of skin is much greater; the pulse quicker, yet not unequal and subject to such decided variations; delirium occurs much earlier, and is much more marked,—indeed, tubercular meningitis may run through all its stages without mental wandering.

In reviewing the maladies with which tubercular meningitis may be confounded, it is incumbent upon us to bear in mind the *inflammatory affections of the lungs*, which, in children especially, are not uncommonly associated with delirium and other symptoms of a deranged nervous system. But the cerebral phenomena take a different course; the febrile excitement is more intense; and an examination of the chest reveals the cause of the disturbance of the brain. Yet we must not overlook the fact that the signs of acute phthisis may be like those of acute bronchitis or of acute pneumonia; that hence it may become a very perplexing subject to determine the precise cause of the disordered res-

---

* I have never seen an eruption in tubercular meningitis; but Barthez and Rilliet speak of fugitive imperfectly-formed rose-spots being present in rare cases.

piration, and the presence or absence of tubercular disease in the lungs. Indeed, if the explanation of the brain symptoms depend solely on the elucidation of this point, the diagnosis at times remains uncertain. In adults the difficulty is far less, because the demonstration of the existence or non-existence of pulmonary tubercle is much easier.

Tubercular meningitis is a very fatal disease. Whether it be invariably fatal, is as yet an undecided matter. But, notwithstanding the observations of Rilliet, the weight of evidence tends in that direction. Cures are said to have been effected by the free use of iodide or of bromide of potassium, and by counter-irritation to the scalp.

Cerebro-spinal Meningitis.—Now and then cases of meningitis are encountered in which the inflammation affects simultaneously the membranes of the brain and of the spine, and in which the symptoms of the cerebral malady are found to be blended with severe pain along the vertebral column, with convulsions, with rigidity of the muscles, with perverted cutaneous sensibility—in short, with the phenomena denoting spinal meningitis. But such sporadic cases are of rare occurrence. Generally cerebro-spinal meningitis is not met with save as an epidemic disease which presents itself at different times in somewhat dissimilar forms, changing mainly as the cerebral or the spinal disturbance prevails, and varying, moreover, according to the predominance of the constitutional or local phenomena.

Let us look at its most common characters. The disease is either gradual in its approach—a feeling of chilliness, succeeded by headache, by pain in the back and joints, and stiffness of the muscles of the neck, preceding its full development; or it begins with a chill, quickly followed by vomiting, by headache, by delirium or stupor, and extraordinary prostration. When the complaint has fairly set in, the headache is intense, and often accompanied by vertigo. The face has a fixed expression, or bears a look of suffering; the head is thrown backward and rigidly fixed. There is pain at the nape of the neck and along the spinal column, not increased by pressure, but much augmented by movements of any kind, felt also in the loins, and shooting into the ex-

tremities.   The patient is restless; he trembles; talks inco-
herently; and when spoken to does not appear to hear; his
pupils are generally dilated, and there may be dimness of
sight, or double vision.   The skin is dry, often very sensitive, or in some parts the sensibility is increased, in others
diminished, and the cutaneous surface is frequently spotted
with a red or a brown eruption, which becomes rapidly
petechial, and wholly uninfluenced by pressure; vesicles, too,
are apt to appear on the lips.   They show themselves from
the third to the sixth day of the disease, while the eruption
is seen either on the first day, or may at all events be detected by the third or fourth day.   The pulse at first is generally either natural or slow; but it becomes rather frequent
and irregular, and commonly remains accelerated throughout the disease.   The tongue is moist or dry, and brown;
the breathing often hurried and shallow, and the urine
slightly albuminous.   The bowels are at the outset constipated, but as the malady advances they become relaxed.
There is very usually persistent irritability of the stomach,
with great thirst, and spasmodic contractions or convulsive
movements in the muscles of the extremities.   With these
symptoms, to which those of exhaustion become plainly
added, the disorder progresses to its close, presenting in
some cases now and then strange and delusive remissions,
soon followed by distinct exacerbations.   In fortunate instances the morbid phenomena gradually lose their violence,
and the patient enters upon a tedious convalescence.

   But though these are the symptoms, which frequently
recur in epidemics, yet, as already indicated, they cannot
always be taken as the standard expression of the disease.
Most of them were observed in the formidable examples of
the malady. which have but recently been encountered in
this country; and they have also been met with in the epidemic cerebro-spinal meningitis not long since prevalent in
Germany.   As regards this epidemic, we are told by a distinguished observer,* that the spleen, early in the affection,
enlarges, but does not continue tumefied; and that the tem-

---

* Wunderlich, Archiv der Heilkunde, No. III., 1865, quoted in the Am.
Journ. of Med. Sciences for Oct. 1865.

perature reaches 106° to 108° Fahr., or even higher, without
there being a proportionate rise in the pulse; or this may
become frequent without a corresponding increase in the
temperature, which, moreover, is not sustained at the same
height. And whether the pulse be rapid or slow, the force
of the heart's impulse is at times found to be singularly
augmented.

The duration of the malady is very various. Patients
may become rapidly comatose, and die within twelve hours,
before any distinctly febrile action has commenced; or sink
in a few days; or, on the other hand, the complaint may
pursue a very chronic course, lasting for weeks, and during
this time deafness and blindness, convulsions, retention of
urine, and partial palsies—though this is very unusual—
may be prominent phenomena. In any case, the prognosis
is highly unfavorable; especially so when the symptoms
from the onset are violent, or the signs of spinal disturbance
preponderate.

Of the cause of the formidable disease we know little.
Many look upon it as modified typhus; and what tends to
support this view is, that the disorder occurs epidemically
under much the same circumstances as typhus. We find it
in crowded jails, in poorhouses, among ill-clad, half-nour-
ished persons. And whether typhus or not, it is certainly a
general disease, not merely an inflammation, and the description of this cerebro-spinal fever here can only be justified on
grounds of clinical convenience.

Cerebro-spinal meningitis is an affection very familiar to
military surgeons. It attacks recruits who have been subjected to unaccustomed fatigue, or have been huddled together in unhealthy barracks or camps. Attention to cleanliness, good food, pure air, sufficient clothing, and, as far as
possible, not overmarching raw troops, are then its surest
prophylactics.

To determine the diagnosis is ordinarily not difficult; the
epidemic character of the malady is a safeguard against
error. The protracted cases simulate *typhoid fever*. They
resemble it in its long duration, in several of the cerebral
symptoms, in the occurrence of an eruption, and sometimes

of diarrhœa. They differ from it in more sudden invasion, or rather in the short time in which the disease reaches an alarming aspect; and in the early stages the violent headache, the constipation, the constant vomiting, the slow or normal pulse, and the cool or but slightly heated skin, are unlike the signs of enteric fever. In those cases in which an eruption appears, it is noticed, at latest, by the third or fourth day, not at the end of a week, as in typhoid fever; nor is the rash, save in extremely rare instances, rose-colored. Later in the malady the traits of distinction become broader and broader. The prominence of the abdominal symptoms in the one disorder; the continued violent headache, the fixed spinal pain, the severe twitchings, or the tetanic rigidity of the muscles in the other, are signs the import of which are not easily overlooked.

The suddenness with which the morbid phenomena occasionally develop themselves, and the lulls that take place in the course of the affection, may cause it to be mistaken for the cerebral variety of *congestive fever*. But the remissions are not so marked as in this pernicious malady, nor are the exacerbations preceded by a long, violent chill. Moreover, congestive fever does not begin with congestive symptoms, but the first attack is like that of an ordinary intermittent or remittent; hence we have the history of the case to instruct us.

From *tetanus* cerebro-spinal meningitis may be distinguished by its epidemic prevalence, and by the signs of mental disturbance, which are very slight or wholly wanting in the former disorder. Generally, too, the cognizance of the exciting cause of the tetanic convulsions, such as their following wounds or punctures, aids in interpreting their meaning.

How can we discriminate between *inflammation of the cord* and of the cerebro-spinal meninges? Thus: in myelitis, as in pure spinal meningitis, mental symptoms are absent; their presence in cerebro-spinal meningitis constitutes one of the marked features of the disease. In myelitis there is an utter absence of convulsions or spasms, or should these happen, they occur in the shape of clonic spasms; but tonic contractions of muscles do not occur unless there be coexisting meningeal inflammation; in cerebro-spinal meningitis, on the other hand, rigidity of the muscles is one of the most striking peculiarities. In myelitis priapism is a frequent symptom; it is scarcely met with in cerebro-spinal meningitis. Myelitis is usually accompanied or followed by paralysis; paralysis is a very rare sequel of cerebro-spinal inflammation, and when it happens, is limited in extent. A complete palsy always justifies the conclusion of myelitis, or, at all events, of considerable pressure on the cord from an effusion.

The ordinary form of *cerebral meningitis*, as well as *tubercular meningitis*, differs from the cerebro-spinal affection by the presence in this of marked spinal symptoms and commonly of an eruption, and by the dissimilar origin and progress of the cases. The likeness of the malady to *typhus fever*, and the relation it bears to it, we shall elsewhere discuss.

Delirium Tremens.—The prominent trait of this complaint is delirium, associated with trembling and with sleeplessness. It occurs in intemperate persons; yet such is not always the case, for we may find an affection identical with mania a potu in those who are not intemperate in the ordinary acceptance of the word, but whose nervous systems have been racked by persistent mental anxiety, or by the use of other than alcoholic stimulants.

Generally, however, delirium tremens is brought on by the abuse of intoxicating liquors. It is a current belief, and one which has found much favor among habitual drinkers, that a diminution or a sudden discontinuance of the accustomed beverage is followed by an onset of delirium. This may perhaps happen; but, if I am to take as a standard the large number of cases of the disorder that have come under my care at the Philadelphia and Pennsylvania Hospitals, I should say that its appearance is most commonly preceded by a long-continued and unusually severe debauch, which finds its winding up in an attack of mania; and hence that this occurs in consequence of an excess, rather than of a diminution of the habitual stimulus.

Let us look a little more closely at the mental wandering.

It is very rarely fierce; nor is the patient taken up wholly with his delusions. He pays a certain amount of attention to surrounding objects, answers, perhaps in a rambling manner, the questions put to him, but fancies that animals are running around on his bed, or are crawling on the walls, and is thereby, or by some equally distressing illusion, kept in horror and dread. Or he imagines himself to be engaged in his ordinary occupations, and gives minute directions as to what he wishes done; tries to get out of bed, yet is quite tractable when thwarted in his efforts. His hands are constantly moving, and his delirium, to use the graphic epithet of Dr. Watson, is a busy one. With it are associated great sleeplessness, a frequent, soft pulse, a moist, coated tongue, and a clammy skin.

How are we to distinguish the malady from one to which it bears a certain resemblance—acute meningitis? Taking clearly expressed examples of each, we find the following marks of distinction: the pulse is different; tense and hard in meningeal inflammation, it is yielding and soft in delirium tremens. The skin and tongue are dry and feverish in the former affection, moist in the latter. Then the characteristics of the delirium are dissimilar: and in the one disease the mental wandering is combined with severe headache, but not with tremors; in the other, with tremors, but not with headache.

Yet in actual practice the diagnosis is not always so easy as it might appear to be at first sight, and we meet here and there with cases presenting symptoms the exact meaning of which it is puzzling to determine. The difficulty is mainly occasioned by extreme cerebral congestion, or by inflammatory action, having been produced by the same exciting cause that has brought on delirium tremens. In this blending of two morbid states, the pulse is, or soon becomes, tenser than in pure mania a potu; the skin is hotter; and I believe the irritability of the stomach is more marked and more persistent. In some instances, convulsions, strabismus, and deep stupor (carefully to be distinguished from the sleep which announces the termination of mania a potu) set all doubt at rest. But when these signs are not present, we have to judge chiefly by the vascular excitement, and by the activity of the fever, of the mischief that is going on within the cranium. Yet caution is necessary in accepting as evidence phenomena which may be of diverse origin; the fever may be the result of an intercurrent or coexisting pneumonia, of a gastritis, of a pulmonary apoplexy.* Only after a thorough exploration of the condition of the internal viscera can we accord to heat of skin and bounding pulse their full value.

There is another point connected with the diagnosis of the malady which it is necessary to mention, and chiefly for the purpose of calling attention to a very common error. The fact that a person known to be of bad habits is affected with delirium, is often received as a sure indication that the mental delusions have been produced by the abuse of ardent spirits. But they may be in reality owing to other causes: to fever; to a visceral inflammation; to acute mania. To avoid being deceived, we must lay stress rather on the special character of the delirium, and on the symptoms with which it is combined, than on its mere presence. In other words, delirium in intemperates is not of necessity the fruit of intemperance. In discussing acute mania we shall return to this subject.

The prognosis of delirium tremens is not unfavorable; at all events, not unfavorable in the first attack. Indeed, if the patient possess sufficient strength of will to reverse his habits, and be disposed to take his first punishment as a warning, it is powerful for good, instead of for evil. But, unfortunately, most attempts at reform do not last long, and sooner or later the drunkard dies a drunkard's death. The fatal issue is occasionally brought on by an intercurrent inflammation, especially of the lung; sometimes, after the subsidence of the urgent cerebral symptoms, the patient dies very unexpectedly, and no morbid appearances in the brain or its membranes account for the abrupt extinction of life. In many instances, however, of these sudden deaths, a large amount of serum is found in the ventricles, or in the subarachnoid spaces.

---

* Case at the Philadelphia Hospital, July, 1860.

Acute Mania.—It would be obviously out of place to attempt to give, in a work on medical diagnosis, a detailed account of any of the forms of insanity; but, in its acute variety especially, it resembles other affections of the nervous system so closely, that it cannot be wholly passed over.

There are mainly two disorders with which acute mania is liable to be confounded—acute meningitis and delirium tremens; and we shall for our purposes best learn the manifestations of acute mania by contrasting it with these maladies.

From acute meningitis mania differs in these essential particulars: the premonitory symptoms of the former are headache, drowsiness, and often a sense of tingling and of numbness in the extremities; these signs are, however, soon succeeded by the severer headache, tense pulse, high fever, and optical illusions of the developed disease The premonitory symptoms of acute mania, on the other hand, have generally existed for a longer time before the marked outbreak; some singular change of manner or of mode of thought commonly precedes the first violent attack of insanity, excepting in those cases in which the overthrow of reason results from a sudden great grief or a violent shock to the nervous system. Further, when the delusions have taken full possession of the mind, the patient attempts to act up to them, and his bodily strength enables him to do so. He has little if any fever; no spasms; his pupils are not contracted; his stomach is not irritable; he does not suffer from headache, or at least does not in any way complain of his head. It is needless to point out how all this differs from acute inflammation of the brain.

There is but little difficulty in discriminating between typical cases of delirium tremens and of acute mania. The anxious and distressed countenance, the alarm, the good-natured loquacity and restlessness of the patient, his moist skin, compressible pulse, and creamy tongue,—are phenomena very different from the ravings and excitement, or stubborn silence alternating with the wildly expressed hallucinations of insanity. Yet there are cases in which it is not easy to tell if the delusions are really due to intemperance: cases of insanity excited by drink in persons predisposed to mania. It may, indeed, at first be impossible to decide upon their nature, and upon the share the drinking has in their production. A few days, however, ordinarily remove all uncertainty; the person who is thought to be merely delirious is seen to become frantic after an intermission of quiet, or, entirely unlike what happens in mania a potu, to be still out of his mind after he has had a good, sound sleep. In one instance, in which much doubt existed as to the diagnosis, the patient solved the doubt by jumping out of bed after having been quietly sleeping for hours, and in a state of wild excitement knocked down the nurse who tried to prevent her from leaving the room.*

Diseases marked by Sudden Loss of Consciousness and of Voluntary Motion.

The chief diseases of this class are apoplexy, sun-stroke, and catalepsy. Epilepsy, too, might assert its claims to be here regarded; but it is more convenient to consider it with the convulsive affections.

Apoplexy.—This is coma coming on rapidly, in consequence of the compression of the brain by extravasated blood. At all events, hemorrhage is the condition by far the most commonly linked to the comatose symptoms; in comparatively rare cases only does the pressure upon the brain result from turgescence of the vessels, or from an effusion of serum.

The malady has sometimes no prodromata; but not·unfrequently it is preceded by great depression of spirits, by attacks of loss of memory, by illusions, by vitiated perceptions, by vertigo, or by odd sensations in the head.

The seizure is generally very sudden, and the coma quickly developed. The patient falls to the ground, bereft of all consciousness. In other instances, before he sinks into the comatose sleep, there will be more or less pain in

---

* For fuller information on the diagnosis of acute mania, see particularly Dr. Henry Maudsley's work.

the head, sickness at the stomach, heaviness and confusion of thought, or even slight convulsions. Such gradual cases, Abercrombie tells us, are more dangerous than those of abrupt origin.

When, whatever its commencement, the attack has reached its height, it presents these well-known features: the patient lies as if in a deep sleep, breathing laboriously and noisily, and each snoring inspiration followed by a flapping of the cheeks in expiration. The pulse is slow, full, at times irregular; the carotids throb violently, and the increased pulsation is particularly noticed in large effusions, whether of blood or of serum; there is difficulty of deglutition; the pupils are immovable, and either contracted or dilated; the eye half open. All thought, all sensation, all volition is suspended; the limbs are motionless, flaccid, and when lifted fall passively and to all appearance lifeless to the ground. Occasionally, not often, their muscles are rigid; but, save when the apoplexy is very extensive, reflex contractions can be excited in them.

If the patient recover from the comatose state, he does so generally in a short time; in a few hours, unless the lesion be very great, the intellectual faculties begin to resume their sway, and all the functions of the body are slowly restored to their natural condition. Yet there is a palpable exception to this in the muscular system. Paralysis of one side is very apt to remain long after everything else presents a normal look; nay, it may be a sequel lasting for years, or even permanently.

One attack of apoplexy is likely, sooner or later, to be followed by another, and the reason of this is, that the predisposing cause is generally of a persistent character—an organic cardiac malady, especially hypertrophy of the left ventricle or tricuspid regurgitation; a disease of the cerebral arteries; or softening of the brain.*

Now, is there anything at the time of the apoplexy, or

---

* The most recent researches have rendered it likely that the extravasation of blood is always due to the same immediate cause, to rupture of miliary aneurisms on the minute arteries. See Charcot and Bouchard, Archiv. de Physiol., 1868; also Charcot, Maladies des Vieillards.

after its most urgent symptoms have passed away, by which
we can recognize whether the pressure on the brain results
from a clot, a serous effusion, or from a turgescence of the
cerebral vessels? And, again, do the morbid manifestations
furnish any clue to the seat of the hemorrhage? With reference to the former question, all clinical experience forces us
to admit that, in any of the states mentioned, the actual
signs may be the same; and that we never can be quite certain of the non-existence of a clot. It is true that when the
apoplectic symptoms abate rapidly; when thought, however
confused, soon returns; when the limbs are not paralyzed,
or are so but imperfectly and for a short time,—we have
strong reason for believing that congestion simply lies at the
root of the disturbance; that, in other words, the case is one
of those called simple apoplexy. But it is never possible to
give a positive opinion, since a clot near the periphery of
the brain may occasion the same phenomena as those
specified.

And with regard to a rapid effusion of serum, the difficulty of distinction is quite as great, or even greater. In
fact, the only differential signs which were formerly claimed
for serous apoplexy, namely, pallor of face and feebleness of
pulse, are now known to be very common in large sanguineous effusions; and when we analyze the symptoms of the
cases recorded by Abercrombie, by Morgagni, by Andral,—
for the descriptions of older authors respecting this affection
are not to be trusted, and most modern authorities seem to
pass it by as wholly unworthy of notice,—we find absolutely
nothing that can be looked upon as even pointing to a diagnosis. In a case which came under my observation some
years since,* the respiration was not noisy, nor was there
flapping of the cheeks, or the least discernible movement of
any portion of the body; yet I am not aware that any of
these points can be regarded as diagnostic.

The *seat* of the hemorrhage can ordinarily be detected
with somewhat more certainty than the cause of the cerebral
pressure; it could be detected with yet greater certainty,

---

* Charleston Medical Journal and Review, March, 1859.

were it not that the extravasation so often takes place into an already diseased brain. In the vast majority of instances, the blood is effused into one of the corpora striata and optic thalami, and we find, in consequence, only one-sided paralysis. If the lesion be in both hemispheres, the palsy is on both sides of the body, although almost invariably more complete on one side than on the other. Yet a double-sided palsy does not justify an absolute opinion that the extravasation of blood into the brain substance is double-sided. It betokens also an effusion into the ventricles. But ventricular hemorrhage is, besides, distinguished by profound coma and by tonic contraction of the muscles.

Hemorrhage into the corpora quadrigemina presents most frequently this combination of symptoms: muscular tremblings, convulsions, impairment of sight and alteration of the pupils. Cerebellar hemorrhage gives rise to very temporary loss of consciousness; to relaxation of the muscles of the limbs without paralysis or impaired sensibility; and to frequent vomiting.* In hemorrhage into one-half of the pons, there is palsy of the extremities on one side, and of the face on the other.† There may also be hyperæsthesia in some parts of the body, and aunaurosis.‡

Hemorrhage limited to the arachnoid, with the blood poured into the subarachnoid spaces, occasions ordinarily pain in the head, somnolency, and profound coma without paralysis, and without anæsthesia or slow pulse, but with relaxation of the muscles, and sometimes with convulsions; and now and then the symptoms assume, to all appearance, a remittent course. It is a very fatal form of apoplexy, occurring chiefly in new-born children, and after injuries to the head, or from the giving way of a diseased and widened artery, or in consequence of a rupture of one of the sinuses of the dura mater.

When the effusion of blood takes place between the dura mater and the arachnoid, it is, as Virchow has of late years proved, generally the ultimate result of an inflammation and

---

* Hillairet, Arch. Gen. de Med., 1858, tome xi.
† Gubler, Gaz. Hebdom., 1858, 1859.
‡ Brown-Séquard.

of subsequent changes of the inner surface of the dura mater. On close inquiry, the precursory symptoms of a disease of the membrane may, perhaps, be traced by the constant and localized pain.

Let us now examine how the diagnosis of apoplexy can be determined, and how this malady may be distinguished from other states which produce rapid loss of consciousness, or sudden paralysis. Not to mention epilepsy—the phenomena of which we shall further on contrast with those of apoplexy, and shall observe to differ chiefly in the prominence of the convulsions; or meningitis—in which fever, headache, and other signs of an acute cerebral disease precede insensibility; or a tumor—which, save in the rarest instances, leads only very gradually to a comatose condition; or uremic coma— marked by peculiar prodromata and peculiar stertor; or sun- stroke—belonging to the same group as cerebral hemorrhage, yet presenting points of contrast, which will shortly engage our attention,—we find these morbid states liable to be mis- taken for apoplexy:

INSENSIBILITY FROM DRINK, OR FROM NARCOTIC POISONS;
SYNCOPE;
ASPHYXIA;
ACUTE SOFTENING;
SUDDEN EXTENSIVE PARALYSIS;
OBSTRUCTIONS OF CEREBRAL ARTERIES;
PROTRACTED SLEEP;
CEREBRAL HYSTERIA;
APHASIA.

Insensibility from Drink, or from Narcotic Poisons.—Both these conditions are sometimes difficult to distinguish from the coma of apoplexy; and if we are not cognizant of the circumstances preceding their development, we have only these points to guide us: in intoxication there is a strong smell of whisky, gin, or whatever liquor has produced it, emanating from the mouth, and the man, although uncon- scious, is not often entirely bereft of all power of motion—he is certainly not paralyzed. Moreover, the pulse is not slow, it is frequent; the eye is injected, and the symptoms become suddenly much ameliorated after the inhalation of ammonia, or after the stomach has been emptied of its contents. In narcotic poisoning, especially if from opium, the pupils are very much contracted; and we are likely to encounter repeated vomiting, and a gradual intensification of the coma. The patient, however, unless death be very close at hand, can be momentarily roused from his deep sleep; and his calm breathing is unlike the stertor of apoplexy. But when the hemorrhage has taken place into the pons varolii, the diagnosis is very difficult, especially if the bleeding be extensive, for we then are apt to have a contraction of both pupils, and the respiration may not be stertorous; nor is there always at first paralysis. Yet this subsequently appears, and thus the detection of the cause of the insensibility is rendered easier.*

Nitrobenzole, which operates as a narcotic poison in vapor as well as in a liquid state, may, in the rapidly fatal cases, produce coma, which may be mistaken for the insensibility of apoplexy. But the poison leads quickly to death when coma has been induced, and is detected by its strong odor, resembling that of bitter almonds.† Poisoning by drinking chloroform, and which gives rise to many of the symptoms of apoplexy, is also discerned by the odor, and by the quick and tumultuous action of the heart which accompanies the stertorous breathing, by the relaxation of the limbs, the deathlike aspect of the face, the widely dilated pupils, and the complete general anæsthesia.‡

Syncope—Asphyxia.—The loss of consciousness in either of these states is as striking as that of apoplexy. But there is this decided difference: the suspension of thought and of volition in a fainting fit is due to failure of the circulation; hence the pulse is hardly, or not at all felt, instead of being full, as it is in apoplexy. Further, the pallor of the face, the quiet respiration, the short duration of the syncope mark plainly the one affection from the other. And with reference to asphyxia: the turgid and livid face, the bluish lip,

---

* See an interesting case mentioned by Dr. J. H. Jackson, London Hospital Reports, vol. i., 1864.

† Taylor, Guy's Hospital Reports, vol. x., 3d series.

‡ As in the case reported in l'Union Médicale, October, 1864.

the distressed and embarrassed breathing preceding the convulsions, and the loss of consciousness, show clearly that the
disturbance affects primarily the lungs, and does not reside
in the brain.

Acute Softening.—This may give rise to symptoms so similar to those of cerebral hemorrhage, that a differential diagnosis is impossible. Especially does this happen if the disease manifests itself suddenly, which Rostan informs us
occurred in one-half of the cases he noted. In those of
more gradual origin, a feeling of numbness, deterioration
of memory, irritability of the temper, slight impairment of
motion, and a vacant, dull look, are noticed for some time
before the attack. Occasionally delirium immediately precedes the loss of consciousness. Now this may be very perfect, or imperfect, or even wholly wanting,—for the patient
may become paralyzed, after being merely confused or feeling distressed, but without losing his consciousness. The
palsy is at times attended with hyperæsthesia and with rigidity
of the limbs.

But it is by the after-symptoms that we most easily separate acute softening from apoplexy. In the latter, after the
shock is over, a gradual improvement takes place, very
obvious as regards the mental faculties and the power of
articulation; in the former, the mind remains obtuse, or
greatly impaired, and there is otherwise but slight amelioration; defects of sensibility are particularly apt to be noticed.
A significant sign, too, of acute softening is an increased
secretion from the mouth and eye.*

Sudden Extensive Paralysis without Coma.—This is not a trait
of apoplexy, although it is a common error to suppose that
a sudden palsy is produced by hemorrhage into the brain.
Sudden extensive paralysis without coma is ordinarily owing
to softening of the brain; but it may be due to hemorrhage
into the spinal column. Palsy from this source, unlike that
caused by cerebral hemorrhage, is almost invariably double-
sided, is accompanied by severe spinal pain, and, if the extravasation have taken place into the meninges, by tonic
spasms, like those of tetanus.

---

* Durand Fardel, Maladies des Vieillards.

Obstruction of the Cerebral Arteries.—If a cerebral artery be suddenly closed by a fibrinoid vegetation being washed into it, apoplectic symptoms arise. We may suspect, for we never can be quite certain, that an arterial obstruction is the cause of the disturbance of the brain, if the patient be laboring under an acute or subacute endocardial inflammation, or a chronic valvular trouble in which fragments of vegetations may be broken off; and if within a brief period of each other several incomplete attacks have occurred before a perfect (and generally fatal) comatose condition sets in. The usual locality of the impaction is, according to Virchow, in the artery of the fossa of Sylvius; and the consequences of the interrupted circulation are at once perceived in the adjacent centre of motion—the corpus striatum. The palsy which ensues in connection with the apparently apoplectic phenomena is one-sided; and the facial paralysis is on the same side with that of the limbs. Other peculiarities of the hemiplegia are, that its onset is not of necessity attended with loss of consciousness, or that this is slight and of short duration; that the palsy is often quickly followed by gangrene of the extremities; or is associated with disturbance of the kidneys, or with enlargement of the spleen and tenderness in the splenic region, due to changes in the organs, produced by an impaction of fibrin. Just as in apoplexy, we may find in obstructions of the vessels, softening as a result of the accident; nor are the symptoms of this sequel different from what they are when softening is owing to more usual causes.* Occasionally the clot is not washed into the brain, but is formed in one of its arteries. The thrombosis may extend thence as far as the common carotid. Hasse, who has placed two such cases on record, mentions that, independently of the cerebral symptoms, they may be recognized by the absence of pulsation in the carotid of the affected side, and its tense, cordy feel.†

---

* But it is possible that we shall learn to look upon thrombosis and emboli as among the ordinary causes of softening of the brain. A recent author, M. Lancereaux ("De la Thrombose et de l'Embolie Cérébrale"), states that of 22 cases he observed, 16 were connected with arterial obstruction.

† Zeitschr. für Ration. Pathol , Band iv. There may be other causes, too,

Protracted Sleep.—While recovering from acute diseases, the sick often sleep profoundly, and for a long time. Yet there is little likelihood of confounding this with the sleep of apoplexy; for the antecedent circumstances reveal the meaning of this restoration of nature. Sometimes, however, persons sink into a deep and prolonged slumber, without any previous ailment. Medical literature furnishes a number of such instances. In one recorded by Dr. Cousins,* the tendency to somnolency has lasted for years. The patient frequently sleeps three, and sometimes five days at a time. When he awakes he is well. In a case which I saw with Dr. S. Weir Mitchell, and which is described by him,† the slumberer was aroused several times by the exciting influence of electricity; but this finally lost its effect, and she relapsed into a sleep from which she awoke no more. These kind of cases may give the impression of apoplexy, yet they do not resemble it very strictly. They are unlike it in the gentle, noiseless breathing, and feeble pulse; in the occasioual motion of the body; and in the protracted unconsciousness.

Cerebral Hysteria.—The actual similitude and the points of contrast between this curious state and apoplexy may be learned from the following sketch:

A married lady, of a remarkably susceptible and nervous disposition, had been for many months suffering from amenorrhœa and from sluggish action of the bowels. She was at the same time troubled with a constant cough, evidently dependent upon a deposition of tubercles in one of the lungs. She had been in very bad health, but by the steady employment of tonics, and the beneficial effects of a sea voyage, her symptoms were much amended. Her appetite improved, and she commenced to gain flesh and to take exercise without

---

of cerebral embolism. For instance, a case of carbuncle ending in embolism of the middle cerebral artery, is described in the Med. Times and Gazette, Feb. 1869. Cases of fat globules in the smaller arteries leading to a fatty embolism have been analyzed by Busch. See Virchow's Archiv, as quoted in Brit. and Foreign Medico-Chirurg. Rev., April, 1869, p. 551.

* Medical Times and Gazette, April, 1863; see also a somewhat similar case, N. Y. Journ. of Med., Dec. 1867.

† Transact. of Phil. Coll. of Physicians, 1856.

fatigue. She was, however, troubled with headache, and with pain at the lower part of the abdomen. On one occasion in the evening I ordered her some cathartic medicine; and in the morning she was better than usual and in the liveliest spirits. A few hours afterward I was sent for, and found her insensible. She had complained of a sudden, sharp cramp near the umbilicus, and had then ceased to speak. She remained unconscious for about twelve hours; yet not wholly so, for every now and then she opened her eyelids, muttered a word or two, a pleasant smile flitted over her countenance; but she soon relapsed into her deep slumber. Her thumbs were drawn inward; she had occasionally convulsive movements; the breathing was rapid, but not noisy; the pulse feeble—at first slow, then frequent; her eyes squinted in the most decided manner. Stimulants and antispasmodics were freely given, but without much benefit, for she recovered from her lethargy only with the setting in of the most violent paroxysmal pains in the abdomen, shooting down the thigh, and accompanied by contractions of the muscles and by exquisite local tenderness. The next day, without much abatement of the suffering, she was perfectly conscious; but still she squinted—nay, was totally blind, and remained so for two days. During this time a menstrual discharge commenced, which in part relieved the abdominal pain. The head symptoms were, if the expression be admissible, a metastasis of hysteria from the ovaries to the brain. It is needless to point out how this display of hysteria differed from apoplexy.

Aphasia.—By this term is meant loss of the faculty of expression of thought, either in consequence of loss of the faculty of speech, or of communicating thought by writing or by gestures. The patient may be deprived of the ability of expressing himself in one of these ways, or in all; the loss of speech is the most common, and is apt to be associated with a very decided impairment of memory and an enfeeblement of intelligence. The disorder is temporary, lasting but a few hours or some days, or it continues for months or years. And during its course the affected person is incapable of recalling words to give utterance to his ideas;

or if he can recall the words to the mind, and thus think, cannot express them. He has lost, to use the language of Trousseau, to whom, more than to any one else, we are indebted for our knowledge of the subject, "at the same time, to a greater or less degree, the memory of words, the memory of the acts by the aid of which the words are articulated, and intelligence; but all the faculties are not equally lost, and, however damaged the intelligence, it is less so than the memory of the acts of phonation, and this less so than the memory of words."

Very often the patient has but a few words at his control; he says "yes" or "no" for everything, and appears angry that he can say no more; or he uses wrong words, knowing perhaps that they are wrong, and sometimes only those of a profane kind; or he confuses merely some syllables in the words he employs; or he may not be able to utter a word. Yet while in this condition there is no defect in the tongue, or lips, or palate, to account for the inability to talk; they are as healthy as usual; the act of swallowing is easily performed; and even where the aphasia is complicated with hemiplegia, it is not difficult to discern that the imperfect articulation and thick speech attending the palsy—which, moreover, are very apt to become greatly ameliorated, or even pass off within a short period after the seizure—are not the cause of the singular disturbance of the faculty of expression; a disturbance which will mostly show itself not simply by the failure to utter words, but also by the inability to recollect them and write them down. Indeed, it is necessary to bear in mind that these states may coexist, but they also may be present separately. Thus, there are persons who can think, but cannot speak or write; there are those who can think and write, but cannot speak; and there are those who can think and speak, but cannot write. For the second group the term aphemia; for the third, that of agraphia has been proposed.* Most patients understand perfectly well what is said to them; some can read to themselves; and unless the general intelligence is very per-

---

* Bastian, Br. and Foreign Med.-Chir. Review, April, 1869.

ceptibly affected, they can express themselves by signs and gestures. In some cases there is rather loss of memory and forgetfulness and confusion; but it is very doubtful whether these defects of memory ought to be included under the general head of aphasia, for when prompted the word is at once spoken.

Aphasia is believed to be dependent upon disease situated in the frontal convolutions, and, by Broca, the lesion is even located in the supposed seat of articulate language, in the posterior part of the third frontal convolution of the left side of the cerebrum. This view receives support from the fact that the hemiplegia which may accompany aphasia is almost invariably right-sided.* Still, even this fact rather favors the lesion being on the left side than being strictly in the convolution mentioned. Indeed, several cases have been obseved—I have myself met with two—in which the part in question was healthy; and, on the whole, I think it rather proves that the trouble is in the left anterior portions of the brain than in a special convolution. As regards the exact lesion in the affected portion of the brain, it is very various. In cases of aphasia of short duration and without palsy, there is probably merely congestion; in protracted cases, and those in which we find coexisting hemiplegia, a clot or softening is likely to be present; deficient tone of the blood-vessels and enfeebled nutrition will perhaps explain the aphasia, which may be noticed during the convalescence from grave acute maladies. This form of the complaint and that consequent upon congestions end in more or less rapid and generally perfect recovery; in the other forms, either no improvement follows, or only a very partial gain of words takes place.

The suddenness with which the attack may set in will

---

* Trousseau, in his Clinique Médicale, records an exception, and several are mentioned by Sanders, in the Edinburgh Medical Journal, June, 1866, and by Hughlings Jackson, in a very interesting paper in the London Hospital Reports, vol. i. The same author notices the concurrence of the loss of speech and hemiplegia with valvular disease of the heart, and traces their connection, in many cases, to embolism of the cerebral arteries, particularly plugging of the middle cerebral artery on the left side.

cause it to be mistaken for an ordinary apoplectic seizure. But we find either not the least deficiency in motion in any part of the body, and well-preserved consciousness; or the disease may become manifest subsequent to attacks of vertigo, or to a paralytic stroke preceded or not by the ordinary signs of an apoplectic fit. Under these circumstances the diagnosis cannot be definitely made, until, after fully returned consciousness, we have an opportunity of examining the state of the mind, and of the tongue and the muscles concerned in articulation, remembering that if there is difficulty in articulation the case is not one of aphasia.

Sun-stroke.—Persons exposed to the scorching rays of the sun in midsummer often become dizzy, and fall to the ground insensible—they have had a sun-stroke. The attack either takes place while the patient is still exposed to the sun; or, in rarer instances, he reaches his home with a staggering gait, giddy, faint, suffering from a dull, oppressive pain in the head, and after some hours becomes unconscious. However the onset, the insensibility which occurs is generally complete, although it may be so but for a few minutes. Associated with it are a frequent, feeble pulse, a skin not deficient in warmth and sometimes very hot on the forehead, stertorous breathing, difficulty in swallowing, and relaxation of the limbs.

When we contrast these symptoms with those of apoplexy, we find the following marks of distinction: the pulse is not slow and full, but feeble; there is more difficulty in deglutition, but a less snoring respiration; the coma does not ordinarily remain as complete for so great a length of time, for soon the patient may, temporarily at least, be partially roused from his deep sleep; and no paralysis, either of the limbs or of the cheek, occurs. The after-symptoms, too, are different: in cerebral hemorrhage, paralysis; in sun-stroke, feebleness of movement, but no paralysis. In the former, no marked, persistent headache; in the latter, headache, more or less chronic, always aggravated by walking in the sun, and often for months accompanied by signs of an exhausted nervous system, and in some instances by epileptic convulsions.

The question with regard to the discrimination of these

morbid states is one of great practical value, as on the conclusion arrived at depends our therapeutic action. Are we
to bleed, and to purge actively? or are we to withhold the
lancet, use purgatives moderately, and trust to cold affusions,
sinapisms, and stimulants? Are we, in other words, to follow
out a treatment of service in apoplexy, or a treatment of service in the majority of instances of sun-stroke? •

These points are, as a rule, readily determined by paying
attention to the variance in the symptoms mentioned. But
it must be confessed that we sometimes meet with ambigu-
ous cases—cases in which the signs of nervous exhaustion
produced by exposure to heat are blended with those of cerebral congestion or hemorrhage excited by the same cause,
and in which, when they terminate fatally, the autopsy shows
not simply a changed blood, or pulmonary congestion, but
turgescence of the cerebral vessels, or an extravasation. The
management of such patients requires great care; we must
stimulate or not, according to which indication the weight of
the symptoms inclines.

The remarks just made refer to the most common form
of sun-stroke—that attended with more or less sudden loss
of consciousness, and therefore simulating apoplexy. But
there are cases in which the abnormal manifestations come
on gradually, and in which the patient at no time becomes
insensible. I have seen a number of the kind; they were
not unusual among officers sent home from the wearing summer campaigns of the late war. The chief symptoms are,
intense headache, nausea, prostration, and inability to perform any work requiring sustained attention. All these
signs appear after protracted exposure to the sun; and they
mend but very tardily. In truth, in the slowly developed
disorder the subsequent nervous exhaustion and the paroxysms of headache seem to be much more persistent than the
same phenomena following what looks like the more violent
form of the malady. Among the sequelæ of these apparently
incomplete attacks are, irritability of the bladder, incontinence of urine, and irregular action of the heart. But nothing is as striking as the loss of mental and bodily energy.

The symptoms of "insulatio," or sun-stroke, may be induced by prolonged atmospheric heat, while the patient is in-doors and not exposed to the rays of the sun. Such cases of heat apoplexy are known to occur in India even at midnight. They may be preceded by a sense of extreme weariness, by inability to sleep, by loss of appetite, by constipation and frequent micturition, and by deficient perspiration; or the signs of exhaustion, followed by more or less complete insensibility, appear without distinct prodromes.

Catalepsy.—This is a sudden suspension of thought, of sensibility, and of voluntary motion, during the continuance of which the muscles retain the exact position they happen to be placed in at its onset. This strange and uncommon complaint occurs in paroxysms, which may last but a few minutes or several hours, and during which the most conplete anæsthesia, not only of the skin, but of the deeper tissues, may occur.* The disorder is met with in females, especially in hysterical females, and alternates with outbreaks of hysteria. But it may also exist in the male sex, and be in either hereditary. It has been even noticed as an epidemic in localities where there are many families closely connected by intermarriages.†

Catalepsy may be mistaken for apoplexy, or even for death itself. It differs from apoplexy by its constant recurrence: and further, during an attack the eyes are wide open ; the pupils, although dilated, are very susceptible to light; and there is an absence of stertorous breathing as well as of the characteristic relaxation of the muscles or of the paralysis of apoplexy,—for the limbs are outstretched, or held in every conceivable annoying or painful position, yet as soon as consciousness is restored, their power of movement fully returns. The pulse is not retarded ; on the contrary, although feeble, it becomes very frequent.

The perplexing affection varies from a kindred state, *ecstasy*, in this: in the latter the loss of consciousness is not complete. The patient is merely insensible to external objects, because he is intensely absorbed in some vision present

---

* As in the case reported by Lasègue, Archiv. Génér de Médecine, tome i., 1864.

† Vogt, Schmidt's Jahrb., Bd. cxx. p. 301.

to his imagination, or in the contemplation of some subject to him of all-engrossing interest.   But he is not statue-like; on the contrary, his countenance is animated, earnest, and he talks, declaims, sings.

There is a curious form of the disorder, which Sir Thomas Watson describes.   It is an imperfect kind of catalepsy called *daymare*, the affected person being at the time incapable of moving or speaking, yet cognizant of all that goes on around her.   These seizures of temporary deprivation of muscular power, without unconsciousness, were thought, by the accomplished physician quoted, to have depended, in the case he cites, upon a diseased state of the blood-vessels of the brain. Were this condition always present in the complaint, it would be a far more serious one than ordinary catalepsy.

Diseases marked by Convulsions or Spasms.

Epilepsy.—Epilepsy is a disease the chief manifestation of which consists in recurring attacks of sudden loss of consciousness, attended with convulsive movements.   The patient falls to the ground without thought, without feeling, without the power of voluntary motion.   He utters often a short piercing cry, then a fearful muscular struggle begins. The legs are stiff, and turned inward; the head is tossed backward, or from side to side; the mouth is distorted, the lips covered with foam; the arms outstretched and rigid, or thrown about with great force; the eyelids are half closed; the teeth are ground together, and the tongue is thrust between them, and often severely bitten.   Gradually the convulsive movements become less violent and cease altogether, and the patient passes into a deep sleep, from which he awakes fatigued and exhausted, and dull in intellect.   But these symptoms disappear, and he returns to his usual state of health.

But every paroxysm does not present the same phenomena, or run the same definite course.   In many the attack is preceded by strange sensations: by a peculiar train of thought; by retching; by the feeling of a puff of air ascending from the extremities to the head.   This "aura epileptica," on which so much stress has been laid, is, however, very far from constant. Yet it may exist, as Brown-Séquard teaches, without hardly being perceived: it may be an unfelt irritation starting from some centripetal nerve in any part of the skin, or from some organ not deeply seated, as the testicle, and its point of departure may be detected by observing, during the fit, in what neighborhood the first, or the most violent, or the most prolonged contractions occur. In very rare instances sudden spasms of the face and chest occur with arrest of respiration, and followed by a clonic convulsion, yet with so little unconsciousness, that it remains doubtful whether the paroxysm has been attended by unconsciousness at all.

Some seizures are very light,—a transient suspension of consciousness, a slight twitching of some of the muscles, a fixed gaze, perhaps a decided impression of vertigo, and all is over. These abortive fits, the *petit mal* of the French, are very apt to precede by some days a severe attack, or several of them may take the place of the more turbulent form of the disorder. And they, too, like the graver epileptic convulsion, may present strange irregularities. They may manifest themselves, for instance, only in bursts of unmeaning laughter, as happened in the extraordinary case recorded by Dr. George Paget;* or in attacks of sudden and intense facial neuralgia, with or without partial convulsions, as in the cases narrated by Trousseau.†

The epileptic paroxysm does not always pass off without leaving some trace of the profound disturbance it has occasioned. It may be followed by hemiplegia, due, it is ordinarily thought, to a congestion of the brain during the fit. Whether this be the explanation or not, it is certain that the palsy, like that following cerebral congestion, is very transient and generally disappears in a few days. Another sequel of the attack is loss of voice; another, abdominal tenderness.

In the intervals between the seizures the patient is not

---

* British Medical Journal, Feb. 1859.
† Clinique Médicale, tome ii.

in reality well. His temper is irritable, and his mental faculties slowly but certainly deteriorate. The loss of memory particularly is very marked; and dementia is not an unusual complication of long-continued epilepsy. In some epileptics, as Herpin so well points out, there is much mental excitement or a curious mental state preceding the seizures, or a violent and dangerous mania may follow the fit.*

Epilepsy is either central or peripheral: that is, the exciting cause is seated in the nervous centres, especially in the brain or medulla; or affects the centripetal nerves, and is by them reflected to the nervous centres. It is thus that the malady originates in injuries of nerves, in diseases of the skin, of the gastro-intestinal tract of the uterus, from the irritation of worms, or in consequence of congenital phimosis.† Now with reference both to the prognosis and the treatment, it is very important to discriminate between epilepsy of centric and of eccentric origin; and to arrive at this discrimination is only possible by a thorough examination of all the constitutional symptoms, and by ascertaining the starting-point and tracing the course of the aura. Another diagnostic separation of great practical value is to determine, after we have concluded the epilepsy to be central, if it be symptomatic of a cerebral disorder—such as of a tumor, of cysticerci lodged in the organ, of a syphilitic affection of the membranes, or of a disturbance of the brain produced by disease of the skull-cap—in fact, of any of those cerebral maladies which are known to engender epileptic seizures; or if it be watery blood, or vitiated blood full of abnormal ingredients, as in diseases of the kidneys, acting injuriously on the nutrition of the cerebral texture; or if it be idiopathic, due to causes we do not fully understand, chief among them, perhaps, if we may look upon the observations of Küssmaul and Tenner‡ and of Schroeder van der Kolk§ as conclusive, to

---

* Maudsley, Article "Insanity" in Reynolds's System of Medicine, vol. ii.
† Althaus, Lancet, Feb. 1867.
‡ On Epileptiform Convulsions. Translated by New Sydenham Society, 1859.
§ Minute Structure and Functions of Spinal Cord and Medulla. Sydenh. Soc., 1859.

a morbid excitation or an affection of the medulla oblongata. During the paroxysms it is impossible to settle the matter; but in the interval we may often do so by close attention to the history of the case, and by noting whether the patient enjoys the usual health of epileptic subjects, or presents signs of a chronic cerebral trouble. Romberg tells us that where affections of the bones lie at the root of the complaint, the fits are readily induced by pressure upon the skull; and further, that if there be disease residing in one of the cerebral hemispheres, the aura affects the opposite side of the body, and is generally confined to the upper extremity.

Much has been said of the distinction between epilepsy and *convulsions*. Now as regards the seizure itself, there is no appreciable difference; the only diversity consists in the recurrence of the attack after intervals of comparative health, and in the non-existence of any disturbance from which convulsions are likely to arise, such as a recent injury to the head, an eruptive fever, the parturient state, inflammation of the brain, a Bright's kidney, teething, or rickets. In children, who, as is well known, are particularly subject to convulsions, the diagnosis may be a difficult matter; but the fits of epilepsy are distinguishable by the dulness of intellect, and the slow mental and bodily development, observable in the intervals. And we are not often called upon to make this differential diagnosis, because of the extreme rarity with which epilepsy occurs in the young; although many insist that it is more frequent than is supposed, basing this assumption on the generally-received fact that the history of epileptics shows them to have suffered greatly from convulsions during childhood.

The diseases which are most apt to be confounded with epilepsy are hysteria and apoplexy. The former—like all the rest of the group now under discussion, like chorea, like tetanus, like hydrophobia—is discriminated by the absence of that perfect suspension of consciousness that takes place in epileptic seizures; and there are other marks of distinction, to which we shall presently refer. In apoplexy, as in epilepsy, we meet with loss of consciousness, sometimes with convulsions. But these are, on the whole, rare, and coma precedes and does not follow them, as happens in epilepsy. Then, stertorous breathing, and a slow, full pulse, are not observed in epilepsy; for the breathing, although irregular and gasping, is not coarse and noisy, and the pulse is feeble, irregular, and frequent. Epileptic patients bite their tongue; this does not occur in apoplexy. In epilepsy the paroxysm seldom lasts longer than from ten to fifteen minutes before consciousness returns, and before the convulsions cease; in apoplexy the insensibility is of much longer duration. Epilepsy is not usually followed by paralysis; apoplexy is commouly.

Epilepsy is often feigned; yet impostors cannot feign it completely. They may bite their tongue; they may imitate the stertor, the foam at the mouth, the convulsions, the thumb drawn inward toward the palm, the confused air on awakening: they may simulate, although they rarely do so, the indifference to pain; but there is one feature of the real attack they cannot copy—the insensibility of the iris. No matter how skilful the dissembler, his pupils must contract when exposed to a strong light; they must dilate when the stimulus is withdrawn.

But, unfortunately, there are several difficulties in making this test an absolute one. In the first place, the pupils, during a fit, cannot always be readily observed. In the second place, not in every case of epilepsy are they perfectly immovable; in some, though sluggish, they react to light. And again, as proved by Dr. Keen, violent muscular motion instantly dilates the pupil, and so long as the movement continues, so long will the iris act dilatorily, even when exposed to a bright light. Thus muscular spasms alone, even when simulated, may cause the pupils to be dilated and inactive. A test, said to be more generally useful, is the administration of ether. When given to an epileptic, its first effect is to increase the violence of the spasm, but eventually the patient passes into the deep sleep produced by ether, without any of the prior cerebral excitement; while in the malingerer this manifests itself by talking and laughing—in fact, in the usual way.*

---

* Keen, Mitchell, and Morehouse, Am. Journ. of Med. Sci., Oct. 1864.

Chorea.—This spasmodic affection is chiefly met with in young persons, especially in girls approaching the age of puberty. It is characterized by irregular clonic spasms of groups of muscles under the influence of the will and mainly of those on one side of the body. But the patient is not deprived of consciousness, and with it of all power of voluntary motion. He knows what he is about, and can in part execute the movements he undertakes; yet his limbs are not completely under his control. They obey only his general directions, but not entirely or at once; for the muscles jerk and pull as seems to them best, taking no heed of the time or the manner in which the will wishes any movement executed. In some cases, not in many, the muscles of deglutition and of respiration become implicated, and difficulty in swallowing and in breathing occurs. A dilated pupil, too, acting very sluggishly in response to light, may be met with among the phenomena of this singular malady.

Chorea is essentially a functional disorder of the nervous centres—at least morbid anatomy has as yet failed to prove its definite connection with any organic lesion. A centric structural cause for the irregular movements has sometimes been found in cerebral tubercles, or in the circumscribed softening of segments of the spinal cord; but these are very exceptional instances.* In a large number of persons the malady is called into existence by an irritation of peripheral

* In an admirable paper by Dr. John W. Ogle (British and Foreign Med.-Chirurg. Review, 1868), congestion more or less complete of the brain or spinal cord was met with in six cases out of sixteen; in one case there was actual softening of the cord; in one softening of certain portions of the brain. In ten out of the sixteen cases there existed more or less fibrinous deposit or granulations upon some portion of the valves of the heart or its lining membrane. A knowledge of this fact had led several pathologists to the belief that chorea is connected with these vegetations being set free and carried as emboli to different organs. Dr Tuckwell (Br. and Foreign Med.-Chir. Review, Oct. 1867) explains thus the cases we sometimes encounter in which wild maniacal delirium, with subsequent rapid emaciation, arises; and Dr. Hughlings Jackson (London Hospital Reports, vol. ii., and Edinb. Med. Journ., Oct. 1868) believes that in chorea plugging of the minute vessels supplying the corpus striatum is the immediate cause of the disease; a one-sided embolism giving rise to but a one-sided chorea. These ingenious views still require substantiation.

portions of the nervous system.   Thus a blow, a wound of a nerve, disorders of the uterus, painful menstruation, pregnancy, or gastric or intestinal affections may act as the exciting causes of the perverted muscular movements.

Chorea is often produced by strong mental emotion, especially by fright.   It may also be the sequence of rheumatic fever.   Indeed, it is the opinion of many eminent pathologists that it usually arises from the same diathesis that attends or occasions rheumatism.   The evidence adduced consists, in the proneness of those of rheumatic constitution to chorea, in the muscular pains, the high-colored, acid urine, in the tendency of both maladies to recur, and the frequency with which in both endocardial affections are evoked.   Yet this view of the subject, although sanctioned by high authority, and now the generally-received one, cannot be accepted as conclusive.   Certainly, in a large number of persons affected with chorea, we fail to detect any proof of a rheumatic diathesis.   And as for the cardiac complication, the presence of which is chiefly deduced from the existence of a murmur, the inference drawn from this sign is hardly a fair one ; for is it not often due to anæmia, or dependent upon spasmodic action of the papillary muscles—the same spasmodic action that is seen in the striated muscles of the face or of the extremities ?

The disease is rarely fatal : but it is not of short duration ; for, although it may be acute, it commonly lasts for months. There are no cerebral symptoms attending it, yet the mental faculties are not in a perfectly healthy state.   The intellect of a choreic child develops slowly, and is evidently enfeebled while the disorder lasts.   In some cases paralysis supervenes ; but it is not permanent, nor indeed of long duration.   But those who have been choreic remain subject to nervous disorders ; and I have known several instances in which the complaint has been, in after-years, followed by epilepsy.

The diagnosis of chorea is generally very easy.   The malady differs from the spasms of acute cerebral disease by the absence of fever, and of delirium or of coma ; from epilepsy, by its continuousness, by the non-existence of unconsciousness, and by the rarity with which the muscles jerk at a time when epileptic convulsions are most frequent, namely, at night; from tetanus, it is chiefly distinguished by not exhibiting tonic spasms.

Paralysis agitans is, like chorea, attended with disturbed muscular movements. But we find weakness and tremor rather than spasmodic contraction, and want of control over muscular motion. Then, as the malady progresses, the propensity to lean forward, or to walk on the fore part of the foot, is very characteristic. The affection is met with chiefly in old persons; though there are forms of it which may happen at any age, and in which the violent shaking movements take place when any muscular action is performed and are entirely beyond the patient's control, but subside when he is at rest and during sleep. This peculiar kind of paralysis agitans, if such it may be called, is nearly affiliated to chorea. Like it, too, it may originate in fright. It differs chiefly in the motions repeating themselves rhythmically and symmetrically on the two sides of the body,* and in presenting nothing of the irregular and rapidly changing character of the true choreic movements.

Convulsive tremor, to adopt the name given by Dr. Hammond† to a paroxysmal affection in which several times in the day severe muscular tremor arises, differs from chorea in not being continuous, as it occurs in attacks lasting from fifteen to twenty minutes, passing off gradually, and leaving the patient in a profuse perspiration. The seizures, moreover, in their sudden onset resemble more an attack of epilepsy, and there is slight headache, with vertigo, and an intense feeling of anxiety, though not unconsciousness. The unrestrainable muscular tremor affects the face, the arms, the trunk, but not the lower extremities, and is associated with increased sensibility of the skin of the disturbed parts.

Mercurial tremor, another variety of tremor, is discriminated from chorea by observing that the trembling and the incessant movements stop when the shaking limb is sup-

---

* As in the case recorded by Sanders, Edin. Med. Journ , May, 1865.

† New York Medical Journal, June, 1867.

ported. And the gradual manner in which the disease appears, its occurrence among persons whose occupations predispose them to the absorption of mercury, the wakefulness, the disorder of the digestive organs and the sponginess of the gums,—form a group of phenomena very dissimilar to those of chorea.

Facial spasm differs from the spasmodic contractions of chorea in being always of equal intensity, and in the grimaces being strictly confined to the same group of muscles, and generally existing only on one side of the face.

The *writer's cramp*, a strange affection in which every attempt at writing at once produces spasmodic action of the muscles of those fingers which are brought into play, is separated from chorea by its occurrence in individuals who have strained their muscles in using a pen continuously and rapidly; by the almost instant cessation of the spasm when the afflicted person ceases to write; and by the ease with which the fingers perform other motions, and are capable of being used for every other purpose excepting for the one which has brought on the disorder. A very analogous complaint is sometimes encountered in seamstresses.

There is a form of chorea, or, if it be a distinct disorder, one closely allied to chorea, which consists in repeated violent bobbings of the head, lasting many minutes at a time. These *salaam convulsions*, as Sir Charles Clarke calls them, are a very obstinate complaint. Although most commonly met with in children, they have been known to occur in adults.*

Hysteria.—This description of hysteria will deal chiefly with the symptoms of an hysterical paroxysm. Most of the local hysterical affections have been, or will be, considered in connection with the disease they ape; and to discuss any questions relating to the nature of this perplexing malady, or to attempt to scrutinize or to interpret all the false and contradictory signals it hangs out, is, in a work of this kind, manifestly impossible.

An hysterical fit may set in suddenly, under the influence of some violent mental emotion; but more generally it is

---

* Levick, Amer. Journ. of Med. Sciences, Jan. 1862.

preceded by altered spirits, by a sensation of pressure, and of constriction at the pit of the stomach, which feeling ascends to the throat, and is likened by the patient to the rising of a ball. She becomes much agitated, sobs, laughs, cries, her muscles contract violently, or she lies motionless, and apparently without the power of motion, until her seeming insensibility is disturbed by something she disapproves of, or fears. The heart palpitates; the breathing is irregular and heaving,—on account, perhaps, of an affection of the larynx, but not of its temporary closure, which, as Marshall Hall tells us, so commonly ensues in epilepsy.

These hysterical outbursts differ from the spasms of chorea by their remissions, the patient remaining at times for months free from the convulsive movements. Moreover, there is not even partial unconsciousness in chorea. It is true that this malady and hysteria are sometimes combined, or rather that chorea happens in hysterical subjects; yet even then it is remarkable how rarely fits of hysteria take place in those affected with St. Vitus's dance.

It is sometimes very difficult to distinguish between paroxysms of hysteria and of epilepsy; and it becomes the more difficult if the epileptic seizures occur in hysterical patients. Yet there are ordinarily many well-marked points of distinction between the two maladies, as will be seen from this table:

Epilepsy.	Hysteria.
Sudden and complete loss of consciousness.	Gradual and only partial, or apparent unconsciousness.
Livid face; escape of frothy saliva from the mouth; eyelids half open; eyeballs rolling; grinding of the teeth; biting of the tongue; more or less insensibility of the pupils to light	Face flushed, or complexion unaltered; no froth on lips; eyelids closed; eyeballs fixed; neither grinding of the teeth nor biting of the tongue; pupils react readily.
Distortion of countenance.	No distortion of countenance.
Patient evinces no feeling.	Patient sighs, or laughs, or sobs.
Aura epileptica.	Globus hystericus.
Convulsions often more marked on one side than on the other; and more tonic than clonic.	No such difference; convulsions clonic.
Paroxysm generally of short duration	Paroxysms generally of longer duration.

EPILEPSY.	HYSTERIA.
Paroxysm followed by a heavy, half-comatose sleep, by headache, and dulness of intellect.	Paroxysm not followed specially by sleep; patient often, after attack terminates, wakeful and depressed in spirits.
Frequently occurs at night	Rarely occurs at night.
No particular connection with uterine disturbance, although a paroxysm often takes place at the menstrual period.	Often connected with disorders of the uterus, or of menstruation.

But hysteria is not an affection merely of paroxysms. In the intervals between them we find peculiar and significant manifestations of the strange complaint, which should be understood lest they be taken as the signs of other troubles. We observe an extreme susceptibility of the nervous system, various hyperæsthesiæ, such as tenderness in the epigastrium, or in the course of the spinal column; that peculiar pain in the left side which distresses so many hysterical and anemic women; and sometimes local anæsthesia. Besides these, we encounter manifold local hysterical ailments, such as hysterical paralysis, hysterical aphonia, hysterical peritonitis, hysterical affections of joints, or hysterical pain in the forehead.

The distinction between these hysterical pseudo-maladies and the diseases they simulate, is far from being an easy task. We have to take into account the patient's age and sex; the existence of any irregularity in the uterine functions; whether or not she has suffered from paroxysms of hysteria; how the pain is influenced by pressure; and the signs of functional disorder of the apparently affected part. We may thus avoid mistaking a phantom for a true disease. Yet there is another and opposite source of error quite as strenuously to be guarded against. The complaint may be really an organic one, occurring in an hysterical patient, and concealed, or exaggerated and complicated by the symptoms of hysteria. In all such doubtful cases we must accord great weight to the extent of functional and constitutional disturbance accompanying the local morbid state.

Hysteria is sometimes feigned—feigned to elicit sympathy, or to procure compliance with wishes or caprices. Nor is

the simulation of the disorder an outgrowth from our civ-
ilization.   The epigrams of Martial prove how common the
feigning of hysteria was among the Roman women.

Tetanus.—A disease of very obscure pathology, but of
clearly defined and thoroughly characteristic symptoms,
marked by persistent rigid contraction of the voluntary
muscles, particularly of those of the jaw.

The distressing malady, as we see it, is generally *traumatic*,
following a wound or an injury; for *idiopathic* tetanus is very
seldom met with in temperate climates.   But in hot countries, or in those in which sudden alternations of temperature
are common, it is not a rare disease, and is indeed frequent
among children.   The cases of idiopathic tetanus we encounter are almost always the result of exposure to cold.

The muscles ordinarily first affected are those of the jaw
and neck; there is a stiffness about them which the patient
is apt to attribute to having caught cold.   Sometimes, however, the disorder exhibits itself primarily in the external
respiratory muscles.   When the malady is fully developed,
most of the muscles are stiff and hard, the jaw cannot be
opened,—whence the common name of lock-jaw,—and there
is much difficulty in speaking and in swallowing.   With
these symptoms we usually find rigidity of the muscles of
the abdomen and of the limbs, and a distressing pain at the
pit of the stomach, dependent upon spasm of the diaphragm.
And besides the permanent contraction of the voluntary
fibres, exacerbations of spasm take place, during which the
muscles become very hard.   These paroxysms are accompanied by intense pain, and recur with increased severity
and frequency as the disease advances to a fatal termination.
When at their height, the body becomes curved, the patient
merely resting upon his head and heels.   This is *opisthotonos;*
while the setting of the jaw, especially when its muscles alone
are affected, is called *trismus.*

Notwithstanding the striking muscular disorder and the
exhausting pain, there is little constitutional disturbance;
the pulse may be quickened, but it preserves its volume
until the last stage is reached; and there is no fever, nor is
the intellect affected.

Tetanus runs an acute or a chronic course. Some eases last three weeks, and when of such long duration are apt to recover. But generally the malady terminates fatally before the eighth day.

Few complaints are likely to be confounded with tetanus; yet these few resemble it closely in many respects. For instance, one of the freaks of hysteria is to take the appearance of tetanus; and tonic spasms dependent upon an affection of the spinal cord or medulla oblongata, strychnia poisoning, or hydrophobia, may accurately simulate its symptoms.

Hysterical tetanus is distinguished from the real disease by being preceded by, or attended with, fits of hysteria; by the age and sex of the patient; by the absence of pain; by the occasional occurrence of clonic instead of tonic spasms; and the intermission every now and then of all muscular rigidity. Moreover, the influence of the mind upon the seeming tetanus is very striking. If within hearing of the patient, the employment of cold to the spine, or the application of the cautery be threatened, or, better still, if the latter instrument be actually made ready for use before her, an extraordinary subsidence of all stiffening and starting of the limbs takes place.

Tetanic spasms *symptomatic* of an affection of the spinal cord are separated from tetanus by the different history; by no violent exacerbations being brought on, as they are in tetanus, by slight movements, or by an attempt at speaking, or by any reflex irritation; by the absence of marked remissions; by the rigidity being almost always limited to the extremities (excepting in the case of meningeal apoplexy, in which, as in tetanus, the head is drawn backward); and by the setting in of palsy before the malady terminates.

In the tetanic spasms which may occur in scarlet fever, in typhus, in small-pox, or in pyemia, and which are the result of an irritation of the cord produced by the poisoned blood, rather than of a disease of its membranes or its structure, the rigidity runs so uncertain a course, appears so quickly, disappears so suddenly, perhaps not to reappear, or only to reappear after a considerable interval, that there is little likelihood of confounding the muscular disorder with tetanus.

Yet another form of symptomatic rigidity requires to be distinguished from tetanus — a local rigidity, owing to the irritation of the nerve supplying the stiffened muscles; as for instance, a spasm from irritation of the peripheral or the central tract of the motor portion of the fifth, the so-called " masticatory spasm" of the face. This curious ailment may be of reflex origin, the exciting cause being a decayed tooth, a wound, exposure to cold; or it may exist in connection with apoplexy, or with an inflammation of the brain. Its main marks of distinction from the trismus of tetanus are, that it is purely local, is often of long continuance, is not painful, has no paroxysms of aggravation, is not combined with impaired deglutition, and is not dangerous.*

The symptoms of *strychnia poisoning* are almost identical with those of tetanus; yet there are some characteristic differences. The spasms from strychnia do not supervene upon exposure to cold, or upon a wound; but follow within about two hours or less the taking of some solid or liquid. They come on suddenly, and with violence; and the tetanoid convulsions affect simultaneously nearly all the voluntary muscles of the body, but with greatest intensity those of the trunk and spine, producing very early — within a few minutes, commonly — a marked opisthotonos, which in tetanus does not appear, if it appear at all, for many hours or for days after the seizure. On the other hand, the stiffness of the jaws, which is among the very earliest signs of tetanus, is not at first perceived in strychnia poisoning; and if it occur, occurs only imperfectly. Further, we do not see the frightful tetanic face, with its knit brow and horrid grin; we do not observe intermissions in the convulsions, or difficulty in swallowing; and in from ten minutes to two hours after the commencement of the attack the patient dies or recovers.†

Finally, let us contrast tetanus with *hydrophobia*. Both

---

* Bright, in the second volume of his Medical Reports, gives the particulars of a case which illustrates many of the difficulties of diagnosis to which the affection may give rise.

† These statements are based on the researches of Taylor (Guy's Hospital Reports, 3d Series, vol. ii.), of Todd, and of Christison.

showing the reflex functions of the spinal cord to be in an exalted condition; both spasmodic affections lasting ordinarily but a few days; both taking place. the popular opinion to the contrary notwithstanding, at all periods of the year; both presenting violent paroxysms of convulsions, which are often excited by the slightest touch or jar to the body; both frequently occasioning torturing pain near the pit of the stomach; both ensuing commonly upon an injury; both usually augmenting in intensity from hour to hour, and scarcely within the reach of therapeutic measures,—these ghastly maladies are yet dissimilar. In the one, deglutition may be difficult; in the other it is next to impossible, all attempts at swallowing, especially of fluids, exciting the most distressing spasmodic dysphagia. In the one, the breathing may or may not be interfered with; in the other, the spasms of respiration are almost as marked a feature as the spasms of deglutition. Then the irritability of temper; the fierce manner of the patient, his rabid, perhaps maniacal paroxysms; the constant thirst; the accumulation of stringy mucus about the angles of the mouth; the vomiting; the acute sensibility of the surface; the trembling of the muscles; the clonic instead of tonic spasms; the strangling sensation in the throat,—are phenomena too strikingly peculiar to render an error in diagnosis very likely.*

Diseases characterized by Gradual Impairment of the Mental Faculties with Paralysis.

Chronic Softening.—This subject displays even more difficulties in its symptomatic relations than it does in its pathological. There are, in truth, no pathognomonic symptoms the presence of which would enable us to declare, without hesitation, that we are dealing with softening of the brain, or the absence of which would justify us in concluding that it

---

* Some of the points here referred to serve also to distinguish hydrophobia from acute mania, and from hysteria. For as in tetanus, so here we find this erratic complaint simulating the terrible disease. (See, for instance, a case referred to in Guy's Hospital Reports, vol. xii. 3d Series, and remarks in Gamgee's article on Hydrophobia, in Reynolds's System of Medicine.)

does not exist. Yet a large number of cases exhibit uniform manifestations which permit us ordinarily to recognize the malady with some degree of certainty.

There are two main forms of softening—the red and the white. The former is inflammatory, and runs an acute course, with symptoms, as we have already discussed, often closely simulating those of apoplexy, but sometimes with signs like those of the chronic malady, and differing in nothing but in their intensity and short duration. The second kind is chiefly dependent upon a change in the nutrition of the brain, and is very often linked to a diseased condition of the cerebral arteries; it may, however, be caused, or at all events accompanied, by an inflammatory exudation infiltrated among the nervous pulp. These briefly are its early symptoms: gradual impairment of intelligence; weakening of memory; headache; vertigo; muscular debility; cutaneous hyperæsthesia or anæsthesia; formication and numbness; and slight and partial palsies, particularly of the muscles of one side of the mouth, or of one eyelid. Then there is not unfrequently defective articulation, with great irritability of temper, nausea and vomiting, extreme sensitiveness to sounds, and painful feelings in various parts of the body. As the local mischief advances, the paralysis becomes more universal, assuming generally the hemiplegic form; and spasms, either tonic or clonic, or epileptic convulsions occur.

The mental decay proceeds steadily, and sometimes shows itself in a constant repetition of the same action or the same phrase. In an old lady whom I attended, this was the most marked symptom: she was constantly complaining of her teeth needing attention, was perfectly satisfied when assured by the dentist that they did not, but soon reiterated her complaint. Beyond this, and most painful sensitiveness to sound and to light, intense headache, nausea, and a progressive deterioration of memory and of the faculty of thought, she presented no signs of cerebral softening. She died without the occurrence of paralysis.

Softening of the brain may be caused by a diseased state of its blood-vessels, or by their obstruction; by long-continued grief; by persistent mental labor; by constitutional syphilis;

by frequently repeated epileptic paroxysms; and by an inflammatory disease spreading from the meninges to the brain. It may also be dependent upon apoplexy. At all events, we frequently meet with it in connection with hemorrhage, and associated sometimes in a manner to make it a very perplexing matter to ascertain if the softening has followed the extravasation of blood, or if the extravasation has taken place into an already diseased brain. We may conclude the latter to have occurred, if signs of deranged intellection or sensation have preceded the attack; if, soon after reaction from the shock, the patient, instead of mending in mind, exhibit unmistakable evidences of progressing mental decay; and if convulsive movements or rigidity of the limbs appear.

And, indeed, it is by this combination of signs alone that we are enabled, whatever the relations of the softening to the hemorrhage, to decide whether, after an apoplectic seizure, softening is present at all; an inquiry practically of much more consequence than to determine whether the cerebral disorganization has or has not existed prior to the bleeding. And let us, in passing, remark that a small clot breaking down the softened cerebral mass, yet not extending beyond the limits of the diseased texture, occasions no special signs —occasions only the signs of a sudden giving way of nerve pulp: paralysis without unconsciousness.

Assuming now the relations of hemorrhage to softening to have been for our purpose settled, we shall next study how various other cerebral maladies, such as congestion, anæmia, abscess, and hardening, may be distinguished from softening.

Congestion is discriminated by its being very rarely a persistent state. An acute attack produces the symptoms of apoplexy; a more lasting congestion is recognized by tracing the cause which has led to the fulness of the vessels,—such as an interference with the circulation, the result of a disease of the circulatory system itself, or of the abdominal viscera, —and by noting that, although the patient suffers from dull headache, from jerking of the muscles, from pulsation of the carotids, from vertigo, these signs are far from being constant, and come and go for a long time without any material disturbance of the functions of the brain being perceptible, either in reference to thought or to voluntary motion.

Cerebral anæmia is a state in which the supply of blood in the brain is diminished, and usually also altered. Occurring suddenly, it produces unconsciousness, or dizziness or stupor, or, if very general, and especially if associated with venous congestion, it may cause convulsions. When more gradually induced, it manifests itself by drowsiness, distressing headache, often more particularly referred to the vertex; by the pale face and uninjected eye with large pupil; by derangement of the special senses, by the vertigo and the other symptoms of cerebral disorder being relieved in the recumbent position; and by the feeble pulse and cool forehead. Then in tracing its history we are apt to find that it occurs in those who have been exhausted by debilitating diseases, or repeated hemorrhages, or by albuminuria. The chief distinction from softening lies in the history of the case; the aspect of the patient, too, and the absence of palsies or their passing nature must be taken into account. But we must not forget that if the morbid condition be long continued, the ill-nourished brain will soften.

Abscess of the brain differs mainly in this from chronic softening: the disease is of short duration. Some cases may run a very rapid course, others may continue for months; yet few, as Lebert* informs us, last longer than eight weeks. Further, we find in abscess, unlike what happens in softening, convulsions in the earlier period, and paralysis late in the malady; and not unfrequently we discover, in analyzing the history, that chills have occurred, or we can detect the clue to the cerebral abscess in a disease of the internal ear, or in an injury to the head, or in the presence of a suppurative process in some distant part of the body.

Hardening of the cerebral substance is a morbid state scarcely to be discerned during life. It appears chiefly in children; in adults it is rarely seen excepting as the result of lead poisoning. The comparatively healthy condition of

---

* Archiv für Path. Anat., Bd. x.; see, also, Gull's paper in Guy's Hosp. Reports, 3d Series, vol. iii.

the general nutrition of the body; the pain in the course, or at the extremities of peripheral nerves; the double-sided palsy spreading from the extremities up; the frequency of convulsions and of muscular tremors; the remissions in the symptoms; the want of prominence of the evidences of deranged sensation or of mental decay,—all serve to distinguish, so far as it can be distinguished, cerebral induration from cerebral softening.

There is yet, leaving tumors out of the question, another affection of the brain which may be confounded with softening: an *exhaustion of brain-power* encountered among professional men, or those engaged in laborious literary undertakings. This sometimes comes on very suddenly, with signs like those of a collapse; at other times it is slower in its development. Its manifestations are, a slight deterioration of memory, and an inability to read or write, save for a very short period, although the power of thought and of judgment is in no way perverted. Nor is the power of attention more than enfeebled; the sick man is fully capable of giving heed to any subject, but he soon tires of it, and is obliged from very fatigue to desist. He passes sleepless nights, is subject to ringing in the ears, cannot bear much exercise, is troubled with irregular action of the heart, with a frequent desire to urinate, and with neuralgic pains in the face or a feeling of soreness in the head; but he does not lose flesh, and his digestion is uninjured.

Many remain in this condition for months, and then slowly regain their health. What the precise disturbance of the brain consists in, I cannot say; it is possible that the nutrition of the organ has been interfered with from overuse, and that the further continuance of mental toil and anxiety would have led to softening. The phenomena differ from those of this serious cerebral disease, by the absence of or at least by the far less permanent and marked headache, by the comparatively unimpaired intelligence, and by the non-occurrence of spasms, or of paralysis of motion or sensation.

To consider now the *diagnosis* of the chief varieties of softcuing. In how far is it possible to distinguish the inflammatory from the non-inflammatory form? The more acute

the symptoms, the greater is the likelihood of their being due
to an inflammatory lesion; and in young subjects this probability becomes almost a certainty. A latency of the affection,
its slow and gradual manifestation, its existence in persons
advanced in life, and in whom we have reason to suspect degeneration of the coats of the arteries, are facts which justify
the conclusion that it is owing to a depraved nutrition of the
cerebral substance, and not to its inflammation.

Tumor.—Tumors of the brain give rise to a great diversity of signs, according to their locality, their size, and their
nature. Let us examine the peculiar symptoms, or group of
symptoms, by which we may infer their occurrence, and then
see in how far an attempt is likely to succeed to distinguish
their seat and precise nature.

The presence of a tumor in the brain is rendered probable
if, in addition to vertigo, to vomiting or a disposition to
vomit, to headache, violent but paroxysmal and neuralgic in
its character, we find impairment or loss of vision, or indeed anæsthesia of any special sense, and epileptiform convulsions not followed by any greater deterioration of health
than previously existed; if with these signs of cerebral irritation the intellect is not at first markedly disordered, nor the
articulation affected; and if paralyses do not show themselves until a very long time after the headache, and are
even then limited to the muscles of the eyeball or of the face,
or to the muscles of the extremities of one side of the body.
Yet before the evidence is considered conclusive, we must
exclude other chronic cerebral troubles, especially softening,
abscesses, and chronic meningitis.

We separate *softening* by noticing that the headache caused
by a tumor is much more violent and paroxysmal, not dull
nor of steady intensity; that the intelligence remains for a
long time intact in all, save, perhaps, a weakening of the
memory; that motor and sensory disturbances are less frequent and prominent, but convulsions far more so. Remissions, or intervals of apparent improvement, occur in both
morbid states; but they are more perfect and of longer duration in tumor than in softening.

The differential diagnosis between tumor and *abscess* is

more difficult. We may conclude the latter to furnish the explanation of the signs of cerebral pressure or disorganization, if the cephalalgia be sudden in its development, and uniform and general, instead of neuralgic and limited. Then, convulsions, drowsiness, paralysis, and coma succeed each other much more rapidly and much more constantly in abscess than in tumor—a malady running a very chronic course, and in which the patient does not remain drowsy or palsied after the epileptiform seizures.* If, moreover, we obtain the history of a severe injury to the skull, or find a discharge from the ear, or pain upon pressure over the mastoid process, or a chronic disease about the head, or albuminous urine, or protracted suppuration in any part of the body, we may safely infer that an abscess, not a tumor, is the cause of the evident cerebral mischief.

Chronic meningitis, an affection sometimes complicating tumor, is discriminated by laying stress on its etiologic relations—such as blows upon the head, diseases of the bones, syphilis, rheumatism; and by observing its frequent yet irregular accessions of fever, the great irritability of temper, the dulness of intellect, the loss of memory, and the nocturnal delirium. The pain, too, is, as a rule, somewhat duller and more diffused than in tumor, though more fixed and constant, and there is more vertigo; but the convulsions, on the other hand, are less distinctly epileptiform in type, yet convulsive movements of some muscles are very common, and may be even followed by incomplete paralysis.

---

* I have mentioned epileptic seizures in these affections because I believe they belong to them. But Brown-Séquard has recently stated (quoted in Am. Journ. of Med. Sciences, April, 1869, p. 531) that diseases of the cerebral substance are incapable of producing epileptic symptoms, and that when these occur they are to be attributed to concomitant lesions of the meninges. However, whatever the cause, the epileptic fits may be absent. Thus they occurred in only 38 cases of abscess of the brain out of 73 collected by Gull and Sutton (see article "Abscess of Brain," in Reynolds's System of Medicine). Again, it must be borne in mind that both affections may be quite latent. Particularly is this the case with cerebral abscess; and the sudden rupture of the abscess may give rise to symptoms undistinguishable from those of hemorrhage, undistinguishable at least unless from a disease of the bones of the skull, or some points in the history of the case, we can infer an abscess.

Thrombosis of the sinuses of the brain may occasion partial palsies, and the symptoms of cerebral pressure like those of tumors, and cannot be distinguished excepting in those instances in which we can find distention of the collateral circulation and injection and œdema of the forehead and eyelids.* Convulsions, further, are scarcely among the symptoms.

The precise *seat* of the tumor, it is impossible to determine. An affection of the special senses points to disease near to, or at the base of the brain; and the probability of this view is much strengthened if there be paralysis of the face on the side opposite to that of the extremities,† and if vigorous inspiration, during which the brain falls and presses the morbid mass against the walls of the base of the skull, cause or increase pain; whereas, so says that high authority, Romberg, in tumors on the upper surface, forced expiration produces a like result.

And what of their *nature*—can we form an opinion regarding it from any of the signs referable to the cerebral disorganization? We cannot: the character of the pain has been thought to be of great significance; but the testimony to prove that it is so, is in the highest degree unsatisfactory. We may sometimes, however, from the history of the case, or from the existence of some of the manifestations of special cachexias, draw a correct inference. For instance, if we find disease of the lungs, or any evidences of scrofula, and the patient is young, we shall probably be right in conjecturing the tumor of the brain to be a mass of tubercle; but if the sufferer is advanced in years, and exhibits tumors in various parts of the body, and further signs of a cancerous diathesis, we may with reasonable certainty presume the tumor within the skull to be cancerous. Other kinds of tumors and deposits can scarcely be said to be within the reach of diagnosis. Cysts seated in the superficial portions of the brain either occasion no symptoms, or they give rise to headache, to attacks of vertigo, to vomiting, and to epileptic seizures, but very rarely

---

* Heubner, quoted in Schmidt's Jahrbücher, No. 1, 1869.

† But as regards the palsy of the face being on the side opposite to that of the body, this depends very much upon the exact position and extent of the lesion, as has been explained while discussing hemiplegia.

to palsies.   The symptoms mentioned are far more apt to be present when the cysts occupy the lateral ventricles; epileptic convulsions especially are very rarely absent.

The symptoms of an aneurism within the cranium are usually those of an ordinary tumor, and the affection is not distinguishable excepting where we find decided indications of disease of the vessels in other parts of the system.*

General Paralysis.—This fatal and obscure cerebral malady resembles softening of the brain—nay, softening is frequently found after death; but there may be atrophy with hardening, or other morbid changes, and the affection is now recognized as a distinct disease by most pathologists.

The disorder is, clinically speaking, marked by impairment of the powers of locomotion; by an inability to articulate distinctly—a symptom which precedes the deranged locomotion; by the peculiar meaningless countenance; and the complete perversion of the mental faculties, amounting ordinarily, in fact, to insanity.

The palsy is very peculiar: indeed, Dr. Skae, who has so graphically described the affection,† says that, in the usual sense of the term, there is no palsy in the limbs at all; there is rather a want of control over their co-ordinate action, displaying itself in a swaying from side to side when the patient attempts to walk.   The impairment of the muscular movement gradually extends: there is a tremulousness in the muscles of expression; the speech becomes more inarticulate, until scarcely a word can be distinguished; and the patient cannot rise without being assisted.   The cutaneous sensibility is greatly diminished or is lost.   The mental derangement is often marked by an exaggerated sense of personal power or importance.   Death is often preceded by convulsive attacks and by coma, or sometimes by painful contractions of the muscles of the trunk or extremities, or by obstinate diarrhœa, or pulmonary troubles.‡

The strange malady differs from other forms of extensive

---

* See an excellent paper by Dr. James H. Hutchinson, Pennsylvania Hospital Reports, vol ii.

† Edinburgh Med. and Surg. Journ., April, 1860.

‡ Calmeil, Traité des Malad. Inflammat. du Cerveau.   Paris, 1858.

general paralysis in being far less of a real palsy. It is certainly far less complete than the extensive paralyses that follow lesions of the upper portion of the spinal cord, or which are consequent upon the poison of lead, or of malaria, or of diphtheria. Its association with marked disturbance of the intellect furnishes, moreover, a differential test of great value, and not merely with reference to the general palsies just mentioned, but also as regards the trembling movements of old age, of progressive muscular atrophy, and of chronic alcoholism.

Diseases characterized by Enlargement of the Head.

Chronic Hydrocephalus.—The signs of dropsy of the brain are, a progressive enlargement of the head, and a perversion or a gradual loss of one or several of the special senses, of the mental faculties, and of the power of voluntary motion. The child cannot bear the weight of its head; the gait is tottering and uncertain. The intellect slowly, but certainly, becomes deranged. As the malady advances, strabismus, partial palsies, epileptic convulsions, vomiting, cutaneous anæsthesia, and loss of sight, smell, and of taste are observable; the bowels become very constipated; and a copious secretion of tears and of saliva is not infrequent.

Before death takes place, which sometimes does not happen for years, the child ordinarily becomes idiotic. A few cases recover: fewer reach adult age with their brain compressed by the accumulated fluid; in still fewer the disease does not develop itself until after childhood. If the patient survive until adult age, the size of the skull is generally immense. I saw, a few years since, a young man, twenty-two years of age, whose head measured fully two feet and a half in circumference. He could walk unaided, but often fell. He was half idiotic, and subject to epileptic fits; yet he had sufficient intelligence to understand what was said to him, and in his childish way to do as he was told.

The skull is sometimes very large without dropsy of the brain existing. The head may be overgrown, and its bones thickened and spongy in rachitis; or it may be large when there is no disease.   These states differ from chronic hydro-cephalus by the absence of cerebral symptoms; and in doubt-ful cases we may call in the ophthalmoscope as a means of diagnosis.   The vessels of the eye, even in the early stages of chronic hydrocephalus, enlarge, and, in proportion as the serum compresses the brain, we find an increase of vasen-larity in the retina with dilatation of the veins, and with an increase of the number of vessels in the retina; its complete or partial serous infiltration; and an atrophy, more or less perceptible, of the optic nerve.   These lesions vary with the age of the disease and the amount of serous effusion; but none of them exist in rickets.*   The size of the head may also be augmented in consequence of meningeal apoplexy, or of hypertrophy of the brain.   The former may be sus-pected, if the distention of the cranium follow, at no very long interval, an attack of convulsions and of coma in a teething child.

Hypertrophy of the Brain.—A strange complaint, in which the brain develops with disproportionate rapidity to the growth of its bony case, which thus becomes too small for its contents.

The symptoms this morbid state occasions, irrespective of the enlargement of the head, are: headache, vertigo, drow-siness, and epileptiform convulsions.   The gait is very un-steady; the mind gradually gives way.   After the paroxysms of headache and of convulsions we often find stupor, which may deepen into fatal coma.   Sometimes delirium, and even mania are noticed.

Hypertrophy of the brain requires to be carefully distin-guished from the *enlargement of the head* which takes place when both the brain and the skull increase rapidly; a hyper-trophy, too, in a certain sense, but not a hypertrophy fraught with danger or occasioning any morbid manifestations.

Equally, or yet more important, is it to discriminate be-tween the augmented brain and *chronic hydrocephalus*.   And, unfortunately, the marks of distinction are not very clearly traced.   Both diseases have much the same symptoms; both

---

* Bouchut, quoted in Br. Med. Journ., 1865, or *op. cit.*

are generally of long duration. There is, however, in many cases, this dissimilitude: in hypertrophy the convulsions are a much more marked phenomenon, and they precede, rather than accompany, the signs of failing intellect and of cerebral pressure. The changes in the special senses are not so common, nor so prominent; there is not, when the fontanelles are touched, the sensation of a tense membrane filled with water, but more that of a solid substance; and the body does not waste as in dropsy of the brain.

Dr. Mauthner* lays great stress on the different shapes of the head. In chronic hydrocephalus, he states, the forehead is the first to enlarge, and the posterior part of the skull does not expand until long afterward; in hypertrophy the reverse takes place. But this is not a sign free from doubt; indeed, it may be looked upon as of very questionable value. The same may be said with regard to the observation of West, that in hypertrophy there is no prominence, but an actual depression of the anterior fontanelle, and that a similar depression is observable at all the sutures.

Diseases characterized by Paroxysmal Pain.

There is a group of nervous disorders characterized solely by pain, which is confined ordinarily to one nerve, and is seemingly seated in it. These nervous pains, unconnected, so far as we know, with disease of structure, bear the generic name of *neuralgia*. They are acute, follow the course of a nervous branch, and come on in paroxysms having distinct exacerbations, succeeded by distinct intermissions. In some cases these intermissions are long, in others short; in some they are complete, in others the pain is lasting and becomes from time to time exalted—more remissions, therefore, than intermissions. Save in the rarest instances, the excruciating sensations are not complicated with heat and swelling. Nor is there tenderness, excepting when the neuralgia is of long continuance; at least there is not tenderness along the aching nerve, though we may find certain sensitive

---

* Krankheiten des Gehirns, etc. Vienna, 1844.

spots, which, in the case of the spinal nerves, are readily detected by pressing on, or to one side of, the spinous process of the vertebra near which the affected nerve emerges, and by examining the points of terminal expansion. These painful spots are often looked upon as proving the presence of what is vaguely called "spinal irritation."

The pain of neuralgia is, then, of a purely nervous character, and exists independently of inflammation, or of any recognizable textural change of the nervous centres or nervous trunks. This we must always bear in mind before concluding the complaint to be neuralgia; seeking carefully for the signs of a disturbance of the nervous centres or of the larger nervous trunks before the morbid excitation of sensibility is looked upon as forming the whole disorder. And it is only when, after a minute search, we can detect no definite organic cause for the local pain, that we may set down our patient as laboring under neuralgia.

From the characteristics of the pain just mentioned, it is evident that it is not very likely to be confounded with that of local inflammation. But there is a kind of local pain for which neuralgia is often mistaken : the pain of subacute or of chronic rheumatism. Yet this is in reality very dissimilar. The rheumatic pain is attended with soreness, is aggravated by movement or by pressure, is more diffuse and irregular, much more constant, much more influenced by alternations of temperature, but not acute nor paroxysmal, and, finally, not limited anatomically to the course of one nerve, but scattered over parts supplied by several.

The source of the neuralgia should always be determined as closely as possible, both on account of the prognosis and the treatment. In many cases it will be found to be connected with anæmia : in others with the poison of rheumatism, of gout, of syphilis, or of uræmia. It is often reflex, the pain being far away from the seat of the disease, and due to irritation reflected through the nervous centres. For instance: an affection of the digestive apparatus, of the liver, or of the kidneys, may give rise to neuralgia in parts quite remote from them. It is evident that if such be the origin of the disorder, and if the malady which lies at its root and

excites it can be controlled, the neuralgia will simultaneously
disappear.   Yet it must be confessed that we cannot always
detect the cause, whether or not it be of the nature just mentioned, and we have often to treat the neuralgia by employing those agents which are suitable to the greatest number
of cases; using local means and anodynes to allay the pain,
and quinine, iron, arsenic, or aconite, to mitigate the severity
of the attacks and eradicate their tendency to return.

Neuralgia may occur in any portion of the body.   It may
shift rapidly from one part to another, as in that peculiar
neuralgia described by Putegnat,* excited by a desire to pass
water and by the act of micturition, beginning with numbness and acute burning or lancinating pain along the urinary
passages, then affecting particularly the nerves of the forearm, especially the ulnar, and disappearing completely after
micturition.   The most frequent seat of neuralgia is perhaps
about the head; and we shall here notice chiefly a few of its
most common kinds.   Most of the other varieties of the disorder, and especially intercostal neuralgia and some of the
abdominal forms, will be elsewhere alluded to.

Facial Neuralgia.—The facial branches of the fifth pair
are very often the site of agonizing pain.   But all the
branches of the nerve are not equally liable : the lowermost
of them is rarely affected.   When the supra-orbital division
is the seat of the ailment, the pain shoots to the forehead,
the eyebrow, and the eyeball.   If the infra-orbital nerve be
disturbed, the pain darts to the upper lip, the upper row of
teeth and the posterior nares, and the cheek tingles, or the
eyelids twitch.   When the pain occurs in the inferior branch,
it radiates to the lips and chin, and is frequently accompanied by a flow of saliva.   Generally the parts around the
point where the affected nerve emerges are sensitive to the
slightest touch.   Sometimes only one, at other times two, at
others all the branches of the fifth are implicated in the
complaint, or they may be seized upon alternately.

The disease is one of those belonging to advancing years.

---

* Gaz. Hebdom. de Méd. et Chir., April, 1864; quoted in Ranking's Abstract, vol. xxxix.

It has the same causes as any other form of neuralgia. Sometimes it is associated with decayed teeth, or with an abnormal state of the bones of the head or face, such as thickening of the frontal, ethmoid, and sphenoid bones. Many of these cases terminate, after months or years of excruciating agony, in apoplexy.*

The intervals between the paroxysms are of very varying length. They may be of six months, or even a year's duration; but so long an intermission is uncommon. Seasons in which sudden changes of weather are frequent generally excite several attacks in those predisposed to them.

The malady is easily recognized. It may be mistaken for, or rather there may be mistaken for it, a disease of the bones of the face. But the local signs of this are different, and the pain is not paroxysmal. Painful anæsthesia of the fifth nerve is discriminated by the insensibility of the painful portions to the touch, or indeed to any irritation. Spasm of the face is distinguished by the absence of pain, from the convulsive twitchings which sometimes take place in tic douloureux.

The *epileptiform neuralgia* described by Trousseau is dissimilar in these peculiarities: whether simple or combined with rapid convulsive movements of the muscles on one side of the face, it is quickly over; it lasts but ten or twenty seconds at a time, never more than a minute. Yet during the short duration of the seizures, the pain reaches an intensity greater even than in ordinary neuralgia. Moreover, in some persons who suffer from this terrible malady—the attacks of which may happen in quick succession by day as well as by night, and then perhaps remit for weeks or months—vertiginous sensations or epileptic fits occur, and thus the diagnosis is facilitated by the history of the case.

Hemicrania.—As in the other forms of neuralgia, the chief symptoms of the disorder resolve themselves into one symptom—the symptom of pain. This is ordinarily limited to the supra orbital and temporal regions of one side, but it may extend to the scalp; and in very rare instances the

---

* Sir Henry Halford's Essays and Orations, delivered at the Royal College of Physicians, page 37 et seq.

cerebral neuralgia is not one-sided, but double-sided. The pain is intensified by sound of any kind, and is commonly accompanied by a sense of weight, and by more or less sickness of stomach. Sometimes, indeed, the nausea and vomiting are very prominent features of the paroxysm, hardly less prominent than the pain. The attack lasts for hours or days. At its termination, the patient feels exhansted, yet soon recovers his usual health, and may remain free from a seizure for a long time. But as the disorder most commonly occurs in women, and usually at their menstrual periods, the interval is not apt to extend beyond four weeks.

Hemicrania is a very stubborn affection. It generally argues a debilitated state of system, and has of late years been explained as a neurosis of the sympathetic. It is a disease the tendency to which diminishes after middle age.

Hemicrania must be carefully separated from the pain in the head which accompanies an organic cerebral affection. The main points of distinction are, that the neuralgic malady is paroxysmal, is attended with the same group of symptoms during each attack, and produces no nervous derangement in the intervals between the seizures; while the other morbid condition is more or less constant, and yields persistent signs of a cerebral trouble.

Rheumatism of the scalp differs from hemicrania in the pain being continuous, dull, and superficial; in occupying generally both sides of the head; in being augmented by moving the affected muscles, and relieved by warmth. Moreover, there is almost always other evidence of rheumatism, and the pain is intensified by pressure; whereas in hemicrania, although the hair may be sensitive to the touch, strong pressure on the forehead, and even on the hairy part of the scalp, does not increase the pain, may indeed afford relief.

In *periostitis* affecting the bones of the head, particularly when occurring in connection with constitutional syphilis, we may find the same violent pain as in hemicrania. But there is considerable tenderness on pressure, and the parts attacked are swollen and less elastic than the healthy portions, and the pain is especially severe at night.

Sciatica.—This is neuralgia following the course of the sciatic nerve. The seat of the greatest suffering is generally the lateral surface of the thigh; thence the pains extend to the popliteal space, and in some instances along the anterior part of the leg. Often, too, the patient complains of an aching near the sciatic notch and in the loins. The pain is more or less steady, but it has its periods of fierce exacerbation; and damp, cold, and pressure augment it.

The disease is obstinate, and lasts for weeks or months. It interferes with locomotion, on account of the distress which movements of the leg and foot occasion. It is rare in children, being most frequent between the ages of twenty and sixty.* Generally it depends upon the rheumatic diathesis, or upon an irritation affecting the nerve before it leaves the pelvis, the result not unusually of pressure from a gravid womb, or from an accumulation of feces in the colon. In some instances it is connected with gout, in others with syphilis; and it may be, although it very rarely is, symptomatic of cerebral disease. Occasionally it is due to reflex excitation of the nerve. Sometimes it occurs after forced marches or long rides; probably in the majority of these cases, however, the sciatica is rheumatic.

It is often a very essential matter to determine whether or not an effusion has taken place within the sheath of the nerve, since it becomes of the greatest importance to adopt local and general means by which the fluid can be absorbed before the pressure on the nerve causes an alteration of structure.

"When," says Dr. Fuller, who has carefully investigated this subject, "a patient who is suffering from sciatica complains of a dull aching and benumbing pain in the limb, causing it to feel swollen; when this sense of numbness and increased bulk has succeeded to pain of greater intensity, accompanied by cramps and startings of the limbs; and when, more especially, in addition to these symptoms, there

---

* Valleix, Fuller. Both of these authors further state it to be more common in men than in women, which is denied by Copland and Romberg.

is more or less inability to move the limb,—the presence
of fluid within the sheath of the nerve may be inferred, and
steps should be taken to obtain its evacuation."*

The disorders which are most likely to be confounded with
sciatica are: rheumatism of the muscles and fibrous sheaths
around the hip-joint; affections of the joint; and pains
caused by irritation of the kidney. The former is very
readily distinguished. It is generally, what sciatica is rarely,
double-sided; and the pain is dull, diffuse, not paroxysmal,
not limited to the course of the sciatic nerve, nor as much
increased on pressure as that of sciatica. But, practically
speaking, this kind of rheumatism is seldom seen unless
associated with rheumatic neuralgia of the sciatic nerve.

In *affections of the hip-joint* the suffering is increased by
standing with the weight of the body thrown on the diseased
leg. Moreover, the pain is usually limited to the hip- and
knee-joints; the aspect of the limb points to the disorganization that is going on; the leg shortens. Yet before admitting this as a mark of difference, it must be ascertained by
careful measurement; for, in consequence of muscular contractions, the affected limb in sciatica may appear to be
shorter than it is. The main points of distinction between
sciatica and the nervous affection of the hip-joint, so admirably described by Sir Benjamin Brodie, are the usual combination of the latter with hysteria, the very superficial tenderness, and the fact that the pain is apt to extend over the
whole thigh.

Irritation of the kidney causes pain shooting down the thigh.
The distress exists, however, in the course of the anterior
crural nerve, is therefore not localized in the sciatic, is unattended with tenderness, but is accompanied by a frequent
desire to pass water, and by other signs of trouble of the
urinary functions.

Sciatica is sometimes feigned, especially by soldiers. But
the copy is rarely a very accurate one. Impostors complain
of pain on pressure and on motion, but are ignorant that the

---

* Rheumatism, Rheumatic Gout, etc.

pain is prone to exacerbate after intervals of comparative quiet, and to increase in violence as night approaches. Their fancied torment is constant, but does not prevent them from sleeping; they wince when the muscles of the thigh are touched, yet, if their attention be diverted, the hand may be pressed along the sciatic nerve without any sign of tenderness being manifested.

CHAPTER III.

THE larynx and trachea form the main portion of the upper air-passages. Let us inquire into their affections, and, on account of their greater frequency, especially into those of the larynx.

There are several symptoms constantly met with in laryngeal diseases which at once direct attention to the seat of the malady. The larynx is the organ of speech; hence changes in the *voice* constitute the most striking manifestations of laryngeal disorders. These changes vary in degree. The voice may be merely hoarse, or so completely lost that the patient is hardly able to speak in an audible whisper. In young children the different tone of the cry corresponds to the altered voice of adults. The alteration of the voice depends almost wholly upon an affection of the vocal cords, and this may be of organic origin, such as from inflammation, œdema, ulceration, cicatrices, and morbid growths; or proceed from perverted or impaired innervation. To the latter class belong most of the cases of "functional aphonia." Very often the hoarseness or loss of voice is caused by diminished tension, and want of certain and prompt action of the vocal cords, whether connected with structural change or not. The same cause gives rise, for the most part, to the modifications of the voice which show themselves as huskiness in speaking, or in the loss of certain notes in singing.

Next to the voice in diagnostic importance stand the character of the breathing and the cough.

The *breathing* is labored and difficult, and is frequently perceived to be noisy, and coarse or shrill—the so-called laryngeal stridor: a sign encountered whenever the orifice through which the air has to pass is narrowed, either temporarily by

(172)

a spasm, or more permanently by any state which gives rise to a constriction of the parts; for instance, by swelling of the mucous membrane.

The difficulty in breathing is in some diseases very slight; in others very great. One of the peculiarities of this laryngeal dyspnœa is its tendency to recur in paroxysms, during which the patient appears to be in imminent danger of strangling. These fits of suffocation are mostly produced by a spasm of the glottis. They occur in pure spasm of the glottis; in croup; in œdema of the glottis; in ulceration, and in polypi of the larynx.

The *cough* of laryngeal affections presents frequently the same peculiarity as the dyspnœa—it happens in paroxysms. Another peculiarity, although not so constant a one, is its harsh and ringing tone. The cough is often short and dry; but sometimes it is followed by a muco-purulent expectoration of roundish shape, or by a blood-streaked sputum, or, as we may find in pseudomembranous laryngitis, by the spitting up of false membrane. It is readily excited by the act of swallowing, and its seat is referred by the patient himself to the windpipe.

Pain is not so usual a symptom of laryngeal disease as either cough or changed breathing. In some of the chronic affections it may be, indeed, wanting. It is very rarely severe; often more a sensation of tickling, of burning, or of uneasiness than actual pain. It is apt to extend down the trachea to the upper part of the sternum. Sometimes it is increased on pressure, as in acute laryngitis and in ulceration of the mucous membrane, and it may be also augmented by the act of swallowing.

By the symptoms, then, of altered voice, cough, dyspnœa, and, in some cases, of local pain and difficulty in deglutition, we recognize a laryngeal affection; and these symptoms reveal more than any physical examination of the organ made by the means ordinarily in use. The stethoscope is occasionally of service; yet, on the whole, it furnishes little information. But of late years, inspection of the larynx has been rendered practicable by the aid of an ingenious instrument, the *laryngoscope*, and our knowledge of laryngeal diseases has

FIG. 4.

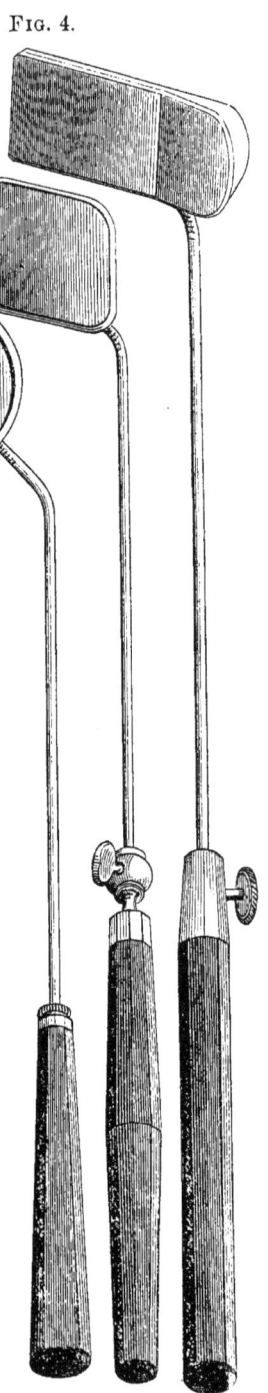

already been revolution-
ized through its powerful
influence. The instru-
ment employed by Czer-
mak*—the physician to
whom we are chiefly in-
debted for the informa-
tion gained by the appli-
cation of laryngoscopy to
disease—is a modification
of the one used by Garcia
in his researches on the
human voice. It consists
of a small mirror fixed on a long stem.

The mirror is best made of glass
backed with silver or with amalgam.
It may be either circular, square, or
oval. The circular mirror occasions
generally least irritation. It may vary
in size from half an inch to an inch
and a quarter in diameter. The larger
the mirror we can employ, the better
is the image.

The mirror is in some cases all that
is necessary to practise laryngoscopy.
It is heated in warm water or over a
spirit-lamp, and then introduced into
the back of the mouth in the manner
presently to be described; the person
to be examined having been placed
with his face toward the sunlight, so
that its rays may strike the laryngeal
mirror.

But examinations by direct light are
only practicable on some days and at
certain periods of the day. Usually we
require a second mirror to illuminate
the throat and the laryngoscope. This

* On the Laryngoscope, etc.   Translated by
the New Sydenham Society.   1861.

Laryngoscopes of various shape;
not quite natural size.

mirror, when sunlight is employed, has a plane surface; when artificial light is used, it is better that the reflector be slightly concave. One of circular form, in size about three inches and a half in diameter, and with a focus of from ten to fourteen inches, answers best. It may be either attached to the head by means of a band, or worn on a pair of spectacle frames, or be placed on a movable stand or affixed to a lamp, or be fastened to a handle which is held in the mouth. The latter plan, that of Czermak, is the one least employed; it is far less convenient than the spectacle attachment introduced by Semeleder.* When this, or the frontal band is made use of, the observer may either place the mirror opposite to one of his eyes, and look through the central perforation, or adopt the easier method of wearing the reflector on his forehead.

Yet another way of obtaining a strong illumination of the fauces is by means of a globe of glass filled with water, as recommended by Stoerck and Walker. The French, following the lead of Moura,† have recourse for the most part to lenses, and concentrate the light directly into the throat. The lamp which I often employ has a concave reflector attached to it on a movable arm, and by means of a bull's-eye condenser light is first thrown on the reflector and thence into the mouth. But a yet better arrangement is obtained by a combination of lenses attached to a metallic frame, which can be fastened to a lamp, as in the now so generally employed apparatus of Tobold.

Supposing that we wish to examine the larynx of a person with the usual instruments, and by artificial light, we should proceed thus: the patient, sitting in an upright position, with his head very slightly inclined backward, is placed near a petroleum- or gas-lamp, burning with a steady brilliant light, and the flame of which is behind and about on a level with his eyes. He is directed to open his mouth widely, to put out his tongue, and to hold it at its point between two fingers enveloped in a soft napkin

---

* Rhinoscopy and Laryngoscopy. Translated, New York, 1866.
† Traité Pratique de Laryngoscopie. Paris, 1864.

or handkerchief. If he cannot accomplish this readily, the observer must hold the protruded tongue, or a tongue depressor be employed. The observer now seats himself directly in front of the patient, and nearly a foot from his mouth. Putting on his spectacles or frontal band, he throws a disk of light into the back part of the mouth; he then rapidly introduces the laryngeal mirror, previously heated in warm water or over a spirit-lamp, and its temperature regulated by touching his own hand or cheek. The mirror, great care being taken not to bring it in contact with the tongue, is placed with its back against the uvula, and it and

FIG. 5.

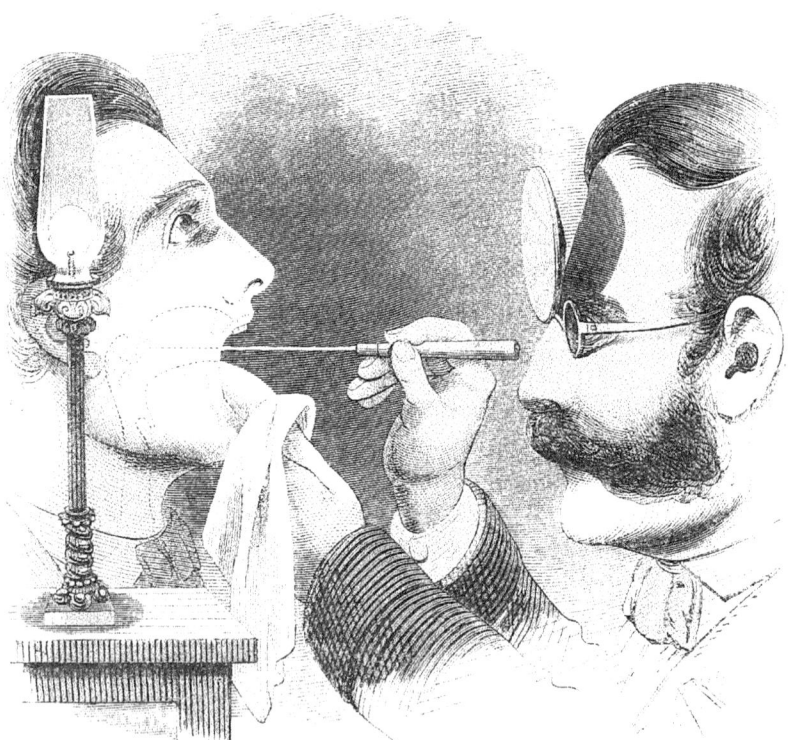

Laryngoscopic examination, as made with the means ordinarily employed.

the soft palate pressed backward and upward; the lower surface of the laryngoscope should be firmly applied to, or if this occasion too much irritation, should be held near the posterior wall of the pharynx. The inclination of the mirror varies with the position of the patient and the parts we wish more particularly to explore. As a general rule, it may rest at an angle of about 45°.

This is the manner in which an examination is made where the reflector is worn by the examiner. Where it is stationary, as for instance with the Tobold laryngoscopic lamp,—a less portable but far easier mode of illuminating, and well adapted for office practice,—the reflector is attached to the lamp by a flexible brass rod, and the light is thrown from it into the mouth, leaving the examiner unembarrassed.

When the mirror has been introduced in the manner described, the laryngeal image is readily perceived. We see the epiglottis, the glottis, the cartilages, the true vocal cords, the superior thyro-arytenoid ligaments or false vocal cords, and in some cases even the rings of the trachea. We may be able to discern each portion of the laryngeal aperture with distinctness, or it may take several examinations to do so.

In health, the color of the various parts is very different. Stoerck has well described it in likening that of the epiglottis, the interior of the larynx below the glottis, and of the cricoid cartilage to the coloration of the conjunctiva of the eyelid; and the hue of the aryepiglottidean folds and the prominences of the arytenoid cartilages to that of the gums.

FIG. 6.

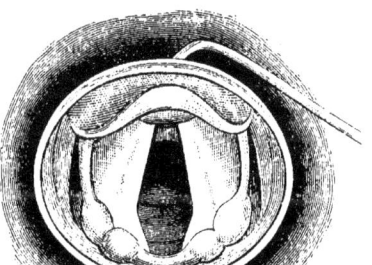

Laryngeal image, as seen in the laryngoscope under favorable circumstances.

The mucous membrane of the trachea between the rings is of a pale pink color; the vocal cords have a white glistening look. Mackenzie takes special notice of the whole of the under surface of the epiglottis being in some cases of a bright-red hue; and Gibb points out that in negroes the cartilages of Wrisberg have a yellowish tinge.

The laryngeal image in the mirror bears this relation to the real position of the parts: the right vocal cord of the person who is examined is seen on the left side of the mirror,

12

and the left vocal cord on the right; or, to state the matter in a form easily to be remembered, the cord which corresponds to the right hand of the patient is the right, that seen toward his left hand is the left. The epiglottis appears in the laryngoscope at the upper portion and toward the front; so do the other structures which lie in front. The arytenoid cartilages appear at its lower portion.

To judge of the movements of the vocal cords, we tell the patient alternately to inspire deeply and to sound, as a high note, a sound like "ah." During this the vocal cords are closely approximated and stretched, and the epiglottis, in fact the whole larynx, elevated; while during a full inspiration the cords are far apart, and hence the glottis is wide open. To obtain a satisfactory sight of the deeper-seated parts, we must bear in mind that the more the surface of the mirror is placed horizontally, the more distinctly they come into view. For the exploration of these structures, and particularly of the trachea, the light must be thrown from below upward upon the laryngoscope.

In some patients laryngoscopy is easy; the instrument causes no irritation, and a conclusive examination may be made at the first attempt. In others, a course of training is required to subdue the sensibility of the fauces, which may be general, or be limited to a very small spot. As a means of overcoming the difficulty, sucking small pieces of ice, or the previous administration of bromide of potassium has been recommended. But the best means is skill in the use of the instrument—its rapid and decisive handling.

In some persons with very irritable throats, I have obtained good views by pressing the instrument against the roof of the mouth, instead of passing it back into the pharynx, and by altering the position of the head a little, tilting it more backward. The epiglottis, and the structures at the entrance of the windpipe, are thus readily enough brought into view; with the deeper parts we do not succeed so well. But in many cases we get sufficient guide for topical applications.

There are some further obstacles, such as a rising up of the tongue, greatly enlarged tonsils, a very long uvula or a pendant epiglottis, all of which at times seriously interfere with our investigations. But in any case we should not endeavor to make the view more satisfactory by constantly altering the position of the mirror. It is always better to introduce it repeatedly, than to shift it often when introduced, or to keep it for any length of time in the patient's mouth.

To acquire dexterity and quickness of manipulation, one of the best means in our possession is *autolaryngoscopy*. We may readily inspect our own larynx by the simple method recommended by Dr. George Johnson,* by employing a toilet glass and throwing the light, with the reflector worn in the ordinary manner, on the image of the fauces as seen in the toilet glass; the laryngeal mirror is then introduced into the mouth.

If the mirror is passed behind the uvula, and the reflecting surface directed upward, the posterior nares may be examined. To practise, however, *rhinoscopy*, the mirror should be small and fixed to the shaft at a right angle. The patient is directed to keep his head erect, or bend it slightly forward, and while his mouth is widely open a strong light is thrown to the back of the throat. But before the rhinal mirror is placed in position, a tongue spatula is applied, with which the back of the tongue is well pressed down. After the spatula has been suitably fixed, it is given to the patient to hold. It is very rarely we can dispense with the use of the spatula, though we may do so by employing, as recommended by Voltolini, a shield of gutta-percha, a part of which is raised up to allow the handle of the mirror to pass through. Yet, whether the spatula be employed or not, a difficulty still remains, namely, to get the uvula out of the way. This is not easily accomplished without a palate hook, by which means the uvula, with a portion of the soft palate, is gently drawn forward and upward; the handle of the hook being held to one side of the mouth. The mirror, with its reflecting surface toward the operator, is now passed along the spatula, until it reaches the posterior wall of the pharynx. By then raising somewhat the handle of the mirror, we obtain a view of the septum; and by slanting the mirror first toward one

---

* Lectures on the Laryngoscope.

side and then toward the other, the posterior nares and the orifices of the Eustachian tubes may be inspected.

The art of rhinoscopy is more difficult than that of laryngoscopy, and demands, to acquire proficiency, constant practice. And though the rhinal mirror aids us in detecting morbid appearances which would otherwise escape observation, it neither does so as readily nor as completely as the laryngoscope. By the aid of this we can discern inflammation of various parts of the larynx; œdema; ulcers, simple or specific; cicatrices; excrescences and morbid growths; irregularities in the shape of the glottis, and in the mobility of the cords; abscesses; diseases of the cartilages, and other abnormal conditions which, without it, could not be recognized, or, to say the least, not be diagnosticated with any degree of certainty. Indeed, any one who attempts a diagnosis of laryngeal diseases without the laryngoscope, attempts to do without the only means which renders the diagnosis at all trustworthy, and is guilty of neglect.

Let us now look at the chief diseases of the larynx. Grouped in accordance with their main features, and without classifying them in strict obedience to laryngoscopic inquiries, they may be arranged as follows:

Acute Organic Diseases.

Inflammation of the mucous membrane of larynx—Acute laryngitis.
Œdema of the glottis.
Acute affections of the larynx and trachea as met with in children. } Spasmodic and pseudomembranous laryngitis—False and true croup.

Chronic Organic Diseases.

Inflammation of the mucous membrane in part, or of the whole—Chronic laryngitis in its various forms.
Destruction of the cartilages.
Growths and tumors of various kinds.
Ulcers, simple and specific.

Affections of the Nerves.

Spasm of the glottis. (Laryngismus stridulus.)
Nervous aphonia. { Functional, or purely nervous aphonia.
Paralysis of the muscles of the cord.

Acute Laryngeal Affections.

Acute Laryngitis.—In its mild form, acute laryngitis is neither an uncommon nor a dangerous disease. In its severer form it is much more uncommon, and very much more dangerous. The inflammation attacks, in either case, the mucous membrane lining the cartilages. When it is slight, it occasions simply hoarseness; a feeling of tickling and irritation in or near the larynx; a trifling though annoying cough, or rather a constant disposition to clear the throat, more than a cough; and, owing in a great measure to a coexisting inflammation of the fauces, some difficulty in swallowing. This is one of the forms of the "bad sore-throat" so frequently seen in winter and in the early months of spring, and which passes off in the course of a few days.

When the inflammation is violent, and especially when it involves the submucous tissues, the symptoms are much aggravated, and the patient's life is in imminent peril. His suffering is very great; for the swollen membrane nearly closes the narrow aperture through which the air is conveyed to the lungs. His respiration becomes seriously impeded, he breathes often, and each time he draws his breath a wheezing or whistling noise is heard. He coughs frequently, yet expectorates very little; and the cough is distressing and painful, and has a harsh sound. The voice is hoarse, or sinks into a scarcely audible whisper. The patient knows the seat of his disease : he feels that it lies in the windpipe, and complains of this being tender when pressed, and of a feeling of constriction in the throat. There is trouble in swallowing, and fever, with a full pulse and flushed face. If the case advance unchecked, the countenance becomes distressed and pale, the lips bluish, the pulse irregular, and death sets in with all the signs of deficient aeration of blood and of strangulation.

The disease in its graver form runs a very rapid course. If, in a few days after its commencement, no improvement show itself, life does not last long. Sometimes death takes place on the first day of the attack. It rarely waits for the sixth.

Acute idiopathic laryngitis is very seldom met with save in adults. Children suffer from an analogous but not an identical disease, croup. Occasionally, however, we do see acute laryngitis in children, and exhibiting the same features as in the adult; but then it has almost always arisen as the consequence of swallowing irritating substances, and not as the result of exposure to cold or wet.

The marked symptoms of the perilous complaint prevent it from being overlooked, and render its discrimination easy. There is fever with dyspnœa in the acute pulmonary affections; but the voice remains unaltered, and they exhibit physical signs which acute laryngitis does not: they show rales, or abnormal respiration sounds; while in laryngitis the murmur of the lungs is that of health, although it is sometimes enfeebled by the impediment in breathing, or obscured by the shrill sound which issues from the larynx. We find difficulty in swallowing and some hinderance in breathing in tonsillitis; but inspection of the oral cavity immediately detects the source of the trouble. There is difficulty in swallowing in pharyngitis, but there is not embarrassed breathing, nor a peculiar voice, nor cough, and the fauces appear dusky and injected, while they are but slightly affected in laryngitis, unless the inflammation of the larynx have supervened upon that of the throat. Croup resembles acute idiopathic laryngitis most nearly; but it is as rare in the adult as acute laryngitis is in the child, and, as we shall presently see, obvious differences in the symptoms exist.

There is a peculiar form of inflammation of the larynx, a *diffuse inflammation of the cellular tissue*, with lymph or pus infiltrated in the submucous tissue, to which attention has been called by Mr. Henry Gray.* It is a very formidable affection, which bears a strong likeness to erysipelatous laryngitis, but, what is not by any means constantly the case in this disorder, the symptoms commence in the fauces and larynx; and, wholly unlike erysipelatous laryngitis, the neck becomes greatly swollen from the effused products around the larynx, trachea, and œsophagus, filling its cellular

---

* Holmes's System of Surgery, vol. iii.

tissue. The disease begins with chills, soreness of throat, and fever, soon succeeded by a hacking cough, by dyspnœa, by a dusky hue of the fauces, by enlargement of the tonsils and of the glands in the neighborhood of the jaw, and by very great difficulty in swallowing. As the complaint proceeds, the neck increases greatly in size, the fever assumes a low type, and the patient either sinks gradually, or dies asphyxiated.

Œdema of the Glottis.—The danger of acute laryngitis of any kind is very much aggravated by the precise seat of the disease. When the inflammation takes place immediately around the glottis, and causes a serous fluid to transude, the peril is greatly increased. The inspiration is audible, noisy, hissing; there is a most distressing sensation of constriction or obstruction in the windpipe, and the patient makes repeated efforts, by swallowing or by hawking, to clear his throat of the substance which seems to him to be clogging it. His difficulty of breathing is intense, and occurs in frightful paroxysms, sometimes of a quarter of an hour in duration, during the whole of which time strangulation appears to be imminent, and often he does perish by strangulation. This grave form of *œdema of the glottis* sometimes follows an extension of the peculiar inflammation of the throat in the exanthemata, or is of erysipelatous origin, and it occasions death quickly, and amid great suffering. But the œdema may arise without preceding acute inflammation, whether this be specific or not. It may result from long-continued pressure on the trachea or larynx, or occur in connection with the external œdema of Bright's disease. Again, an effusion of serum may cause death most suddenly and unexpectedly in a person who has been laboring under a chronic laryngeal disorder. Such cases of œdema of the glottis are distinguished from those produced by active laryngeal inflammation by the absence of fever, of local tenderness, and of marked difficulty of deglutition. It is true that, if the edematous affection ensue upon a chronic inflammation of the larynx, tenderness and an impediment in swallowing may be observed. But the history of the malady and the non-existence of fever leave little room for error.

The diagnostic sign which some have proposed as the proof of the presence of œdema of the glottis—the swelling of the epiglottis, as ascertained by the touch—cannot be relied upon, because this swelling does not always exist to an obvious degree, and even when it does exist, is not readily determined by the finger.

Croup.—Croup is inflammation of the larynx and trachea; but it is something more. It is a spasmodic action of the muscles of the larynx, which spasmodic action gives rise to much of the peculiar cough, the stridor, and the paroxysms of dyspnœa, so characteristic of the disease. As croup is thus an affection composed, as it were, of several distinct elements, it differs somewhat according as one or the other of these elements preponderates.ʹ Thus the inflammation may be comparatively slight, yet the spasm play a very prominent part; or the inflammation may be very severe, and result in the formation of a false membrane. To the first class belongs the disorder known as false croup, catarrhal croup, stridulous laryngitis, spasmodic laryngitis; to the second, the true croup, or pseudomembranous laryngitis.

False croup.—This is one of the most common diseases of childhood. Its seizures happen chiefly at night; and the child that has gone to bed well, or perhaps a little fretful from teething, or with a slight catarrh, wakes up suddenly in a great state of alarm, breathing with much difficulty. It coughs with violence and at short intervals, and the cough is noticed to be loud and ringing and hoarse; and so are the voice and the cry. Each inspiration is attended with that shrill, "croupy" sound, which, once heard, is never forgotten. The face is flushed, the pulse frequent, and the skin hot, or, to speak more accurately, heated, for, in the majority of cases, the fever is not of a very active character. The paroxysm continues in this manner for about an hour; the breathing then becomes quiet, the child falls asleep, and rests well until toward morning, when the attack is apt to be renewed. The little patient may, however, escape this altogether, and keep well; or else the paroxysm recurs the next night, or for several nights in succession. In the intervals the voice and respiration are natural, there is little or no fever, little or no cough. Yet sometimes a cough remains, which has every now and then a croupal sound; and the voice, too, is slightly hoarse, but not smothered or extinct, as in true croup.

False croup most frequently follows exposure. It is very rarely fatal; hence we are not conversant with its morbid anatomy. The few cases which have been examined, presented signs of inflammation in the larynx and trachea, inadequate, however, in themselves to account for death. Yet such inflammation probably always exists to a greater or less degree. Cases in which it is extensive and severe, without having led to a plastic exudation, approach in their persistency and in the character of their symptoms closely to true croup. Indeed, one form of the complaint may run into the other, which is far from astonishing, since they are not two diseases, but only two forms of the same disease.

The main element in the production of the symptoms of false croup is undoubtedly *spasm of the glottis*, and this is the reason why this affection is so frequently described by authors as identical with the first-named malady. But without entering into the much-vexed question of pathology; without discussing whether or not the laryngismus stridulus, as spasm of the glottis is called by many, is due to enlargement of the thymus gland, or of the cervical and bronchial glands; whether or not it is caused by an organic disease of the cerebro-spinal axis, or is simply a reflex phenomenon,—it seems undoubted that the spasm, while it may complicate any affection of the larynx and trachea, may also exist independently. It may, therefore, form a distinct disorder, which differs from false croup by the absence of all inflammation and by several circumstances which unmistakably proclaim its non-identity, such as its occurrence in adults as well as in children, and especially its frequent association with other convulsive symptoms—with distortion of the face, spasmodic contraction of the hands and feet, and general convulsions.

As in croup, the seizures are most apt to take place at night. Generally the child has been fretful from teething, or from gastric or intestinal irritation, when suddenly an attack of difficult breathing occurs, accompanied by several loud, crowing inspirations, and by an appearance of the most manifest distress and of threatening suffocation; yet the paroxysm is not associated either with cough, or with fever, or with an altered voice or a materially changed cry. A fit of this kind may be repeated twenty or thirty times a day. It may terminate fatally in a short time; usually, however, the paroxysms are spread over weeks, or even over a longer period. Thus, in addition to the frequent combinations with other convulsive symptoms, the protracted duration of the disease, and the absence of febrile disturbance, of hoarseness, and of cough, point out the distinction between spasm of the glottis and spasmodic laryngitis.

True croup.—True croup is a formidable affection, in which there is not only inflammation, but inflammation which results in the formation of a false membrane. The plastic exudation is found lining the larynx, extending into the trachea or down into the bronchial tubes, and is seen in the fauces and on the tonsils.

The symptoms of this dangerous malady are: the same brazen cough, the same stridulous breathing as in false croup; and a decided change in the voice, dyspnœa, and fever. But all these symptoms do not show themselves at once. The disease usually begins with, or rather is preceded by, slight fever and catarrh, and some hoarseness. This may last for a few days, when the symptoms peculiar to croup manifest themselves. The cough attracts attention by its ringing sound, and at the same time, or shortly after, the characteristic croupal respiration is perceived. High fever and difficulty in breathing soon set in, and, although exhibiting exacerbations and remissions, only cease when the disease ceases. There is much thirst, no appetite; but what is taken is readily enough swallowed. The voice is changed almost from the onset. It is hoarse and whispering, and as the disease advances, often becomes totally suppressed.

The child remains in this condition for several days: restless, with its head thrown back, its respiration labored, and the croupal sound never completely disappearing. Sometimes, but far from always, solid masses of membrane are coughed up. Finally, the cough may stop altogether; the intervals between the paroxysms of dyspnœa are effaced; the face becomes livid; the skin loses its sensibility; the extremities grow cold; and, unless relief be afforded, either by medicinal means or by an operation, the little sufferer dies comatose or suffocated. The fatal termination is not unfrequently hastened by an intervening attack of bronchitis or pneumonia—a fact which teaches us not to neglect examining the lungs in cases of croup, so as to be sure that no disease is there silently running its course with its symptoms masked by the tracheal malady. In this respect, auscultation affords us important information, much more important than any it yields as to the exact seat and the extent of the affection of the windpipe.

Still the application of a stethoscope to the larynx or trachea is not without value. It may enable us to judge of the position of the exudation, for we may occasionally hear a vibrating sound, as if a membrane were being tossed to and fro by a current of air. In a case that came under my notice several years ago, this sign was perceived with great distinctness at the lower part of the trachea, and toward the commencement of the left bronchial tube; and at the autopsy, at exactly this point was found a thick layer of membrane lying unattached in the tube.

Croup is a disease not apt to be mistaken. Yet we must be cautious not to attach too much weight to any one of the symptoms; we ought rather to judge of the existence of the disorder by their grouping. Thus the ringing cough is in itself by no means diagnostic, for it may occur in some chronic laryngeal affections, and it is met with in children suffering from intestinal irritation. The stridulous respiration is also heard, or at all events there is a tolerably close copy of it, in simple spasm of the glottis, and sometimes when foreign bodies have found their way into the larynx. The paroxysms of apparent suffocation happen equally in œdema of the glottis. Not even the symptom considered of all the most pathognomonic—the expectoration of false membrane—is strictly so, since this may come from the bronchial tubes or from the throat. But when we take the symptoms collectively: the ringing cough, the peculiar respiration, the dyspnœa aggravated in paroxysms, the changed voice, the fever, the expectoration; when we regard the comparatively short duration of the disease,—there is but one interpretation of the phenomena possible, and that is, the existence of true croup.

It is, of course, of the utmost consequence to distinguish between false croup and pseudomembranous laryngitis. The main difference consists in this: in the former, the invasion is usually more sudden; we do not find the pharyngeal exudation so often seen in true croup; there is little fever, or this disappears with the paroxysm; and so does the croupal breathing, and, to a great extent, the hoarse voice and loud, barking cough. The disorder lasts rarely more than two or three days, the attack usually occurring at night; whereas in true croup the duration is seldom less than from four to six days, and the disease progresses steadily, and the voice and respiration show at all times the nature of the affection. Then in the latter we find expectoration of false membrane. This is, indeed, the most absolute proof; yet the absence of membrane in what is coughed up or vomited is not a positive sign that the case is not one of membranous croup. The membrane may be retained in the larynx; and we meet, indeed, with instances in which it is impossible to say whether the inflammation has or has not produced a plastic exudation; whether, in other words, the case is a severe one of false croup, or one of pseudomembranous laryngitis.

The disorders which, next to false croup, are most likely to be mistaken for the formidable malady under consideration, are: acute laryngitis, œdema of the glottis, pseudomembranous sore-throat, and retropharyngeal abscesses.

Acute laryngitis is, like croup, a disease of short duration, and, like croup, attended with a changed voice, with a harsh cough, and with dyspnœa. But it attacks adults, not children. It presents difficulty in swallowing, for which the slight marks of inflammation in the fauces are insufficient to account; whereas, in croup, in spite of the pharyngeal exudation, there is little or no difficulty in swallowing. A form of laryngitis, however, happens in children, which is very liable to be considered as croup; it is the secondary laryngitis of the exanthemata, especially of variola. Attention to the history of the case, and to the circumstance of the inflammation having spread from the throat downward, will go a great way toward forming a correct opinion of the disease. Yet the diagnosis is sometimes one of extreme difficulty, and, if the characteristic expectoration of croup be absent, the most accomplished physician may be deceived.

Œdema of the glottis resembles croup in the dyspnœa, the fits of suffocation and of coughing, the altered voice, and the noisy inspiration. It resembles it further in the fact that most of the symptoms do not disappear in the intervals between the paroxysms. Here is certainly a strong likeness. But the cough has not the croupal, brazen sound; there is no fever, unless the œdema occur in the course of an acute affection; and, above all, œdema of the glottis is a disease of adults, and unattended with the pharyngeal exudation and the peculiar expectoration. Again, the history of the case often guards against error, for œdema of the glottis happens frequently, perhaps most frequently, in those who have been long laboring under ulcerative laryngitis.

Pseudomembranous angina, or diphtheria, may present the same expectoration as croup; the walls of the pharynx, and the fauces, too, are coated with false membranes. But we know that the windpipe is not the seat of the complaint by the absence of paroxysms of cough and of difficulty in breathing, and by the voice being unchanged or somewhat nasal, but not husky or extinct. And there are some other points of difference which we shall further on inquire into.

Retropharyngeal abscesses share with croup the dyspnœa, the stridulous respiration, and the altered voice. They do not, however, share with it the expectoration of false membrane or the peculiar cough; and further, in croup there is not that trouble in swallowing, nor that evident tumefaction and stiffness of the neck, nor can a tumor be recognized by the touch, as it can when an abscess is seated behind the walls of the pharynx. Moreover, the dyspnœa and the voice present somewhat different characteristics. In the case of abscess, the former is greatly augmented, or paroxysms of it are brought on by attempts at deglutition, and it is frightfully aggravated by the horizontal position; whereas in croup the patient seeks relief by throwing back his head, and although he loses his voice and speaks in a hardly audible whisper, still the words are sufficiently distinct; while an abscess gives a nasal or guttural tone to the voice, which makes it impossible to understand what is being said.

Croup may further be mistaken for tonsillitis, for capillary bronchitis, for hooping-cough, and for the presence of foreign bodies in the larynx or trachea; but to any but the most careless observer the points of distinction are evident. In tonsillitis the breathing is not at all or but very slightly impaired; and looking into the mouth is sufficient to reveal the real nature of the malady. In capillary bronchitis there is dyspnoea, as in croup; but the dyspnoea is unremitting and associated with fine rales in the lungs, and not with a ringing cough, a harsh tracheal breathing, a hoarse voice. In hooping-cough paroxysms of coughing and of obstructed respiration occur; but then follows the distinctive hoop; and there is no fever, the voice is not husky, the child does not suffer between its coughing spells. Foreign bodies in the windpipe give rise to stridulous breathing and to cough, but they do not often mimic croup closely enough to deceive; and the absence of the peculiar cough and of fever, and the history of the case prevent error; so also does attention to the fact that the signs vary as the foreign body shifts its position.

Chronic Laryngeal Affections.

Of the chronic diseases of the larynx, chronic inflammation of the mucous membrane and the changes produced in it by inflammation, viz., thickening and ulceration, are the most common.

Chronic Laryngitis. — This affection has as its main symptom an alteration of the voice; but it is also accompanied by cough and an uneasy feeling in the larynx. The cough is at first dry, but when of any standing is followed by a yellowish opaque expectoration. It either presents nothing peculiar in its tone, or else it is harsh and barking.

The breathing is very little, if at all, embarrassed, excepting when the mucous textures are greatly thickened or ulcerated. In that case there is dyspnœa, the respiration is apt to be noisy and the voice completely lost, because the vocal cords have also suffered. There is, moreover, considerable pain on pressure; the sputum is muco-purulent, or else purulent and streaked with blood; and sometimes, if the cartilages also be involved, fragments of them are expectorated, and by the touch we recognize the changed state of the tube.

The symptoms of chronic laryngitis are purely local. It is only when there is considerable ulceration or a progressive alteration of structure in the affected part that the general health gives way. Yet chronic laryngitis is frequently found to be connected with a broken constitution, because the inflammation of the larynx, both in its simple and ulcerated forms, is often combined with the tubercular diathesis, or with syphilis. In every patient, therefore, who places himself under our care, suffering from chronic laryngitis, we must endeavor to ascertain, by careful inquiry, whether either of these morbid conditions is present. Many a time what has been considered as a case of pure chronic laryngitis turns out, on thorough examination, to be laryngitis linked to a serious pulmonary trouble: or we detect ulcers in the pharynx associated with those in the larynx, and are enabled to trace clearly the ravages of constitutional syphilis.

Chronic laryngitis is liable to be mistaken for an aneurism of the aorta, or, more strictly speaking, an aneurism of the aorta is liable to be regarded and treated as a case of chronic laryngitis. The distinction, as will hereafter be shown, is mainly made by attention to the physical signs.

Cases of functional or *nervous aphonia*, too, are sometimes confounded with chronic laryngitis, and it is by no means always easy to avoid this error. The loss of voice may be either partial or complete. It not unfrequently comes on without any previous warning, and this fact aids us greatly in diagnosis. So does the absence of cough, of expectoration, of local pain, and of all trouble in breathing; for none of these symptoms are commonly observed in aphonia which is solely nervous. One of the causes of this singular disorder is overstimulation of the vocal nerves, by straining the voice in singing or in speaking. We also meet with it as occasioned by narcotics or by lead poisoning, and perhaps most frequently as a reflex manifestation, due to irritation of the intestines by worms, or to a disorder of the uterine system. In these instances of nervous aphonia the voice suddenly disappears and as suddenly reappears, a phenomenon not unusual in the aphonia of hysteria. It is evident that in all cases of nervous aphonia the laryngoscope will assist us greatly in diagnosis, as it will show us the true condition of the parts, both as regards their structure and their mobility. It also aids us in distinguishing these laryngeal disorders from cases of aphonia due to want of strength in breathing, —to want of power in expiration.

Enlarged bronchial and cervical glands and an aneurism which paralyzes the vagus and the recurrent nerve, also produce hoarseness, and ultimately complete loss of voice. Under such circumstances, the trachea is insensible to pressure; there is a short cough, attended often with loud tracheal rales; and we observe attacks of dyspnœa, with a noisy, hissing respiration. The practical lesson which all such cases teach, is to remember that the symptom considered most characteristic of chronic laryngeal inflammation—the altered voice—may occur when no laryngitis exists.

Now, with reference to the nervous forms of aphonia just alluded to, the loss of voice, with the exception of those caused by pressure, is due to deficient power, and the cords move sluggishly or not at all. When the disorder reaches a high degree we perceive, on looking into the laryngeal mirror, that the vocal cords do not approximate as the patient attempts to say *a* or *o*. But, besides these cases, owing to general want of force, we find cases of absolute paralysis of individual muscles, as of one adductor of a cord ; or of one or both posterior crico-arytenoids, or abductors; or of the crico-thyroids, or tensors. In some of these there is considerable dyspnœa, with noisy breathing; in all the laryngoscope affords the only means of diagnosis.*

---

* See Morell Mackenzie, London Hospital Reports, vol. iv.; also Oliver, Am. Journ. of Med. Sciences, April, 1870.

Chronic laryngitis, or rather its chief symptom, loss of voice, is at times feigned; and the deception may be kept up for an indefinite period. Yet we possess, in the use of anæsthetics, the means of detecting the fraud at any moment. Just before the impostor falls into the deep sleep produced by ether, or as he is recovering from the insensibility it occasions, his will no longer controls his voice, and he speaks in his natural tone, or even screams violently.

Now, under the term chronic laryngitis, which formerly for want of more precise knowledge was made to embrace most kinds of chronic diseases of the larynx, many different morbid processes are embraced, the exact nature and seat of which we may discriminate by the laryngoscope. Thus the disorder may be wholly, or nearly wholly, confined to the *epiglottis.* We may find this structure very highly congested and enlarged; we may be able to note that it is pendant, almost completely covering the glottis; and it is frequently the seat of ulceration. The attending symptoms in any case are those regarded as characteristic of a greater·or less degree of laryngeal inflammation. In instances of ulceration, there is soreness with pain in swallowing, hoarseness and irritative cough, followed at times by blood-streaked expectoration. The ulceration may terminate in total destruction of the epiglottis.

When the *vocal cords* are affected, we recognize in the laryngeal mirror either their reddening in part or entirely, or their induration and thickening, or we observe edematous swelling in and around them, or their ulceration; and we can usually detect during breathing and phonation their impaired action. Now all these conditions are generally combined with very marked aphonia; the voice indeed may be reduced to the merest whisper. And in making our diagnosis we must always be careful to find out if the laryngeal phenomena be not secondary, forming part of a general morbid state, such as dropsy, tuberculosis, syphilis, or changes in the blood.

Diseases of the cartilages and of the perichondrium are still more frequently occasioned by the conditions alluded to; tuberculosis, syphilis, and low forms of fever are at all events the states with which they are most commonly combined. The affection often commences in the submucous tissue, and the ulceration spreads until the cartilaginous parts of the larynx are involved. The arytenoid cartilages are generally the ones first attacked; and portions of these cartilages may be thrown off and expelled. At times pus is formed which gives rise to swellings which can be recognized by the aid of the laryngeal mirror; sometimes a displacement of the cartilages takes place, before any portion of them is completely separated, and the most distressing and dangerous attacks of suffocation result; or the perichondritis may lead to the development of bone substance and a constriction of the tube. In some instances, the purulent collection presses on a vocal cord, which, when the laryngoscope is used, may, as Tuerck* has recorded, be seen to be immovable. This instrument reveals very often the ravages the disease has committed; and we are thus generally enabled to form an opinion as to how far the destruction or the "laryngeal phthisis" has progressed, and which of the soft parts as well as of the cartilages are involved. The symptoms attending this terrible complaint are difficulty in breathing and in swallowing, local pain and soreness, a greatly altered; or a lost voice, a distressing, harsh cough, which is followed at times by a purulent expectoration.

Respecting *tumors* of the larynx, cancerous or otherwise, and polypoid growths in its interior, we do not know as yet sufficient to distinguish them with any certainty, by their symptoms alone, from chronic laryngitis. Their most trustworthy signs, irrespective of the cough, altered voice, and the other manifestations of chronic laryngeal inflammation, are a steadily increasing difficulty in breathing and attacks of suffocation, for which nothing in the lungs, or heart, or great vessels accounts. The detection, at the seat of the larynx, of a growing tumor, accompanied by a severe cough, by a sanious sputum, and by emaciation, would, in addition to the symptoms just enumerated, warrant the diagnosis of cancer, whether or not much pain were present. *Polypi* in the larynx may sometimes be seen by depressing and drag-

---

* Clinical Researches. Translated, London, 1862.

ging forward the tongue until the epiglottis is brought into view. At least they have been thus discovered, and even successfully operated upon.* But as regards any form of morbid growth, and particularly as regards polypi, we possess in the laryngoscope the most certain, usually the only certain, means of detecting them, and even of aiding us in removing them, as is now being constantly done. These laryngeal growths vary much in size; they are often seated at the anterior free edges of the true vocal cords, or still more generally just above or just below the origin of the cords. I have seen numerous instances of the kind; and they are, as a rule, very readily discerned. Sometimes they may exist for years, merely producing changes in the voice and some cough, but no very great distress; or they may lead to fits of strangulation and to sudden death.

Before concluding these remarks on diseases of the larynx, it may be thought necessary to point out the differences between them and diseases of the *trachea*. But affections of the trachea need not be separately considered. Lying between the larynx and the bronchi, the trachea commonly shares in their disorders. Thus we have seen croup to be a malady in which both larynx and trachea are involved. Slight inflammation of the trachea occurs constantly in slight attacks of laryngitis or of bronchitis. Ulcers in the trachea may exist without ulceration of the larynx; but then they usually escape detection. Sometimes, however, they reveal themselves by a constant pain at the lower portion of the neck and upper part of the sternum, joined to all the symptoms of ulceration of the larynx excepting the impaired voice. Morbid growths, too, occur in the trachea, as they do in the larynx, and the tube may be altered in form and in structure. We can make use of the laryngoscope to assist us in the diagnosis of any of the forms of tracheal disease referred to. Yet the instrument is not always available; for it is only under very favorable circumstances that the entire extent of the trachea can be seen.

---

* Horace Green, Polypi of the Larynx Also, Ehrmann, Histoire des Polypes du Larynx: Strasbourg, 1850. Buck, Transact of Amer. Med. Association, vol. vi.

CHAPTER IV.

An examination of the diseases of the chest must be prefaced by a description of those methods of investigation which have given to their diagnosis such certainty. The same methods may be applied in the study of the maladies of other parts of the body, but they are of special service in the recognition of thoracic disorders, and will be here, therefore, most appropriately considered in detail.

The discrimination of disease by the eye, the ear, the touch, in fact by the direct aid of the senses, is called *physical diagnosis;* the signs thus ascertained are connected with perceptible alterations in the material properties or physical nature of structures—such as alterations in their form, their density, or their sounds—and are known as *physical signs.*

Physical signs are, then, the exponents of physical conditions, and of nothing more. But as the same physical conditions may occur in various diseases, so may the same physical signs occur in various diseases. An isolated sign is, therefore, not diagnostic of any particular malady. It reveals usually an anatomical change; but it does not determine the disorder occasioning this change. The tendency to ascribe to each thoracic affection, and even to each stage of an affection, a pathognomonic sign, has greatly retarded the usefulness of physical exploration. By presenting a never-ending list of specific signs, it has frightened many from attempting to become acquainted with the most serviceable of all the means of diagnosis, and many more, by the unnecessary complications introduced, have been disheartened at the very threshold of their studies. The subject may be much simplified by laying less stress on individual signs, and by grouping them together according as their association becomes distinctive of certain well-marked physical states. Morbid anatomy then

(196)

steps in with its teachings, and tells us in what diseases these states are commonly found. It is in conformity with these views that I shall attempt, in the following pages, to delincate the signs of thoracic affections.

But physical signs cannot be acquired from books; they must be learned at the bedside. Their value can be ascertained by reading; yet to distinguish them with readiness requires constant cultivation of the eye, the ear, and the sense of touch. And it is of great importance to have clear ideas regarding the structure of the parts to be investigated, and of their action in health. It must, for instance, be borne in mind that the lung is covered by a serous investment; that it consists of tubes more or less rigid, the bronchial tubes, of their numerous ramifications, and of their termination in an elastic parenchyma, the air-vesicles, or the pulmonary tissue proper. It must further be borne in mind that the organ is separated into lobes, and that it contains air which is constantly shifting, and that locked up with it in the same cavity is the main organ of circulation.

For the sake of convenience, the surface of the chest has been mapped out into regions. Various arrangements of these have been made by different authors. The simplest division of the chest is into anterior, posterior, and lateral surfaces. The regions into which the anterior surface may, for practical uses, be subdivided, are: an upper region, extending from just above the clavicle to the fourth rib, and a lower region from the fourth rib downward. Posteriorly, also, there are an upper and a lower part of the chest to be specially examined. It is hardly necessary to say that all these regions are double—the same on each side of the chest. Many more divisions are usually made; but they are perplexing to the student, and of very doubtful value. The artificial boundaries generally laid down are, indeed, too minute and yet not minute enough; they are too minute for ordinary purposes, not minute enough when it is desirable to localize a physical sign. Whenever this is requisite, instead of resorting to the names of the regions usually employed, I think it preferable to designate the seat of the sign with reference to some fixed anatomical point. This may be done for the an-

terior part of the chest by indicating the distance above or
below the clavicle, or near what part of the sternum, or at
which rib, or spreading over how many intercostal spaces,
the sign in question is perceived. At the posterior part of
the chest, the spinous ridge of the scapula, its lower angle,
and the spinal column, serve as landmarks. For most clinical purposes, it is only needed to study the region above the
spinous process of the scapula, as separate from the space
below. But in some instances it may be necessary to notice
the region between the scapulæ (inter-scapular) or that extending from the lower angle of the bone to the limits of the
chest (infra-scapular).

Let us now examine the different methods of physical
diagnosis, and particularly in their relation to pulmonary
diseases.

SECTION I.

DISEASES OF THE LUNGS.

The different Methods of Physical Diagnosis, and the Physical Signs of Pulmonary Diseases.

INSPECTION.

If the chest be examined with the eye, we obtain an idea
of its form, size, and movements. In health this inspection
shows us that the two sides of the chest are, to a great extent, symmetrical in form, as well as in size and movement.
Both sides rise equally during inspiration and sink equally
during expiration. On both sides the motion of inspiration
is longer than that of expiration, and the pause between
them extremely slight.

This *respiratory movement* is visible over the whole thorax.
In males it is most distinct at the lower portions of the chest;
in females it is most discernible at the upper. This difference in the breathing of the two sexes becomes the more
manifest, the more hurried the respiration. In healthy adults
the lungs expand with regularity from sixteen to twenty times

in a minute. In certain pulmonary affections, especially in pneumonia, the number of respirations often exceeds fifty in a minute. But hurried breathing and changed movements of the thorax occur independently of diseases of the lung. The heaving of the chest in a hysterical paroxysm is a sight familiar to every practitioner. Where the diaphragm does not descend, as in consequence of peritonitis, or of abdominal dropsy and tumors, the breathing is much more rapid, and is perceptible at the upper parts of the chest. Again, the thoracic movements may be distinct on one side and hardly noticeable on the other, as in pleurisy, in pneumothorax, or in hemiplegia. Lastly, as happens in some cerebral lesions, the motions of the chest may be very slow and labored, or irregular, or they may have apparently ceased, and the breathing be altogether abdominal.

The *form* of the chest is sometimes strikingly altered by disease. Congenital malformations and curvatures of the spine modify it; so do intra-thoracic affections. Frequently the chest presents a retracted, or an expanded look. Retraction denotes diminished size of the lung, and, if one-sided, is usually indicative either of chronic changes in the lung tissue, particularly those owing to tubercle, or of false membranes which bind down the lung. Expansion of the chest is met with in emphysema and in pleuritic effusion. A local or partial expansion, or bulging, may be encountered in the latter disease; but is more often associated with the former, or it may depend on thoracic tumors, on pericardial effusions, or on hypertrophy of the heart.

The *size* of the chest can be only approximatively judged of by the eye. Where accuracy is required, measurements must be resorted to.

MENSURATION.

To measure the circumference of the chest or of the abdomen, or to ascertain the distance from one portion of the surface to the other, a graduated tape is all that is required. To attain the former object, the spinous process of a vertebra is chosen as a fixed point, and the tape is thence passed round the body to the median line, first on one side, then on the other, taking care that it be applied evenly to the skin, and that the level of the measurement be the same on both sides. This level, if the examination be recorded, should always be noted, that we may have a uniform standard of comparison. And for the same reason, it is best to adopt the plan of always making our measurements, as nearly as possible, on the same line; for example, in determining the circular width of the thorax, we can, as a rule, select a line immediately above the nipple, or draw the tape around the chest toward the sixth costo-sternal joint, and, therefore, on the level of the sixth rib near its attachment to the cartilage.

In estimating the size of the chest in disease, it must be borne in mind that even in health its two sides vary widely. The half circle on the right side is, in right-handed persons, at least half an inch larger than the half circle of the left. But the measurements, to be trusted, must be performed while the patient is holding his breath in expiration. If it be desirable to ascertain in how far the respiratory acts modify the dimensions of the chest or of the abdomen, this may be readily effected

FIG. 7.

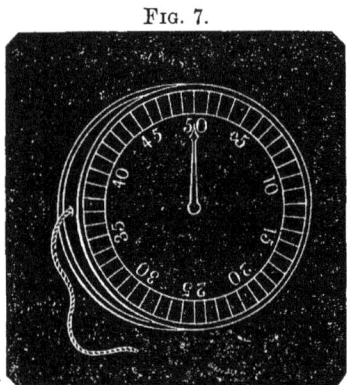

The stethometer of Quain. The box is placed on the sternum and the string carried around the chest. One revolution of the index, which is moved by a rack attached to the string, indicates an inch of motion in the chest.

by the ingenious "chest-measurer" of Dr. Sibson, or by the "stethometer" of Dr. Quain or of Dr. Carroll,* all of which instruments register accurately the movements of breathing; or the respiratory curves can be traced and studied by the atmograph of Burdon Sanderson, or by the anapnograph, an instrument made use of by Bergeon and Kastus, and similar to the sphygmograph.†

The transverse diameter of the chest may be determined by means of a pair of callipers; and the curves or flatness of the surface, should it be necessary, by Dr. Alison's stetho-

---

* New York Medical Journal, 1868.

† Gazette Hebdom., sér. 2, V. 1868.

goniometer (Fig. 8); but it is rarely necessary. In truth, these minute measurements, however interesting to the physiologist, have, as yet, not been made available to the physician. Inspection teaches us the same as mensuration. What it

FIG. 8·

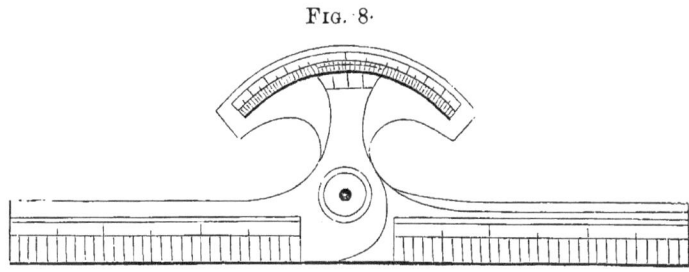

The stetho-goniometer of Scott Alison.

teaches with less precision can be learned for purposes of diagnosis with a graduated tape.

Mensuration may be employed not only to judge of the size of the chest and of its movements, but also to ascertain the amount of air which is received into the lungs. The instrument used for this object is the *spirometer*, an invention of Dr. Hutchinson (Fig. 9); and since his time numerous modifications of the instrument have been made : for instance, the ordinary dry and the wet gas meter have both been adapted to the purposes of spirometry, and an instrument small enough to be carried in the pocket has been suggested. The results the spirometer has yielded are of great value in a physiological point of view; in a clinical, there are too many sources of fallacy and too many drawbacks to render its use of much importance; and not the least of these drawbacks is, that it takes considerable practice to learn how to blow. The spirometer may indicate that a large quantity of air enters the lungs, and thus become a rough test of their normal condition. But when less air passes into the organ than the spirometric standard requires, this leads in itself to no conclusions; certainly not to any concerning the disease which occasions the diminished vital capacity. In estimating results arrived at by the spirometer, it must be remembered that sex, weight, age, and height have to be taken into account. To the latter Dr. Hutchinson assigns much importance, since he enunciates the law that for every inch above five feet, eight cubic inches are to be added to the healthy standard. For the height of five feet, the breathing volume is one hundred and seventy-four cubic inches. But these calculations are not exact; they only approximate the truth.

To determine both the expiratory and inspiratory power, the hæmadynamometer (Fig. 10) may be employed. Dr. Hammond* lays great stress on the indications furnished by testing the inspiratory power as regards the health of the individual, and recommends the use of the instrument in the examination of recruits. According to his observations, men of five feet eight inches possess the greatest amount of inspiratory power. They raise the column of mercury about two inches by inspiration, and about three inches by expiration.

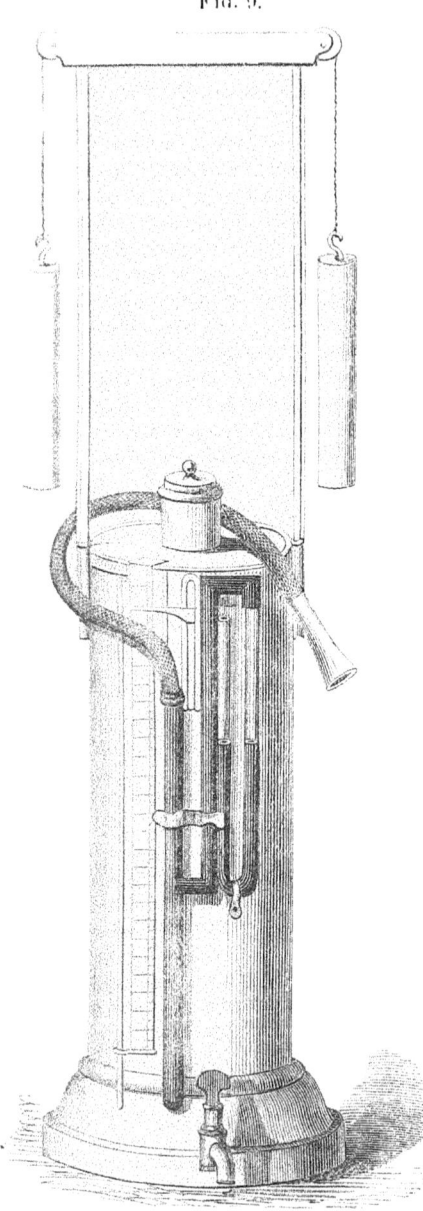

Fig. 9.

Dr. Hutchinson's spirometer.

PALPATION.

Palpation, or the application of the hand, confirms the results obtained by inspection and mensuration as to size, form,

FIG. 10.

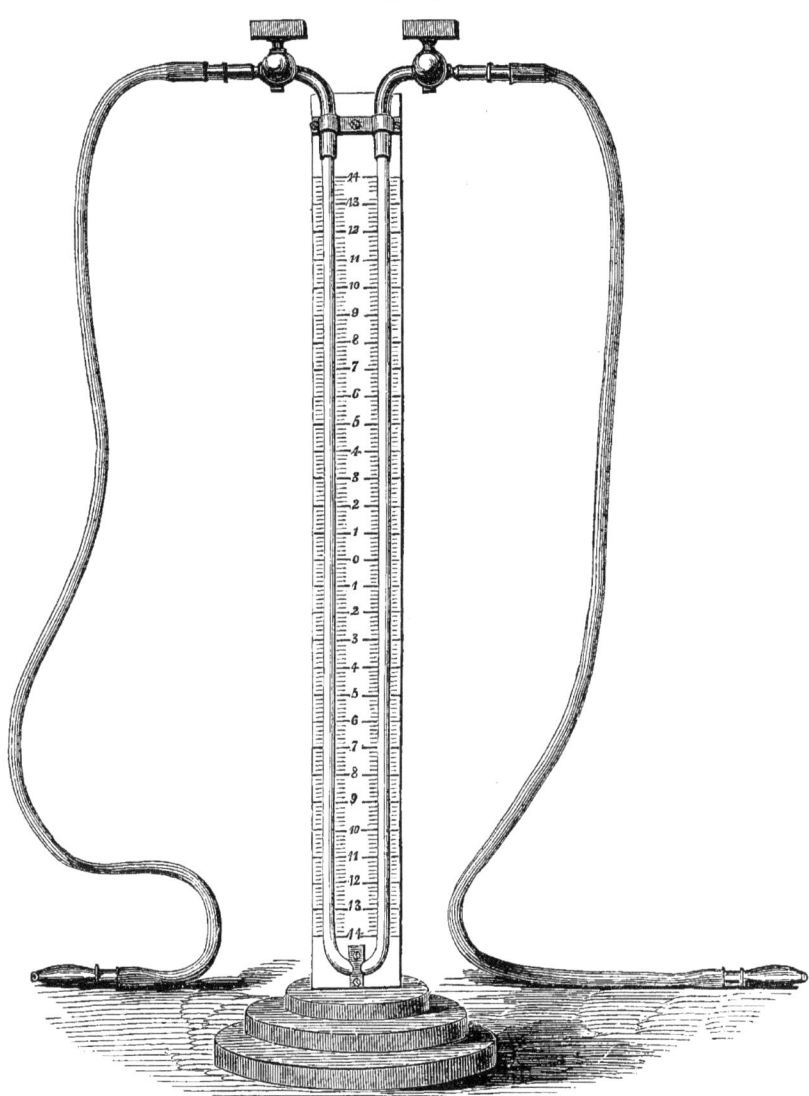

The hæmadynamometer, as adopted by Hammond for examinations of the lungs. Mercury is
poured into the glass tube until the zero on both scales is reached. Upon expiring into the apparatus, the mercury is forced to rise in the opposite portion of the tube, and is correspondingly
depressed on the side to which the elastic tube made use of is attached. When the act of inspiration is performed, reverse movements of the mercury occur. Care must be taken to exert only
the muscles of the chest, and not those of the mouth and cheeks.

and movements. It may, in addition, be employed to determine spots of soreness, the density and condition of tumors, the state of the thoracic walls, the frequency of the breathing, and the action of the heart. The hand may further be of service as a means of distinguishing vibrations produced by rhonchi (rhonchal fremitus), or by the voice (vocal fremitus): or it may detect fluid by the sense of fluctuation it imparts, or a roughened serous membrane by the friction fremitus. When both fluid and air are present in a large hollow space, by shaking the patient a distinct vibration of the parietes is felt, accompanied by a splashing sound, known as the Hippocratic or succussion sound.

Palpation is to be practised by applying the palmar surface of one or of several fingers evenly, and without too much pressure, on the part to be examined.

PERCUSSION.

By percussing or striking bodies we elicit sounds by which we judge of their composition. That a solid body sounds differently from a hollow one, was probably familiar to every artisan from time immemorial; but the application of this well-known fact to the study of the diseases of the human frame is a discovery of Avenbrugger, a Viennese physician of the last century. He and the brilliant editor of his work, Corvisart, practised percussion by striking directly with the hand over the organs to be explored; a method which, although serviceable to ascertain marked differences, or to obtain an idea of the general resonance of a part, is inferior to the one introduced by Piorry, of mediate percussion. The media used to receive the blow are various: a disk or plate of ivory, of wood, or leather; a piece of india-

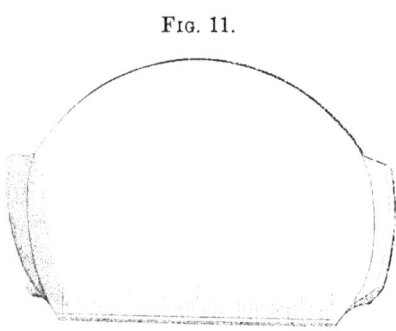

FIG. 11.

The pleximeter; about natural size. It may be conveniently made of hard rubber.

rubber; or the middle finger of the left hand. The finger answers best for percussion of the chest; for abdominal percussion a pleximeter is preferable.

When the finger is employed, it ought to be applied with its palmar surface firmly pressed against the chest, and as parallel as possible to the ribs. One or two fingers of the other hand may then be used to tap with—for the finger is, for ordinary purposes, quite as good as, if not better than, any of the percussion hammers invented—the greatest attention being paid to the circumstance that the percussing finger strikes perpendicularly whatever pleximeter be used, and not slantingly, as is too generally done. The whole movement should proceed from the wrist, and only from the wrist, and ought not to be too rapid, or unequal, or of great force. If all of these apparently unimportant points are attended to, the results obtained may be relied upon; if not, the want of manual dexterity invalidates the conclusions. No fault is so often committed by the beginner as the raising of the finger used as a pleximeter from the surface —thus obtaining the sound of the finger, and not that of the organ he wishes to percuss—unless it be the fault of striking with great force, as if the object were to break into the cav-

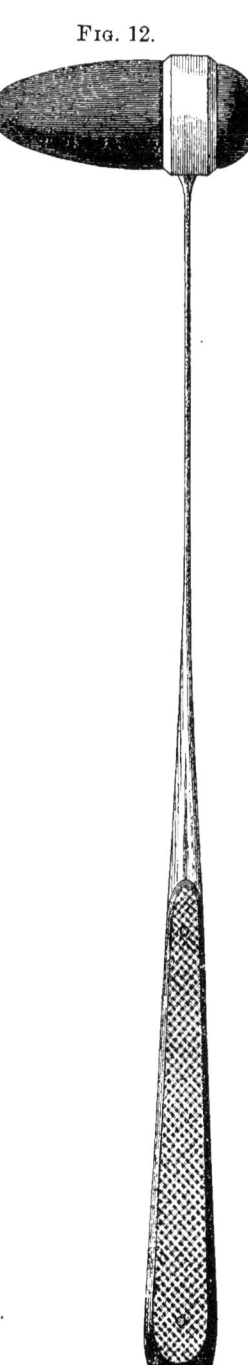

FIG. 12.

FIG 12.—A serviceable model of a percussion hammer; not quite natural size. The india-rubber is screwed to the ring, which has a diameter of five-eighths to three-quarters of an inch. The metallic ring is attached to a steel stem with a very decided spring. The pointed portion of the india-rubber is used to strike with on the pleximeter.

ity of the chest. Forcible percussion is only of use when the sound of deep-seated organs is to be brought out.

The main sounds elicited by percussion may be designated as dull, clear, and tympanitic. Of course these, like all other sounds, may differ in strength, in duration, and in pitch.

A *dull* sound denotes absence of air. It is the sound both of fluids and of solids. It is, thus, the sound sent forth from the airless viscera: from the liver, spleen, and heart. When it takes the place of the pulmonary sound, it bespeaks consolidation, or the presence of something which checks the normal vibrations of the lung texture. Dulness is always associated with an increased sense of resistance to the percussing finger.

A *clear* sound is produced by a series of marked and unhindered vibrations which are emitted from a substance containing air. As thus defined, a clear sound is evidently yielded by percussing any air-containing organ. But custom has restricted the employment of the term clear to denote the peculiar resonance obtained by striking over pulmonary tissue. When, therefore, a clear sound is spoken of, it means a sound having the nature of that of the lungs, or of normal vesicular, or pulmonary resonance.

A *tympanitic* sound, on the other hand, is a non-vesicular sound, having the character of that of the intestine. Wherever heard, it indicates the presence of quantities of air in conditions similar to that contained in the intestine, namely, inclosed in walls which are yielding, but neither tense nor very thick. When elicited over the chest, it may be only the transmitted sound of a distended stomach or colon. But generally a tympanitic sound over the seat of the lungs is expressive of emphysema or of pneumothorax, or sometimes of a cavity. Many find difficulty in distinguishing between the clear sound of the pulmonary tissue and the tympanitic sound. The more ringing character of the latter, and its higher pitch, constitute its essential properties.

As modifications of the tympanitic sound may be viewed the *amphoric* or *metallic* sound, and the *cracked-pot* or *cracked-metal* sound. The first of these is a concentrated tympanitic sound of raised pitch, and denotes a large cavity with firm, elastic walls. The second is not unfrequently found associated with it. It requires for its development a strong, abrupt blow of the percussing finger while the patient keeps his mouth open. The condition usually occasioning the sound is a cavity communicating with a bronchial tube. It is, however, also met with uncombined with an excavation, as in the bronchitis of children, in pleurisy above the seat of effusion, and in emphysema. Indeed, any disorder in which the chest walls remain very yielding, and in which a certain amount of air contained in the lung and in uninterrupted connection with the external air, is, by sudden percussion, forced into a bronchial tube, will occasion this cracked-metal sound.

In addition to the character of all these sounds, we may advantageously study their *degree*, or amount of fulness: such changes as are expressed by the words "more or less," "diminished or increased." Thus, a clear sound may be increased, owing to stronger vibrations and a larger quantity of air, and yet not lose its distinctive pulmonary character, as, for instance, often happens when the air cells are dilated; the sound of the large intestine is fuller, more tympanitic than that of the small intestine, and so forth.

With changes in fulness or volume of sound go hand in hand changes in its *pitch*. Increased volume is linked to lowered pitch, diminished volume to higher pitch.

To sum up the chief results of percussion, as above described:

QUALITY, OR CHARACTER OF SOUND.

CLEAR:—Presence of air—as in the lung tissue.

DULL:—Solidification or compression.

TYMPANITIC:—Certain amount of air inclosed in a structure or cavity the walls of which are not too tense.

Metallic:—Large hollow space, with firm but elastic walls.

Cracked-metal sound:—Usually a cavity communicating with a bronchus.

DEGREE, OR INTENSITY.

Any of the sounds mentioned may be *diminished* or *increased* in intensity as the conditions which produce them are modified.

If it be desirable to obtain a more distinct idea of the character or of any alteration of sound than can be done by the ordinary method of practising percussion, it may be accomplished by resorting to *auscultatory percussion*—a method introduced by Drs. Cammann and Clark, and which consists in listening, with a stethoscope applied to the parietes, to the sounds elicited by percussion. It is a very serviceable means of determining with accuracy the boundaries of various organs, as of those of the lungs and heart, or of the liver or spleen. I have found it yield particularly exact results, when carried out with the double stethoscope further on described: by the aid of which differences in the pitch and intensity of sound are very readily detected.

Percussion of the Healthy Chest.

The sound elicited by striking a healthy chest differs in accordance with the part percussed. The *anterior* portion of the chest renders a clearer sound than the posterior, on account of the slighter thickness of the thoracic walls. But the pulmonary resonance is not, even anteriorly, alike at all parts. The portion of lung above the clavicle yields a sound which becomes somewhat tympanitic as the trachea is approached. Percussion is difficult in this region, as it is almost impossible to apply the finger or pleximeter properly to the surface; hence arise errors in diagnosis if too much value be attached to trifling differences between the two sides. Over the clavicle the sound sent forth is clear and pulmonary at the centre of the bone; at its scapular extremity it is duller; toward the sternum it becomes of higher pitch, and mixed with the sound of the bone. In the region bounded above by the clavicle, and below by the upper margin of the fourth rib, the resonance is very marked. In fact the sound of this region may be taken as a type of the pulmonary sound: it is very clear and distinct, and but little resistance is offered to the percussing finger. Yet a slight disparity generally exists between the two sides. On the right side the sound is somewhat less clear, shorter, and of a higher pitch than on the left. From the fourth rib downward, on the right side, the resonance of the lung, on strong percussion, is found to be slightly deadened; near the sixth rib the perfectly dull sound indicates that the liver has been reached. On the right side, during full inspiration, the liver is pushed downward for the space of an inch or more; and the dull sound on percussion begins, therefore, lower down, and on a line corresponding to the displacement of the organ.

On the left side the heart deadens the sound from the fourth to the sixth rib, and, in a transverse direction, from the sternum to the nipple. This dull sound is lessened in extent during inspiration, and in cases of emphysema; indeed, under any circumstances in which the lung more completely covers the heart. Lower down, owing to the liver reaching over to the left side, and to the presence of the spleen and a portion of the stomach, the sound rendered on percussion consists of a mixture of the dull sound of the solid viscera and of the clear sound of the lung with the tympanitic sound of the stomach. The latter character of sound predominates when the stomach is empty. Over the upper part of the sternum, to the third rib, the percussion sound is slightly tympanitic; at the lower part, the heart and liver cause this tympanitic or tubular character of sound to give way to a dull sound.

At the *posterior* portion of the chest the sound varies materially according to the part percussed. Directly on the scapulae the sound is duller than between the bones, or than below their inferior angles. Beneath the scapulae a clear sound is emitted as far as the lower border of the tenth rib; here, on the right side, the dulness of the liver begins. Strong percussion, however, causes the dulness to become manifest higher up. On the left side, below the angle of the scapula, the percussion sound may be tympanitic if the intestine be distended; or, on the other hand, it may be rendered slightly dull by the spleen. In and under the axilla the sound is very clear. But on the right side, at the lower border of the sixth rib, dulness becomes perceptible; at a corresponding situation on the left side, the sound is clear or tympanitic from distention of the stomach; and at the ninth or tenth rib, distinct dulness and a sense of resistance to the finger disclose the presence of the spleen.

14

AUSCULTATION.

Auscultation, or listening to sounds, informs us of the play of organs, and furnishes us with the most trustworthy means of studying their action. It is of a very signal service in diseases of the chest. Indeed, any one who reflects upon the certainty with which cases of thoracic disease, which would have set at defiance the skill of a Sydenham or a Cullen, are now capable of being detected, even by comparative tyros, will gladly acknowledge the heavy debt of gratitude we owe to the genius of Laennec.

The method of listening he practised was the *mediate*, or by the stethoscope. Another method has since his time grown up—the *immediate*, or the direct application of the ear to the chest. Much controversy has arisen as to which is to be preferred; a controversy which has only tended more and more to prove that both are good and that both are to be learned, since a person unaccustomed to the use of a stethoscope hears but indifferently with it, even when the habit of immediate auscultation has made him familiar with the sounds in the chest. For ordinary purposes, the direct application of the ear is best; but where it is desirable to analyze circumscribed sounds, as in diseases of the heart, the stethoscope is preferable.

Stethoscopes are made of various materials and of different shapes. One of moderate length, with an earpiece which fits the pavilion of the ear, and with the extremity not too much expanded, is the best. The material it is made of is of far less importance. Of late years double stethoscopes have been introduced. The ingenious instrument invented by the late Dr. Cammann, of New York, consists of two tubes, the extremities of which are placed into the ears. It possesses the advantage of rendering sounds louder: its great drawback is, that it indiscriminately intensifies all sounds, whether in the chest or not, and its use is, therefore, at first very confusing. With practice, however, this objection

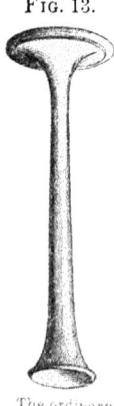

Fig. 13.

The ordinary stethoscope.

lessens, and the double stethoscope is in many cases extremely available. A similar, but not identical kind of stethoscope is the differential stethoscope of Dr. Alison, by which each ear receives simultaneously the sound from a different region.

FIG. 14. FIG. 15.

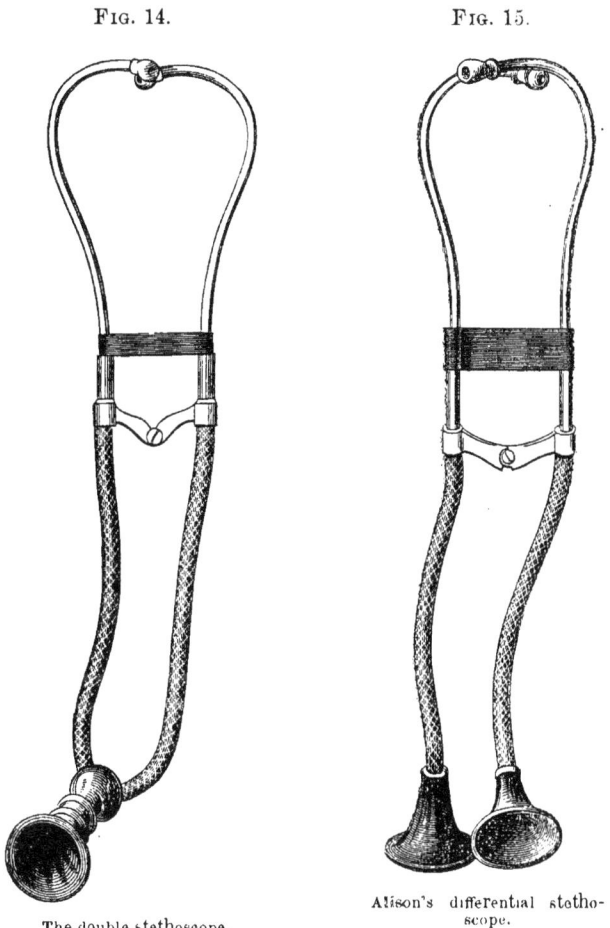

The double stethoscope.

Alison's differential stethoscope.

In auscultating, the following rules are to be borne in mind:

1st. Place yourself and your patient in a position which is the least constraining, and permits of the most accurate application of the ear or stethoscope to the surface. Above all, while auscultating, avoid stooping, or having the head too low.

2d. Let the chest be bare, or, what is better, covered only with a towel or a thin shirt.

3d. If a stethoscope be employed, apply it evenly and closely to the surface, but abstain from pressing with it. This may be obviated by steadying the instrument, immediately above its expanded extremity, between the thumb and the index finger.

4th. Examine, repeatedly and with care, the different portions of the chest, and compare them with each other while the patient is breathing quietly. Making him cough or draw a full breath is at times of service; especially the former, when he does not know how to breathe.

Sounds of Respiration in Health and in Disease.

The ear applied over the trachea of a healthy person, and subsequently over the lungs, discriminates two dissimilar sounds, which may be severally taken as starting-points.

The first is plainly blowing, both in inspiration and expiration. It is heard over the larynx and trachea; and in a slightly modified form, as a less intense and hollow sound, at the upper part of the sternum; and sometimes, owing to the closeness of large bronchial tubes to the surface, it is perceived between the scapulæ, on a level with their ridges. It is occasioned by air passing through the tubes, and is known as the tubular or the *bronchial* sound.

The sound over the lung tissue is very different: it is much softer, more gradually formed, of lower pitch, mainly inspiratory, and almost immediately followed by a shorter and far less distinct expiration. This is the *vesicular* murmur—produced in the finest bronchial tubes and air-cells by their expansion and contraction. The expansion gives rise to the distinct breezy inspiration; the noiseless contraction of the elastic walls of the vesicles and the passage of air back into the smaller bronchial tubes cause the indistinct, sometimes almost inaudible expiration. But the vesicular murmur is not exactly alike at different parts of the lungs. It is, as a rule, better marked over the upper lobes than over the lower, and more clearly defined anteriorly than posteriorly. Nor is the sound of the two lungs precisely the same; a disparity may generally be noticed at the apices. Most authors describe the vesicular murmur as more intense on the right side. Investigations instituted to determine this point lead me to agree with Dr. Flint,* that the reverse is the case. More expiration, a higher pitch, therefore more of the bronchial element, is presented by the upper portion of the right lung. But a stronger, more vesicular inspiration belongs to the left lung.

The murmur of the air-cells, then, is the sound which the ear encounters when it is placed over the greater part of the chest. Bronchial respiration is constantly engendered in the tubes of the lung: but either because it is overpowered by the sounds of the myriads of expanding air-vesicles; or because the pulmonary tissue is a bad conductor for a deep-seated sound; or perhaps because the sound requires consolidated tissue for its perfect production,—bronchial breathing is not heard over the chest (excepting at the very limited space indicated), unless, for the time being, the action of the air-vesicles has been suppressed.

Disease, however, gives rise not only to changes as absolute as suppression of the vesicular murmur and its substitution by a bronchial respiration, but also to certain modifications of the murmur, which serve as valuable guides in the diagnosis of morbid conditions of the lung. Thus the vesicular murmur may be abnormal in its intensity, in its rhythm, or it may have lost some of the elements of its distinctive character, such as its softness.

Changes in the Vesicular Murmur.—The changes of the murmur which are of importance, may be summed up as follows:

ALTERATION IN INTENSITY... {
Increased, or puerile breathing;
Diminished, or feeble respiration;
Absent respiration.
}

ALTERATION IN RHYTHM..... {
Divided and jerking respiration;
Alteration of length of expiration relatively to inspiration.
}

ALTERATION IN CHARACTER. {
Harsh respiration.
}

---

* Physical Exploration of Diseases affecting the Respiratory Organs.

Intensity.—An increase of the vesicular murmur is called *supplementary* respiration, or, from its resemblance to the breathing of children, *puerile* respiration. It depends upon an increased action of the air-vesicles; more air, or air with greater force, entering them. The sound is simply a loud, distinctly vesicular respiration; both inspiration and expiration being augmented in duration and loudness, but retaining as near as may be their relative length.

Puerile breathing is not in itself a sign of any disease. It indicates rather greater activity and energy of the part over which it is heard, which activity makes up for the deficient action of other parts. In this manner effusions compressing one lung, one-sided deposits, or obstruction of the bronchial tubes by secretions, necessitate a supplementary respiration in the healthy portion of the same lung, or in the other.

A diminution of the vesicular murmur, or *feeble* respiration, consists in a lessening of the whole sound without change in its character. But the relation of inspiration to expiration does not remain in the weakened murmur quite the same as in health. In the large majority of instances the inspiration suffers most, and the expiration does not diminish in proportion : a circumstance readily explained by reference to the states which occasion the diminished vesicular murmur. These are varied; but their causes may be reduced to four.

1st. Any cause which obstructs the passage of air and prevents it from fully reaching the pulmonary tissue. Foreign bodies lodged in the trachea or bronchi; affections of the larynx; considerable thickening of the mucous membrane of a bronchial tube; its compression, or the accumulation in it of secretions, or its contraction by a spasm,—all diminish the quantity and force of the air which reaches the vesicles, hence reduce the strength of the murmur.

2d. Deficient respiratory action. This may arise either from general debility; or from impairment of the nervous force, as in paralysis; or from local pain, as in pleurisy or pleurodynia.

3d. Causes which interfere mechanically with the free expansion of the air-cells. Pleuritic effusions, by compressing the lung tissue, will of course diminish the vesicular murmur; so, too, will morbid growths, or malformation of the chest. Comparatively slight deposits in the pulmonary tissue of tubercle or of lymph obliterate some, and prevent other air-cells from unfolding, and by having impaired their elasticity, diminish their sound. The same loss of elasticity happens in emphysema: the overdistended cells cannot expand much more, they are rigid and more or less fixed; the vesicular murmur is therefore feeble.

4th. The respiratory murmur may be imperfectly trans-mitted to the ear, owing to intervening fluids or solids. To this category belongs the enfeebled murmur so constantly met with in fat persons.

As so many conditions may occasion a feeble respiratory murmur, it is evident that it is only by association with other phenomena that it acquires much importance. Taking the diseases in which the sound is most frequently found, it may be stated that if a feeble respiratory murmur be com-bined with dulness on percus-sion, it signifies a tubercular deposit, or a pleuritic effusion: the former, if at the upper, the latter, if at the lower part of the lung. If it be connected with increased clearness on percussion, distention of the air-cells is its cause. A vesic-ular murmur, feeble through-out both lungs, with the percussion sound unaltered, arises

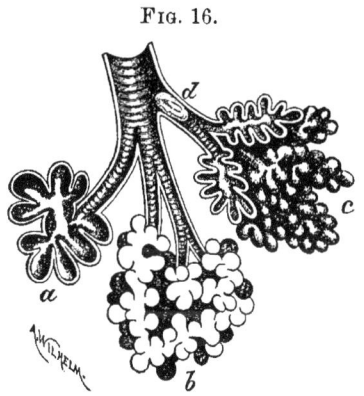

FIG. 16.

Diagram illustrative of the main forms of feeble respiration. *a*, from distention of the cells in vesicular emphysema; *b*, from deposits in the pulmonary texture; *c*, from a solid body (*d*) lodged in a bronchial tube, which has led to partial, or, in some spots, to complete collapse of the air-vesicles.

from general debility, or from obstruction of the upper air-passages. Where the feebleness of the murmur is found to change from place to place, it is dependent upon a loose foreign body which is shifting its position in the bronchial tubes. Joined to unwillingness to expand the lung (on account of the pain thereby brought on), feeble respiration denotes pleurodynia or commencing pleurisy.

In absence of the vesicular murmur is produced by the same causes, carried a step further, which occasion feeble respiration. Complete obstruction of the tubes by foreign bodies, extensive deposits in the pulmonary tissue, or its compression by large pleuritic effusions, arrest the vesicular murmur. But, practically speaking, there is only one complaint in which we are apt to find it entirely wanting, and that is, when associated with flatness on percussion it attests the presence of a large collection of fluid in the pleura. Extensive deposits in the lung tissue, tubercular or lymphous, also suppress the sound of the air-cells; but they do not suppress all sound. The noise of the tubes, the bronchial respiration, then takes the place of the vesicular murmur, and denotes the perfect consolidation of the pulmonary tissue.

Rhythm.—The inspiration and the expiration may be altered as regards their rhythm. The inspiration may be broken up into little puffs—jerking respiration—or both inspiration and expiration may be lengthened or shortened. But neither lengthening nor shortening of the inspiratory murmur has a distinct clinical value: and *jerking inspiration*, met with as it is in spasmodic affections, in hysteria, in pleurodynia, and in tubercular infiltrations, is present under too many different circumstances to have by itself much diagnostic significance. But if limited to the apex, it may serve to excite, or aid in corroborating, a suspicion of tubercular deposit. One modification of the rhythm is, however, of decided importance,—a marked increase in the duration of the expiratory murmur while the patient is breathing quietly.

Prolonged expiration denotes that the air has difficulty in getting out of the lung. It is detained either in consequence of loss of elasticity of the cells, or of an obstruction in the bronchi. The former state may be occasioned by overdistention of the air-vesicles, as in emphysema, or by deposits which impair their contractile power. In the first case, the prolonged expiration is associated with augmented clearness on percussion; in the second, with impaired clearness. Where the prolonged expiration is met with at the apex of the lung, in connection with dulness, it is for the most part caused by a tubercular deposit.

But a prolonged expiration from tubercular or any other kind of deposit, is not simply the pure prolonged expiration of deficient elasticity of the air-cells. It is something more. The solid material conducts a portion of the sound of the bronchial tubes to the ear; and bronchial breathing is nearly always best and earliest perceived in expiration. Thus a prolonged expiration, when joined to dulness on percussion and to an inspiration still vesicular, is a sound partly vesicular, partly bronchial, and may be interpreted as consolidation of the lung tissue; consolidation not sufficient to have obliterated all the air-cells, but sufficient to have obliterated some, and to have impaired the contractile power of others.

The obstacle to the exit of the air may reside wholly in the bronchial tubes. Such is the source of the prolonged expiration when the mucous membrane of the bronchi is swollen. Not only does this condition cause the air to be retained longer in the air-cells, but the resistance to the exit of the columns of air brings out more of the bronchial sound. On the whole, then, an accurate study of the expiration is of decided value; and it is of great importance to impress on young auscultators the advantage of becoming accustomed to inquire into the expiration separately from the inspiration.

Character.—The distinctive character of the vesicular murmur is its softness. From the moment it loses this, it commences to pass into the bronchial sound. That form of the respiration which is wanting in softness is termed *harsh* or *rude* respiration, or, very slightly to modify a term introduced by Dr. Flint, *vesiculo-bronchial.* Harsh respiration is, in truth, a union of the vesicular and the bronchial sounds: it is a vesicular sound mixed with some of the qualities of a bronchial sound—a rough inspiration devoid of all the softness of the normal respiratory murmur, with a prolonged, somewhat blowing expiration. Any affection which, without destroying the murmur of the vesicles, causes the sound in the bronchial tubes to be produced with greater intensity, or to be better transmitted, will occasion harsh breathing. Thus it exists when the bronchial membrane is swollen, as in bronchitis, and still more frequently in diseases which are

attended with compression of the lung tissue, or with partial condensation, such as some stages of phthisis or of
pneumonia. Being a transition murmur from vesicular to
bronchial, harsh respiration shares the properties of the latter
in having its expiration more developed than its inspiration.
It is true, the inspiration alone may be harsh, and the expiration not be materially changed; but this is uncommon.
Harsh respiration may be confounded with puerile respiration, with sonorous rales, and with bronchial breathing.
From the first it varies by its higher pitch, its roughness, its
more distinct and blowing expiration; from sonorous rales,
by the absence of all vibrating or musical character. From
bronchial respiration harsh respiration differs merely by degrees: it is mixed with more of the vesicular sound, is less
blowing in inspiration, and, when produced by condensation,
is not associated, owing to the smaller amount of deposit
which gives rise to it, with so much dulness on percussion.

Bronchial Respiration.—A purely bronchial respiration
may exhibit the same modifications as the vesicular murmur
as to rhythm and intensity. But neither its rhythm nor its
intensity is of much significance; its character is. To hear
a well-defined bronchial respiration is, in the large majority
of cases, to meet with *complete* consolidation of the pulmonary
tissue. It is thus that in extensive tubercular infiltrations
and in hepatization of the lung we find the bronchial or
blowing breathing so marked; particularly so in the latter
morbid state, for the most distinct blowing or tubular respiration is heard in pneumonia.

The bronchial breathing encountered in disease resembles
more that heard in health over the larynx or trachea, than
that heard over the larger bronchial tubes. It entirely replaces the vesicular sound, which has for the time being
ceased to exist. It differs from the normal vesicular murmur
by its higher pitch; its occurrence equally in inspiration and
expiration; its blowing character, especially in expiration;
and by the pause between inspiration and expiration. Harsh
respiration resembles it most; but this or vesiculo-bronchial
respiration is, as already stated, a transition from vesicular
to bronchial breathing.

Whether bronchial respiration be owing, as Laennec taught, to a better transmission of the sound of the tubes through the solid lung; or whether wé hold, with Skoda, that it is produced by consonance,—is not of much consequence for diagnosis. The important practical fact connected with this form of respiration is, that it happens when the pulmonary tissue is condensed, which, in the large majority of cases, takes place from deposits; in a small proportion only, from compressions by growths or effusions.

As a variety of bronchial respiration, at least so far as the quality of the sound determines the point, is to be regarded that very significant sign, *cavernous* respiration. This is essentially a blowing sound; yet it is not always distinct during both inspiration and expiration, being often only perceptible in the one, and mixed in the other with a gurgling sound. The question whether it can always be distinguished from bronchial breathing, has given rise to much dispute. That cavities may exist without cavernous respiration being perceived, and, on the other hand, that, owing to peculiar physical conditions, cavernous respiration occasionally may have been heard where no cavities were present, cannot be denied. But that a sound is met with which is less diffused, much more hollow, and, above all, of a much lower pitch than ordinary bronchial respiration; that connected with it other signs of a cavity are often found; and that, under such circumstances, a post-mortem examination proves an excavation to have existed at the spot where during life the sound was detected,—are facts which equally cannot be denied. The peculiar sound occurs, and may be discerned by the ear. And no theory, however cautious it may make us in our conclusions, can put aside the evidence of the senses.

Cavernous respiration is, then, a blowing sound of a low pitch, circumscribed, alternating with gurgling, and deriving its chief character from the cavity in which it is formed. Hollow spaces of any kind—from abscesses, from gangrene, from bronchial dilatation, or from softening tubercle—give rise to it. How it is to be distinguished from bronchial respiration has already been indicated. A student learns this sooner than he does to discriminate between cavernous

breathing and the vesicular murmur; the best proof that
the ear recognizes a difference between bronchial and cavernous respiration, since the later, as a sound of lower pitch,
is more like the vesicular murmur. It is only necessary to
recall, with reference to the distinction from the sound of the
air-cells, that this murmur is entirely devoid of all blowing
quality.

Amphoric respiration is a blowing respiration engendered
in a large cavity with firm walls.. Its peculiar character is
owing to an echo from the walls of the cavity. It may be
humming and of low pitch, or decidedly ringing and metallic.
An imitation of the sound, but only an imperfect one, is
effected by blowing into an empty jar.

Amphoric or metallic respiration is always indicative of a
large cavity. The sound is rarely met with in phthisis; much
oftener is it heard over the cavity which is formed between
the layers of the pleura, by the entrance of air, and in which
fluid collects. Yet the presence of liquid is not necessary for
the production of amphoric breathing.

New, or Adventitious Sounds.—These consist of sounds
which have no analogue in the healthy state, and which cannot, therefore, be considered as modifications of the normal
respiration. Of this kind are the rales; the sound known as
crackling; the friction sound.

Nearly all *rales*, or rhonchi, are sounds which are generated in the air-tubes by the passage of air through them
when contracted or when containing fluid. In the first case
are occasioned dry, in the second, moist rales. Rales may
occur in inspiration or in expiration, or during both acts.
They may obscure or entirely take the place of the natural
murmurs. They may have their seat in the upper air-tubes,
or in any division of the bronchi. When in the larynx or
trachea, they are called tracheal rales; of these the death-
rattle is an example. When in the bronchial tubes, they are
designated bronchial rales: and as this is their most frequent
situation, the term rale means a bronchial rale, unless the
location be specially indicated.

Dry rales are, for the most part, produced by the vibration
of thick fluids which the air cannot break up, and which tem-

porarily narrow the calibre of the tube. When this narrowing exists in the smaller bronchial tube, the sound which results is high pitched—*sibilant;* when in the larger, unless the calibre be very much altered, it is low pitched, more musical—*sonorous.* A similar difference, caused by the varying size of the tubes, is observed with reference to the moist or bubbling sounds. When the fluid is thin, whether it be mucus, or blood, or serum, and breaks up into large bubbles, large bubbling sounds are occasioned; when it separates into small bubbles, small bubbling sounds are the consequence. And the latter, for obvious reasons, generally take place in the smaller bronchial tubes.

FIG. 17.

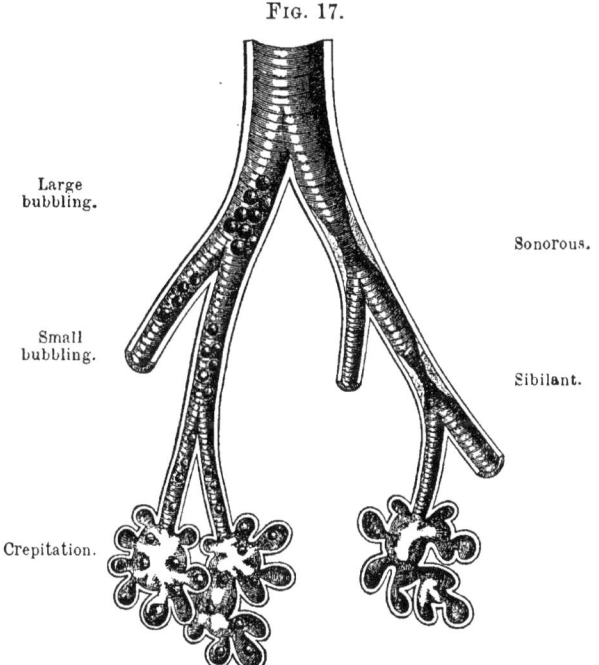

Large bubbling.

Sonorous.

Small bubbling.

Sibilant.

Crepitation.

Diagram illustrative of rales. The narrowing in one division of the tube gives rise to dry, the fluid in the other to moist rales. The rales at the termination of the tube and in the air-vesicles are the crepitant or vesicular rales.

Neither dry nor moist rales are persistent, but vary in intensity, or shift their position, as the air drives the liquid which gives rise to them before it. Dry rales are particularly prone to be dislodged by coughing. When they are unin-

fluenced by the act of breathing or of coughing, they do not
depend upon the presence of secretions, but upon a narrowing
of the air-tubes from the pressure of surrounding tumors or
from a fold of thickened mucous membrane, or by a spasm.

It has just been stated that rales are, for the most part, produced in the bronchi by the passage of air through fluids there
contained. This is their most frequent seat; but they are
not limited to the tubes. Similar conditions may give rise to
rales in other places. We find liquids in cavities breaking
up into large, sharply-defined, bubbling rales, the so-termed
cavernous rale—*gurgling;* and again, the presence of fluid in
the air-cells occasions a minute rale—the *crepitant.*

This vesicular rale, or *crepitation,* is a very fine sound, or
rather a series of very fine sounds, occurring in puffs and
limited to inspiration. It resembles the noise occasioned by
throwing salt on the fire. Its name indicates its seat. It is
caused by the agitation of fluid in the air-cells, or in the
finest extremity of the bronchial tubes; or, to adopt a view
now held by many, by the forcing open during inspiration of
the air-cells agglutinated by the exuding lymph. The first
stage of acute pneumonia is the state in which this rale is
mostly engendered.

The rales, including crackling, may be thus grouped:

BRONCHIAL RALES. {
  Dry or vibrating sounds. { Low pitched (sonorous).
                            { High pitched (sibilant).
  Moist or bubbling sounds. { Large bubbling (mucous).
                            { Small bubbling (subcrepitant).
}

VESICULAR RALES. { Crepitation.
                 { Crackling?

RALE OF CAVITIES. { Hollow bubbling, or gurgling.

Crackling is a sign closely connected with rales, and although
its mechanism is undecided, is usually regarded as a rhon-
chus. It consists of a few fine and readily-discerned crackling sounds which happen generally in cases of tubercle of
the lungs, of which, therefore, they are considered a diagnostic sign.

The distinction between crackling and the crepitant rale is
one most puzzling to a beginner. Nor is there, in reality, any

difference, excepting in the number of the sounds. Crackling is a few fine sounds limited to inspiration, and heard commonly at the apex of the lung. Crepitation is a number of fine sounds limited to inspiration, but more diffused, and heard generally at the base of the lung. The sound is similar because the conditions giving rise to it are similar. Both, so far as we know, depend upon tenacious fluid in the ultimate structure of the lung: in the one case it is tubercle, in the other usually the lymph of beginning inflammation. The crackling which indicates softened tubercle—called by some authors moist crackling, by others clicking—is a succession of sounds like small moist rales, only less liquid than these, because breaking up tubercle is not very fluid. The fine or dry crackling of the earlier stages of phthisis corresponds, then, to a vesicular rale; the coarser, or moist crackling, to the small bubbling sound. When the bubbles become larger and larger, and cavities form, and the fluid matter in them is agitated by the ingress and egress of air, the large bubbling ringing rale of cavities, or gurgling, is occasioned. Dry crackling, moist crackling, gurgling accord then with the crepitant rale, small bubbling, and large bubbling sounds, and happen in the progressive stages of infiltration and softening of deposits, and generally in those of a tubercular nature.

Pleural friction, or the sound due to the rubbing together of roughened pleural surfaces, consists of a number of abrupt superficial noises heard in inspiration and expiration, rarely in expiration alone. Its seat is not usually very extended, for it is, as a rule, only audible over portions of the lower part of one side of the chest. Sometimes it is so creaking and intense as to be distinctly perceptible to the hand as well as easily recognizable by the ear. But it may be so much like crepitation that even long practice in auscultation does not enable us to determine at once whether the fine sounds we hear are the friction of a roughened pleura, or the vesicular rales of an inflamed lung. It is easy to lay down in books the distinguishing mark of greater superficiality; but at the bedside the difficulty remains the same, and is only removed by attention to the physical signs and symptoms accompanying the doubtful sounds.

Nor is it, in some cases, less perplexing to discriminate between line friction sounds and fine moist rales. By the sound alone it is often impossible; concomitant phenomena must be taken into account. A friction sound is mostly confined to a smaller space, and is uninfluenced by cough; while cough changes the position and the distinctness of rales. Yet even this rule is not absolute. A fine friction sound may be temporarily increased during the deep breathing which follows the act of coughing; and on the other hand, the influence cough exerts on the small moist rale is not so great as on the larger bubbling sound. As for the more marked character of moisture which a rale is said to possess, that only aids us in some cases. Where the secretions are viscid, it would require a sense of hearing more delicate than belongs to the majority of mankind to judge, by the application of this test, whether the sound we perceive is formed in the lung or on its covering. As the result of investigations undertaken to ascertain whether there is any positive difference, so far as the ear can detect, between some of the finer kinds of friction and fine moist rales, I have come to the conclusion that frequently little or none exists; and still less is there between crackling and the crackling variety of friction sound, or between this and the vesicular rale. The features most at variance are: that the friction phenomena are not so strictly limited to inspiration as the vesicular rales, and are not seldom coarser in expiration than in inspiration; that they are less uniform; and that their seat is more circumscribed. Their production closer to the ear may assist us in the diagnosis, but does not always.

The reason why some of the finer friction sounds resemble so closely fine moist rales or crepitation, is apparent when we reflect that the irregularities in the pleura may be very slight, and be surrounded by fluid which keeps them moistened.

The creaking or grating varieties of friction are much easier of recognition than the finer forms. Their discrimination from rales is readily effected by noticing the distinctly rubbing and harsh character they possess.

Auscultation of the Voice.

Attention to the voice, as heard over the chest, is by some auscultators regarded as very important in examinations of the lungs. The one, two, three, which patients are made to pronounce, may be almost daily heard resounding in clinical amphitheatres. Yet the information derived from a study of the thoracic voice is very small, and next to valueless, unless confirmed by other physical signs.

When the ear is applied to the thorax of a healthy person who is speaking, a confused hum is perceived, most distinct in adults who are possessors of a deep voice, but very tremulous in the aged. Now the normal *vocal resonance*, for by that name the ill-defined vibrations are called, is more marked on the right than on the left side, and corresponds to the vesicular murmur. Over the bronchial tubes a more concentrated sound strikes the ear. This, termed *bronchophony*, accords with bronchial respiration, and when detected over the lung, denotes, with rare exceptions hereafter to be referred to, the same as bronchial respiration, namely, increased density of pulmonary tissue caused by pressure or by deposit. Any normal vocal resonance which is augmented, passes by degrees into bronchophony, and has a meaning similar to bronchophony.

Of the sound known as bronchophony there are several varieties: the *simple bronchophony* just explained — observed in pneumonia, or in tubercular consolidation; the hollow, *cavernous voice*, or pectoriloquy; and the bleating variety, or *egophony*. The latter, indicative of a thin layer of fluid between compressed lung and the ear, is a sign generally too transitory to be of much diagnostic value; and pectoriloquy, if by this be understood what Laennec meant—complete transmission of articulated words,—is of no special significance, as it may be met with where no cavity exists. But if the term be applied to a well-defined chest-voice, of hollow character, and heard as such over a comparatively limited space, pectoriloquy is a distinct physical sign, and really deserves the name of cavernous voice. This is particularly true of *whispering* pectoriloquy. Over large cavities the voice is peculiarly ringing and *metallic*. The conditions which produce amphoric or metallic voice are the same as those which occasion any of the amphoric or metallic phenomena. Be the respiration metallic, be the voice metallic, be the rales metallic, they are all caused by a cavity large enough and with walls firm enough to reflect, to echo the sound.

Bronchophony and amphoric voice are instances of increase and change of character of the normal vocal resonance. A *diminished vocal resonance* occurs when the lung is compressed by air or fluid, as in pleuritic effusions, or in pneumothorax; or when it is greatly distended with air, as in extreme cases of emphysema. Clinically speaking, the sign is most frequently encountered in pleuritic effusions.

The vibrations of the voice may be *felt* as well as heard. The vibration detected by placing the hand over the thorax when the patient speaks, or, to designate it by the name it bears, the *vocal fremitus*, is, like the voice, increased by all consolidations of pulmonary tissue, and diminished by fluid or air in the pleura. Its relations to the voice are, however, not uniform; and sometimes with increased density of the lung tissue there is no increased fremitus, although increased voice. In women the sign is valueless; and, indeed, its main importance is derived from noting *its absence* in cases of pleuritic effusions. Just as the voice, it is most marked on the right side.

The Combination of the Physical Signs, and the Examination of Patients affected with Disease of the Lungs.

In the preceding pages isolated physical signs have been discussed. But if in the investigation of disease we were to trust solely to isolated signs, incomplete and unsatisfactory indeed would be our conclusions. All the methods of physical exploration must be employed; the results obtained compared with each other; and the attending symptoms carefully inquired into and brought into connection with the physical signs, before a diagnosis is made, or a treatment instituted.

A patient presents himself for examination. After having obtained the history of the case, it is well to look at his general appearance; to scan the expression of his countenance; to feel the skin and the pulse; to inquire into the state of his digestion, into the nature of the cough and the expectoration; to determine the existence or non-existence of pain. The character and frequency of the breathing are then noted. Next we proceed to a physical exploration. The chest is narrowly watched; its movements, its size are carefully inspected—if necessary, measured. Percussion is employed, and finally auscultation.

The manner of investigating by these different methods has been already detailed; it need not here be repeated. But what may be repeated is, that there are two lungs, and not one; that it is incumbent always to examine both, and as we proceed, to compare the action of one with that of the other. Nor, even when the pulmonary affection has been made out, ought the examination to be stopped. The state of other organs and of the system must be inquired into, so as not, in the pursuit of a few physical signs in the lung, to pass by accompanying disorders of the heart, or liver, or stomach; so as not to overlook vital conditions, compared with which, as respects the treatment, the physical phenomena often sink into insignificance. There are acute and chronic diseases of the lung. The physical signs of both may be the same; but the general symptoms and the constitutional state attending them are not always identical. In truth, these are at times, in the same malady, so different, as to render a remedy which is of use in one case, useless or worse than useless in another.

As many of the signs elicited by the various methods of physical diagnosis depend on the same physical conditions, they may be studied in groups. The following will be usually found to be associated:

Association of Physical Signs.

Percussion	Auscultation of Respiration.	Auscultation of Voice.	Vocal Fremitus.	Physical Condition.
Clear.	Vesicular murmur or its modification.	Normal Vocal resonance.	Unimpaired.	Lung tissue healthy or nearly so; at any rate no increased density of lung tissue from deposit or from pressure.
Dull...	{ Bronchial, or harsh respiration.	Bronchophony	Increased.	Solidification of pulmonary structure.
	Absent respiration.	Absent voice.	Diminished or absent.	Effusion into pleural sac.
Tympanitic..	Cavernous or feeble, according to cause.	Uncertain; cavernous or diminished.	Uncertain; mostly diminished.	Increased quantity of air within the chest, or air confined in particular points; states commonly due to a cavity, or to overdistention of the air-cells.
Amphoric or metallic. .	Amphoric or metallic.	Amphoric or metallic.	Mostly diminished.	Large cavity with elastic walls.
Cracked metal sound..	Cavernous respiration.	Cavernous voice.	Uncertain.	Generally a cavity communicating with a bronchial tube.

In adults these phenomena are commonly combined. In children, however, their connection is not so constant nor so apparent. Owing to the extreme elasticity of the thoracic walls, and the naturally clearer sound of the lungs, the relations of percussion to auscultation are in them not the same as in the adult. Dulness, even where the condition exists for its production, is rarely as marked; nor is comparison between the two sides of the chest as valuable, since most of the acute pulmonary affections of childhood are more often double than those of grown persons. Again, the diagnosis of the diseases of the lung in children requires some knowledge of the disorders to which they are peculiarly liable, and, above all, great care and patience. Yet, no matter what trouble be taken, the information gained will amply repay for it. When we consider the very great frequency of affections of the respiratory organs in youth; when we reflect upon their danger, upon the tendency of the main fevers of childhood, such as scarlatina and measles, to involve the bronchial mucous membrane or the lung structure proper; when we take into account the valuable information gained in the diagnosis of the disorders of other organs, as of the brain, by watching the movements of the thorax,—no care appears too much, and the advice to examine the chest and the manner of the respiration in every sick child, as we would feel the pulse, or inquire into the state of the skin, or into the discharges, will not seem far fetched or ill judged.

Among some of the peculiarities of the respiratory function, before the age of puberty, may be mentioned the greater frequeney in breathing. Infants between two months and two years breathe irregularly, and about thirty-five times in a minute. Between the age of two and six years the average number of respirations in the same space of time is twenty-three. The breathing is also of a different type from that of the adult: it is abdominal, and can be more readily counted by noting the rising and sinking of the abdomen than by watching the slight movements of the chest.

Of the methods of physical exploration, auscultation is in children the most applicable. It is far more so than percussion, and is to be practised first, since percussion causes the child to cry. The voice as well as the breathing may be advantageously listened to; and although the fretful patient will not or cannot speak, it can and does cry. From the cry, when studied with the ear applied to the thoracic walls, we may obtain the same indications as from the vocal resonance.

The back of the lungs should be invariably examined. It is there where the mischief is mostly seated. Fortunately, also, this investigation does not occasion the same fear or struggling on the part of the little sufferer; hence it is better not to place the ear to the anterior portion of the chest until the posterior has been listened to. The position, too, in which the child is auscultated should vary with its age. Very young children may be examined either in a lying or sitting posture on the lap of their nurses, or may be held in the arms of an attendant, who is directed to present the different parts of the thorax successively to the ear of the physician.

Before proceeding to the discussion of the symptoms of pulmonary diseases and of the diseases themselves, let us group the latter according to their anatomical seat.

DISEASES OF THE LUNGS AND THEIR COVERINGS.

BRONCHIAL TUBES.
- Inflammation, or Bronchitis;
  - Acute
    - Of large-sized tubes
    - Of capillary tubes.
  - Chronic
- Dilatation;
- Narrowing;
- Diseases of bronchial glands;
- Spasm of muscular fibres, or asthma.

LUNG TISSUE.........
- Congestion;
- Hæmoptysis;
- Apoplexy;
- Œdema;
- Collapse;
- Inflammation, or pneumonia;
- Induration;
- Cirrhosis;
- Gangrene;
- Emphysema;
- Tubercle, or phthisis;
- Cancer;
- Deposits, such as syphilitic, typhoid, melanic, etc.

PLEURA...............
- Inflammation, or pleurisy;
- Empyema;
- Hydrothorax;
- Hæmothorax.

PLEURA AND LUNG.
- Pneumothorax;
- Perforations and fistulous openings.

WALLS OF CHEST...
- Pleurodynia;
- Intercostal neuralgia;
- Abscesses, etc.

The Principal Symptoms of Diseases of the Lungs.

After having in general terms described the physical signs; after having alluded to the methods pursued to ascertain the existence of pulmonary affections,—it is necessary to inquire into the more prominent symptoms they occasion. At the same time, several of the disorders which are mainly recognized by these symptoms, and the physical signs of which are comparatively unimportant, will be dwelt upon.

Yet of the symptoms about to be mentioned, not one belongs exclusively to pulmonory diseases. We have met with some of them in studying laryngeal complaints; we shall meet with them again in examining the affections of the heart. And in investigating them here we shall not view them simply with reference to morbid states of the lungs, but shall indicate their general relations to diseased conditions, even at the risk of discussing what might in part be more appropriately elsewhere discussed.

The symptoms which it is proposed more specially to sift, are dyspnœa, cough, and hæmoptysis.

Dyspnœa.—Dyspnœa means difficulty of breathing. It is mostly accompanied by a sense of uneasiness and suffocation, and by an increased frequency of the respiratory acts. But, strictly speaking, it is not correct to apply the term dyspnœa to mere increased frequency of breathing, for accelerated respiration and difficult respiration do not of necessity go hand in hand. The breathing may be slower than natural, and yet very laborious; it may be very quick, and not impeded. Pneumonia furnishes often an example of this kind of respiration.

Dyspnœa depends upon various causes. Feeble persons are sometimes troubled with it after the slightest exertion. It may be temporarily produced by any bodily or mental excitement. It is observed when the play of the diaphragm is interfered with, and the lung cramped in its expansion. This is its cause in ascites, in abdominal tumors, and in pregnancy. It may occur in perverted innervation, as in hysteria, or in connection with cerebral affections, from a want of power in the respiratory muscles, or be due to morbid conditions of the blood, as in anæmia, scurvy, and pyæmia. It is, however, most frequently met with as a prominent symptom of the disorders of the larynx and trachea, or of the heart, and in the various diseases of the lung and pleura, whether idiopathic or secondary. Being common to so many morbid states, it is not diagnostic of any.

Dyspnœa is usually aggravated by position. When the patient lies on his back, the respiration becomes more difficult. The form of dyspnœa in which the sufferer is obliged to remain in the erect posture in order to breathe, is termed *orthopnœa*. This is mostly witnessed in hydrothorax, in œdema of the lung, and in affections of the mitral or tricuspid valves.

In phthisis there is rarely marked dyspnœa. In capillary bronchitis the trouble in respiring is very great; so, too, is it in pneumothorax, in emphysema, and in pleurisy, if the lung be extensively compressed.

Dyspnœa may come on in paroxysms, and constitute the only, or certainly the main symptom of disease. This is the case in asthma.

Asthma.—Asthma consists in a spasmodic narrowing of the bronchial tubes, caused by a contraction of their circular muscular fibres. Its chief symptom is great distress in breathing, occurring in paroxysms, and attended with distinct wheezing. These spasms may be preceded by a feeling of suffocation, or they may come on suddenly. The patient wakes up out of his sleep, finds himself wheezing and with a fit of the disease fully on him. He continues to respire with great difficulty, sits upright in bed, or walks about the room gasping for breath. His look is wild and anxious, the face pale, the skin cold, and the color of the lips shows that the blood is not properly aerated. In spite of the struggle to get air into the lungs, the chest moves but little; and when the ear is placed on it, no vesicular murmur is heard—simply the same loud wheezing which is perceptible to the by-standers; or sonorous and sibilant rales are detected, due to the narrowing of the bronchial tubes, and disappearing with the spasm. At the end commonly of several hours the fit passes off with a copious expectoration, and as suddenly as it came. But it may last for days, ameliorating in the daytime, exacerbating at night, and only ceasing gradually.

The exciting causes of these bronchial spasms are very various. In some persons there is no apparent reason for the attack; in others it is brought on by the inhalation of irritating fumes or of disagreeable vapors. In some it is preceded by digestive troubles, or by inflammation of the bronchial mucous membrane; in others, again, an interruption to the free circulation in the lung, or a disturbance in the sexual organs, or in the urinary secretions, seems to occasion it. It is not unusual to find, on closely questioning patients, that for some time prior to the asthmatic paroxysm they have passed a dark-colored, heavy urine.

Now, whatever be the exciting agent that calls the bronchial spasm into existence, the symptoms of the attack of asthma are the result of that spasm. And yet asthma is not often a purely nervous disease. The seizure itself is the expression of perverted nervous action; but there are generally permanent conditions present, such as diseases of the brain or medulla oblongata, of the heart, or of the lungs, which act as constantly predisposing causes to these seizures, and lead to attacks either by direct irritation of the pneumogastric nerves or through the medium of the reflex system. Emphysema especially is a fruitful source of spasmodic asthma.

The detection of the causes inducing an asthmatic fit may be at times very difficult; but the diagnosis of the fit itself is not so. No disease of the lungs or bronchial tubes is likely to be mistaken for it, because no disease of either gives rise to the same symptoms. The dyspnœa of pleurisy or bronchitis is not paroxysmal, nor is it attended with wheezing. Some of the affections of the larynx and trachea bear a nearer resemblance; yet they, too, announce themselves by different symptoms. Asthma may be distinguished from croup by the entire absence of fever, and by its lacking the peculiar hoarse voice and cough which appertain to both forms of this malady. The age of the patient is also very different: asthma is as rare in a child as croup is in an adult. Œdema and spasm of the glottis differ from asthma by the much more markedly paroxysmal nature of the difficulty of breathing, by the shorter duration of the seizures, and the absence of the loud and continued wheezing. The sensations of the sufferer, further, indicate correctly the seat of the obstruction. A large goitre pressing on the trachea may give rise to dyspnœa and to a noisy sound in breathing; but the cause of both is easily traced to the tumor in the neck.

The most deceptive condition is when the glands of the neck enlarge suddenly and press on the trachea. I had, some time since, a young man under my care for acute bronchitis. He was progressing favorably, when one day he presented himself, breathing with great difficulty, and each respiration attended with a noise like the wheeze of asthma. It is very probable that I should have been deceived, and should have regarded him as having been attacked with asthma, had I not, in looking at his neck, detected the group of enlarged glands. Such cases are extremely rare, and belong more to the curiosities of medical practice.

Very marked dyspnœa may be occasioned by the pressure of an aneurismal tumor, or by an organic disease of the heart. But it is hardly necessary to enter here into a detailed description of the distinctive character of either of these forms of troubled breathing. The stridor and the persistent difficulty of respiration in the first, aggravated though it may become in paroxysms, and the constant want of breath in the second, are not likely to be taken for the wheezing and the paroxysmal dyspnœa of asthma. True asthmatic seizures may both produce and be produced by a disease of the heart. But what is called cardiac asthma is not always a spasm of the bronchial tubes: it is usually only a temporary increase of the dyspnœa, dependent upon a decided obstruction to the circulation in the lungs, and not accompanied by wheezing.

There is a very peculiar form of difficulty of breathing connected with a *loss of power in the diaphragm*. The patient, when the disorder is fully developed, cannot make even the slightest effort, without his being seized with a feeling of suffocation and his respiration being very greatly accelerated. He cannot take a long breath, and often his voice is very much enfeebled. But the most significant sign of paralysis of the chief respiratory muscle is, that during inspiration the epigastrium and the hypochondria are depressed, while the chest dilates; and the converse takes place during expiration. If there be merely a lessened power of the diaphragm, these phenomena are only observed during forced breathing; a paralysis of one-half of the muscle occasions them on one side only. Duchenne adds another important diagnostic test, by which we may distinguish a paralyzed state of the diaphragm, namely, that if the phrenic nerve be galvanized, the diaphragm acts again with proper strength, and, during inspiration, the abdomen rises simultaneously with the thoracic walls. To discriminate the cause of the impaired or lost muscular force,—whether this be due to a lesion of the nervous system, to inflammation of the muscle or of the adjacent textures, whether produced by rheumatism or by lead poisoning, or having its origin in progressive muscular atrophy,—we have to rely chiefly upon the history of the case. In rheumatism of the diaphragm, an absence of the vesicular murmur over the lower portions of the chest; a respiration effected by the upper ribs exclusively; tense, hard abdominal walls; want of power to strain so as to aid the bladder or intestines in expelling their contents, with darting, stabbing pain from the spine to the margin of the ribs on each effort to inspire,—have been particularly noticed.* In fatty degeneration of the diaphragm, which often coexists with a fatty heart, we find, in its last stage, great distress and difficulty of breathing, and death may rapidly follow the markedly embarrassed breathing.†

From the foregoing remarks it will have become obvious that there is no treatment directly applicable to dyspnœa. We must aim at removing its cause; and if this be possible, the difficulty of breathing ceases. The laborious respiration of a fit of asthma is relieved by relaxing the spasm which has caused it.

Cough.—Cough is a spasmodic effort, consisting in a sudden and violent expiration, and having usually for its objcet the expulsion of some annoying substance from the air-passages. But it may be purely nervous, and unconnected with the presence of any irritating matter in the respiratory organs. There are several kinds of cough: according to the amount of expectoration which follows the act, a cough is dry or moist; according to its origin, it is laryngeal, tracheal, bronchial, sympathetic, etc.

A *dry* cough is indicative of irritation. This is often seated in the larynx, trachea, or in their vicinity, or in the bronchi, or the lung itself. An elongated uvula, and many of the diseases of the larynx or pharynx, give rise to a dry cough : it happens, too, in pleurisy and in the earlier stages of phthisis. In disorders of the larynx and trachea the cough is

---

* Chapman, Boston Med. and Surg. Journal, July, 1864.
† Callender, London Lancet, Jan. 1867.

attended with a peculiar shrill noise, or a hoarse sound. But the irritation may not be situated at all in the respiratory system. Affections of the liver, of the stomach, the intestine, the uterus, or the brain, will occasion an obstinate dry cough. It is also produced by dentition, by the presence of worms in the intestinal canal, and by diseases of the organs of circulation. Again, it may be strictly nervous. The brazen cough of hysteria is dry; indeed, nearly all sympathetic coughs possess a dry character.

A *moist* cough may succeed to a dry cough. The moist cough is rarely associated with any diseases but those of the respiratory apparatus. It depends, for the most part, on the presence of fluid in the bronchial tubes or the lung structure. It attends bronchitis with free secretion, œdema of the lung, the more advanced stages of phthisis, and pneumonia when the exudation is breaking up. It is generally accompanied by a free expectoration, which varies in appearance and amount with the morbid state causing it.

Cough is frequently preceded by a sensation of tickling in the larynx, to which the patient is apt to refer his whole trouble. It is much affected by position. Lying down often increases its intensity. Sometimes a cough occurs in severe paroxysms. In various laryngeal affections, in abscess of the lung, in consumption, and in bronchial phthisis, such fits of coughing are observed. But in no complaint are they so constant as in hooping-cough.

Hooping-cough.—This is essentially a disease of childhood, and the result of an epidemic influence, or of contagion. The peculiar spasmodic cough succeeds to a catarrh of more than a week's duration. During the paroxysms the eyes fill with tears, the child's face is injected and anxious, and its whole appearance shows how it is suffering for want of breath. The air in the lungs is expelled by a series of abrupt spasmodic expirations, when a long-drawn inspiration, attended with a hoop, temporarily puts a stop to what appears to be threatening suffocation. The rest is, however, very short. The cough recommences, and is again followed by the loud hooping inspiration. It continues in this manner until after a copious expectoration of stringy mucus, or after vomiting, the paroxysm ceases, and a more lengthened calm ensues. These fits of coughing repeat themselves at varied intervals during the twenty-four hours. They are especially frequent at night. Yet the child's health remains good, in spite of the violence of the attacks and the length of time they are spread over. The spasmodic cough lasts for weeks; the hoop then ceases, the cough loses its ringing sound, and gradually leaves entirely. It is only in comparatively rare instances that it persists, and is followed by the development of tubercles in the lungs; just as it is only in exceptional cases, or in certain epidemics, that bleeding from the nose or convulsions happen during the violent coughing.

An affection of so long duration, marked by such a peculiar sign as a hoop, is easy of diagnosis. Yet there are certain conditions with which occasionally it may be confounded. In its first stage, before the characteristic cough sets in, it may be mistaken for catarrhal bronchitis. There is, indeed, at this period, no means of distinguishing between the two disorders, except by taking into account whether or not hooping-cough be prevalent as an epidemic; for it is only very seldom that the cough possesses from the onset a decided ring. And bronchitis is in fact the most frequent complication, or, to state it more accurately, almost an essential element of the malady. It is usually present in a mild form at the onset; it outlasts the paroxysmal stage. At the height of this, a severe attack of acute bronchitis or of broncho-pneumonia may mask the special traits of pertussis. Yet whenever these are detected, we know that the complaint before us is not pure catarrhal bronchitis. It is true that occasionally acute bronchitis may exhibit paroxysms of spasmodic cough. But the want of the nervous element in the disease, the absence of the hoop and of vomiting, the dyspnœa between the paroxysms, the decided fever, the presence of many rales indicating abundant secretions in the lung, the greater violence, and the shorter duration of the disorder,—do not permit us to be long in doubt.

A disease less easy to discriminate from hooping-cough is tuberculization of the bronchial glands, or *bronchial phthisis*. It, too, produces a ringing paroxysmal cough. It, too, occurs

in children. There is, however, this difference: the enlarged
bronchial glands are apt to press on the surrounding parts.
This becomes manifest by the engorgement of the veins of
the neck, by the lividity and puffiness of the skin, by the
trouble in breathing or in swallowing. The character of the
voice, also, may change; and yet, as at times happens in hooping-cough, there may be no abnormal physical signs in the
chest. But often there is dulness on percussion between the
scapulæ, where the swollen bronchial glands lie, and impaired
respiration in portions of the lung. The symptoms are those
of pulmonary phthisis, with which the disease, indeed, may
be associated: there are emaciation and the same loss of
strength, the same sweating at night, the same hectic fever,
the same tendency to diarrhœa. Now when we compare
these phenomena with those presented by hooping-cough,
we miss the hoop, the vomiting accompanying the fits of
coughing, the epidemic or contagious origin, and the distinct
periods, first of catarrh, then of spasmodic cough, then of
gradual decline. We see, on the contrary, an affection of
more gradual and uniform progress, and which often proves
its existence by special signs.*

When emaciation, hectic fever, and marked cough are met
with in the last stage of hooping-cough, it is always highly
probable that this has been followed by a tubercular deposit.
It is not likely that such cases will be mistaken for those instances of pulmonary consumption in which violent paroxysms of coughing occur. The age, the origin, the history
are so entirely different. Equally dissimilar are the history
and the symptoms in other spasmodic coughs, such as that
of hysteria, or of some laryngeal affections.

Hæmoptysis.—Sputa are streaked with blood in bronchitis, intimately admixed with blood in pneumonia; yet we
do not call this hæmoptysis. It is only when a certain quantity of pure blood is expectorated that the complaint is re-

---

* Refer, for cases of diseases of the bronchial glands, to J. C. T. Tice,
Medico-Chirurg. Transact., vol. xxvi.; P. H. Green, *Ibid* , vol. xxvii.; and
Barthez and Rilliet, Maladies des Enfants, tome iii.; and De Mussy, Gaz.
des Hôp., No. 67, 1868, where also instances of the disease in adults are
analyzed.

garded as hæmoptysis, or hemorrhage from the lungs. Now, a pulmonary hemorrhage may be an idiopathic affection; but it is not often so. It is mostly symptomatic of a grave disease of the lungs or heart, and usually of consumption. It is at times, although rarely, a discharge which takes the place of a suppressed flow of blood from another part of the body. Some females have these vicarious hemorrhages from the lungs at their menstrual periods.

It is a matter of dispute among pathologists where the blood springs from. It would seem, in some cases, to proceed from the capillaries and finer arterial branches of the bronchial mucous membrane and lung tissue; in others, from larger vessels that have been laid open. But what interests us mainly as diagnosticians, is to ascertain whether it flows from the lung at all, and subsequently why this organ is so disordered. Now, when called to a person who has been spitting blood, we have first to solve the question, Where does the blood come from? It may issue from the nose or mouth; from the trachea; from the œsophagus or stomach; it may stream from an aneurism which has burst into the air-passages; or it may be that the lung is bleeding.

When in *epistaxis* the blood, instead of flowing out of the nostrils, flows backward, it is coughed up. But on the patient inclining forward, it will issue from the nose. The color of the blood is not florid; and it can be seen trickling down the pharynx. Inspection is of equal service when the blood comes from any part of the *oral* cavity; especially if it proceed from the gums. Their swollen state, their spongy appearance, and the readiness with which they bleed when pressed, point out at once the source of the hemorrhage.

Loss of blood from the *larynx* and the *trachea*, or from the *œsophagus*, is exceedingly rare: and when it does occur, it is dependent upon some local lesion, or the presence of some foreign substance which has been swallowed. By attention to the history, then, we can recognize the cause and the seat of the hemorrhage. The blood itself furnishes no certain mark of distinction.

When blood is vomited from the *stomach*, it is preceded by a feeling of weight and uneasiness in the epigastric region, and sometimes by decided nausea. The ejected matter consists of a dark grumous blood, thus altered by the gastric juice; and is often mixed with broken-down food. Its dark color is invariable, excepting where an artery has been laid bare by an ulcer, in which case a sudden discharge of florid blood takes place. There is not commonly more than one act of vomiting; the blood which remains in the stomach passes into the intestines, and goes of with the stools. Hæmatemesis is attended with tenderness at the epigastrium. It is usually symptomatic of an organic affection of the stomach, of the liver, intestine, or spleen; it may, however, depend upon the swallowing of irritating poisons; or happen in fevers or in scurvy; or as a substitute for suppressed discharges.

The blood which gushes out of the mouth when an *aneurism* opens into the air-passages, is red and arterial. It spurts out in jets, and the patient rarely long survives the hemorrhage. Should this not prove quickly fatal, we are seldom at a loss to determine the cause of the bleeding; for the physical signs of the aneurismal tumor in the chest assist us in arriving at a correct understanding of the case.

But when the blood comes from the *lungs*, it presents characters, and is connected with symptoms, totally different from any of those just mentioned. The bleeding is preceded by a sense of weight and of uneasiness in the chest. The patient perceives a saltish taste in the mouth and a tickling sensation in the larynx, when suddenly, and without any effort, the mouth fills with blood, or after a very slight cough he expectorates a quantity of light-red and frothy blood. His anxiety becomes very great; the skin is covered with a cold sweat; the pulse is quick and full, and bounds under the finger. He spits up more blood, and this continues to come up at varying intervals and in changing quantities all day, or for several days, or even for a very much longer period. It is at first pure blood, or mixed with the sputum; is red and not coagulated, and frothy, except when the hemorrhage is very profuse. But after one or two bleedings, the matter which is coughed up contains dark clots, being the blood which has been retained somewhere in the air-passages since the previous attack. The blood is never, at the onset of the hemorrhage, dark and grumous; still, in rare cases it has more of a venous than of an arterial hue.

The amount which is brought up at one bleeding ranges from one to two drachms to as many pints; but the quantity that comes out of the mouth is by no means an index of the quantity extravasated. The blood may be effused into the pulmonary structure, and but little be expelled. This happens in *pulmonary apoplexy.*

After the description above given, it is not necessary to point out the marks of discrimination between blood ejected from the lungs and from other parts. The symptoms are different; the blood itself is different. And listening to the chest detects bubbling sounds in the air-tubes; still, to find these is not requisite for the diagnosis of pulmonary hemorrhage, and indeed, while the bleeding is going on, the patient's welfare forbids an accurate and extended thoracic examination. But as soon as circumstances permit, that examination becomes of immense value by teaching us with what morbid state the hemorrhage is connected. Auscultation alone can determine whether the bleeding is symptomatic of a disease of the heart or lungs, or whether it depends upon neither. It is, however, mostly owing to an affection of the heart or lungs; and is exceedingly prone to be repeated.

Yet the lungs may bleed frequently without there being an organic lesion within the chest to account for the hemorrhage. I had, some years ago, a patient under my care, who had been spitting blood daily for five years. Although enfeebled by the loss of blood, his general health remained good. His lungs and heart appeared to be sound. Another patient had pulmonary hemorrhages at varying intervals for eighteen months. He finally died of exhaustion; but he never presented any physical signs of thoracic disease. It is, however, likely enough that latent tubercle existed in the lungs. An examination of the body was, unfortunately, not permitted.

In these instances the hemorrhages recurred often. But we meet with cases in robust persons, in which the loss of blood follows active exercise or exertion, and is not apt to be protracted. In such cases, of which I have seen a number in soldiers sent to hospitals after the fatigue of a long march or the excitement of a battle, simple congestion of the lungs is probably the cause of the disorder.

Except under the circumstances mentioned, hæmoptysis may be looked upon as a grave symptom. It is not dangerous as regards its immediate termination, but dangerous because it is, for the most part, the index of a serious malady. Few die as the direct consequence of the hemorrhage, but many die of the disorder of which the hemorrhage is the consequence.

Diseases in which Clearness on Percussion is met with and constitutes a Valuable Sign.

Some of these ailments are acute, others chronic; and nearly all have as their prominent symptom a cough, and are affections, or follow affections of the bronchial tubes.

Acute Bronchitis.—This is an acute inflammation of the bronchial tubes, which occurs idiopathically, or happens as a secondary complaint in the course of fevers, of rheumatism, and of cardiac disorders. Let us examine the manifestations of the idiopathic malady.

Bronchitis varies considerably according to the size of the tubes involved. When the smaller tubes are affected, a disease called capillary bronchitis, or suffocative catarrh, is established, the prognosis of which is very grave, and the diagnosis of which presents points for special consideration.

The forms of bronchitis, dissimilar as they are clinically, do not differ much in their anatomy. Whatever portion of the membrane the inflammation attacks, swells, becomes injected and relaxed, and may undergo partial softening. Its surface is either dry, or covered with cast-off epithelium, muco-pus, and exudation matter, which, if it collect in the smaller tubes, blocks up their calibre. In ordinary bronchitis, the pulmonary texture is undisturbed; likewise in capillary bronchitis, unless the inflammation have here and there run into the lung parenchyma and solidified some of the lobules.

The symptoms of acute bronchitis of the *large and middle-sized tubes* are, a sensation of tickling in the throat, soreness or pain behind the sternum, a slight oppression in breathing, rather hurried respiration, and a paroxysmal cough. Let us add to these pain in the limbs, coryza, and a fever of slight or of moderate intensity, and we have the main phenomena met with during the onset and at the height of an attack of ordinary acute bronchitis. The fits of coughing in the earlier stages are followed by a clear, frothy expectoration, which, as the cough becomes looser and less fatiguing, changes from an almost transparent fluid to a yellowish or greenish sputum. This may be uniform, or streaked with blood; it may be small in amount, or in large quantities. The fever soon leaves, but long after it has ceased, the patient still has a cough and expectoration, both of which only gradually disappear.

The physical signs may be inferred from the lesions. As there is no condensation of pulmonary tissue, there is no dulness on percussion, the thickening of the bronchial mucous membrane and the injection of its texture not being sufficient to modify materially the normal resonance. But these very conditions must alter the respiratory murmur. They bring out more of the bronchial element of sound, hence more expiration with the coarser inspiration—in other words, a harsh respiration; or the swelling obstructs the entrance of air into the air-vesicles, and enfeebles the vesicular murmur. Again, new sounds, the rales, are produced: first dry, then, as the disease advances, moist. This succession of the rales is, however, not absolute, and depends, to a great degree, on the density of the fluid in the bronchial tubes. Dry rales, mixed with moist, may be perceived even in the latter stages of acute bronchitis, and long after the febrile signs have ceased. In fact, the tenacity alone of the exudation determines the nature of the rales, and even somewhat their exact character; for every dry rale is not precisely like every other dry rale; nor every moist rale equally moist. With reference to size, the sonorous rales and the large bubbling sound prevail when the disorder attacks the larger tubes. Sometimes, when the bronchial inflammation is severe and extensive, we find a sound which seems to be neither a dry nor a bubbling rale, but rather a compound of both—a dry sound, yet not continuous, giving the idea of its being caused by the breaking up of fluid. Or, there may be a mixture of the sounds of respiration with the rales, occasioning a very peculiar kind of breathing—one in which the most practised ear can recognize neither a distinctly vesicular, nor a distinctly bronchial element, nor a well-defined rale. All these states are dependent upon the amount, and, above all, upon the condition of the exudation in the bronchial tubes. But they indicate nothing beyond the fact that there is an exudation present which is unusually large in quantity and tenacious in character. When the sounds are of the indeterminate nature just alluded to, the vibrations produced in the tubes are apt to be transmitted to the parietes of the chest, occasioning with each respiration a marked fremitus, the so-termed rhonchal fremitus.

The diagnosis, then, of acute bronchitis is determined by the cough, the fever, the expectoration, and the signs of clearness on percussion, diffused rales, or harsh respiration. From all those diseases of the lung which result in the consolidation of the pulmonary tissue, such as pneumonia and tuberculosis, we distinguish bronchitis by the absence of dulness on percussion. Some cases of acute consumption, on account of the sudden invasion of the malady and of the general diffusion of the physical signs, are liable to be mistaken for acute bronchitis; but the different progress of the disorder usually clears up all doubt. Error in diagnosis is more likely to arise from the habit, when the signs of bronchitis have been made out, of not looking further; forgetting, in the attention to the disease within the thorax, the various morbid states which bronchitis may accompany, and partienlarly its frequent association with fevers.

Capillary Bronchitis.—This is essentially a disease of the aged, and of young children. It begins with an acute inflammation of the larger bronchi; or the disorder may from the onset affect the smaller tubes. In either case, signs of obstructed circulation soon manifest themselves: there is lividity of the lips and cheeks, with hurried breathing, a rapid pulse, an anxious countenance, great restlessness, a skin the temperature of which is either natural or but little warmer than natural, and a cough, followed by viscid expectoration. As the malady advances, the color of the skin and the mucous membranes shows more and more the want of properly aerated blood; the sputa diminish or cease with the failing strength; and in old persons delirium and coma, in young children convulsions, mark the closing struggle.

The physical signs are those of ordinary bronchitis, but modified by the seat of the malady. High-pitched whistling sounds, accompanied or superseded by very fine moist rales, denote the smaller size of the tubes involved. The resonance on percussion is clear, or very slightly different from that of health. When materially duller, it indicates that the pulmonary tissue itself shares in the inflammation, or that it has been exhausted of its air and has collapsed.

The parts of the lung which the physical signs prove to bear the brunt of the disease, are the lower lobes. In the upper there may be large rales and some fine ones; but it is low down and at the posterior portion of the chest that the fine sounds are always most abundant. Yet where the inflammation is extensive, and the accumulation of secretions and morbid products great, quantities of small rales are heard at every part of the chest.

From this description, brief though it be, of the signs and symptoms of capillary bronchitis, it will be apparent that it differs from the ordinary acute bronchitis by the greater tendency to prostration and to suffocation, by the signs of imperfect aeration of the blood, and by the fineness of the rales.

Like the more usual kind of acute bronchial inflammation, capillary bronchitis is liable to be mistaken for acute lobar pneumonia and for phthisis. And in the majority of cases the same rules serve for its discrimination: the absence of percussion dulness and the diffusion of the morbid sounds are here again of the utmost value. The rapidity of the attack and the signs of suffocation might mislead into the supposition of œdema of the glottis, of laryngitis, or of croup; errors in diagnosis which the detection of fine rales, by the application of the ear to the chest, will prevent.

Capillary bronchitis is apt to be confounded with *lobular*

pneumonia—a form of inflammation of the lung occurring mainly in children, and which, as it is limited to the lobules, yields but imperfect signs of consolidation. The bronchial breathing is rarely very marked; the minute rale indicative of exudation into the air-cells is not usually perceived, or can scarcely be distinguished from the small bubbling sounds of capillary bronchitis; and, from the usual association of the malady in question with inflammation of the fine bronchial tubes, it is in individual cases often difficult, nay, it is impossible, to say whether portions of the lung tissue are consolidated, or whether the inflammation is limited to the tubes. Theoretically speaking, broncho-pneumonia may be distinguished from bronchitis by the dulness on percussion; but practically, this aids but little. Dulness on percussion is in children difficult to elicit; and again, a dulness may be temporarily produced in capillary bronchitis by collapse of the pulmonary tissue. There are, therefore, no trustworthy signs of difference. Still, we may suspect that the inflammation has consolidated the lobules if the breathing be very rapid, the fever severe, and if in addition to rales, not very diffused, spots of dulness, which do not change their seat, be discerned. On the other hand, when there are signs of deficient aeration of blood; when the symptoms point more to prostration than to activity of febrile action; when the child seems to suffocate from want of power to expectorate; when multitudes of fine dry and moist sounds are heard at every part of the chest, and little or no corresponding impairment of the natural resonance on percussion is detected,—we know that the capillary bronchi are extensively filled with pus and morbid secretions, and that a graver disease than bronchopneumonia usually is, that true suffocative catarrh is threatcuing life.

The two forms of acute bronchitis considered, furnish somewhat different indications for treatment. There is too much prostration in the capillary variety of the disorder to admit of any depressing agents, and carbonate of ammonia, beef tea, and wine are more often called for.

Chronic Bronchitis.—The symptoms and signs of chronic bronchitis are not very different from those of the ordinary form of acute bronchitis. The duration of the complaint and the absence of marked fever are the chief distinguishing elements. Yet the cough, although on the whole chronic, is far from being constant. It may disappear almost altogether, and then reappear with more than its previous severity; and this state of things may go on for years; undue exposure and change of season aggravating the disorder..

The sputa vary even more than in acute bronchitis in tenacity and quantity. There may be merely a small quantity of yellowish matter expectorated in the morning, or an almost continued flow from the bronchial tubes—*bronchorrhœa*. The physical signs differ accordingly. A harsh or feeble respiration, and few or many, either dry or moist, rales are present, in conformity with the state of the bronchial mucous membrane and of its secretions. The sound on percussion is clear. Excessive secretions somewhat impair the pulmonary resonance; but only temporarily; for with the shifting secretions shifts the slight dulness.

One of the most important points iu the diagnosis of chronic bronchitis is to attend to the manner in which it arises. It may follow a seizure of acute bronchitis, or be the result of recurring attacks of subacute character; it may appear as a primary affection; or it may follow the exanthemata; or again it may complicate some previously existing disorder, as Bright's disease, rheumatism, gout, psoriasis, or eczema, and be directly traceable to the constitutional taints of these maladies; and its symptoms will vary and be influenced by those of the general malady to which it is subordinate.

In the ordinary idiopathic malady the general health, as a rule, suffers but little. In some instances, however, emaciation takes place, and the disease simulates phthisis.* The resemblance becomes still greater, when superadded bronchial dilatation produces physical signs like those of phthisis. Ordinarily, the chronicity of the cough, the occasional sub-

---

* This is particularly the case in the bronchial affections among knife-grinders and coal-miners, also in that of potters. See Parson on *Potters' Bronchitis*, Edinb., 1864; also a Lecture on Bronchitis from Mechanical Irritation, in Greenhow's work on Chronic Bronchitis, London, 1869.

acute exacerbations, the small amount of constitutional disturbance, the post-sternal pain, the diffusion of the signs
discerned on auscultation, and the clearness on percussion,
constitute a group of phenomena which do not permit an
error.

A chronic *catarrhal inflammation of the mucous membrane of
the nose* may be mistaken for chronic bronchitis, with which,
indeed, it may coexist. But when occurring uncombined,
there are no rales in the chest, or altered breathing sounds
indicative of disorder there, though there may be a cough,
from the throat being also affected. The secretion, too, from
the nose is very copious and of muco-purulent character, the
upper part of the nose looks somewhat flattened, and the
sense of smell is impaired,—not one of which signs is met
with in chronic bronchitis.

The treatment of chronic bronchitis is not always the
same. Different remedies suit different cases. In selecting
our therapeutic agents, the amount and condition of the discharge from the membrane, and the general state of the
patient and the attending complications must be taken into
account. The acute exacerbations of the obstinate disorder
require the same treatment as acute bronchitis.

We meet occasionally with a form of bronchitis in which
the expectorated matter is solid. This *plastic bronchitis* presents all the usual signs and symptoms of bronchial inflammation. It may be chronic, or it may be acute. It is,
perhaps, most frequently chronic, with occasional acute or
subacute exacerbations. The disease extends in this way
over weeks, months, or even years, and is apt to end in complete recovery. But in its acute form it is a complaint of
great danger, and accompanied by much dyspnœa. Males,
as we find by looking at the cases which Dr. Peacock* has
collected, are more often attacked than females. The same
carefully-collated observations show that the disorder affects
more commonly the upper than the lower part of the lungs.
As regards the physical signs, Fuller,† who has met with a

---

* Transactions of the Pathological Society, vol. v.; Medical Times and
Gazette, vol. ix.

† Diseases of the Chest.

number of well-marked examples of the complaint, states that there is weakness or entire absence of breathing over the affected portions of the lungs; and that, from attending collapse, complete and rapidly developed dulness on percussion may ensue. But the only absolutely diagnostic phenomenon is the peculiar membranous material expectorated. In form this may either be in thin shreds, or it may be moulded into an accurate cast of a bronchial tube and its ramifications. The expectoration of the firm bodies is sometimes attended with copious hæmoptysis.

The little round solid pellets which phthisical patients or even some persons in excellent health cough up, from time to time, are the result of a plastic bronchitis on a very limited scale.

Emphysema.—A distention of the air-cells is a frequent sequel of chronic bronchitis. It may happen in only one lung; but the air-vesicles of both are usually distended. The effect of this is to obliterate some of the capillaries, and to interfere with a flow of blood through the lungs. From this proceed, to a great extent, the feeling of constriction and the dyspnœa; from this, further, result the anxious look, the bluish lip of emphysematous patients, and the tendency the disease has to produce dilatation, or dilated hypertrophy of the right side of the heart.

Emphysema is essentially a chronic malady; but in its course, subacute attacks of bronchitis occur which much augment the difficulty of respiration. The trouble in breathing is, indeed, the most prominent of the symptoms. It is not so much the difficulty of getting air into the lung, as it is of getting it out, which annoys the patient. He breathes as if he had no object in life but that of forcing the air out of the pulmonary tissue. And this task is often aggravated by spasmodic narrowing of the bronchial tubes. In fact, nothing is more common than to meet with the loud wheezing of asthma in those whose air-cells are permanently dilated.

The physical signs of emphysema are easily deducible from the pathological conditions. The distention of the lung tissue explains the great prominence and fulness of the

chest, and the displacement of the liver or heart. The ringing clearness on percussion—at times, in fact, almost tympanitic in its character—and the increased resistance to the

FIG. 18.

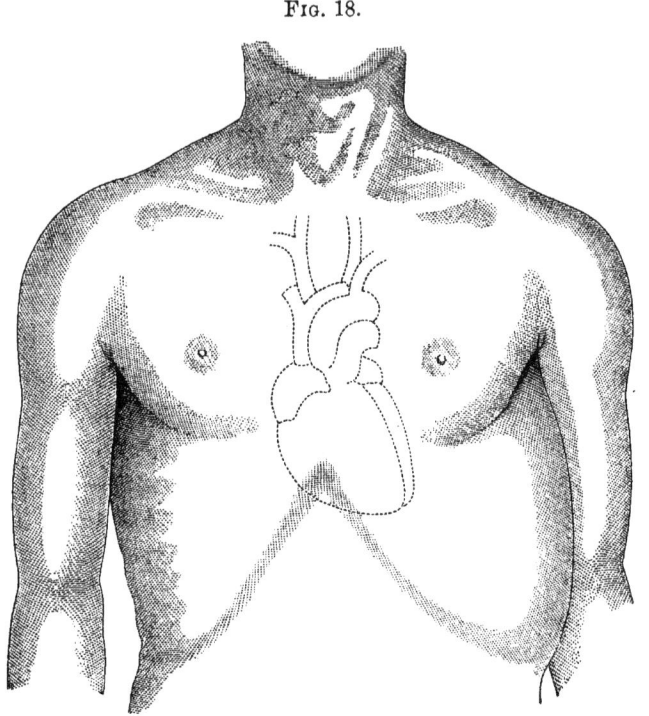

Appearance of the chest in a patient suffering from a high degree of emphysema.
The heart is displaced. The other physical signs are extreme percussion clearness;
a feeble, hardly audible inspiration; a very prolonged expiration.

finger have the same cause. Nor is it difficult to understand
how the loss of elasticity in the dilated air-cells will give
rise to a prolonged expiration, and to a feeble inspiratory
murmur. If bronchitis coexist, the signs on auscultation are
necessarily somewhat altered. The respiration is harsh, or
intermixed with dry and moist rales. The former especially
assume great prominence, and are heard as sonorous, or still
oftener as sibilant rales, during the prolonged and labored
act of expiration. When the emphysema is partial, all these
signs are limited; when more general, they are diffused.

If the upper lobe of the right lung or the lower lobe of the left, which, as Louis* tells us, are the parts most frequently affected, be emphysematous, the visible local bulging might mislead into the idea of the prominence being due to an aneurismal tumor, or to the presence of fluid in the pleural cavity. Any doubt that may have entered the mind will, however, be dispelled by a careful examination of the chest. The dulness over an aneurismal tumor, its pulsation, and its sounds, are different from the exaggerated clearness on percussion, and the changed respiratory murmur of an emphysematous lung. Pleuritic effusions produce a bulging at the lower part of the thorax. But, although there may be a very clear, or rather a tympanitic sound above the fluid, the absolute dulness *over* it shows that the prominence of the chest is not caused by distended air-vesicles. Where the emphysema is very extended and general, there is little or no action of the diaphragm, and the complaint gives rise to displacement of the liver or heart; and this circumstance, taken in connection with the dilatation of the chest and the dyspnœa, brings the malady into a category of affections which will hereafter be more especially examined into. When considering this group, we shall return to emphysema, and point out its distinguishing marks from the disease for which it is most likely to be mistaken, namely, pneumothorax. Let us only add here that in its general forms it is apt to be associated with marked signs of impoverished blood and of cachexia.

But a few words on a special variety of the complaint, one more closely corresponding to what surgeons term emphysema:

An effusion of air may take place into the areolar tissue uniting the lobules of the lungs. There are no physical signs peculiar to this *interlobular emphysema;* they are exactly the same as those furnished by dilatation of the air-cells, except that a dry friction sound and a large, dry crackling (both of which occur occasionally in vesicular emphysema), are very much more common. Nor are there any general circumstances specially indicative of the disease, save its suddenness, and the external emphysema which follows. The latter

---

* Memoires de la Soc. Méd. d'Observat., tome i.

is detected under the jaw, or at the base of the neck, and yields a peculiar crepitation. Yet the extravasation of air into the areolar tissue of the neck is not a constant attendant on the extravasation of air in the lung. Besides, the possibility of a crepitating swelling in the neck being due to a rupture of the bronchial tube or of the larynx, must be borne in mind.

The rupture of the air-cells which gives rise to interlobular emphysema is brought about by any severe effort, by violent coughing, by laughing, or by the throes of parturition. It has also been known to have happened in the course of pneumonia or of pulmonary hemorrhage, and to have caused sudden death. Its most frequent association, however, is with hooping-cough.*

In all of the disorders which have just been treated of, the resonance on percussion has been dwelt upon as a most valuable sign. Before proceeding to consider the diseases in which dulness is encountered, a few words may here find their place on a morbid condition in which clearness rapidly gives way to dulness, and dulness changes quickly back into clearness. As, moreover, the complaint to which I allude—*collapse of the lung*—bears a close connection to bronchitis and emphysema, and has been made to play an important part in the explanation of some of their symptoms and complications, its consideration is at this time most fitting.

In noticing that dulness on percussion sometimes appears in the course of a case of capillary bronchitis, it was remarked that this does not of necessity show that the inflammation has extended to the lobules; it may be owing to the air in the lung being exhausted, and the pulmonary tissue collapsing. Collapse of the lung is thus a return of the organ to a condition akin to its fœtal state, and takes place throughout a large portion of the lungs—diffused collapse—or it is lobular. Formerly the lobular collapse was invariably mistaken for lobular pneumonia; and indeed it is still often so regarded by those who are unwilling to admit that many, it

---

* Roger, Rev. de Thérap. Médic., April, 1862.

may be the larger number of cases of so-called lobular pneumonia, are really cases of bronchitis in which parts of the lung have been deprived of their supply of air and have closed.

The aspect of the lung in lobular pneumonia had attracted the attention of pathologists long before MM. Legendre and Bailly inflated the supposed hepatized lobules, and demonstrated their essential difference from the recognized features of hepatization by restoring them absolutely to their normal condition. This discovery enhanced the importance of bronchitis, and lessened that of lobular pneumonia; for it was soon found that an accumulation in the bronchial tubes was the most frequent exciting cause of that condensation of the pulmonary tissue which had previously been regarded as a sure indication of an inflammation.

These accumulations occasion collapse by shutting up the tube through which the air reaches the air-vesicles. No fresh air can enter; the residual air is gradually exhausted, and the disordered portion of lung is reduced to a state as if it had never breathed. But although in the majority of instances this condition of things is brought about by catarrhal secretions in the bronchial tubes which cannot be expectorated, it would be a mistake to suppose that these are always present. Any want of power to fill the cells of the lung with air may lead to their collapsing. In some of the typhoid forms of acute and chronic diseases, in the pulmonary congestions of the aged and enfeebled, and in those occurring just prior to death, large portions of the lung tissue may collapse simply from inability to breathe with sufficient force.

Such is a sketch of collapse of the lung from a pathological point of view. But when we come to inquire whether the diagnostic signs of this condition are so clearly defined that we can always make out a collapsed state of the pulmonary tissue, we have to admit that our knowledge of the pathological phenomena as yet exceeds our power to recognize them in the living. The physical signs are not very satisfactory; the symptoms vary with the conditions producing the disease. There is dulness as in the other forms of condensation, as in pneumonia, as in pleurisy. Neither voice nor respiration is characteristic. The most usual physical sign is dulness on percussion, with an absence of all respiration, or with a blowing sound, which is faint and not so distinct as in pneumonia. The dulness is, on the whole, not very great, and in cases dependent upon inspissated mucus may disappear suddenly, or nearly suddenly, when the obstructing cause is removed. Yet it must not be forgotten that collapse of the lung is at times a state of long duration. Great stress is laid by some on the signs of emphysema which surround the dulness of the condensed tissue.

When collapse takes place, the breathing becomes very difficult. The patient makes intense efforts at inspiration. Dr. George A. Rees tells us that, owing to the non-expansion of the lung during this inspiratory effort, the ribs move inward and recede, instead of moving outward, as in ordinary respiration. This sign, the suddenly increased dyspnœa, and the appearance of dulness unaccompanied by marked bronchial breathing, are, in a case of bronchitis, the most trustworthy indications that collapse of the lung tissue has taken place. Yet where the collapsed lobules are small and scattered through the lung, these signs are not all present, and the diagnosis is very uncertain. The dulness is wanting; and the peculiarity in inspiration may not be observed.

When collapse affects a large portion of lung, it much resembles lobar pneumonia and pleurisy, from both of which, however, it may often be distinguished by the phenomena indicated, and, still more positively, by the history and the absence of that *group* of symptoms and physical signs which characterizes inflammation of the lung or pleura.*

---

* See, on the subject of collapse, besides the writings referred to of Legendre and Bailly, Archives Génér. de Médic., 1844; Fuchs, Bronchitis der Kinder, Leipsic, 1849; Gairdner, Month. Journal of Med. Science, Edinb., 1850, Brit. and For. Med.-Chirg. Review, April and July, 1853, and Jan. 1854, etc.; Rees, Essay on Collapse, London, 1850; Barthez and Billiet, Maladies des Enfants; and West, Diseases of Childhood.

Diseases in which Dulness on Percussion occurs.

The diseases of the lungs in which dulness on percussion is met with, are all those in which compression or consolidation of the pulmonary tissue takes place. Especially, however, do we find dulness, and the physical signs which accompany it, in tubercular infiltrations, in pneumonia, and in pleurisy.

Phthisis.—Phthisis presents itself in a chronic and in an acute form. The chronic variety is by far the most frequent. It is essentially "the consumption," which is such a scourge to the human race. Beginning usually with a short and insidious cough, with a feeling of lassitude, and a decline in general health; attended at times from its onset with a pain in the affected lung and a somewhat quickened circulation; or giving the first indications of its existence by the occurrence of a hemorrhage; or developing itself after severe bodily or mental fatigue; or traceable to some neglected cold,—the disease becomes fully established, with symptoms which hardly need a detailed description. The harassing cough by day and by night; the impaired appetite and disturbed digestion; the loss of blood from the lungs; the steadily augmenting debility; the short breathing; the exhausting night-sweats; the hectic fever; the deceptive blush which this imparts to the cheek; the increased lustre of the eye; the singular hopefulness; the temporary improvements; the relapses; and the greater vividness of the imagination, so strongly contrasting with the waning frame,—are phenomena with which sad experience has made not only every physician, but many a fireside familiar.

The most constant of all these symptoms are the hemorrhage, the cough, and the emaciation. The *cough* of phthisis is at first dry, and followed by a frothy expectoration. As the disease advances, the sputa thicken. They become greenish in color, streaked with yellow, and "nummular," consisting of large greenish masses of a rounded form, or sometimes rounded yet with jagged edges, which masses do not sink in the cup containing them, but float imperfectly in a condensation, as in pneumonia, as in pleurisy. Neither voice nor respiration is characteristic. The most usual physical sign is dulness on percussion, with an absence of all respiration, or with a blowing sound, which is faint and not so distinct as in pneumonia. The dulness is, on the whole, not very great, and in cases dependent upon inspissated mucus may disappear suddenly, or nearly suddenly, when the obstructing cause is removed. Yet it must not be forgotten that collapse of the lung is at times a state of long duration. Great stress is laid by some on the signs of emphysema which surround the dulness of the condensed tissue.

When collapse takes place, the breathing becomes very difficult. The patient makes intense efforts at inspiration. Dr. George A. Rees tells us that, owing to the non-expansion of the lung during this inspiratory effort, the ribs move inward and recede, instead of moving outward, as in ordinary respiration. This signifies suddenly increased dyspnœa, and the appearance of dulness unaccompanied by marked bronchial breathing, or, in a case of bronchitis, the most trustworthy indication that collapse of the lung tissue has taken place. Yet where the collapsed lobules are small and scattered through the lung, these signs are not all present, and the diagnosis is very uncertain. The dulness is wanting; and the peculiarity in inspiration may not

When collapse affects a large portion of lung, it much resembles lobar pneumonia and pleurisy, from both of which however, it may often be distinguished by the phenomena indicated, and, still more positively, by the history and the absence of that group of symptoms and physical signs which characterises inflammation of the lung or pleura.[*]

[*] See, on the subject of collapse, besides the writings referred to above, Gairdner, Archives ... in Medic. Sept. ... Kinder, London, 1850; Gairdner, Month. Journal of ... Phys. Soc. and For. Med. Chir. Review, April ... 1851 etc. ; Spec. Essay on Disease, London ... Maladies des Enfants, and the disease of ...

thin serum.   This "money-like" expectoration is, however, by no means pathognomonic of the malady.   Cases of phthisis occur without it; and, on the other hand, it is occasionally encountered in chronic bronchitis.   In the last stages of consumption, the sputa are often homogeneous, and have a dirty-grayish, decidedly purulent aspect.   Examined microscopically, they show fragments of the structure of the lung, many pus-cells, exudation-globules, and those peculiar granular bodies which are regarded as characteristic of tubercle.   Yet the microscope does not aid us very much in the diagnosis of phthisis.   The only appearances in the sputum at all distinctive, are the fragments of the pulmonary fibrous tissue and the so-called tubercle-corpuscles.   But, though from the presence of the former we are sometimes enabled to suspect the existence of consumption before the physical signs of even its early stages are well defined, we can never be quite certain that the breakage of the lung texture is due to tubercular disease,   And as regards the so-called tubercle-corpuscles, they are always very difficult to distinguish from shrivelled pus-cells, and their absence in the expectoration does not disprove the possibility of the lungs being filled with tubercles. An excellent way of finding the lung tissue is by the plan proposed by Dr. Fenwick*—to liquefy the sputum by means of pure caustic soda, when any particles which may be contained in it fall to the bottom of the vessel, and can be readily removed and placed under the microscope.

In another manner, too, has it been proposed to make use of the sputum for diagnostic purposes.   Taking as a starting-point the discovery of Villemain, that tubercular matter can be inoculated from man to animals, Dr. William Marcet† suggests the inoculation of the expectoration of persons considered as phthisical.   From his experiments on guinea-pigs, he found that these animals die of tubercular disease, or on being killed thirty days after inoculation, exhibit tubercles in their organs, when inoculated with tubercular sputum.

In rare instances, the cough remains slight throughout the malady; but generally it is a very distressing feature of the

---

* Medico-Chirurg. Transactions, vol. xlix.   † Ibid , vol. l.

complaint, and is particularly worrying at night. Sometimes its violent paroxysms bring on vomiting.

Among the less constant and distinctive symptoms of pulmonary consumption are a troublesome and rebellious diarrhœa, chronic laryngitis and pharyngitis, and the red line around the border of the gum. In some persons this gingival line is a mere streak; in others it is more than a line in breadth; in none is it a certain indication of phthisis. A sign which has a much more definite connection with tubercular disease of the lungs is the strange appearance of the nails. The end of the finger is somewhat clubbed; the nail is curved, prominent in the centre, depressed at the sides, its surface slightly cracked, its appearance bluish. This peculiar condition of the nails is not always present; yet it is tolerably constant, and is sometimes met with even in the earlier stages of the disease. A similar nail is, however, seen in chronic pleurisy and in diseases of the heart.

Another symptom of phthisis of significance is the heightened temperature as ascertained by the thermometer. Ringer,* who in an able essay has drawn attention to the subject, states, indeed, that the temperature may be greatly elevated for several weeks before we find physical signs indicative of the deposition of tubercle, or of an undoubted increase in the already existing deposition. It is furthermore maintained, that the rise in the heat of the body closely corresponds to the activity of the deposition of the tubercle. If the temperature be decidedly and permanently elevated throughout the day, there is active deposition; if normal, or nearly so at one period, though at another it rises to considerable height, the deposition is less active; and it is slow if the rise be far less marked. When the animal heat is normal, the deposition in the lungs has ceased, and the tubercular process is arrested or retrogressing.

These statements are clinically of importance; but, I think, from repeatedly examining into the matter, that they are not to be trusted absolutely. They only represent a general truth, and do not aid us much, for instance, in lingering lung

---

* On the Temperature of the Body.   London, 1865.

complications in febrile states, nor in affections intercurrent in phthisis, nor in certain forms of persistent non-tubercular consolidations.

The symptoms which precede a fatal termination are various, and depend on the precise manner in which the formidable malady ends. Patients may go on failing for years; or an attack of acute phthisis, of pneumonia, or of inflammation of the brain or of the intestinal tract may at any time result in death.

But at no stage of the disease do we derive as exact knowledge from a study of its symptoms as we do from a study of its physical signs. Before explaining these, it is necessary to recall briefly some facts connected with the general laws governing tubercle.

Tubercle is an unorganized substance, the deposits of which are at first isolated, then accumulate, and lead to consolidation of the part. The tendency of tubercular matter is to soften and to destroy the textures among which it is infiltrated. It may undergo at any period in its course a retrogressive development, by shrivelling up, or by passing into a calcareous state. When situated in the lungs, it seeks the apices by preference; it is rarely limited to one lung, although one lung is usually the most diseased, and often at the beginning of the malady alone affected. It is not merely a local complaint, but it stands in connection with a peculiar, tainted state of the constitution; hence the symptoms of phthisis are not solely the expressions of the condition of the lungs.

These pathological facts are all of the greatest importance. They tell us where to seek for the earliest indications of a deposit. They explain to us its signs. They teach us to look further than the lungs, and prepare us for finding lesions in other organs. They point out the path which alone promises to lead to any result in treatment.

In accordance with the laws affecting tubercular depositions, we have three stages of phthisis, which run, however, by almost imperceptible degrees into each other. They are:

1. Incipient stage, or commencing deposition;
2. More complete deposition, occasioning consolidation;

3. Stage of softening and formation of cavities.

1. A few scattered tubercles do not change the normal percussion resonance; nor do they appreciably alter the natural breathing sounds heard on auscultation. But as soon as the deposit is at all sufficient to impair the elasticity of the lung tissue or increase its density, a relative loss of clearness on percussion on one side, and modifications of the vesicular murmur, such as feeble or jerking inspiration, or a prolonged expiration, may be ascertained. The dulness is most readily detected by percussing the patient with his mouth open and during a fixed expiration. To find it at the upper part of the chest posteriorly, the position recommended by Dr. Corson,*

FIG. 19.

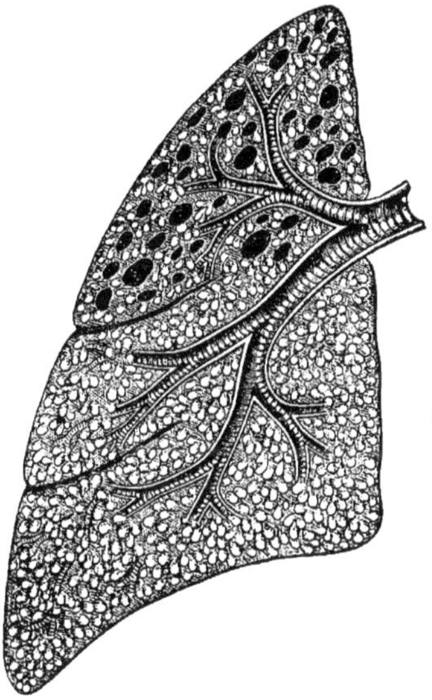

Slight percussion dulness.

Feeble or harsh respiration.

Prolonged Expiration.......

Exaggerated respiration.

Commencing infiltration; masses of tubercle have accumulated, but the intervening lung tissue is still healthy.

of crossing the arms and clasping the shoulders, is very advantageous. In a certain number of cases, with the slight dulness on percussion and changed breathing is associated a blowing sound in the subclavian or in the pulmonary artery. A mur-

* New York Journal of Medicine, March, 1859.

mur is, indeed, at times present in the pulmonary artery long before any other physical indication of tubercle is discernible. All these physical signs may be accompanied by rales of various kinds. What makes them significant is, that they occur at the upper portion of the lung, whether anteriorly or posteriorly. If, therefore, any modification of the vesicular murmur, or any adventitious sound limited to the apex, exist; if there be a slight dulness on percussion above or under the clavicle, or in the supra-spinous fossa; if this coincide with flattening of the anterior surface of the chest, especially on one side, with defective expansion of the thorax and shortness of breath, with a cough and falling off in general health,—the diagnosis of commencing tubercular disease is almost positive.

2. As the infiltration advances, the signs become more decidedly those of consolidation. Greater dulness on percussion at the upper portion of one or of both lungs; more resistance to the percussing finger; stronger vocal resonance; a sinking in of the side most affected, and often soreness to the touch over the diseased part; a very harsh murmur; or, when the infiltration surrounds the bronchial tubes, a distinct blowing respiration,—are all present in varying degree, and all denote consolidation. And chronic consolidation at the apex has, in the large majority of instances, but one interpretation: phthisis. In the second stage, as well as in the first, we often meet with superadded signs of bronchitis which occasionally mask the respiratory sounds, and with friction sounds from local pleurisies, or with fine crackling.

3. The diseased organ now passes into a state of softening, or rather some portions of the lung begin to soften while others remain indurated, and in yet others fresh infiltration takes place. Moist crackling or persistent moist rales indicate that softening has begun. The broken-down material may be expectorated, and the malady for a time be stayed; but such is not often the case. The area of the softened mass widens; cavities form; and in addition to the moist rales, to the physical phenomena of the second stage, and to the increasing debility, night-sweats and hectic, the signs indicative of a cavity are noticed. What these are, may be learned from

the engraving on this page. But the hollow, cavernous respiration may be caught only in expiration, or it may be

FIG. 20.

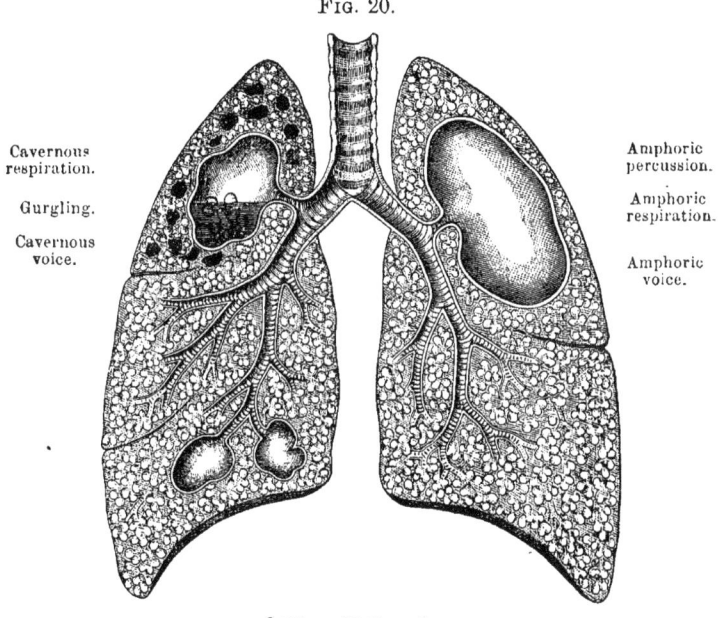

Cavernous respiration.

Gurgling.

Cavernous voice.

Amphoric percussion.

Amphoric respiration.

Amphoric voice.

Cavities of various sizes.

temporarily superseded by very large bubbling sounds—gurgling. Again, over small or over very deep-seated cavities none of these sounds may be perceived; and, in truth, even when they exist, their limitation to a particular locality is an element in the diagnosis of a cavity almost as important as their presence.

The results of percussion over an excavation are not always the same, nor can they be relied upon. They depend too much on the thickness and the state of the walls of the cavity. If dense, percussion yields a dull sound; if thin, a tympanitic, or its varieties, a cracked-pot or metallic sound. If only a certain amount of indurated tissue intervene between them and the surface of the chest, a singular sound, a mixture of dull and tympanitic, is produced. If healthy lung tissue form the walls of the excavation, the sound is clear, or nearly so. Moreover, in all cases the pitch, and, to some extent, the character, of the sound are changed by percussing over the cavity while the mouth is kept open. When it is shut, the sound elicited is of lower pitch. Another sign by which we may judge of the existence of a cavity at the upper part of the lung, is the extraordinary clearness with which the heart sounds are heard at that point, and the perception of a waving impulse in the second intercostal space.

Such, then, are the physical signs which indicate the varied structural conditions of the lung in the three stages of phthisis. With these signs are associated, as symptoms: cough, increasing quickness of breathing, progressive debility, hectic fever, digestive disorders, and emaciation—symptoms the occurrence and severity of which mark also, though not very accurately, the periods of the malady. But irrespective of these three stages, some have admitted a stage preceding the deposition of the tubercles. That such a pretubercular stage exists, is not improbable; that to be able to recognize it would be one of the most important and valuable gifts to practical medicine, is undoubted; but whether it be recognizable, is another matter. It does not seem to me that the advocates of the possibility of detecting phthisis at this stage have clearly proved their point. On the one hand, they lay claim to signs, such as diminished expansion of the chest, decreased vital capacity, a murmur, feeble and remaining feeble on forced breathing, hæmoptysis, even slight dulness on percussion—a combination which we are accustomed to regard as evidence that tubercle already exists; on the other hand, they assert that defects of temperature, lessened muscular power, improper assimilation, emaciation, sorethroat, and slight, dry cough, are prodromic symptoms. Yet all of these may be associated with a temporary derangement of health, and all of these are far more frequently so associated than with threatening consumption. And to say that they become of value only when coexisting with the physical signs alluded to, is but saying that they are the clinical phenomena which, thus grouped, we are in the habit of accepting as proof of the first stage of the disease. But without entering further into this question, it may be stated that the deposition can generally be detected at a very early period by careful explorations of the chest, and by connecting the physical signs with other sources of information, such as the symptoms and the history of the case.

Let us now examine the disorders with which phthisis, in its various stages, is likely to be confounded. They are, to speak of thoracic affections only:

CHRONIC BRONCHITIS;

CHRONIC PNEUMONIC CONSOLIDATION;

CHRONIC PLEURISY;

PULMONARY CANCER;

SYPHILITIC DISEASE OF THE LUNGS;

BRONCHIAL DILATATION;

PULMONARY ABSCESS;

PULMONARY GANGRENE.

Chronic Bronchitis.—The first stage of consumption is particularly prone to be mistaken for chronic bronchitis. Nor is the diagnosis always easy. Distinct dulness on percussion at the apex is of much aid in discrimination, especially if it be on the left side. On the right side it is of far less value, unless marked alterations of the vesicular murmur correspond to it. When the dulness is not discernible, we have to depend, in our efforts at a separation of the two diseases, on the history of the case, the limitation of the physical signs to the apex, and the proofs of increased activity of the surrounding lung. Cough and expectoration are common to both affections. But they are associated, in chronic bronchitis, with physical signs more or less diffused through both lungs, and unaccompanied by much constitutional disturbance; while from the onset of phthisis, the falling off in general health is out of proportion to the local lesions. Yet until crackling or some dulness on percussion is perceived, no absolute diagnosis is possible. These indications of beginning consolidation settle the diagnosis against bronchitis. And this view of a case will be strengthened, if hemorrhage have occurred without any other more certain cause to account for it than the tubercles which are presumed to exist, and if the phenomena are present in a person born of a family in which consumption is hereditary.

Where the deposition is at all extensive, an erroneous diagnosis of bronchitis is with ordinary care impossible, unless, as isi always highly improbable, phthisis should be complicated with emphysema, or the tubercles be quiescent and so diffused as not to impair the resonance on percussion. Under the latter circumstances especially, the occasional tympanitic character of the sound over the seat of the tubercular deposition is very liable to be misconstrued into increased clearness on percussion, and into an absolute disproval of the existence of phthisis. When tubercle and emphysema coexist, the percussion note may really be pulmonary and like that of healthy lung. We would then have to judge of the one disease following the other mainly by the respiratory sound, which becomes much feebler; generally, too, the dyspnœa is increased. Perhaps the thermometer, as Ringer suggests, by showing a higher temperature than in pure emphysema, may assist us in the diagnosis.

In the stage in which the signs of consolidation become well defined, phthisis may be mistaken for any of those conditions which occasion the physical signs indicative of greater density of the lung tissue, and which are accompanied by cough and by loss of flesh. Such are particularly pneumonic consolidation, pleuritic effusion, and cancerous deposits.

Chronic Pneumonic Consolidation.—Chronic pneumonic consolidation, or, as the affection is commonly called, chronic pneumonia, gives rise to many manifestations which simulate consumption. These are cough, emaciation, and the local signs of chronic pulmonary condensation—increased voice and fremitus, sinking in of the chest wall, feeble inspiration and prolonged expiration, or a fully-developed bronchial respiration. But in pneumonic consolidation the history usually points to an antecedent acute affection; the health is not so much impaired; there has been no hemorrhage, although, owing to an intervening acute bronchitis, the sputa at times may have been streaked with blood; and the dulness on percussion and the other physical signs of consolidation are, for the most part, perceived over the lower lobe of *one* lung.

This position of the physical signs is of great importance. Yet there are two sources of fallacy which may arise. On the one hand, tubercles may, by way of exception, be seated in the lower lobe; on the other, chronic pneumonic induration may affect the apex. When an infiltration of tubercle takes place in the lower lobe, its distinction from chronic pneumonic condensation is very difficult. Our only guides are the evidence furnished by the graver constitutional symptoms of phthisis, and attention to that pathological law which teaches that consumption is not met with in an advanced state in one lung alone; hence we must examine accurately and watch carefully the other lung. While it is not involved, there is certainly reason to conclude against the tubercular character of the deposit. In like manner, by ascertaining the one-sidedness of the disease, and by noting the want of those serious symptoms which go hand in hand with the physical signs of phthisis, we may determine the real nature of the case when an inflammation of the upper lobe has resulted in its persistent induration. To adduce a few instances, by way of illustration:

A gentleman has been under my care for years, in whom, after pulmonary inflammation, signs of condensation remained in the upper part of the right lung. He does not suffer at all, excepting from attacks of acute bronchitis, to which he is very liable. During these he loses flesh; but when they pass off he rapidly regains it. He has a chronic cough, but it is slight.

In another case, with a similar history, I found dulness on percussion, prolonged expiration, and a friction sound limited to the apex of the right lung. There had been a continuous cough, but very little constitutional disturbance, in fact next to none, and no hemorrhage. The abnormal signs lasted for a year, and then almost disappeared under a succession of blisters, and the cough ceased.

In both cases the signs were entirely confined to the summit of one lung. I had some time since under observation a patient affected much in the same manner, a man of seventy-five years of age, in whom the dulness at the right apex had for years remained stationary. I might cite further examples; but these are sufficient to justify the conclusions that can be drawn from the facts mentioned. And ought not such instances to make us careful in our deductions?

Ought they not to have their full weight when estimating the cures of supposed cases of consumption by cod-liver oil, or by any other remedy?

But to return to the points of difference between chronic induration of the lung and phthisis. They may be thus summed up: when the signs of consolidation, whether existing at the upper part of the lung or not, are out of proportion to the general symptoms, there is reason to believe that they are not the result of tubercular infiltration. The non-occurrence of hemorrhage would tend to strengthen such an inference. But the most important information is drawn from watching whether the physical signs undergo changes indicative of a deposit in the hitherto healthy portions of the pulmonary texture. And it must be confessed that minute and accurate examinations having reference directly to this point are sometimes the only means through which anything like a positive opinion can be reached. Hence time and repeated observations are important elements in the diagnosis.

In so close a manner, then, may phthisis be imitated by chronic pneumonic induration. It is true, this disease is a rare one; yet we meet with it more frequently than authors on diseases of the chest imply, who, for the most part, ignore induration of the pulmonary tissue, excepting as a local attendant on cancerous or tubercular depositions.

But a great and complicating difficulty in the differential diagnosis remains to be mentioned. It grows out of the circumstance that tubercular disease may be devoloped in a lung which is in a state of chronic induration. I cannot enter here into the question whether latent tubercle may not have preceded the pneumonia which has lapsed into the chronic malady. Be that as it may, the fact cannot be disputed that we find persons in apparently excellent health, and without a trace of any pulmonary disorder, seized with an inflammation of the lung, which is followed by persistent consolidation, and in the course of time by undoubted phthisis. I have noted a number of such instances, and I cannot but believe that many of the reported cases of tubercle affecting primarily the lower lobe of the lung are, in reality, cases of tubercle following chronic pneumonic consolidation.

The history of these patients is usually as follows: a person previously in all respects healthy is attacked with an acute pulmonary affection. He recovers from it, but with a trifling cough, with a persistent dulness on percussion, and a feeble respiration, heard over one of his lungs. He continues ailing, yet is not positively sick, when, without any apparent cause, after a time varying from a few months to years, his cough increases, the expectoration augments greatly in quantity and becomes decidedly purulent, and he commences to emaciate rapidly. Profuse night-sweats occur; and the physical signs, which have been stationary for a long time, now begin to change. The dulness extends; and instead of the enfeebled respiration, a harsher, blowing respiration is perceived over the affected part, and moist crackling and the signs of a cavity follow. Doubt may still exist as to the nature of the malady, but the advance of the disease clears it up. True to the laws of tubercle, a deposit takes place in the lung previously sound, and not at the lower portion, but at its apex.

Hemorrhage may or may not occur. In the patient from whose case the above description is drawn, it did not happen; and in others, too, it was wanting. Its presence is, therefore, strongly in favor of the fact that tubercles have been developed; its absence does not positively prove the contrary.

I leave these remarks as they were originally written. Of late years a school of pathologists, with Niemeyer at their head, have endeavored to re-establish the old doctrine that consumption of the lung and the formation of cavities are most frequently the result of chronic inflammation. According to this view, the kind of cases just discussed belong to that grand group of phthisis in which the pneumonic process terminates in caseous degeneration and destruction of tissue. This group, the most common form of consumption, presents somewhat different traits according to the rapidity of its development. It differs from the true tuberculous consumption, due to a tubercular deposit, in this: the latter has no precursory catarrh, the fever and the emaciation are not deferred until the expectoration becomes profuse and purulent, the patient first wastes, and then begins to cough and expectorate. At first the physical examination of the chest gives negative results, and even at a later period the solidification is not so extensive as in the first form of consumption,—that following inflammation. Of this, however, it is assumed as one of the dangers, that it may become tuberculous, though even then the morbid process appearing at an advanced stage of the phthisis has but little to do with disorganization of the lungs. How the tubercle arises is not certain, but it has some indirect connection with the cheesy changes of the products of the inflammation.

Chronic Pleurisy.—A persistent cough attended with emaciation and with dulness on percussion is common to chronic pleurisy and to phthisis, and is a cause of many errors in diagnosis. But with care such errors may be avoided; certainly by those who pay any attention to physical diagnosis. The seat of the dulness at the lower part of the thorax; its much more absolute character; the almost entire cessation of all sound of respiration; the diminished or absent vibration of the chest walls when the patient speaks; the dilatation of the affected side,—are in striking contrast with signs most manifest at the apex, with the distinctly-prolonged expiration, with the rales and the evidences of commencing softening. Nor are the symptoms of a pleuritic effusion as grave as those produced by phthisis. Even where the fluid filling the chest is pus, we do not find hectic fever so intense, emaciation so great, or night-sweats so constant and exhausting. And the patient coughs less, and never spits up blood.

In those cases of chronic pleurisy in which the side, instead of being dilated, is retracted, the diagnosis is more difficult. Attention to the seat of dulness being at the lower part of the chest, to the diminished respiration, voice and fremitus, and to the shrinking affecting only one side of the thorax, will, however, serve as the foundation for a correct conclusion.

Tubercle may complicate pleuritic effusions. We suspect this by the occurrence of hemorrhage, and by the marked emaciation and hectic. We can only be sure of it by finding signs of deposit on the non-affected side, which deposit, in accordance with the custom of tubercular disease, will take place first at the apex. Chronic *double* pleurisy is very apt to be associated with a tubercular affection of the lungs.

Pulmonary Cancer.—Cancer of the lung has many symptoms which it shares with tubercle. Emaciation, cough, night-sweats, hemorrhage, gradual wasting belong to both diseases, as do also the signs of pulmonary consolidation. But cancerous formations are usually limited to one lung. Only one side of the chest is, therefore, flattened; the other looks distended. Over the cancerous lung the percussion dulness is very great. There is either very loud, blowing respiration, or, if the mass have obliterated a bronchus, enfeebled or absent breathing. We find no rales; but all the signs of consolidation are much more perfect than in tubercle. Owing to a cancerous deposit in the mediastinum, the dulness at times extends beyond the median line. Cancer in the lung may soften; yet the signs of softening are very rarely as manifest as they are in tubercle. The sputa are purulent, or like currant-jelly. Further, a cancerous tint of the skin may be present; and again, cancerous tumors in other parts of the body become next to absolute evidence in favor of a deposit in the lung being cancerous, since with rare, very rare exceptions, cancer and tubercle do not coexist. The different character of the pain must also be taken into account. In tubercle, it is transitory and shifting; in cancer, it is much more constant, and usually much more severe.*

Syphilitic Disease of the Lungs.—Syphilis may lead to tubercular disease of the lungs. But it will also occasion a specific form of bronchitis, preceding the syphilitic eruption; or produce gummata, which may soften and be eliminated, and which, according to Ricord, form in the lungs toward their periphery and base. When syphilis manifests itself in the pulmonary structures, it gives rise to most of the phenomena of phthisis. The chief differences are, that the nodules affect generally only one lung, and principally the base or the lower part of the upper lobe, that they remain circumscribed, not spreading to the surrounding textures, and occasion, as a rule, neither hæmoptysis, nor fever, nor decided

---

* Compare, on this subject, the cases collected by Bennett in his Clinical Lectures; by Hughes, Guy's Hospital Reports, 1st Series, vol. ii.; by Stokes, Dub. Journ. of Med., vol. xxi.

emaciation. Still, the syphilitic affection can only be distinguished with certainty by the history of the case, and by the thickening of the periosteum of the head of one or both clavicles. Milroy,* in his investigations on soldiers, also lays stress on the thickening of the perichondrium of one or more of the upper cartilages, with frequently a tumefaction of the soft parts between them and the skin. To these tests may be added that recognized by Broderick†—substernal tenderness as a means of diagnosis of acquired syphilitic taint. In all cases, we must be careful that the thickcuing at the upper part of the chest walls and the altered resonance thus occasioned be not looked upon as a sign of a tubercular consolidation.

The preceding diseases are most likely to be confounded with the stages of consumption prior to softening and the formation of cavities. Next, to review those affections which, like phthisis, occasion the signs of excavation, and which, therefore, may be mistaken for its third stage: they are, chiefly, bronchial dilatation, abscess, and gangrene of the lung.

Bronchial Dilatation.—A dilatation of the bronchial tubes takes place in two forms: either the tubes are uniformly dilated and like the fingers of a glove, or else they form cavities by undergoing a saccular enlargement. The former variety furnishes the symptoms and physical signs of a case of chronic bronchitis, attended with copious expectoration. The percussion clearness may be slightly lessened, owing to the condensation of the surrounding pulmonary tissue; the respiration be more strictly bronchial; but otherwise, both symptoms and signs are those of chronic bronchial inflammation.

In the globular form of dilatation, however, we meet with all the sounds of tubercular excavations: the hollow, blowing respiration; the hollow, well-transmitted voice; gurgling; even metallic tinkling. Yet all these phenomena are in strange contrast to the almost unimpaired health, and to the

---

* British Army Medical Report, quoted in Annals of Milit. and Naval Surg., vol. i., 1863.

† Madras Medical Journal, July, 1865.

non-occurrence of hemorrhage, of night-sweats, and of emaciation. Hence when we find the signs of a cavity, and when the general symptoms do not indicate that profound constitutional disturbance with which consumption is always associated, we may suspect a bronchial dilatation. This suspicion becomes a certainty, if the cavity be at the middle or lower portion of the lung, and if the resonance on percussion be but little impaired. For it is settled beyond doubt that, in bronchial dilatation, the dulness over the seat of the disease is very slight; certainly not nearly so great as that yielded by the dense walls of a tubercular excavation. It is also true that the dulness on percussion, for the most part, follows, and does not precede the auscultatory phenomena of a cavity. And we find further evidence of the affection not being tubercular, in the stationary character of the physical signs: for months they do not change; whereas in phthisis they continually alter with the advancing malady. The expectoration of bronchial dilatation, too, is generally more abundant than that of consumption, and in very chronic cases fetid, suggesting, indeed, at times, the probability of the existence of gangrene. Nor does it look like the sputum of phthisis, for it is much more fluid, and in the watery secretion small masses of pus float, far less coherent and compact than the nummular sputum of phthisis. As regards the cough of dilated bronchi, it is much more persistent, being constant by day and night, and only at times relieved by expectoration, which then varies in copiousness according to the size of the sac.*

Skoda† describes, as a peculiar physical sign present in sacculated bronchial dilatation, a large and coarse crackling, called by him the large bubbling, dry crepitant rale. In a case which came under my observation, the diagnosis was made by this auscultatory sign. The patient, a boy aged twelve years, had swallowed a bone, which lodged in a bronchial tube, and gave rise to bronchitis and bronchial widening. He died subsequently of acute meningitis, and the

---

* Skoda, Allgem. Wien. Mediz. Zeitung, 1864, No. 26.
† Perkussion und Auskultation.

bone was found firmly imbedded on one side of the globularly-dilated bronchial tube.

Pulmonary Abscesses.—The circumstance that cavities or abscesses in the lung tissue are so generally caused by softening tubercles, makes physicians overlook the fact that abscesses of the lung occur unconnected with tubercular disease. Such abscesses may form in the course of acute pneumonia, but are not then likely to be mistaken for chronic phthisis. Different is it with abscesses which are developed three or four months after an attack of pneumonia, and where the lung texture has remained partially consolidated. I have seen not a few examples of chronic induration of the lung terminating in this way. A man who was shot through the lung was seized, soon after the injury, with inflammation of that organ. Percussion dulness and blowing respiration continued at the lower part of the left lung, notwithstanding all efforts to remove the lymph which caused them. One day, after exertion, he suddenly expectorated a considerable amount of pus. The signs of a cavity were detected at once; but they have since disappeared, and perfect recovery has taken place. In another case of pneumonia, the disease in like manner lapsed into a chronic state. Five months after the acute attack, the evidences of an excavation became manifest at the edge of the right scapula, and existed there for two months; then, so far as physical signs could prove, the cavity closed. Instead of the hollow, blowing respiration and gurgling, only a somewhat roughened vesicular murmur was perceived.

Such is, however, not always the termination. The abscess may grow larger and larger, until the entire lung, as proved by post-mortem examination, is destroyed.

These abscesses differ from bronchial dilatation in not being permanent and fixed. They have this in common with tubercular excavations—they change. They increase like these; but further, they do, what tubercular cavities do not, they decrease. Their physical signs are in every respect like those of all cavities, and vary with the size of the excavation. Sometimes metallic respiration and voice may be heard over it; or perforation of the pleura produces the signs of pneumothorax with effusion. In fortunate instances the pus is expectorated, or the abscess opens externally, and a cure is thus established. But very large abscesses are apt to wear out the patient. Hectic fever, and occasional hemorrhage, attend them; yet neither is so constant a symptom as it is in consumption. The sputa are usually copious, purulent, and very fetid, differing in this respect from the expectoration of phthisis. Again, abscess of the lung may be distinguished from tubercular disease by being ordinarily situated at the base of the organ; by its following—although there are exceptions to this rule—pneumonic consolidation; by the occurrence of copious expectoration being often, not constantly, sudden; but, especially, by its limitation to one lung. The other lung remains perfectly healthy. It may enlarge, and its murmur be more distinct; but all its movements and sounds denote its texture to be in a normal condition.

The small amount of constitutional disturbance which pulmonary abscesses sometimes entail is very remarkable. In several patients, in whom I have noticed abscess of the lung consequent upon chronic pulmonary consolidation, the physical signs of a large cavity were in strange contrast to the regular pulse, the easy breathing, the slight cough, and the healthy complexion.

To tabulate the differences between a tubercular excavation and a pulmonary abscess:

PULMONARY ABSCESS.	CAVITY FROM PHTHISIS.
Signs of cavity usually at the lower lobe.	Signs in the upper lobe.
Copius and purulent sputa.	Sputa less copious; and at first nummular.
Comparatively small amount of constitutional disturbance.	Graver symptoms, and a different history.
One lung affected.	Usually both lungs affected.

Pulmonary Gangrene.—Another disease which yields the signs of an excavation, and which, like phthisis, is attended with wasting of the body, here claims attention. Gangrene of the lung occurs either as diffused or as circumscribed gangrene, after pneumonia, from blows on the chest, or from

18

poisoned blood. The physical signs are those of a cavity, seated usually in the lower portion of the lung. The symptoms are: great and increasing prostration, dyspnœa, a very pale face, a quick pulse, hemorrhage, emaciation, and a cough, followed by profuse purulent sputum of a greenish or brown color. But nearly all these symptoms happen also in phthisis. What is characteristic of gangrene, is the extreme fetor of the expectoration and of the breath. The sickening odor is not perceived during each act of breathing, but mainly after coughing, and, as it were, in jets. It is the symptom by which, especially if taken in connection with the signs of breaking up of the pulmonary tissue, gangrene is with certainty recognized; and without it, a diagnosis is impossible. Some authors lay stress on the fact that a cavity is found in only one lung, and at its lower part. This is unquestionably of aid in discriminating between phthisis and gangrene; but it does not distinguish between a gangrenous excavation and a simple abscess of the lung. The only positive proof of gangrene of the lung is, as just stated, that the signs of breaking down of the pulmonary tissue are accompanied by a most disgusting and more or less persistent fetor of the expectoration and of the breath. I say persistent, because local gangrene, on a small scale, occurring around tubercular cavities or in bronchitis, may give rise to temporary extreme fetor of the breath. But it is only temporary, and therefore not liable to lead to fallacious inferences. The expectoration may be fetid in cases of bronchial dilatation or of abscess of the lung, but is never brownish, as in gangrene; and neither it nor the breath has that peculiar gangrenous odor which makes the patient as unbearable to himself as to his attendants.*

---

* But what that odor is, is very difficult to define. Dr. Laycock (Edinb. Med. Journ., May, 1865) states that there are three distinct kinds of pulmonary fetor—that of ozæna, that of feces, that of gangrene. The latter, due to putrescent decomposition of pulmonary tissue, is characteristic of true gangrene. The ozæna odor is connected with chronic tissue changes of rheumatic origin, as with fibrinous exudation and degeneration. It is found chiefly in fetid bronchitis and bronchorrhœa, and in fetid fibroid vomicæ. The fecal odor may also be observed under these circumstances, and has, too, probably a rheumatic origin. In rare instances pleurisy with

The complaints just considered exhibit thus, all of them, points in which they are similar, and all of them points in which they are dissimilar, to pulmonary consumption. Others might be added which are sometimes mistaken for this malady, such as dyspepsia, chronic diarrhœa, chronic laryngitis, chronic pharyngitis, and thoracic pains. But each of these, although it may accompany tubercular consumption, and even mask some of its symptoms, lacks, when it is present as an idiopathic affection, those local evidences of deposition and softening, lacks that profound constitutional disturbance which forms as much a part of phthisis as the disease in the lungs. Throughout, then, the wide range of affections with which this fatal malady may be confounded, we find invariably appearing as landmarks those pathological laws which impart to the complaint a distinctive character, and which teach us:

That pulmonary tubercle is not merely a disorder of the lungs, but is accompanied by a special train of vital symptoms, in their gravity often out of proportion to the local lesions.

That tubercular matter is usually deposited at the apex of the lung.

That it invades in its progress both organs.

And clinically speaking, we find that while not a symptom, hardly a physical sign, is strictly peculiar to the disease, yet that in no other malady do they appear in exactly the same combinations.

In the above remarks on the diagnosis of pulmonary consumption, the complaint has been assumed to be progressive; but in rare instances it retrogresses. Now before dismissing the subject of phthisis, the signs by which such retrogression can be discovered may be alluded to. They are not very fixed. In those cases in which many tubercles undergo a cretaceous transformation, calcareous particles are coughed up; the signs of softening cease; the apex flattens; and a

fetid effusion may occasion a fecal smell of the expectoration and breath, which is gradually lost, as happened in the case reported by Dr. William Moore (Dub. Quart. Journ , May, 1865).

feeble murmur, with prolonged expiration, or a harsh respiration, with slight dulness on percussion, is all that remains to indicate that tubercular disease has existed. It is hardly necessary to say that the cough stops, and that flesh and strength return. These phenomena may be noted even when large cavities have existed. But, unfortunately, it is not often that we have opportunities to make such observations.*

We meet occasionally with instances in which the physical signs of an infiltration into the lung tissue depart with tolerable rapidity. They occur in those who have a decidedly scrofulous aspect, enlargement of the glands of the neck, or a scrofulous inflammation of the eyes. In accordance with the generally acknowledged identity of scrofula and tubercle, we should be forced to admit that the disease in the lungs is tubercular. Yet the connection with the enlarged lymphatics; the circumstance that the diminution in size of the glands is often followed by distinct evidence of increased pulmonary deposits; that these depositions are very beneficially influenced by treatment; that they disappear sometimes altogether, or only reappear months afterward,—all make it a question whether there be not a *scrofulous* disease of the lung independent of a tubercular, and one, moreover, which presents a much more favorable prognosis. Among the scrofulous children who throng our public institutions, cases like those alluded to are not uncommon. The disorder certainly differs from the ordinary forms of pulmonary tuberculosis, and it is not bronchial phthisis. It does not present the paroxysmal cough, the signs of pressure on the trachea or large bronchi, and the dull sound on percussion between the scapulæ, which are the common accompaniments of enlarged and tubercularized bronchial glands.

Some years since I had an opportunity of inspecting the

---

* Observations illustrative of this subject are furnished by Walshe, in his Treatise on Diseases of the Lungs; by Bennett, in his work on Pulmonary Tuberculosis; by Flint, in the American Journal of Medical Sciences, January, 1858; and by Lawson, in his work on Phthisis.

lungs in one of these instances of supposed pulmonary scrofula. I was treating a little girl for this affection, when she received a severe injury which resulted in her death. She had, when first seen, an eruption on the scalp, sore eyes, and enlarged cervical glands. She was also very much troubled by a cough; and marked dulness on percussion was discerned at the upper portion of the left lung. Here, as in fact throughout the whole of the left lung and the upper part of the right, the respiration was harsh. But for two weeks before her death the symptoms and signs had strikingly improved under cod-liver oil and iodide of iron. She was rapidly losing her cough and gaining strength. The dulness on percussion was diminishing, the respiration becoming less and less rough. At the autopsy the greater part of the left lung and a portion of the right were found to contain yellowish, cheesy deposits, which exhibited under the microscope a large quantity of granules and some shrivelled cells, without distinct nuclei.

It would be out of place to pursue here this intricate subject any further. I will only add that there are no phenomena which will serve as a foundation for an absolute diagnosis of a scrofulous in distinction to a tuberculous infiltration. But the rapid fluctuation in the physical signs, their occurrence in those who present a strongly scrofulous aspect, and the course of the disease, may furnish a clue by which to separate, so far as they can be separated, cases of these kindred disorders. Perhaps the absence of hæmoptysis from among the symptoms may turn out to be a matter of much importance in a diagnostic point of view. Certainly hemorrhage did not happen in any of the cases of pulmonary scrofula which have come under my observation.

The Acute Affections of the Lungs accompanied by Dulness on Percussion.

In continuing the consideration of the diseases in which dulness on percussion is a marked sign, let us glance at a group of *acute* affections, in the distinction of which dulness and the physical sounds which correspond to it hold an important part.

The acute diseases affecting that portion of the respiratory apparatus which lies within the chest are bronchitis, pneumonia, pleurisy, and acute phthisis. They have some signs and many symptoms in common. They all present fever; they are all associated with more or less dyspnœa and thoracic pain; they all occasion a cough. If, therefore, a practitioner meets with an acute disease of the chest, and finds the heart healthy, his mind is forcibly directed to the disorders mentioned, and he asks himself, Is the malady acute bronchitis? is it acute phthisis? is it acute pneumonia? is it acute pleurisy?

Now, the symptoms and signs of acute bronchitis have already been discussed. It has been pointed out that the want of intensity of the fever, and particularly the unimpaired resonance on percussion, separate bronchial inflammation from all affections which occasion consolidation or compression of the lung tissue. Its further consideration among diseases accompanied by dulness on percussion would be, therefore, evidently out of place; and we may proceed to examine the other acute pulmonary affections.

Acute Phthisis.—When phthisis runs its course rapidly, it constitutes the malady known as acute phthisis, or galloping consumption. This formidable complaint is met with at the close of other diseases, especially of fevers; but exposure, never-ending toil, and anxiety are also among the exciting causes of acute tubercular formations.

Acute phthisis shows, more even than chronic pulmonary consumption, that the disease is not simply one of the lungs. The lesions found by the knife of the pathological anatomist are for the most part insufficient to account for the early exhaustion and the emaciation, and indicate a constitutional affection, of which the tubercles in the lungs are but the local expression.

The disorder often begins with a chill: fever follows; at first like any inflammatory fever with thirst, anorexia, quickened pulse, parched lips, and hot skin, but soon accompanied by exhausting night-sweats and rapid emaciation, which, in connection with the intense restlessness and prostration, and the frequent supervention of delirium, may cause the febrile disturbance closely to resemble typhoid fever. The symptoms which point to the thoracic malady are the accelerated breathing, the cough, the copious expectoration, the pain in the chest, and the spitting up of florid blood.

The physical signs are not always the same. If the tubercles be scattered through the lungs, no signs are perceived but those of diffused acute bronchitis. More commonly the signs are like those of chronic phthisis, and associated with the fever and prostration we find the percussion dulness of a deposit or the evidences of the breaking up and destruction of the pulmonary tissue, furnished by coarse, moist rales, and cavernous breathing.

When the malady assumes the form resembling chronic pulmonary consumption, the diagnosis from bronchitis is not perplexing; but when its phenomena are similar to those of acute bronchitis, the recognition of the tubercular affection is often impossible. This remark applies particularly to the distinction of the miliary form of acute phthisis from capillary bronchitis; since the slight constitutional symptoms and the coarseness of the rales of ordinary bronchial inflammation are too unlike the phenomena of acute consumption to occasion commonly much difficulty in their discrimination. But from bronchitis of the finer tubes the diagnosis can only be effected by taking into account that emaciation and profuse sweats are wanting in the bronchial affection; that the skin is not hot but more livid; that the rales are more abundant, and more perceptible at the lower part of the chest; and that, perhaps, the breathing is usually not so hurried. Yet none of these are convincing proofs. The presence of dulness on percussion, or the sinking in at the upper part of the chest, the occurrence of hemorrhage, and the longer duration of the case are alone conclusive evidence in favor of the existence of acute phthisis. Hemorrhage is, however, by no means so constant in the acute as in the chronic form of the malady.

When the dulness on percussion is well defined, acute phthisis might be mistaken for acute inflammation of the lung. But the signs of deposit and of softening in both lungs, and the seat of the lesions at the apices, show differences from a disease which, in the large majority of instances, is one-sided and at the lower part of the lung, which exhibits a characteristic sputum, and in which breaking up of the pulmonary tissue is so rare.

Yet there are cases of acute phthisis that display symptoms and signs very puzzling, and strongly simulating those of pneumonia.

A person in perfectly good health is seized, after exposure, with cough and fever. It is accompanied by dyspnœa, and soon we find signs of consolidation of the lower lobe, or of the entire lung. The dulness on percussion does not disappear under treatment; and a hollow, blowing respiration and gurgling, usually first perceptible at the angle of the scapula, gradually appear, and indicate the formation of a cavity. Emaciation, which commenced from the onset, progresses more rapidly, and goes hand in hand with extreme prostration and profuse perspirations. The sputa are copious and purulent, but at no time mixed with blood. The other lung is carefully examined; all its sounds are normal. The case remains in this condition for several weeks, the patient temporarily improving under stimulants, yet, on the whole, growing weaker and weaker. A slight roughening of the inspiratory murmur, or dry rales at the apex of the unaffected lung, attract attention, and dulness on percussion and the signs of deposition become there more and more manifest. A post-mortem examination exhibits nearly the whole of one lung converted into a uniform yellowish or grayish mass of tubercle, and containing one or several large excavations; not a vestige of healthy lung structure is to be seen. Scattered tubercles are found in the other lung, and mainly at its apex.

The case just described is one of a group which every practitioner must have met with. Whether the disease commences as tubercle, or as pneumonia, is next to impossible to say. Perhaps the tubercle has lain dormant in the lung, and has been roused into action by the inflammation. Perhaps the inflammation was of a kind to predispose to the formation of tubercle. These questions, however interesting, need not be here mooted, since they do not materially concern us. What, however, does concern us, is to know that the occurrence of rales and of subsequent dulness on percussion at the upper part of the previously unaffected side, the persistence of the disease and the prostration and sweats which accompany it, permit us to foretell the tubercular nature and the fatal termination of the disorder.

I may, in this connection, again revert to the views of those who, like Niemeyer, accord to inflammation and the degeneration of its products the chief place in the production of consumption. Such cases as just described would be classed as acute galloping consumption, the result of caseous infiltration of the pulmonary tissues and the disintegration of the cheesy infiltration. On the other hand, in true acute tuberculosis an eruption of miliary tubercles in the lungs and in most other organs takes place, and there are repeated chills, the febrile symptoms run very high, the dyspnœa is intense, but the physical signs are usually more those of an extensive bronchitis.

Acute phthisis may simulate other affections besides those of the chest. It has at times the delirium and prostration, the dry tongue, and the bronchial rales of typhoid fever. The diarrhœa and the abdominal symptoms are, however, wanting. Yet simultaneous deposition of tubercles in the intestine may cause these; and in this case the only mark of difference, from typhoid fever, is the absence of an eruption; unless, even under these circumstances, we are aided by the fact pointed out by Dr. Fox,[*] namely, that unlike the persistent high temperature of typhoid fever with its regular diminution when the disease declines, the thermometric record in acute phthisis shows great and sudden variations of animal heat, bearing no regular relation to the number of respirations or to the beats of the pulse. The temperature may vary many times in the course of the disease to the extent of six or seven degrees. Acute phthisis lacks the wild eye, the gastric disturbance, the convulsions of meningitis;

---

* St. George's Hospital Reports, 1869.

or the active delirium it occasionally produces might be attributed to inflammation of the membranes of the brain.

Acute phthisis sometimes progresses with extreme rapidity. I have seen a case terminate in thirteen days. It is almost invariably fatal. Yet it has its periods of deceptive improvement: the tubercular disease may proceed speedily toward softening, and then remain for a time stationary.

Acute Pneumonia.—Inflammation of the lung is the type of the acute pulmonary affections. The hot, dry skin, the flushed face, the quickened pulse, the extremely rapid breathing, the thoracic pain, the cough, and the peculiar expectoration point out at once the acute nature of the attack and the organ which is disturbed. Beginning commonly with a chill, or with flushes of heat, the disease progresses with the symptoms indicated. A few of these require a more detailed description.

The expectoration is very characteristic. It consists at first of a dry, glairy mucus; soon it becomes more viscid, and acquires that significant appearance dependent upon the admixture of blood with the mucus and exudation matter, to which the term rusty-colored has been given. This rusty sputum is pathognomonic of the disorder; yet it is well to be aware that cases of pneumonia run their course without it. The expectoration is sometimes like prune-juice, or it is purulent. Both augur badly; both indicate that destruction of the lung tissue has commenced.

The shortness or increased frequency of breathing is another very marked symptom. The patient draws from forty to eighty breaths a minute; but the pulse, although rapid, does not quicken in proportion. Pneumonia, therefore, forms an exception to the rule, that with greater frequency of breathing the pulse rises. This perverted *pulse respiration-ratio*, on which Dr. Walshe dwells, may be made an important element in the diagnosis of the disorder. The febrile symptoms are ordinarily very severe; still they are not associated with decided cerebral disturbance. Headache is common, but delirium rare, and when it occurs, is indicative of great danger. The heat of the skin is burning; and the flush on the cheek so decided, that by this and the hurried breathing alone the disease may often be recognized. The flush on the cheek is not accidental. It is sometimes very dark, and, according to Bouillard, it is most obvious when the inflammation affects the apex of the lung.

The urine is high colored, and that of fever. A notable circumstance about it is, that nitrate of silver does not precipitate its chlorides. They commonly disappear during consolidation of the lung, and their reappearance shadows forth returning health. The vanishing of the chlorides from the urine happens also in other acute affections; but in pneumonia it is, perhaps, most constant, and most absolute.

The *physical signs* which denote that the lung tissue has become the seat of an acute inflammation may be deduced from a knowledge of the effects which the inflammation occasions. In the first stage, or that of engorgement, occur increased vascularity and commencing exudation in the air-cells, into which, however, the air is still capable of entering. There is, therefore, only a very slight impairment of the normal resonance on percussion. The vesicular murmur is at first somewhat altered; it may be feebler or harsher. But soon are heard with each act of inspiration, and *limited to the inspiration*, numerous equally and rapidly-evolved, very fine, crackling sounds, the "crepitant" or vesicular rales.

As the exudation becomes firmer, and the tissue of the lung solidifies by occlusion of the air-cells, the stage of red hepatization is before us. Now all the signs of complete consolidation are discerned. We find decided dulness on percussion; blowing respiration in all its purity, high pitched and tubular sounding; bronchophony; and increased vocal fremitus. Rales from the accompanying bronchitis are heard with extreme distinctness through the solidified tissue (Skoda's consonating rales); and so are the sounds of the heart. A crepitant rale is still here and there perceptible, or the ear catches a friction sound—a sure sign that inflammation has involved the pleura. When the exudation is reabsorbed or expectorated, the signs of consolidation become less and less perfect. A vesiculo-bronchial respiration succeeds to the bronchial breathing. The dulness on percussion lessens; crepitant rales—not, however, so fine as at the

onset of the affection, and mixed with larger moist rales—
return; the cough increases; the expectoration becomes

FIG. 21.

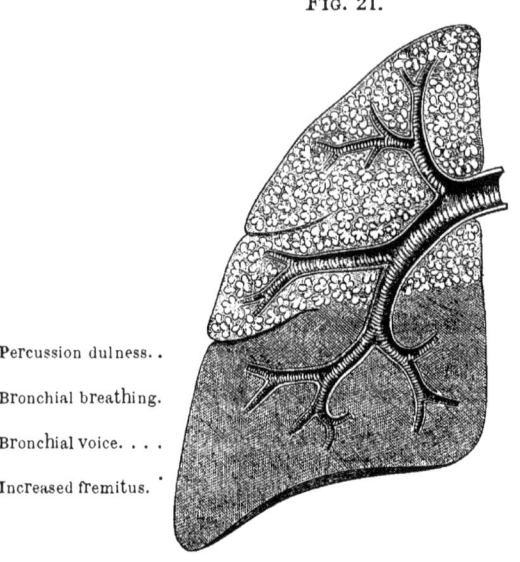

Percussion dulness..

Bronchial breathing.

Bronchial voice. . . .

Increased fremitus.

Diagram illustrative of perfect pulmonary consolidation, such as happens in the
second stage of pneumonia.

more copious, loses its tenacity and rusty color, and contains, when microscopically examined, broken-down exudation corpuscles and a large quantity of fat; the dyspnœa
diminishes,—all phenomena indicative of the breaking up of
the exudation, and of the return of air into the vesicles. If,
instead, the exudation be converted extensively into pus,
and the lungs soften, the physical signs are the same as in
the second stage. The rarity of excavations of sufficient
size explains why gurgling and the signs of a cavity are not
perceived. We suspect the mischief that is going on within
the chest from the protracted dyspnœa, the increasing rapidity of pulse, the purulent or brownish sputa, the pinched
features, the dry tongue, and the mental wandering. Recovery may take place even then. This third stage is indeed not so much an abrupt, suddenly established process,
as it is the extension and greater diffusion of a state that
may be found in portions of the lung which to the eye have
all the appearance of red hepatization. In every instance of

red hepatization the microscope shows that in parts the lung tissue is infiltrated with granules and is undergoing soften-ing, and it is probable that this breaking down occurs, even though on a small scale, in all cases of pneumonia which recover. And these minute appearances explain why com-plete gray hepatization is so rare; why, further, it is often so difficult or impossible to fix the limits of the second stage, and determine that the third stage has arrived; and why death may take place long before the lung presents the con-dition which pathologists term gray hepatization. It is in-deed a great mistake to suppose that a case does not end fatally until gray hepatization has become established, for long before it is fairly developed death may ensue. And with reference to the diagnosis of this third stage, it can safely be affirmed that we may suspect, in fact we may feel sure, from the symptoms, that the pulmonary tissue is seriously dam-aged. But we can never know it, unless we find the physical signs of extensive softening; and in the large majority of cases this cannot be done.

To recapitulate. The morbid phenomena, physical signs and symptoms of the malady correspond usually in this manner:

PNEUMONIA.

I. Stage of engorgement and commencing exudation.	Crepitant rale; slight percussion dulness.	Cough; beginning dyspnœa and fever.
II. Stage of solidifica-tion of lung tissue (red hepatization).	Percussion dulness; bronchial respiration; bronchophony.	Rusty-colored sputum; dyspnœa; cough; high fever.
III. Stage of soften-ing (gray hepati-zation).	The same physical signs as in the second stage; unless large abscesses have formed.	Chills; prostration, etc.; purulent or brownish sputum.

Here, then, is a disease which presents such striking symp-toms and signs in nearly all its phases, in which the sputa are so peculiar, the hurried breathing so evident, the physi-cal signs so distinct, that error is, with ordinary care, difficult. It becomes still more so, if a few of the pathological peculiarities of pneumonia be borne in mind: the fact that it is rarely double; that it comparatively seldom affects the upper lobe of the lung, and that it is often accompanied by the signs of slight pleurisy or bronchitis.

But to contrast pneumonia with the various diseases with which it may be confounded. In its first stage, on account of similar signs, the acute inflammatory disorder is sometimes mistaken for œdema of the lung, or for the pulmonary engorgement which takes place in some fevers; and still more frequently, these morbid states are mistaken for it.

Pulmonary Œdema.—Œdema of the lung consists in the transudation of serum into the air-vesicles. It may be acute, the result of sudden congestion, such as that following injuries of the brain, or irritation of the par vàgum; or arise at the termination of acute affections of the lungs. It is more usually, however, chronic, and is seen as a dropsy of the air-cells, associated with dropsies elsewhere, and in connection with organic disease of the liver, heart, or kidneys. The characteristic manifestations of œdema—be it acute or chronic—are embarrassed breathing, expectoration of frothy serum, and crepitating and very fine bubbling sounds diffused over both lungs, and dependent upon the fluid in the air-cells and small bronchial tubes. It presents, thus, many points of similarity to the first stage of acute pneumonia. The dyspnœa, the crepitation in the lung, may well mislead; but we cannot err, if the frothy sputum, the general distribution of the rales, their somewhat coarser character, the bluish lip, the noisy breathing, and the absence of fever be taken into account. In acute œdema these phenomena are but the precursors of death. In chronic œdema the rales are persistent, and so is the difficulty of respiration. The patient has usually to be propped up with pillows, or he cannot breathe at all.

Pulmonary Engorgement in Fevers.—In fevers of a low type a crepitant rale, which might be supposed to be a proof of commencing inflammation of the lung, is often heard at the back part of the chest. The sound is probably the result of pulmonary congestion. It is ordinarily perceived over both lungs; and this fact, taken in connection with the history of the case, and with the circumstance that the rale is not followed by decided shortness of breath, by dulness on percussion, and blowing respiration, shows that it is not dependent on inflammation of the pulmonary tissue. It is very necessary to be aware that these fine rales may occur in fevers without being due to a true pneumonia; as otherwise the patient is apt to be treated for a disease of the lung which has really no existence.

In its second stage, owing to the cough and dyspnœa, and in part, also, to some similarity in the physical signs, acute pneumonia may be confounded with pulmonary apoplexy, acute pleurisy, acute phthisis, and acute bronchitis.

Pulmonary Apoplexy.—An effusion of blood into the texture of the lung is a rare affection. When met with, it is generally, although by no means invariably, accompanied by external hemorrhage and by difficulty of breathing. Over the effused blood there is dulness on percussion, and the ear hears an enfeebled or bronchial respiration. Around the seat of the mishap it encounters moist rales. Now here are signs bearing some resemblance to those of pneumonia. But we miss from among them the fever. We find, on the other hand, not blood intimately mixed with the expectoration, but pure blood, florid or sooty looking;* and on close scrutiny a grave disease of the heart is generally detected to explain why an extravasation of blood into the pulmonary structure has taken place. Again, the dyspnœa is different. In pneumonia it augments from the beginning to the height of the malady. In pulmonary apoplexy it is greatest when the blood is extravasated, and after that it declines. Yet we must bear in mind that the two affections sometimes coexist. The blood acts as a foreign body, and around it is lighted up an inflammation of the lung structure.

Of the other diseases mentioned which resemble pneumonia, the distinguishing points need not be here fully described. *Acute pleurisy* will be further on more partienlarly studied. With regard to *acute phthisis*, it is only neces-

---

* Walshe, Treatise on Diseases of the Lungs.

sary to repeat that cases are encountered, apparently of
pneumonia, in which, after the symptoms of acute inflammation of the lung pass off, those of phthisis come into
the foreground.   With reference to *acute bronchitis*, I will
merely recall that the dyspnœa is not so great, and that no
percussion dulness is yielded by an inflamed bronchial membrane.

Percussion is thus of signal value in the diagnosis of pneumonia.   In fact, when bronchitis complicates pneumonia, and
loud, dry rales take the place of the blowing respiration, it is
our only trustworthy guide.   A single tap on the chest which
elicits an absolutely dull sound, tells the difference between
pure bronchitis and the inflammation of the bronchial mucous
membrane which accompanies inflammation of the parenchymatous structure of the lung.

The form of pneumonia most liable to be mistaken for
bronchitis is undoubtedly the pneumonia of childhood, the
lobular pneumonia.   It would be obligatory here to dwell on
its special characters, its diffusion, its relations to capillary
bronchitis and to collapse of the lung, were it not that, in
treating of these disorders, it has been described with them.
To enter into particulars at this place would, therefore, be a
tiresome repetition.   But there are two other forms of inflammation of the lung which have not been elsewhere considered, and which, as they present somewhat peculiar symptoms, require to be explained.   They are typhoid pneumonia
and bilious pneumonia.

Typhoid Pneumonia.—Inflammation of the lung may be
from its onset attended with extreme prostration.   This form
of the disease has been made a matter of very warm controversy, both as to the symptoms which characterize it and as
to the relation it bears to other varieties of the malady.
Now, any one who reads the dissimilar descriptions given of
it by different authors will become convinced that, under the
term typhoid pneumonia, the most various disorders have
been ranged together.   On the one hand, it has been applied
exclusively to the inflammation of the lung which may complicate typhus or typhoid fever; on the other hand, it has
been made to include an idiopathic fever in which the affec-

tion of the respiratory organs is occasionally wanting. It is evident that to neither of these diseases ought to belong the name of typhoid pneumonia, since in both the inflammation of the lung is but an incidental, although a grave, accompaniment.

Typhoid pneumonia is pneumonia with symptoms of a typhoid type, and marked by rapid failing of the vital powers. The inflammation of the lung arising in the course of typhus or typhoid fever will of course be apt to present this character: but the malady is also noticed as a consequence of phlebitis; as supervening in cases of erysipelas, of Bright's disease, and of delirium tremens; or as the sole apparent affection. It happens not unfrequently in epidemics, and is very often observed among negroes. Its ravages on the plantations of South Carolina and Georgia are sometimes frightful. Often, too, it is very fatal among troops in the field, serving in unhealthy localities and placed under unfavorable hygienic conditions.

The physical signs are those of the sthenic form of the disease, except, perhaps, that the crepitant rale is less frequent. Most of the same symptoms, too, show themselves: cough, short breathing, and pain in the chest. All of these may be very marked, or so trifling as hardly to direct attention to the lungs. There is, however, one symptom characteristic and constant, and but one, and that is the great tendency toward sinking. As regards the expectoration, it may be rusty colored; yet occasionally, even in the early stages of the complaint, it consists of pure blood. The pulse is always quick, but weak. Dark sordes often collect on the teeth and gums, as they do in typhoid fever. Pain is absent in some cases, and extremely acute and of a radiating character in others. Concerning delirium, we know that it is much more common in this asthenic form than it is in the sthenic variety of pulmonary inflammation. Some authors mention the occurrence of an eruption. It is, however, questionable whether the cases which came under their notice were not rather instances of typhus or typhoid fever, in the course of which pneumonia appeared. The flush on the face in the low type of the malady under consideration is usually of a

19

dusky hue, but not invariably: a pink-colored blush, extending sometimes all over the body, seems to have specially attracted the attention of several observers. The disease is always dangerous, and often lingering. Dr. Stokes* writes of the typhoid pneumonia he met with in Dublin, that although it is generally developed with rapidity, its resolution is extremely slow. Chronic hepatization, with or without a low hectic fever, or a lurking congestion, may continue for many weeks.

The symptoms of typhoid pneumonia are at times strangely mixed up with those produced by other conditions. In many districts, in which the complaint is very prevalent, it bears the distinct impress of malaria. Again, articular symptoms seem to predominate in some regions of country, and in some epidemics. Dr. Gibbes† speaks of an acute pain in the back part of the eye, in the ears, or side of the neck, attended with stiffness of the muscles; and of a swelling of the tonsils, the submaxillary and sublingual glands, which he states to be of evil augury. And Dr. Dickson,‡ drawing his description of the disease from a large number of cases observed in and around Charleston, portrays several forms, the most common of which exhibits a respiration hurried, uneasy, and irregular; deep and heavy sighing; a feeling of weight at the precordial region, with nausea, gastric distress, and vomiting; and a tongue clean, but red. Delirium is present from the beginning, and does not subside until recovery takes place. The duration of such attacks averages from six to ten days. In another form, there are at the onset great gastric oppression and vomiting, and signs of vascular excitement. But muscular prostration and debility soon happen; and lividity of the countenance, petechial spots, and coma are symptoms which usher in dissolution.

Bilious Pneumonia.—Jaundice and other indications of hepatic and gastric derangement are not usual in ordinary sthenic pneumonia. They may be occasionally caused by the inflammation spreading to the liver, or be noticed where

---

* Diseases of the Chest.
† Amer. Journ. of Med. Sciences, 1842.
‡ Elements of Medicine.

no evidence of such an occurrence exists. But in the pneumonia so general in spring and autumn in the miasmatic regions of some of the Southern and Western States, these symptoms are very common, and mark a special type of the disease, known as malarial pneumonia, bilious pneumonia, or by the more familiar name of "bilious pleurisy."

This form of inflammation of the lung is simply pneumonia, sthenic or asthenic, on whose features the stamp of malaria is imprinted. The chill with which it begins is usually very protracted, and is followed by pain in the side, by fever, by hurried breathing, by cough, and by tenacious, rusty-colored expectoration. The pain in the side, which depends upon accompanying pleurisy, is sharp and severe, and renders the respiration irregular. The sputum is at times rusty colored, while at others a frothy and bloody serum or pure blood is expectorated. The fever shows the type of the disease. It is much more paroxysmal than in the other varieties of the malady. This peculiarity, and the obvious symptoms of hepatic and gastric disorder, are indeed the only absolutely distinguishing traits of bilious pneumonia. The febrile exacerbations are stated by Dr. Manson, a physician of North Carolina, to be preceded, during the morning hours, by an insensible chill—a coolness of the ends of the nose, fingers, and toes, which, in grave cases, extends over the entire extremities.* The same writer dwells on the irritability of the intestinal canal, and the occurrence of greenish-black, viscid and inodorous stools. This, and the diminution of the dyspnœa, diaphoresis, and a copious secretion of urine, point to a favorable issue of the disease. On the other hand, it may terminate fatally with symptoms indicative of great prostration.

The physical signs are those of ordinary acute pneumonia. Bronchial breathing and bronchophony are said to be more often absent, or to appear and disappear rapidly. It is cer-

---

* Virgin. Med. Journ , Sept. and Oct. 1857; see also an excellent essay on the subject by W. F. Howard, North Carol. Journ., Feb. 1859; Ramsay, Charlest. Med. Journ., vol. vi.; Merrill, New Orleans Med. and Surg. Journ., July, 1851; and Drake on the Diseases of the Interior Valley of North America.

tain, if this be true, that in these instances the malady could not have been inflammation, but was more probably a collapse of the pulmonary tissue. Any one, indeed, who compares the various statements made with reference to the disease, must have been struck with the fact that cases of congestive fever in which the lungs have become simply engorged, or perhaps collapsed, and cases of inflammation of the lung arising in the course of remittent fevers, are included in the same description with true cases of idiopathic bilious pneumonia.

The nature of an inflammation of the lung bearing so decidedly the livery of malaria has given rise to warm controversies. Regarded by some as nothing more than a special form of remittent or intermittent fever, in which the lungs are made to bear the burden of the disease, it is by others held to be simply a variety of pneumonia, occasioned by the ordinary causes of this affection, but owing its peculiar symptoms to its happening in those in whose systems the poison of malaria has been slumbering.

Acute Pleurisy.—Acute pleurisy has been so often incidentally mentioned, that a description of its main points will here suffice. The first effect of the inflammation is to redden the pleural membrane; an exudation of a soft, grayish, and easily-detached lymph then takes place. This constitutes the first or dry stage of the disease; and if the two inflamed surfaces unite, the disorder does not pass beyond this stage. Often, however, along with the exudation of lymph occurs an effusion of serum, which produces a special train of phenomena, and gives rise to the second stage, or that of liquid effusion.

The physical signs of the *dry* stage are impaired movement of the chest, a feebler respiration, and a friction sound of varying extent and intensity. The first two signs are caused by the patient instinctively recoiling from expanding the lung, because of the pain it occasions. The mechanism of the friction sound, its nature, its superficial character and want of uniformity have been pointed out in a previous part of this chapter. In the stage of *effusion* the physical signs differ somewhat, according to the amount of fluid the pleural

cavity contains. A moderate quantity of liquid only con-
stricts the lung texture, and leaves the bronchial tubes intact:

Fig. 22.

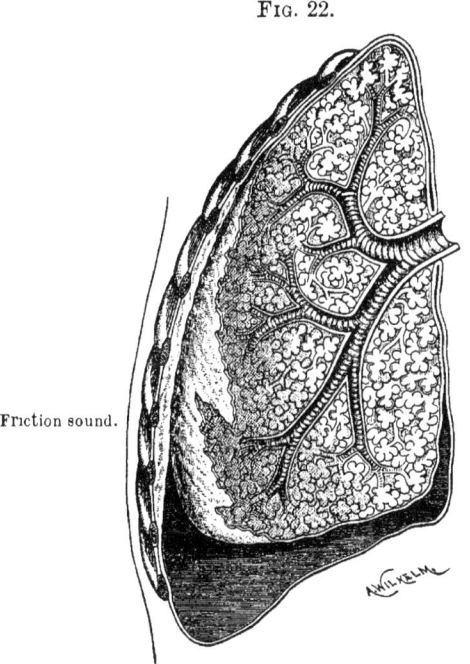

Friction sound.

Roughening of the pleura from inflammation; a small amount
of fluid has begun to collect.

a large accumulation compresses everything; it drives all air
out of the lung, pushes it into a small space against the vertebral column, and displaces the liver or heart. Wherever
the fluid accumulates there is dulness on percussion. When
the patient is in the erect posture, the flat sound on striking
the chest and the sense of resistance to the finger are marked
at the lower part of the thorax, since the fluid naturally set-
tles there. The line of dulness is, however, not the same in
front as it is behind. It is mostly much higher behind, and
alters, of course, with the changing quantity of effusion, and
somewhat with the position of the patient. When he lies
upon his face the fluid gravitates, if not circumscribed by adhesions, toward the anterior chest walls, and the percussion
dulness becomes posteriorly far less perceptible.

Where the effusion is at all extensive, the intercostal

spaces are widened and their depressions effaced.   The side
appears to the eye distended, and, owing to the absolute

FIG. 23.

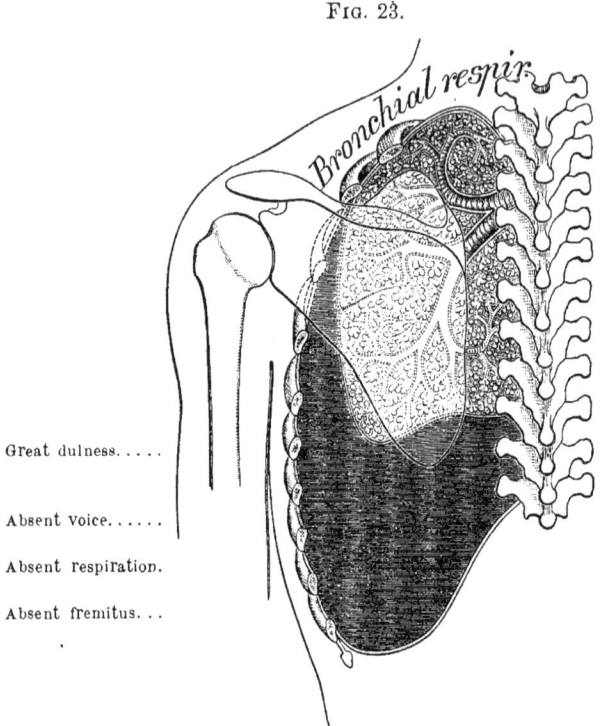

Great dulness. . . . .

Absent Voice. . . . . .

Absent respiration.

Absent fremitus. . .

Examination of the posterior portion of the chest while a large effusion is
occupying the left pleural cavity.

compression of the lung, no sound is heard over the chest
when the patient breathes, or speaks, or coughs.   In more
moderate collections of fluid, the cessation of sound is not
so absolute.   There is an ill-defined, deep-seated respiration,
and the voice reaches the ear with tolerable distinctness,
and occasionally with a peculiar bleating resonance attending it.   But as large collections of fluid are more common
than small ones, the former set of phenomena are, at the
height of the disease, more frequent than the latter.

Above the liquid there is mostly increased resonance on
percussion, or a tympanitic sound.   Various explanations
have been given of this phenomenon.   It has been attributed to the complete compression of the lung: it has been

thought to be due to its slight condensation. Whatever be the true explanation, the fact of its occurrence is undeniable. This tympanitic sound is more manifest at the upper part of the chest in front than behind; it may, indeed, sometimes be found in front when it does not exist at all behind. In many cases the sound has a decidedly amphoric, in others a cracked-metal character. When the ear is applied above the line of percussion dulness, it recognizes occasionally a friction sound; and near the spinal column posteriorly, where the compressed lung lies, it perceives often—were I only to take my own notes as a basis, I should say almost invariably—a distinct bronchial respiration.

When the fluid begins to be absorbed, the voice becomes more audible over the seat of the effusion, the vocal vibrations may be felt by the fingers, and the respiration too is again heard. But for a long time it continues enfeebled, and its character is indeterminate; it is neither vesicular, nor purely bronchial. As more and more of the fluid disappears, the voice becomes more and more distinct; a friction sound finally shows that the roughened surfaces come in contact; and the dulness on percussion is replaced by a far clearer sound. False membranes now unite the two pleuræ; the intercostal spaces resume their normal shape; and the chest is either restored to its natural size, or is left permanently somewhat contracted. The bronchial breathing near the vertebral column persists for a long time, since a lung that has been compressed unfolds but very slowly.

Such are the different physical signs which inflammation of the pleura exhibits. They have been discussed first, and at some length, because I wished to make it apparent that these signs are the most important elements in the diagnosis of the disease. The symptoms, indeed, often hardly attract attention; and if we trusted to them, we should be constantly groping in the dark. Pleurisy mostly begins with a chill, followed by fever and by a dry, irritating cough. The most distinctive, though not a constant symptom of the first stage, is the sharp, acute pain, the "stitch in the side." It is commonly felt under the nipple or in the axilla, and is somewhat increased on pressure. Its seat by no means always corresponds to the seat of the friction sound. As the effusion takes place the pain disappears, dyspnœa becomes evident, and the patient ordinarily lies on the affected side. The febrile symptoms and dry cough continue; yet neither is very marked, and both disappear long before the fluid is entirely absorbed.

Pleurisy may be idiopathic, or occur as an attendant upon other diseases, such as affections of the lungs, measles, scarlatina, typhoid and typhus fevers. It may be caused by wounds of the thoracic walls, or by Bright's disease, by rheumatism, gout, pyæmia, and by many other morbid states.

The malady with which acute idiopathic pleurisy is most likely to be confounded, is acute pneumonia. Both are affections occasioning dyspnœa; both are, in the majority of cases, one-sided; both present, in their most advanced stages, dulness on percussion. But the dulness in the latter disease is far less absolute than in the former; nor do we, save in very rare instances, meet with a tympanitic or amphoric percussion sound in pneumonia, while in pleurisy, as we have just seen, it is far from unusual above the level of the fluid. In those few cases in which an amphoric or a tympanitic sound is perceived in pneumonia,—a condition of things, it may be mentioned in passing, which has not as yet received a satisfactory explanation,—the peculiar tone is most obvious over the consolidated tissue.*

The other physical signs of the two diseases show still less similitude. The absence of respiration, of vocal resonance and of thrill, are in striking contrast with the loud blowing respiration, the strong chest-voice and increased vocal thrill of pneumonia. There are, however, exceptional cases of pleuritic effusion, in which bronchial breathing is heard all over one side of the chest. Especially does this happen if pneumonic consolidation accompany the effusion; but even

---

* Dr. Flint suggests that the line of flatness may serve as a dintinguishing mark. In pneumonia, if the disease be limited to the lower lobe, the line follows the situation of the inter-lobar fissure, crossing the chest obliquely from the fourth or fifth cartilages to the spinal extremity of the spinous ridge of the scapula.

in simple compression of the lung, and where the collection of liquid is not extensive, bronchial respiration may be perceived. The difficulty of distinguishing such cases of pleurisy (in which probably the lung tissue is compressed around the bronchial tubes, but these are not encroached upon) from pneumonia is great. As aids in diagnosis, we seek for the dilatation of the chest; we note the peculiarities of the breathing, which, although blowing, is mostly fainter than, and unlike the high-pitched, brazen respiration of pneumonia; we observe that the voice is less strong and ringing, and has, perhaps, a bleating tone; and we take into account the appearance of the sputum and the character of the fever. But leaving these cases out of consideration—and they do not often occur—the diagnosis between the two affections is easy. It may be thus summed up:

PLEURISY.	PNEUMONIA.
Sharp pain; friction sound; dry cough; impaired chest motion.	Dull pain; crepitant rale; cough, followed by expectoration.
In stage of effusion, obliteration of the intercostal spaces; enlargement of the side; displacement of several viscera.	In stage of hepatization, none of these signs are manifest.
In the large majority of cases, dulness, with enfeebled or absent respiration, voice, and fremitus.	Dulness, with marked bronchial respiration; distinct thoracic voice; increased vocal fremitus.
Decubitus is often on the affected side.	Decubitus not peculiar; sometimes on the sound side.
Sputa frothy; rarely any rales in the chest.	Sputa rusty colored; rales from accompanying bronchial inflammation common.
Febrile symptoms usually slight.	Febrile symptoms severe.

In the first stage of pleurisy the pain might cause the disease to be confounded with pleurodynia or intercostal neuralgia. In all three pain is the prominent symptom. Let us see how it differs.

Pleurodynia.—Pleurodynia is generally described as a form of muscular rheumatism. But frequently it is pleurisy, which does not pass beyond the dry stage. Of this nature are most of the fugitive chest-pains from which phthisical patients suffer. Yet there are cases in which no signs whatever of pleurisy exist, which are attended with the same or with more pain than pleurisy, but which have little or no fever, and are devoid of the rubbing indicative of the motion of roughened pleuræ. The pain of pleurodynia is often excessively severe; the patient refrains from breathing with the affected side, since every motion of his chest, voluntary or involuntary, increases his suffering. The pain is augmented by movements of the arm and by pressure, and is very generally associated with tenderness. Pleurodynia shares with pleurisy the feeble respiration and the want of action of the affected side. It differs from it by the absence of friction sound and of fever; by the shifting tendency of the pain; by its attacking often both sides; and by the greater tenderness of the walls of the chest.

Intercostal Neuralgia.—In anemic women and in consumptives acute thoracic pain is not uncommonly the result of an intercostal neuralgia. The same want of expansion of the chest and enfeebled breathing, as in pleurodynia, are here noted, also the same absence of fever and of pleural friction. The distinguishing marks of intercostal neuralgia are: its intermittent character; its frequent association with uterine disturbance, especially with leucorrhœa; and the limitation of the tenderness to special points in the course of the affected nerve. Valleix has drawn attention to three painful spots which are tender to the touch: one at the exit of the nerve from the spinal column, the second in the axillary region, and the third near the sternum or in the epigastric region. It is on the left side that we are most apt to find intercostal neuralgia, and between the sixth and ninth ribs that the painful places are usually detected.

Pain occurs also in diseases affecting the lung texture. There is pain of a dull nature in pneumonia, of a more severe character in cancer. But the pain is so dissimilar, and the coexisting symptoms so unlike, that the error of confounding these maladies with pleurisy, on account of the pain, is not likely to be committed.

Diseases presenting Dilatation of the Chest, Displacement of the Liver or Heart, and Dyspnœa.

A group of diseases may here be studied, all of which occasion more or less dilatation and prominence of the chest, and all of which are attended with decided shortness of breath. In bronchitis and pneumonia a slight increase in the diameters of the chest may take place; but it is not a sign of any diagnostic importance. In the recognition of emphysema, pneumothorax, and pleuritic effusions, the dilatation of the thorax forms one of the main elements; moreover, it is often combined with marked dyspnœa and with displacement of the liver or heart. These affections, then, may be examined in the same connection, and compared with each other, and incidentally with several less common diseases which present similar manifestations.

The history and signs of emphysema were given when treating of the diseases accompanied by clearness on percussion. It was there mentioned that in many instances the prominence of the chest was circumscribed. Such cases cannot be mistaken: the bulging is too limited. But when the emphysema is more general, and an entire side of the chest or the whole chest becomes dilated, or when the inflated lung displaces the liver or heart, the affection comes into the group under consideration. A patient seeks advice for shortness of breath. His chest is inspected, and looks enlarged. The physical signs prove that the disease is not one of the heart. What, then, is it? Is it an effusion into the pleura? is it pneumothorax? is it emphysema? A tap on the chest goes far toward showing whether it be the former. If the sound rendered be resonant, it is not liquid in the chest that is producing the disturbance: the disorder is either pneumothorax or emphysema.

Pneumothorax.—Of all thoracic maladies, pneumothorax is the one the similarity of which to extensive dilatation of the air-cells is the greatest. In both, the large quantity of air occasions increased clearness on percussion; in both, there is considerable and persistent difficulty of breathing; in both, the distention of the chest and displacement of organs may be very obvious. The symptoms and signs are, however, in pneumothorax, associated with different conditions, which reveal themselves on close inquiry. Pneumothorax is an accumulation of air in the pleural cavity; but it is something more: the entrance of air is soon followed by the effusion of liquid.

Air is let into the cavity of the chest by the pleura being perforated by wounds, or, as is more common, by its partial destruction consequent upon disease of the lung. It is in this way that pneumothorax originates in the course of tubercular softening, of gangrene, pneumonia, or from the bursting of a distended air-vesicle, or of a dilated bronchial tube.* In the large majority of instances it occurs in tubercular patients.

When air passes from the lung into the pleura, it usually happens during a paroxysm of coughing. The pain which ensues is mostly intense; and the frightful, though suddenly developed dyspnœa, and the anxious expression of face, soon show how seriously the respiration is interfered with. If death does not take place, symptoms of pleurisy with effusion begin to manifest themselves; and, as in pleurisy, the patient lies ordinarily, but not invariably, on the affected side. Saussier,† in analyzing the position of fifty-six patients, notes that twenty-eight lay on the affected side, nine on the opposite, and nineteen in various postures.

The absolute and distinctive marks of pneumothorax are furnished by its physical signs. The ingress of air into the pleural cavity widens the chest, effaces the depression of the intercostal spaces, and occasions an extremely clear, or, more correctly speaking, a tympanitic sound on percussion. The air prevents the lung from expanding; hence there is an enfeebled or absent respiration, excepting near the spinal column where the compressed organ lies, and where the breathing is bronchial. The hand, if laid on any other portion of the chest, feels, when the patient speaks, no thrill, and no vocal vibration is detected by the ear. When the perforation

---

* Case recorded by Taylor, Prov. Med. Journal, vol. i., 1842.

† Recherches sur le Pneumothorax. Paris, 1841.

has not closed, and the air rushes into the artificial cavity produced by the separation of the two surfaces of the pleura, the respiration is amphoric, or it, the voice, and the rales are all accompanied by a distinct metallic ring. Drops of fluid falling into the cavity, or the bursting of bubbles on the surface of the liquid in the pleura, are also echoed to the ear with a metallic sound, and are often heard as a clear, silvery tinkle.

The presence of the fluid in the pleural cavity gives rise to a dull sound on percussion at the lower part of the chest, and to a splash, perceptible to the ear and to the finger when the thorax is suddenly shaken. This continues until the effusion increases, and until the opening in the membrane closes, the air disappears, and the case resolves itself into one of chronic pleurisy—the most favorable termination of pneumothorax.

Now let us compare these physical signs with those produced by emphysema. The sound on percussion in both is very clear, or is tympanitic: more so, however, in pneumothorax, which, in addition, exhibits dulness at the lower part of the chest. The respiration in both is feeble. But it is feebler in pneumothorax, and not accompanied by a long, laborious expiration; besides, it is often amphoric, and attended with metallic voice and tinkling—phenomena which dilated air-cells cannot occasion. Moreover, there can be no splashing sound in emphysema; and, on the other hand, the displacement of the heart is generally much greater in pneumothorax, and the dilatation of the chest is more apt to be one-sided. Yet too much stress has been laid on the latter point as a means of differential diagnosis, for emphysema may be one-sided; and, on the other hand, pneumothorax, as the cases of Stokes and of Reynaud* prove, may occur on both sides. In some cases we are aided in the discrimination by noticing that distinct bulging is perceptible over the displaced heart, and that a metallic echo follows the cardiac sounds.

The physical signs of the two diseases are thus very differ-

---

* Journ. Hebdomad., tome vii., 1830. I saw last winter a case of double-sided pneumothorax.

ent; so, too, are many of the symptoms. Difficulty of breathing exists in both. But in emphysema it takes more the form

FIG. 24.

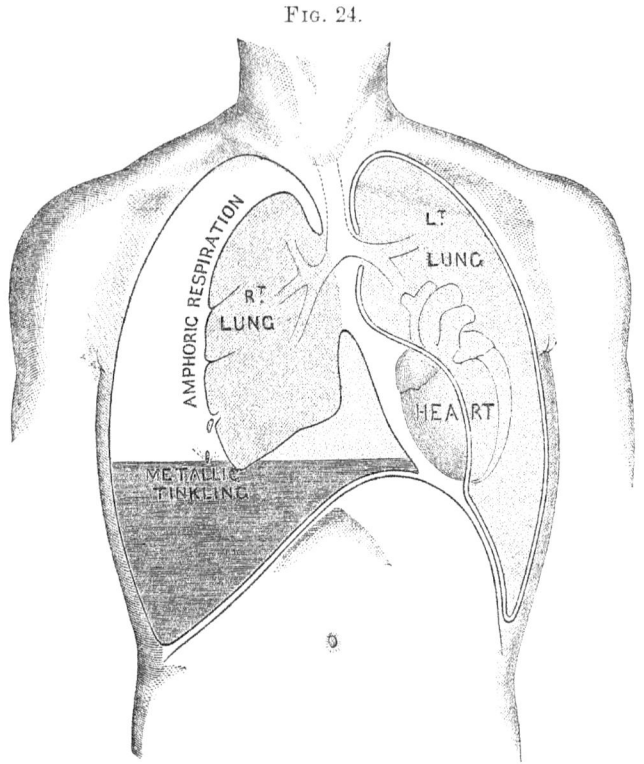

Physical signs in pneumothorax on the right side. The heart is observed to be displaced toward the left, as actually happened in the case from which the outline was
taken. The percussion resonance on the right side was tympanitic, extending somewhat over the left margin of the sternum; the fremitus was annulled; the voice
metallic.

of attacks of asthma; besides, whether spasmodic or not, it
does not set in suddenly and with great intensity, and remain
intense. In pneumothorax the patient remembers to have
been seized with a pain in his chest, since which period he
has been continuously very short of breath.

Yet there are exceptions to this: there are cases in which
the symptoms occasioned by perforation of the pleura are
from the onset so slight as not to attract the least attention.
Such cases cannot be recognized, save by their physical signs.
Among these, dilatation of the chest, with the widened intercostal spaces, the displacement of the liver or heart, and the

exaggerated and altered resonance on percussion are most valuable in preventing the disease from being confounded with some affections which otherwise give rise to many of the same phenomena. In large cavities, for instance, the respiration and voice may be metallic; metallic tinkling, nay, even a succussion sound may occur.* But the prominent chest, the extremely clear, tympanitic, or metallic sound on percussion, bordered by the line of absolute dulness due to the effusion, are not met with. The history also is different, and the dyspnœa is not so great. The same dissimilarities will prevent us from mistaking for pneumothorax a pneumonia in which, by way of exception, the percussion sound over the consolidated lung is tympanitic or amphoric. And a study of the physical signs, too, will at once enable us to discern whether the difficulty in breathing, though it be suddenly developed, and apparently under circumstances which make the swallowing of a foreign body seem likely, be due to this cause, or to perforation of the pleura and pneumothorax.†

There is, however, a morbid condition which exhibits nearly all the signs and many of the symptoms of pneumothorax, and which, were it more frequent, would be the source of constant errors of diagnosis—*diaphragmatic hernia.*

Of this rare affection we know but little. Yet, thanks to Dr. Bowditch,‡ what we do know of it teaches us that a protrusion of the abdominal organs through the diaphragm will generally dilate one side of the chest, compress the lung, and displace the heart. It will do more: it results in dyspnœa; and as the stomach or intestines are, for the most part, the viscera which find their way into the chest, metallic tinkling and a tympanitic sound on percussion are detected. These are all also signs of pneumothorax. And there is no mode of separating the two diseases, excepting by attention to the history of the case, by noting that the dyspnœa of the former suddenly appears and as suddenly disappears; that it has

---

* Cases cited by Gendrin, Gaz. des Hôpit., No. 113, 1847; and Wintrich, Krankheiten der Respirations Organe, page 367.

† As in a case of the disease communicated to me by Dr. Walter F. Atlee.

‡ Buffalo Med. Journ., June and July, 1853.

often existed from birth; and that the metallic phenomena
happen when the patient is not breathing, and are mixed up
with the rumbling sound arising in the stomach or intestine.

It has been made a question whether we can distinguish
ordinary cases of pneumothorax from these very rare ones,
which are supposed to occur *without perforation.* Now, even
admitting that such cases really happen, for instance, as a
sequence of decomposition in pleuritic effusions, there are no
diagnostic signs by which we can recognize them with any
certainty. It has been claimed for them that there is no antecedent history of a chronic pulmonary trouble, particularly
of phthisis, that there is not that suddenly occurring severe
pain and extreme dyspnœa, that the sputum and breath are
not offensive, that metallic tinkling is absent, or very rare
and inconstant, and that the amphoric breathing is not so
well developed or so clearly defined. If in a case of perforation, however, the opening has closed, the physical signs, it is
granted, are the same.*

Chronic Pleurisy.—Chronic pleurisy is the third of the
group of more usual affections which is characterized by
dilatation of the chest, by displacement of the intra-thoracic
viscera, and by shortness of breath. It is true that acute
pleurisy in the stage of effusion would, strictly speaking, find
here a place; but the acute symptoms bring it into another
class with which it has been more conveniently described.

Chronic pleurisy is established if the fluid, after an acute
attack, be not absorbed, or if an accumulation of liquid take
place gradually, in consequence of subacute inflammation
of the pleura. The disease has no constant symptoms, and
is often remarkably latent: the patient frequently does not
remember to have had acute pleurisy. He is not commonly
troubled with much cough, nor is the want of breath so great
as might be expected : he is not capable of talking for any
length of time, or in a loud voice, but does not really suffer
from dyspnœa. His general health may remain good, and no
emaciation occur. In some persons, on the other hand, the
loss of flesh, the quickened pulse, the sweats, the paroxysms

---

* Boisseau, Archiv. Génér. de Méd., vol. ii., 1867.

of hectic fever are so marked as to produce a close resemblance to the last stages of tubercular consumption.

While the differing symptoms rather hide the pleurisy from detection, the physical signs render it easy of recognition. What these signs are, need not be repeated. They have been fully studied in describing the effusion in acute pleurisy. It is only necessary to recall that the most significant are absent respiration and voice, a flat sound on percussion, with a vesiculo-bronchial or a bronchial respiration above the seat of the liquid. The intercostal spaces are obviously widened; their depressions are effaced. They are, indeed, sometimes convex, and the finger pressed on them detects a distinct fluctuation. During the act of breathing, the diseased side is almost motionless, presenting a strong contrast to the obvious play of the healthy side. The lung which is not disturbed increases in size. Its murmur is more intense, sometimes harsher; and the percussion sound over it is exceedingly clear. In some cases it becomes emphysematous. The heart or liver is displaced. A lateral curvature of the spinal column is apt to take place, and the shoulder, as Dr. Corson points out, remains fixed and stiff during the respiratory acts.

Effusions into the pleural sac may last for a long time, and lead to death by progressive exhaustion; or the patient may recover by the fluid being absorbed, or by its finding a vent through the bronchial tubes or thoracic walls. But the chest is rarely restored to its former state. The lung was too much compressed, or is still bound down by too firm adhesions, to resume its full share in the function of respiration. The walls of the chest sink in around it, and the side is flattened, sounds duller on percussion, and presents a feebler breathing than the other lung, which remains somewhat enlarged. The heart generally returns to its normal position, but the shoulder on the affected side is apt to show a permanent depression.

Notwithstanding the decided character of the physical signs in all its stages, it is astonishing how frequently chronic pleurisy is overlooked. The only explanation of this is, that so little attention is paid to the signs. Were the chest more often carefully explored, we should cease to hear of patients whose pleural cavity is filled with pus being pronounced incurable consumptives, because they are emaciating and have hectic fever and clubbed nails; or being treated for disease of the heart, on account of the displacement of that organ, and of dyspnœa and œdema; or being dosed with mercury, for an imaginary disorder of the liver; or subjected to long courses of quinia and arsenic, to check a rebellious ague which the chilly sensations and paroxysms of fever at times simulate.

These physical signs are the same, whether the fluid be serum or pus. The character of the fluid produces, indeed, no distinctive changes, either in the signs or in the symptoms. We suspect empyema if the emaciation be great and accompanied by a quick pulse and hectic fever; but we cannot be sure of it. ·

When we come to inquire into the thoracic diseases with which chronic pleurisy is likely to be confused, we shall find that, although many have some signs in common, few, if any, present the same association of signs. Leaving out the malady which is most commonly mistaken for it—pulmonary consumption—since the points of difference have already been fully discussed, the affections with which chronic pleurisy, while the pleura is full of liquid, and the chest consequently enlarged, is liable to be confounded, are:

EMPHYSEMA AND PNEUMOTHORAX;
INTRA-THORACIC TUMOR;
ENLARGEMENT OF THE LIVER;
ENLARGEMENT OF THE SPLEEN;
ABSCESS IN THE THORACIC WALLS;
PERICARDIAL EFFUSION;
HYDROTHORAX.

Emphysema and Pneumothorax.—These, although distinct diseases, are grouped together because they agree in possessing physical signs indicative of an increased quantity of air within the chest; and they give rise, like chronic pleurisy, to a dilated chest, and to displacement of the liver or heart. But the other signs above pointed out, which are due to the presence of air, are so striking, that an error in diagnosis can only be the result of carelessness.

Intra-thoracic Tumor.—A tumor within the chest may occasion the same distention of its walls, the same displacement of organs, the same dulness on percussion, and absent respiration as an effusion of liquid into the pleura; yet the signs are not exactly alike. There is no fluctuation in the bulging intercostal spaces; the vocal fremitus is not so constantly abolished; and the level of the dulness is not changed by altering the patient's position. Nor is the flat sound so uniform nor so strictly limited as that produced by fluid. Amid the dulness may be detected here and there a spot yielding a clear sound on percussion. A tumor in the chest, moreover, presses on the nerves, or bronchial tubes, or great vessels, and thus gives rise to severe pain, and to dyspnœa and signs of interrupted circulation far more evident than are caused by a pleuritic effusion. It frequently grows into the mediastinum, and then leads to prominence of the sternum, and to dilatation of *both* sides of the chest. These phenomena are found, whatever be the nature of the morbid growth. As most of the thoracic tumors are cancerous, we are often much assisted in our diagnosis by discovering a cancer in other parts of the body, and by noting the severe pain in the chest, the harassing cough, and the expectoration of blood, or of a peculiar jelly-like substance. Yet these evidences, while they aid us in establishing the fact of a morbid growth in the thoracic cavity, do not by any means determine its situation. We cannot go a step further and say, with certainty, whether the abnormal formation be situated exclusively in the lung, or in the pleura, or affect both.

In those cases in which an effusion into the pleura complicates an intra-thoracic tumor, attention to the history and to the signs of pressure alone apprises us of its presence. Yet both signs and symptoms may be so closely like those of chronic pleurisy as to render a differential diagnosis impossible. Nay, friction sounds, a stitch in the side, and fever may be produced by a cancer of the pleura, and be apparently so rapidly developed as to cause the disease to be re-

garded as an acute or subacute inflammation of that membrane. Cancer of the pleura, like tubercle of this structure,
has, therefore, no pathognomonic signs. The most certain
sign of cancer of the pleura is probably the one mentioned
by Trousseau, namely, that the fluid which is evacuated by
paracentesis consists of a bloody serum.

It is at times equally impossible to distinguish a circumscribed pleurisy from a tumor in the chest. In those rare
cases in which adhesions bound the liquid effusion and encyst
it, we observe all the marks of a tumor—a restricted bulging
and percussion dulness, and an absent respiration. Several
cysts may form as the result of successive attacks of pleurisy,
and may exist at any portion of the chest. The fluid may
be collected in the mediastinum, or between the lobes of the
lung, or anywhere between the surfaces of the pleural membrane. The purulent contents of the sac sometimes find
their way into the bronchial tubes, and are expectorated, or
give rise to a distinct fluctuation in the intercostal spaces,
and then discharge through the thoracic parietes. In such
cases the diagnosis is not difficult. But where these phenomena are not present, the dissimilar history of the case
and the absence of symptoms of pressure are the only means
of distinction from a tumor in the chest. Fortunately for
the diagnostician, encysted pleurisy is a rare disease; were
it frequent, it would be a fruitful source of error. The same
remark applies to those cysts known as hydatids, and which
may occasion all the signs of a circumscribed pleurisy.*

Enlargement of the Liver.—An enlarged liver usually descends into the abdominal cavity; yet it may be forced upward as far as the fourth rib, and, by encroaching upon the
lung, may give rise to many of the physical signs of a pleuritic
effusion. The surest diagnostic test is, that during full inspiration and expiration the line of dulness descends and
ascends; while the flat sound of a pleuritic effusion is not

---

* See the observations of Vigla, Archiv. Générale de Médic., Sept. and
Nov. 1855, and of Roger, ibid., Nov. 1861; also cases quoted in Schmidt's
Jahrb., No. 10, 1869; and compare the cases of circumscribed pleurisy in
Blakiston's Practical Observations on Diseases of the Chest, and in Durrant's
paper, Prov. Med. and Surg. Journ., 1849.

affected by the play of the lungs. This test will always be applicable, excepting where the liver is firmly adherent to the walls of the abdomen. As circumstances to assist in discriminating between the enlargement of the abdominal organ and the presence of liquid in the chest, may be mentioned that the heart, if at all displaced, is pushed upward, and not toward the side; that the dulness of an enlarged liver extends higher up anteriorly than posteriorly, which is the reverse of what takes place in a pleuritic effusion. Moreover, the respiration at the lower portion of the lung posteriorly, although enfeebled, is still audible.

Enlargement of the Spleen.—An enlarged spleen is attended with prominence and with dulness on percussion at the lower part of the chest on the left side, and might, therefore, mislead into the idea of a pleuritic effusion. Error in diagnosis is prevented by attention to the fact that the dulness extends also downward and toward the median line. Again, the heart is not laterally displaced, but tilted upward; the respiration is feeble, but not absent; and the vocal vibrations are mostly unimpaired.

Abscess in the Thoracic Walls.—This, too, leads to local tumefaction and fluctuation; but we can always ascertain whether a fluctuating tumor in the intercostal spaces communicates with the pleural cavity or not—whether, in other words, it is or is not the result of an effusion which is pointing externally—by watching how pressure and the acts of respiration affect it. For, unless the diaphragm has become immovable from the extent of the effusion, a bulging which is in connection with the pleura is diminished during a full inspiration, and becomes more prominent when the diaphragm ascends in expiration. The swelling, moreover, can be made to disappear to some extent by pressure. It is not so with an abscess seated in the walls of the chest. It is not reducible, and does not recede during inspiration.

Pericardial Effusion.—An effusion into the pericardium cannot be, certainly ought not to be, mistaken for an effusion into the pleura. The first induces prominence and increased dulness on percussion over the region of the heart; the second, dulness and prominence over the back part as well as over the front of the lung. A few cases are, however, recorded in which an enormously distended pericardial sac produced a flat sound posteriorly, and gave rise to signs of compression of the lung. But in these attention to the feeble impulse of the heart and its muffled sounds permitted it to be foretold that fluid had accumulated in the pericardium, and not in the pleura.

Hydrothorax.—A dropsy having its seat in the pleural cavity is called hydrothorax, or water on the chest. The term is, in truth, sufficiently significant, the fluid which is poured out being mostly very thin and watery. The physical signs of hydrothorax are the same as those of an effusion due to inflammation; but as the dropsy results from an organic disease of the liver, heart, or kidneys, the serum collects in both pleural sacs. Now, an effusion caused by an inflammation of the pleura is nearly always one-sided. Even where both pleuræ are filled with fluid—a rare condition, excepting in tubercular pleurisy—one is affected before the other. This does not happen in hydrothorax. Thus the double-sided effusion, and its usual association with dropsies in other parts of the body, are matters of much significance. Besides, in forming a diagnosis of hydrothorax, we may lay some stress on the absence of friction sounds; on the smaller quantity of fluid; on the history of the malady; and on the presence of a structural lesion of the liver, kidneys, or heart.

These, then, are the diseases with which chronic pleurisy, when it produces dilatation of the chest, may be confounded. I have entered into the subject somewhat at length, because, in view of the frequency of the operation of paracentesis, it is important to know what affections besides chronic pleurisy may lead to prominence of the chest and to compression of the lung. It is well to be able to prove that none of them are present before a trocar is plunged through the intercostal spaces.

Diseases in which Retraction of the Chest occurs.

Chronic Pleurisy.—We may here continue the description of chronic pleurisy in the stage of absorption, since it is under these circumstances that the most marked retraction of the walls of the chest takes place. This shrinking of the thoracic parietes is not a sudden, but a very gradual act, and instances are therefore constantly met with in which the upper part of the chest is flattened and the lower, owing to its still containing fluid, bulges. The contraction of one side of the thorax attains its highest degree when the effusion in the pleura is discharged through the chest walls and external fistulous openings are established.

The symptoms in the stage of retraction are those of chronic pleurisy with dilatation of the chest, and present, therefore, the same variability. But œdema of the affected side, which is sometimes so striking a symptom of chronic pleurisy where the effusion is considerable, is here not noticed. The physical signs alter somewhat, according to the presence or absence of fluid in the pleural sac. When none exists, respiration is heard all over the lung as a feeble inspiration with prolonged expiration, or as an indistinct blowing. Now and then a friction sound may be caught by the ear. Where the pleura still contains liquid, these signs occur at the upper portion of the chest, and a much more absolute dulness on percussion, an absent voice and vocal fremitus at the lower part denote that fluid has there accumulated. The heart is found either in its normal position or still displaced. The force with which contraction takes place may pull it over to the side on which the shrinking is going on.

Now, it is evident that chronic pleurisy, when leading to retraction of one side of the chest, cannot be mistaken for diseases attended with thoracic distention; but it may be mistaken for affections like pulmonary cancer, tubercle, and chronic consolidation, which also occasion a flattening of the chest walls.

From *cancer* we distinguish it by the absence of the peculiar expectoration, and of hemorrhage; by the want of signs of perfect consolidation; by the dissimilar history. From *tubercle*, by the diminution of the chest in the latter not being confined to one side; by the physical signs indicative of deposit and softening at the upper portions of the lungs; by the presence of rales; by the occurrence of hemorrhage; and by the greater emaciation.

Chronic pneumonic consolidation presents, on the whole, most ever, recorded in which a enormously distended pericardial sac produced a flat sound posteriorly, and gave rise to signs of compression of the lung. But in these attention to the feeble impulse of the heart and its muffled sounds permitted it to be foretold that fluid had accumulated in the pericardium, and not in the pleura.

Hydrothorax. — A dropsy having its seat in the pleural cavity is called hydrothorax, or water on the chest. The term is, in truth, sufficiently significant, the fluid which is poured out being mostly very thin and watery. The physical signs of hydrothorax are the same as those of an effusion due to inflammation; but as the dropsy results from an organic disease of the liver, heart, or kidneys, the serum collects in both pleural sacs. Now an effusion caused by an inflammation of the pleura is only always one-sided. Even where

pleura are filled with fluid — a rare condition, excepting in tubercular pleurisy — one is affected before the other. This not happen in hydrothorax. Thus the double-sided effusion and its usual association with dropsies in other parts of the body, are matters of much significance. Besides, in forming a diagnosis of hydrothorax, we may lay some stress on the absence of friction sounds; on the smaller quantity of fluid; on the history of the malady; and on the presence of a structural lesion of the liver, kidneys, or heart.

These, then, are the diseases with which chronic pleurisy, when it produces dilatation of the chest, may be confounded. I have entered into the subject somewhat at length, because, in view of the frequency of the operation of paracentesis, it is important to know what affections besides chronic pleurisy may lead to prominence of the chest and to compression of It is well the able to prove that none of them before a trocar is plunged through the intercostal

Diseases in which Retraction of the Chest occurs.

Chronic Pleurisy. — We may here continue the consideration of chronic pleurisy in the stage of absorption under these circumstances that the most

points of resemblance. But there is this difference: the shrinking of the side in chronic pneumonia is less marked, and is confined to the part involved—usually the lower lobe of the lung. The retraction is much more general in chronic pleurisy; or where it is partial, it is the upper segment of one side of the chest which is flattened, and the lower is prominent, sounds very dull on percussion, and yields the ordinary physical evidences of fluid. In the former malady the blowing respiration, or the enfeebled inspiration and prolonged expiration, and the distinct voice are heard only over the consolidated lobe; in the other lobes the breathing is distinctly vesicular. In chronic pleurisy the same abnormal signs are either manifest over an entire side, or they are perceived over the narrowed portion of the chest, and below, the respiration, voice, and fremitus are abolished.

In that form of chronic pulmonary induration attended with dilatation of the bronchial tubes, to which the name of *cirrhosis* of the lung has been given,* the flattening of the affected part is as obvious as it is in pleurisy; and, as in this complaint, the heart may be drawn to the diseased side. The only traits of difference consist in the signs indicative of bronchial dilatation and of copious bronchial secretion; in the sound afforded by percussion being less dull, or at times tympanitic; and in the well-defined and harsher bronchial respiration, mixed often with coarse rales.

A *collapsed* state of the lung, resulting from a plug of mucus in the bronchial tubes, may, in rare instances, yield the manifestations of chronic pleurisy with partial retraction. No signs distinguish such cases, except the more limited depression; the absence of any disease above the flattened spot; the want of friction sound, and of tenderness on pressure; and the rapid disappearance of the physical phenomena after an effort of coughing has removed the obstruction.†

Where external *fistulous openings* exist, the shrinking of the side, as already stated, is carried to the highest degree.

---

* Corrigan, Dublin Quart. Journ., vol. xiii.

† An interesting instance of this kind is related by the late Prof. Pepper in the American Journal of the Medical Sciences for April, 1852.

These fistulæ, whether produced artificially or by nature, may close after they have served the purpose of evacuating the fluid in the pleural cavity. But they often persist for months or years, and keep on discharging offensive, purulent matter. The patient emaciates under this continued drain, yet not so quickly as might be imagined. More or less troublesome cough annoys him, but it is not ordinarily accompanied by much expectoration. Every now and then, however, he discharges for days a quantity of fetid, purulent sputum. It is difficult to understand why this happens. It seems certainly, so far as physical signs can prove, not the liquid in the pleura which is being voided through a perforation of the pulmonary tissue, for the physical signs of pneumothorax are absent.

The clubbing of the nails is often extremely marked, and may exist to an extent far greater than in phthisis. The nail is rounded and bluish, and the whole end of the finger looks enlarged. This appearance is even more striking than the curve of the nail. The nails and last joints of the toes show the same alteration.

The fistulous opening is situated ordinarily in the intercostal space below the nipple. It may, however, be seated at the back of the chest, and communicate by a tortuous sinus with the intestine and other abdominal viscera. If it pass into the lung, the physical evidences of pneumothorax are present; but the side is still retracted, and striking the chest elicits a mixture of a dull and a tympanitic sound. Where merely an external opening exists, no signs of pneumothorax occur, because no air finds its way into the pleural cavity.

A fistulous opening into the pleura is not difficult of diagnosis. It is easy to establish the fact that the fistula is not simply produced by caries of the rib, for a probe may be run into the chest for two, three, or four inches.

I base these statements on several instances of chronic pleurisy attended with external fistula which have come under my notice. The seat of the opening near the nipple; the peculiar nail; the occasional flow for days of a most offensive sputum from the bronchial tubes, without any traces of pneumothorax; the ease with which the fistula could be probed, and its depth; the gradual emaciation; and, I may add, the decided improvement under the persistent use of tonics,—belonged to them all and justify the description given.

SECTION II.

DISEASES OF THE HEART.

The diagnosis of affections of the heart turns so completely upon a knowledge of its anatomy and physiology, that it will be necessary, before we study its diseases, to recall some of the more important anatomical and physiological facts connected with the organ.

The heart is a hollow muscle employed in forcing blood into all parts of the body. It is kept from rolling about in the chest by the great vessels which spring from its base, and by the attachment to the diaphragm of its membranous covering—the pericardium. It lies obliquely in this membrane, with its long axis directed downward and toward the left. Its broad end, or base, points backward and upward toward the right shoulder; its under side rests upon the central tendon of the diaphragm. The interior of the heart is lined by a serous membrane—the endocardium—which is reflected over the valves guarding the inlets and outlets for the blood. These valves all lie in close proximity to each other, and within a space of less than an inch square.

The relations the different parts of the organ bear to the chest walls are as follows: the auricles are on a line with the third costal cartilages; the right auricle extends across the sternum to the right side of the chest. The right ventriele is placed partly under the sternum, and partly to the left of it Its inferior border is on a level with the sixth cartilage. The left ventricle lies within the nipple, between the third and fifth intercostal spaces. The apex is seated between the cartilages of the fifth and sixth ribs, to the inner side of, and from an inch and a half to two inches below the left nipple. The base of the heart corresponds posteriorly to the sixth and seventh dorsal vertebræ, from which it is separated by the aorta and œsophagus. The greater portion of the anterior surface of the heart is removed from the thoracic walls by the lungs. The right lung extends to the middle of the sternum. The left lung spreads out as far as the fourth cartilage, and covers the whole of the left ventricle, excepting the apex. The part of the heart which remains exposed consists thus mainly of the lower portion of the right ventricle; it presents the shape of a rude triangle.

FIG. 25.

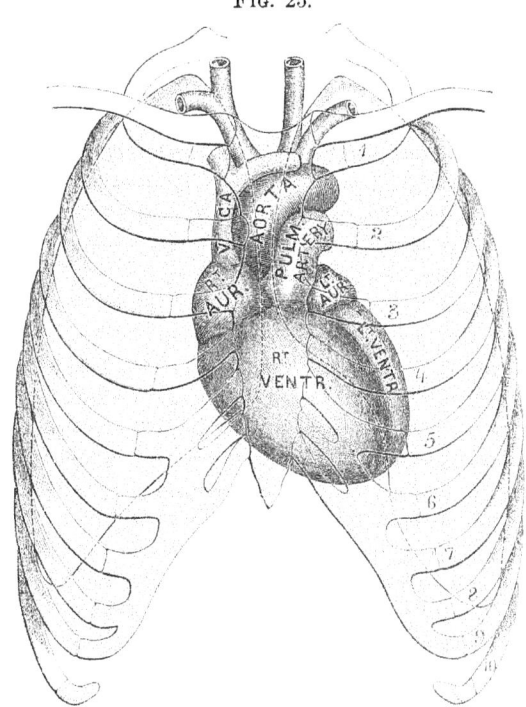

Topography of the heart. The relations of each portion of the heart to the walls of the chest are shown. The dotted lines mark the lungs. The figure may, I think, be relied upon: it is based upon several careful dissections

The position of the valves can be learned by running needles into the chest before the viscus is taken out. In this manner it is ascertained that at the left border of the sternum, on a level with the third intercostal space, lies the mitral, and in front of this, more directly under the sternum, and but a few lines lower down, the tricuspid valve. The pulmonary orifice is seated opposite the junction of the cartilage of the third rib with the left edge of the sternum. Near it, very slightly lower, but placed more obliquely, are the aortic valves. The aorta then proceeds from left to right, and ascends to the upper border of the second costal cartilage on the right side; thence it crosses, under the sternum and in front of the trachea, to the left side. The pulmonary artery is found in the second intercostal space on the left side, inclosed in the pericardium, and passes to the cartilage of the second rib, where it bifurcates.

The size of the heart is about that of the closed fist. Bouillaud estimates its mean weight in adults as between eight and nine ounces. Only in very large persons does it exceed this.

This organ, so essential to life, exhibits, when in action, a wonderfully perfect mechanism and regularity of movement. Its cavities contract on both sides at the same time, and distend on both sides at the same time. It then rests for a short period. This process is repeated about seventy times in the course of a minute. The contraction of the ventricles occasions the impulse which is seen and felt in the fifth intercostal space. While the blood is flowing in and out of the heart, the valves are kept in constant motion. Their play makes itself known by two distinct sounds of unequal length, which are produced mainly by their opening and closing. The first long and dull sound is caused by the forcible closure of the valves at the auriculo-ventricular openings. Yet it is not a purely valvular sound. The stroke of the heart against the walls of the chest, and the muscular contraction itself, aid in its formation. The first sound corresponds, therefore, to the impulse of the heart, to the opening of the valves at the orifice of the aorta and of the pulmonary artery, and to the passage of blood along the arteries.

The second sound is short, abrupt, and ringing. It results from the sudden closure of the semilunar valves. During its occurrence the blood rushes in through the opened mitral and tricuspid valves, and dilates the ventricles.

This seems to be the simplest explanation of the sounds of the heart. At all events, it is the one best supported by physiological proofs, and most in harmony with those manifestations of disease by which nature teaches us, more certainly than vivisections do, her great truths. Yet I cannot dismiss the subject without adverting to the probability of the view of Skoda, that other causes may concur in producing the sounds of the heart; that, in other words, the aorta and pulmonary artery at their origin, and even the ventricles at times, may severally assist in occasioning both sounds. There are certainly phenomena which are met with in some instances of disorders of the valves that do not seem capable of being explained in any other way.

Examination of the Heart by the Different Methods of Physical Diagnosis.

Before proceeding to examine the heart, it is best to inquire into the history of the case, and into such symptoms as the expression of the face; the appearance of the eye; the condition of the capillary circulation; the presence or absence of dropsical swellings and of cough; the state of the breathing; the character of the pulse; and the frequency and violence of the palpitations. By the time these points have been ascertained, the agitation arising from the proposed exploration is somewhat calmed down, and the heart itself may be more advantageously interrogated. First, the cardiac region is scrutinized by the eye and by the hand; then the size of the organ is estimated by percussion; and lastly, its sounds are studied by the stethoscope. These different methods are most conveniently practised when the patient is in an easy position, leaning back in a chair or propped up with pillows in bed. To examine them more in detail:

INSPECTION.

Inspection detects on the chest of some healthy persons a slight protrusion over the seat of the heart; yet this is far from being constant or even the general rule. When the heart is hypertrophied, or when fluid has accumulated in the pericardium, we perceive a marked prominence in the precordial region. A depression at the lower part of this region may be natural; a very evident depression is almost always the result of an attack of pericardial inflammation.

Yet neither prominence nor depression is a very important sign. One much more so, which inspection shows, is the *impulse* of the heart. This is seen where the apex beats against the walls of the chest: between the fifth and sixth ribs, about an inch inward from the nipple and two inches downward. It is for the most part confined to this point, and appears as a brief raising of the integument, occurring with great regularity of succession. In lean persons it is very distinct; in fat persons it is generally not at all perceptible. Its seat, even in those who are in perfect health, is not always exactly the same. It is changed by different positions, and by the distention of the stomach after a full meal or by flatulence. It is, however, most modified by the acts of respiration. During a long-drawn inspiration the expanded lung sweeps the heart inward, and the impulse becomes discernible in the epigastrium. During a fixed expiration the beat moves upward, and appears more extended and weightier. The changes produced in its situation by disease, both thoracic and abdominal, are many. It is tilted upward and outward by the left lobe of an enlarged liver. It is displaced by diverse affections of the lungs and pleura. It is forced up, as Walshe so accurately notices, by a pericardial effusion. It is visible lower down and over a larger surface in enlargements of the heart; but even then it is most distinct at the apex.

The alterations in the character and force of the impulse are as diversified as those of its seat. But they are more readily appreciated by the hand than by the eye.

PALPATION.

Palpation is, as far as the exploration of the heart is concerned, much preferable to inspection. Many an impulse can be felt which cannot be seen. The rhythm of the motion is changed by a large number of cardiac affections, both functional and organic. So are the extent and force of the beat. Both are temporarily increased by any powerful excitement; both are permanently augmented by hypertrophy. In dilatation and pericardial effusion, the extent over which the stroke is felt is greater than in health; but the impulse is feeble, and in the latter disease irregular and wavy. Softening of the texture of the heart, diseases of the brain, some morbid states of the blood, and a low condition of the system will also enfeeble the beat.

The hand, when laid on the precordial region, perceives at times *two* impulses. This double impulse is often recognizable in health, especially in thin persons. It becomes still more evident in hypertrophy with dilatation of the ventricles. One of the beats is systolic; the other corresponds to the diastole. Bouillaud cites examples in which the diastolic stroke was double. Such cases must be uncommonly rare. The systolic beat is occasionally split into several parts when the pericardium adheres to the heart.

All these modifications of the impulse stand in direct connection with the action of the ventricles. The auricles, save in some rare instances in which they are dilated and their walls thickened, give rise to no perceptible movement.

Besides the impulse of the heart, other phenomena may be studied by placing the hand over the cardiac region. The sounds of the heart can be analyzed by means of the touch. They will be felt: the one as a long and dull, the other as a short and distinct vibration. The motion is due to the play of the valves, and disappears with their destruction.

The fingers applied over the heart perceive at times a peculiar thrill, or a rubbing movement. The first—called by Laennec, from its resemblance to the pur of a cat, the purring tremor—is nearly always indicative of a valvular lesion. The second is caused by the to and-fro motion of a roughened pericardium.

A more accurate means of studying the varying impulse than is afforded by the fingers, has been sought to be attained by instruments to record the beat of the heart. The cardioscope of Alison was invented for this purpose, and the sphygmograph of Marey has been used for the cardiac impulse as well as for the pulse. How this ingenious instrument is made applicable to the study of diseases of the heart has been mentioned in another part of this volume, and its tracings, so far as they have been proved to be of real diagnostic value, will be examined in connection with individual maladies.

PERCUSSION.

Percussion affords the readiest means of judging of the size of the heart. But to percuss a heart is not easy; it requires care and some skill. The patient is placed in a recumbent position; then, by a series of moderately strong taps, we proceed downward from near the middle of the clavicle, until a dull sound, accompanied by decided resistance, tells that we are striking over a solid organ. The point at which this dull sound begins is over, or immediately at, the lower border of the fourth cartilage. It corresponds to the upper limit of the portion of the heart which is left uncovered by the lung.

The superior border of the dulness having been thus ascertained, we next percuss on the right side of the sternum, on about a level with the fifth rib, and progress across the bone. At, or very near to, its left edge we find marked resistance and a duller sound. Here we draw our second line, and continue to strike straight across the cardiac region up to the point at which a clear, full note demonstrates that the pulmonary tissue is resounding. This determines the transverse diameter of the heart; at least so far as it can be mapped out on the chest. The apex of the organ and its inferior surface remain yet to be fixed. The first is readily done by advancing in an oblique direction from the already ascertained right border. But we can save ourselves this trouble by feeling for the impulse or listening for it with a stethoscope.

The inferior surface is exceedingly perplexing to circum-scribe. It can only be accomplished by prolonging the line of the dulness on percussion of the upper border of the liver, and then judging by the greater amount of resistance and the fall in pitch that the heart has been reached. These are not easy to appreciate; nor is it indeed often necessary to define the contiguous edges of the left lobe of the liver and of the heart. If the other boundaries have been correctly drawn, the size of the heart can be accurately estimated,— accurately enough, at least, for any practical purpose. But the dulness elicited by percussing the cardiac region is not so absolute as that of the liver or of some other solids. It is mixed up with the sound of the lung tissue, or with the resonance of the sternum. Nor is it a representation of the size of the entire organ. It simply portrays the more super-ficial portion, which is uncovered by the lungs.

In women it is particularly difficult to define these limits. It can only be done by having the mammary gland drawn to one side while percussing. It is equally difficult in children, as the space over which the dulness is perceived is very small. Indeed, so unsatisfactory are in them the results of percus-sion, that, were we to trust only to this method of investiga-tion, we should often have to conclude that the heart was wanting. In adults the dulness ordinarily spreads over two, or nearly two, intercostal spaces. Its transverse diameter in a grown person of medium size is about two inches and a half. In tall, broad-chested men it is upwards of three inches. Such at all events is the result of measurements I have made. It does not agree with the statement of a dis-tinguished clinical teacher, Dr. Bennett: that if, as a general rule, the transverse diameter of the dulness measure more than two inches, the heart is abnormally enlarged.

The range of the dulness is changed by a number of causes, physiological as well as pathological. A full inspira-tion alters it materially, by bringing the lung down over the heart, and by displacing the organ itself. The upper border of the percussion dulness shifts to the extent of an inter-costal space. Below the nipple, between the fifth and sixth ribs, the sound becomes clear; but over the dislodged lower

21

part of the heart, the beat of which is distinctly seen under
the cartilages of the ribs, at a point varying from three-
fourths to one and a fourth inch from the median line, there
is dulness with resistance to the finger.   A full expiration
produces, for the most part, converse phenomena.   It enlarges the boundaries, especially in an upward and transverse direction.   The dulness reaches nearly, or even
entirely, across the sternum.

The area of dulness is diminished in emphysema.   It is
increased by a shrinking of the left lung, and by diseases of
the heart and of its membranes.   Prominent among these
stand hypertrophy, dilatation, and an effusion into the pericardial sac.

AUSCULTATION.

When the ear or a stethoscope is applied over a healthy
heart, it detects two sounds of very dissimilar character : the
first is long, dull, heavy, and corresponds to the impulse
against the walls of the chest ; the second is short and flapping, and occurs after the impulse.   These sounds are audible
at all parts of the precordial region, but not everywhere with
equal distinctness.   The first being more ventricular in origin,
is best heard over the lower part of the heart ; the second, a
more strictly valvular sound, is more defined at the base.

The causes of these sounds have been already explained.
It has been stated that they are, to a great extent, produced
by the play of the valves.   Each of these forms a separate
sound, or at least a portion of one.   Now, experience teaches
that there are points at which the sounds of the several parts
of the heart may be isolated.   Some of these accord with
the anatomical seat of the valves ; others do not.   None do
so very closely ; and the proximity of the valves to each other
is such as to make it desirable that the localities selected for
listening to them should be some distance apart.

Clinical observation sanctions the following : the sounds
of the aorta are to be studied at the right edge of the sternum, in the second intercostal space.   From there the stethoscope may be carried to the second costal cartilage of the
right side, the "aortic cartilage," and down to the left edge

of the sternum opposite the third intercostal space; that is, not far from the seat of the aortic valves. The pulmonary orifice lies very close to them; but the artery itself ascends to the second costal cartilage on the left side. Its sound may, therefore, be isolated in the second intercostal space, near to the left edge of the sternum. The mitral is listened to immediately above the beat of the apex. The sounds of the tricuspid and of the right ventricle may be sought for in the vicinity of and somewhat above the ensiform cartilage.

FIG. 26.

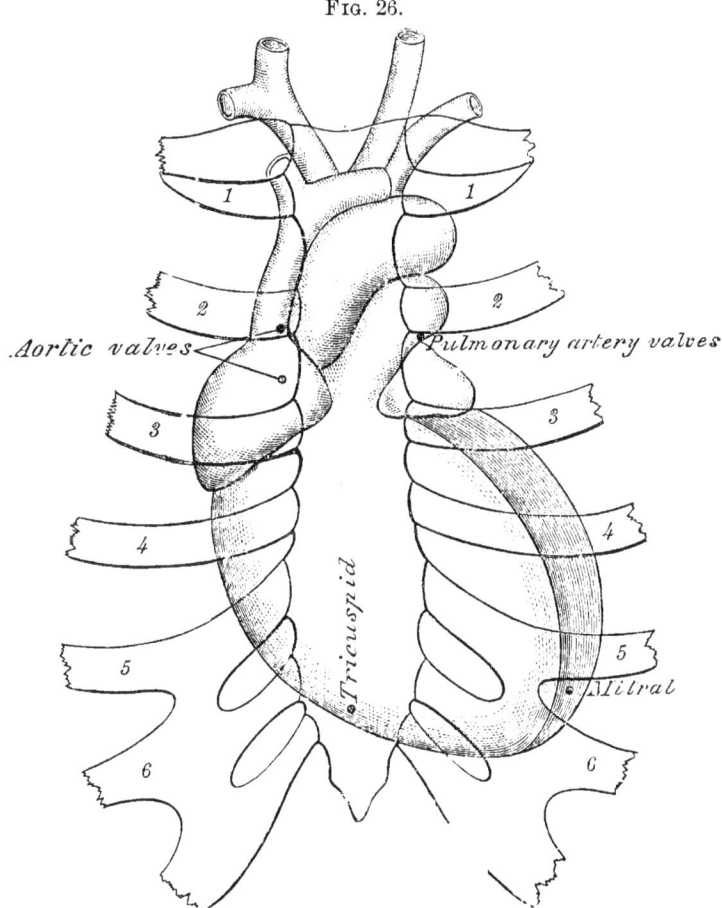

Diagram showing the points at which the separate valves may be listened to.

Both sounds are discerned at each of these points. But the same sound varies in different situations. The first sound over the left ventricle near the apex of the heart is dull, heavy, and prolonged; that over the right ventricle is clearer, shorter, and of higher pitch. The second sound heard there presents no constant and appreciable variance from that of the left ventricle; yet it is less ringing and distinct than the second sound of the pulmonary artery and aorta. Even these two are not precisely alike. The second sound of the latter, when compared with that of the former, is found to be sharper and more accentuated. The first sound, however, does not differ materially from that of the pulmonary artery. But the first sound of both does differ most materially from that over the ventricles. Compared with the first sound over the right ventricle, the first sound of the pulmonary artery is much duller, more indistinct and like a vibration, and not of so high a pitch. Compared with the first sound at the apex, the first sound of the aorta lacks the weighty, prolonged character which belongs to the ventricular sound.

These statements are based on a series of observations made, some with an ordinary stethoscope, some with a double stethoscope. They certainly would seem to favor the view of Skoda, that the first sound, as heard over the great vessels, is not merely a transmitted sound, but is one which is partly, if not entirely, generated by the arteries themselves when the blood rushes into them.

The sounds just considered undergo various modifications, both when the heart is affected and when it is free from disease. They may be audible over a larger space of the chest than usually; they may be changed in character and rhythm. Their transmission over a larger space is an unimportant sign. They are undoubtedly perceived over a more extended surface when the heart is enlarged; but they are equally or more diffused when the surrounding tissues are condensed. And even in the most perfect health their range is very diversified.

During a full inspiration, the sounds at the interspace between the second and third costal cartilages on the left side disappear almost entirely, and become faint at the aortic cartilage. The first sound at the apex lessens also very much in distinctness, but it is better heard at a new point of impulse, visible toward the median line and just below the cartilages of the ribs. During a full expiration, the extent over which the heart sounds are perceived is increased.

The sounds grow in loudness in any functional disturbance of the heart. When the organ is palpitating violently under strong nervous excitement, they may become short and sharp, and sometimes so loud and ringing as to be audible to the by-standers. They are often permanently louder than in health, and shorter and more clearly defined when the walls of the heart are thinned. This is particularly the case with the *first* sound. When the walls of the heart are thick, the first sound over the hypertrophied portion is apt to be exceedingly dull and prolonged. The first sound is weakened if the structure of the heart be softened; hence it is feeble in some low fevers, and in fatty degeneration of the organ. It is also less distinct when there is a want of tone in the muscle, or when the mitral and tricuspid valves are thickened.*

The *second* sound is not so liable to be changed as the first. It is rendered somewhat duller by a thickening of the semilunar valves, and, on the other hand, more ringing when they are thin, and in some cases of great functional excitement of the heart. The sound becomes more distinctly accentuated if the column of blood return on the valves and close them forcibly. This occurs in some cases of hypertrophy of the ventricles. It also takes place where a decided obstruction exists to the passage of blood through the lungs. It is then over the pulmonary artery alone that this accentuated second sound is audible.

Both the sounds are occasionally obscure, and seem to

---

* To determine whether a dull first sound heard at the apex be due to an injured mitral valve, or to an alteration of the muscular power of the heart, Dr. Flint, in his Essay on the Heart Sounds in Health and Disease, advises to place the stethoscope over the apex of the heart, and then on the outside of the left nipple. The element of impulsion and the valvular element which unite to form the complex first sound may thus be isolated and turned to practical account. If there be a marked impulsion over the apex, but if by means of the stethoscope placed to the left we perceive no sound at all which possesses a valvular character, or but a faintly valvular sound, the inference is that the mitral valves are more or less damaged.

arrive at the ear from a distance. This happens when fluid has accumulated in the pericardium. The sounds may be changed in their relative proportion to each other, and the pauses between them be lengthened or shortened, or else the sounds may intermit from time to time. From this perverted rhythm we do not derive any definite instruction as to the condition causing it. It serves only to show that the heart is acting irregularly, and thus directs our attention to the state of the organ. It is apt to be associated with organic disease; but it can exist without it. The same may be said of that curious phenomenon, the reduplication of the sounds of the heart. The second sound is the one which is more generally split. Yet both of them may be doubled, or one may be doubled over one part of the heart and not over another; so that four or three sounds are counted to each beat of the pulse. The cause of the reduplication is, so far as we know, the want of synchronous action of the two sides of the heart. The direct value for diagnosis of the altered movement is not great; but indirectly it teaches a most important lesson: it tells us that each side of the heart forms its own sounds, and that, to arrive at accurate conclusions, each side has to be separately examined.

Such, then, are the modifications which the healthy sounds present. At times we meet with sounds which do not in the least resemble those naturally heard, and which overshadow them or take their place. They are called *murmurs*, and are mainly produced either within the heart or on its surface.

Those that are *endocardial* have all a common quality: they are all more or less blowing. Yet the sound is not always of the same character or pitch. It may be low toned, it may be high pitched; it may be soft, it may be harsh; it may resemble the blowing of a bellows, it may be musical; or it may be filing, or rasping, or sawing. The ingenuity of every listener exerts itself in tracing a similarity to some familiar noise; but all to no practical purpose. These different sounds have not been proved to have a significance beyond that of a blowing sound. They teach us nothing certain as to its source. They are, moreover, not at all times the same in the same case, since the heart, when excited, may emit a sound different from that which it does when it is beating quietly.

A blowing sound originates in the altered relation of the blood to the part over which it moves. This general statement opens the way to the consideration of the specially acting elements, both in the blood and the heart itself.

Most usually a cardiac murmur springs from a change at one of the orifices. This may be either a narrowing or roughening, which interposes a local obstruction to the flow of the blood, or it may be an insufficiency to close the opening. In the latter case the blood regurgitates, and a murmur is occasioned by the deviation of the direction of the current and the establishment of another. This subversion of the course of the circulating fluid, added to its increased velocity and force, is one of the sources of those temporary blowing sounds not unfrequently perceived when a heart is violently excited, while both its valvular apparatus and muscular texture are perfectly healthy. But we meet every now and then with instances where none of these causes are present, and where altered blood is the foundation of the murmur.

Thus, to sum up the subject, we find murmurs which depend upon organic change, and murmurs which are unconnected with any structural alteration; and these inorganic murmurs are either due to an unnatural condition of the blood, or to temporarily perverted action of the heart—in other words, they are either hæmic or dynamic.

The murmurs, however caused, have different effects on the sounds of the heart. They either accompany the sound throughout its whole or part of its duration, and thus obscure it, or else they take its place, and hinder it from being generated. In time of their occurrence they correspond to the contraction or to the dilatation of the heart, and therefore to the first or second sound. At any rate, they do so as far as we can ascertain practically. It is true, they may immediately precede or succeed either, and fill mainly the intervals of silence between the sounds; but attention to such minute divisions is, for ordinary purposes, unnecessary, and indeed they cannot be often readily recognized at the

bedside. In point of fact, it is often difficult enough, and
sometimes even impossible, to say whether the murmur we
hear is systolic or diastolic.

The readiest· method of judging of the time of the production of a murmur is to feel for the impulse with the
finger while listening with the stethoscope. The blowing
sound which agrees with the beat of the heart is systolic;
the one which takes place between the beats is diastolic.

When a murmur is once established, it attends each motion
of the heart that can give rise to it; but it is not always
equally perceptible. It may become very faint, or disappear
entirely by the patient changing his position. It is sometimes
only manifest when the heart is acting strongly. Indeed, it
always requires a certain force and velocity in the passage of
the blood, to generate a murmur. Yet overaction of the
heart may be as destructive of its distinctness as diminished
action. This is, however, a matter that, should it be desirable for diagnosis, we can control by the administration
of medicines like digitalis, aconite, or veratrum viride, provided their use be not contraindicated by other considera-
tions.

A murmur is sometimes heard by the patient himself, or is
audible before the ear is placed over the heart. It may be
perceived as an abrupt blowing sound, apparently coming out
of the mouth. A gentleman, whose mitral valves permitted
of regurgitation, was under my charge. When he held his
breath and kept his mouth open, he, as well as I, could detect
an abrupt blowing sound issuing from the oral cavity. This
sound, when the heart's action was at all excited, aecom-
panied regularly each impulse.

Posture exerts a very decided effect upon murmurs. A
blowing sound distinct in the recumbent position may become
very faint or disappear when the patient stands erect; and
the reverse equally holds good. Its nature—whether organic
or inorganic—does not seem to influence the readiness with
which it is affected by change of posture. Pressure, too,
has an influence upon the abnormal cardiac sound; it notably augments it, and often raises its pitch. Yet, pressing
the stethoscope firmly against the chest does not occasion

as much change in endocardial as it does in pericardial sounds.

A murmur may be obscured by the respiratory sound; but this is not apt to be a cause of error in diagnosis. It is not nearly so fruitful a source of mistake as considering the natural sounds of the lungs to be blowing sounds in the heart. Certainly the resemblance is often very great, and we must be aware of it to avoid blunders, which may be readily done by listening to the heart while the patient suspends his breathing.

Having ascertained positively the existence and the time of occurrence of an endocardial murmur, the next thing is to determine its exact seat, and, if possible, its immediate cause. The *seat* of the murmur is judged of by the place of its greatest intensity, and the relation this bears to one of the four points for the clinical examination of the heart above described. If it be most distinct at or near the apex of the heart, it is produced at the mitral orifice; if immediately above or at the ensiform cartilage, it is generated in the right ventricle and at the tricuspid opening. If we hear it most plainly at the sternum, somewhat toward its left border on a level with the third intercostal space or even the fourth rib, and with equal or nearly equal distinctness at the second costal cartilage on the right side, we are enabled to decide that it is developed at the origin of the aorta. The pulmonary artery is not often the seat of a murmur. When it is, this is clearly perceptible in the second intercostal space on the left side, and extends, if the valves be diseased, to the junction of the third left cartilage with the sternum.

Each of these situations may be the site of a distinct murmur occupying only one sound of the heart, or produced in both,—one murmur taking place with, the other against the current of blood. Yet it rarely happens that the murmur is strictly limited to one of these positions; it will mostly extend from its point of intensity in various directions, growing fainter and fainter as this is left. A blowing murmur thus transmitted may drown the natural sounds of the heart at the parts not diseased. But when one orifice only is affected, we can usually find the sounds at the other valves. They may be obscured, but still they exist; and it is a vast aid when they are heard, since they set the limits to the disease. How important is it, then, to examine each portion of the heart separately, as much for the purpose of saying what is not as what is deranged!

If satisfied as to the seat of the murmur, we naturally turn to inquire into its origin. Is it caused by an alteration of the valves? Is it unconnected with any appreciable change of structure in the heart? There is nothing in the murmur itself which will tell us positively. As a rule, it is true that a harsh murmur results from organic disease, and a soft murmur is inorganic; but there are a fair number of exceptions. We judge with much more certainty by the time of the occurrence of the blowing sound and by the accompanying phenomena. A murmur attending the distention of the heart shows that the orifices are injured. A systolic murmur may be either organic, or it may indicate simply a change in the state of the blood, or of the force and velocity with which it is circulating. In the latter case, however, the abnormal sound is temporary, and disappears with the excitement. If arising from an impoverished state of the blood, it is generally soft, of low pitch, is perceived over the base of the heart, and is accompanied by a humming sound in the veins of the neck. But we shall further on examine this question more in detail.

Throughout the consideration of the endocardial murmurs, they have been treated as originating at the seat of the valves. In truth, it is there where they are formed. Still they are occasionally due to morbid states in the body of the ventricle, or in the auricle. But in either case they are clinical curiosities. As regards the auricles, they yield no appreciable sound in health, nor are they in disease but very rarely the source of either sound or murmur.

A blowing sound is not of necessity limited to the heart; it may be transmitted all over the arterial system. Yet it would be a great mistake to suppose that every murmur heard over the arteries is connected with a disease of the heart. It is often but the sign of impoverished blood, or a sound dependent upon local roughening or narrowing of the tube. The latter may be temporarily produced by the pressure of a stethoscope; a fact of which it is well to be aware. It is even stated that pressure over a healthy heart may generate a murmur; but I confess that I have never been able to satisfy myself of the truth of this statement. It is certainly incorrect as a general rule, and depends, when it happens, much more likely upon the condition of the blood and the force with which it circulates.

Let us now examine the sounds which originate on the outside of the heart. These *pericardial murmurs* have all a common source: they all result from irregularities on the membrane. Like the pleura, the smooth serous covering of the heart moves noiselessly in health; but when it is roughened by a deposit of any kind, the friction of its surfaces gives rise to a sound which may be single, but which is more usually double. The character of this sound is very variable. It may be a distinct to-and-fro rubbing murmur, or it may be grazing, or scratching, or creaking, or whistling, or clicking and resembling the valvular sounds. It has but one quality which is constant, and that is, its superficiality. By this superficiality; by the strict limitation of the sound to the region of the heart; by its altering from time to time its precise seat; by its greater extent and intensity when the patient bends forward; by its occasional increase, and even change of character on external pressure; by its following, rather than occurring with, the movements of the heart; and by the sensation of friction which it communicates to the finger,— we know that the sound heard is produced on the surface, and not in the inside of the heart. Yet in spite of this array of points of difference, it is often difficult enough to distinguish an endocardial from a pericardial murmur.

A friction sound is prone to mask the natural sounds of the heart. At times, although heard over the cardiac region, it is not due to inflammation of the pericardium. The exudation may be on the surface of the pleura adjacent to the pericardium, and the murmur be caused solely by the movements of the heart. Sometimes, again, the sound heard in the cardiac region is in reality the rubbing of an inflamed pleura.

If any doubt exist, let the patient be told to suspend his breathing. As this is stopped, the pleural sound ceases.

Such is a brief description of the different physical signs met with in examining the heart, both in health and disease. Their importance for diagnosis it is difficult to overestimate. A knowledge of the physical signs is the solid foundation, without which any structure that may be raised will soon tumble to pieces.

The General and Local Symptoms of Diseases of the Heart.

It is not easy to say what are and what are not the symptoms that belong to diseases of the heart. There are vital manifestations directing attention to the heart which are not associated with any change in its structure; and most serious changes in its structure may occur without any of these vital manifestations. Yet we often find a significant group of symptoms which accompany an affection of the heart. Some . of these attest directly to the organ disturbed, such as pain in the cardiac region, and palpitation. Others are the indirect and more remote expressions of its derangement, such as cough, dyspnœa, hemorrhages, dropsy, disorders of the brain and nervous system, engorgement of the abdominal viscera, a peculiar state of the arteries and veins, and the aspect of the face. It is unnecessary to do more than mention some of these, since several have been already described in connection with pulmonary complaints, and there is nothing in the cough or in the shortness of breath by which we can absolutely determine it to be caused by a disease of the heart. The same with respect to the hemorrhage; there is nothing characteristic about it. It simply proves the efforts of the blood-vessels to relieve themselves of the strain which the disturbance in the flow of the blood has put on them. The capillaries and the smaller blood-vessels give way first; partly from the reason just assigned, and partly from the altered state of their nutrition, which a disordered circulation brings in its train. These hemorrhages are prone to happen from the bronchial tubes and the lung, and the blood is expectorated; but they may also take place directly into the pulmonary tissue, or into or from any part of the body. Their danger is in proportion to the amount, to the importance of the function of the structures into which the blood is effused, and to the possibility of its finding an outlet. It is hardly requisite to state that the peril is greatest when the circulating fluid has been poured out into the brain or into other parts of the nervous system.

Cardiac Dropsy.—The dropsy caused by a disease of the heart is met with in different situations: in the cellular tissues, in the peritoneal and pleural cavities, in the pericardium, in the ventricles of the brain, and under the arachnoid, in the air-cells of the lungs—in fact, in any part where fluid can exude, and where there is a space which can receive.

In anasarca dependent upon a cardiac lesion, the dropsical swelling commences about the ankles and feet; hence œdema beginning in this situation is regarded as among the surest of the symptoms of a disease of the heart. The accumulation is much influenced by position: the feet are more puffy toward evening, when the patient has been all day in the erect posture, and least so when he gets up in the morning.

What the condition of the heart is that gives rise to dropsy, has been made a matter of much dispute. It has been held to be uniformly connected with dilatation of the right side of the heart. It has been thought not to happen, unless a tricuspid regurgitation was also present. It has been taught to be invariably linked to a valvular affection. Clinical experience shows us that it may or may not exist where these states are present. The dropsy is most constantly found to be associated with an impediment to, or disturbance in the flow of the venous blood, and, therefore, with disorder of the right side of the heart, particularly with a dilatation of the cavities. It may be permanent or not. Its extent certainly does not bear a constant relation to the extent of the cardiac disease. It bears a more constant relation to the amount of venous congestion, and to the impoverishment of the blood.

Derangement of the Circulation.—Unmistakable evidence of the obstruction to the flow of the blood through the veins is afforded by their prominence in different por-

tions of the body. This is specially manifest in the superficial veins of the neck, which, moreover, when the tricuspid
orifice is permanently open, exhibit a distinct pulsation with
each beat of the heart. The turgid condition of the venous
system is rendered equally obvious by the livid tinge of the
skin and the bluish color of the lip, and by those ramifications of fine bluish vessels which strike the eye at once. But
the arterial system may also be gorged, and we may find the
capillaries and the smaller arteries seemingly ready to burst.
The conjunctiva is then highly injected, and the cheek has a
coarse, red look. This change in the color and appearance
of the face, the thickening of the eyelids, and the prominent
eye, make up the peculiar physiognomy of a chronic cardiac
malady. The state of the larger arteries is very variable, and
mainly according to the nature of the disorder. The pulse
may be small and tense; it may be full; it may be rebound-
ing; it may be very irregular; and it is often out of all proportion to the forcible action of the heart. But these are
matters to which we shall return.

The derangement of the circulation of individual parts manifests itself by special symptoms. It shows itself in the brain
by violent headaches, by vertigo, by apoplectic seizures. We
see evidences of the congestion of the nervous system in the
disturbed dreams; in the sudden starting up from sleep; in
the irregular action of certain muscles; in the spots which
float before the eye. It is possible that the strange sense of
insecurity, and the irritability of which patients afflicted with
a cardiac malady complain, are produced by the same cause.
At any rate, whether produced thus or not, they are remarkable symptoms. There is no disease which unnerves more
than a disease of the heart. Indeed, mere fear of its presence gives rise to restlessness and gloom, and breeds timidity
in those who would look any danger boldly in the face.

The disordered flow of blood through the abdominal viscera occasions organic changes and a disturbance of the functions of the several organs. Thus the liver increases in size,
or undergoes other alterations which interfere more or less
seriously with the elimination of the bile; or the kidneys no
longer secrete as in health, but drain off the albumen of the

blood, and finally pass into a state of disorganization; or the spleen sustains textural transformations. These states all tend to give rise to more and more dropsy, and hence to more and more suffering.

The symptoms which point most directly to the heart itself are palpitation and irregularity of action, and pain. These symptoms always, or nearly always, imply that the function of the organ is disturbed, or that its innervation is in some manner deranged; but they imply nothing more. They are, therefore, common to functional derangement which occurs associated with structural changes in the heart, and to purely functional derangement which occurs dissociated with such changes.

Cardiac Pain.—Pain in or over the heart is met with both in acute and chronic diseases; yet it is not a regular or well-defined symptom of either. When we reflect that the heart may be pinched, may be torn, without exciting any suffering, it will be readily understood why its disorders do not occasion much pain. Indeed, many a case of enormous enlargement of the heart, or of profound textural alteration of its walls or valvular apparatus, is unaccompanied by pain. This is, perhaps, the general rule; but, like every general rule, it has its exceptions. We sometimes meet with instances in which a distress at the heart and uneasy sensations of various kinds are among the more marked symptoms of a chronic cardiac lesion; and we even find persons complaining of a persistent pain in the heart, which extends to the left side of the neck and arm, in whom this symptom has preceded the signs of a disease of the heart, or of its great vessels.

In the acute cardiac affections pain is a not inconstant symptom. Uneasy sensations, not amounting perhaps to absolute pain, are complained of in endocarditis. Actual pain is among the vital manifestations of inflammation of the substance of the heart, and of the pericardium. In the latter disorder it is usually increased by pressure, and is frequently very severe. But no suffering in the cardiac region is as harrowing as that which happens in the obscure malady termed angina pectoris.

Angina Pectoris.—Although the nature of the complaint

may be hidden, the symptoms are obvious enough. We do
not know what the precise causes of this angina are; but we
do know that the disease occasions paroxysms of the most intolerable anguish. These paroxysms come on suddenly, and
pass off as suddenly. Their main feature is an agonizing pain
in the præcordia, as if the heart were being firmly grasped by
an invisible hand, or as if it were being torn to pieces. The
pain is, however, not limited to the cardiac region; it radiates
in various directions, shooting to the back, to the neck, and
especially down the left arm. But this is not all: worse than
the pain are the intense anxiety and the feeling of impending
death. The heart palpitates during the fit; and yet, if we judge
by the character of the pulse, its movements are not always
materially disturbed. The beat of the artery at the wrist
may be small, may be weak, may be irregular, may be accelerated; but it may also be full, be strong, be regular, and not
increased in frequency. The face is generally pale. Difficulty in breathing, contrary to what might be expected, is not
a prominent symptom, and is, in fact, often wanting.

The duration of the fits is as uncertain as the causes which
excite them. They may cease in a few minutes; they may
last upwards of an hour. They come on rapidly, without any
assignable reason; they are reproduced by bodily ailment, or
by exertion, or mental irritation. However provoked, they
are always dangerous. The heart may stop beating during
the paroxysm. " My life is in the hands of any rascal who
chooses to annoy and tease me," was a saying of John Hun-
ter's. And in truth, after he had suffered for years from
these seizures, his ungovernable temper brought on one in
which he expired. It happens sometimes that the second
attack follows the one by which the disease first declares
itself at a short interval, and proves fatal. Dr. Latham* narrates the history of two cases of this kind. In the one, life
ceased in a fortnight after the first seizure; in the second, in
ten days. Nay, it may be cut short even in the midst of the
first manifestation of this strange malady. Such was the
death of the esteemed Arnold, of Rugby.†

---

* Lectures on Diseases of the Heart, vol. ii.
† Stanley, Life and Correspondence of Thomas Arnold.

The immediate conditions on which the symptoms of the attack depend are veiled in obscurity. Whether they be or be not produced by a temporary increase of weakness in an already enfeebled organ ; whether a cardiac spasm occur or do not occur ; whether the sensation of approaching death be or be not caused by a distention of the heart with blood,— we do not know. All we do know positively is, that the excessive pain abruptly appearing and disappearing points to what we are content to call deranged innervation. Yet we can go a step further: we can say with certainty, what our forefathers were not aware of, that angina pectoris is very rarely a purely nervous disease. Modern research, which has taught us what dilatation of the heart is, and what softening, and what fatty degeneration; which explains to us that the heart may be in a state of profound alteration when it looks healthy,—has also taught us, or, to speak more guardedly, has rendered it more than highly probable, that these so-called spasms of the heart are always, or nearly always, linked to some structural change. This structural change, so far as we can now see, is, however, not at all times the same. The list of disorders of the heart and arteries which angina pectoris may accompany, is indeed very long. There is hardly an affection of the walls or cavities of the heart, scarcely a morbid condition of the arteries that nourish it or spring from it, with which the distressing malady has not been observed to have been associated. It has been found as an attendant on ossification of the coronary artery ; on every form of valvular disease ; on thinning of the parietes of the heart; on their fatty softening; on fungoid growths springing from the apex of the organ.* It is possible that, combined with all of these states, is fatty degeneration, which thus would be at the root of the angina. Such is the opinion of Dr. Watson, and such would also seem to be the result of the observations of Dr. Quain.† And whether this view be correct or not, it is undoubted that fatty degeneration is more frequently conjoined with angina than is any

---

* B. Travers, Med.-Chirg. Transact., vol. xvii.
† Med.-Chirg Transact., vol. xxxiii.

other organic disease.	Yet fatty degeneration occurs often
without angina, and we are thus forced to admit that, however frequent the association, some unknown element is still
here, as in all cases, the determining cause.

· ˙ Angina pectoris is easy of recognition.	It may be a question
whether those severe pains in the region of the heart, which
are apt to occur in feeble persons after unaccustomed exertion, or which are brought on by the excessive use of tobacco,*
or which happen in rheumatic or gouty subjects, especially
while suffering from indigestion, are real angina, or may be
separated from this affection.	They differ from it, irre-
spective of being far less violent and less radiating, by the
circumstances leading to an attack, and by their constant as-
sociation with palpitation.	Intercostal neuralgia with palpi-
tation might be mistaken for angina; but the painful spots
in the course of the affected nerve, and the comparatively
slight suffering, distinguish it.	In truth, it is a complaint
seated only in the thoracic walls, and referred by the patient
to the heart.	Great irritability of the heart, attended with
pain, due perhaps to neuralgia of the cardiac plexus, is discriminated from angina by the palpitations, and by their connection with pain which never rises to the anguish of angina
pectoris.	Often, too, this apparent angina is found in per-
sons who are subject to neuralgia, or who are laboring under
a disorder of one of the abdominal viscera.	And again it
must be admitted that the distinction may be rather one of
degree than of kind; for the cardiac plexus is precisely the
point particularly involved in angina, and it is thought by
several recent observers, that the disturbance of the heart in
this painful malady occurs through the influence of the sympathetic fibres which meet in the plexus.†

Palpitation.—This arises in various diseases of the heart.
It happens at the commencement of acute affections; it is an
unfailing accompaniment of some chronic lesions.	It is es-
pecially distressing when the cavities are dilated and the walls
of the organ thinned.	But it bears no positive relation to

---

* Beau, Journ. de Méd. et Chirurg., July, 1862.
† Eulenberg and Guttmann, Pathologie des Sympathicus.	1868.

any special cardiac malady; and is therefore not diagnostic of any. So too with irregular rhythm of the heart's action, with which palpitation is in truth often combined. It tells us nothing more than that the regular movements of the heart are disarranged. Frequently, however, this disarrangement is due to a serious change of the valves or of the muscular structure. But palpitation, with or without irregular rhythm, may take place in a perfectly sound heart—sound, at least, so far as our means of investigation enable us to determine.

Often the pulsations of the heart become stronger, more extensive, and more perceptible from mere nervous excitement. But it is not necessary to detail the symptoms of a purely nervous palpitation. Every one has experienced them. Every one knows that there is a feeling of slight constriction about the chest, with a hurried breathing, and a strange sensation as if the heart were leaping from its place. Every one is also aware that the organ is felt thumping against the walls of the chest, and that with a force which shakes them. The popular notion, that the heart is the seat of the emotions, is based on these striking evidences of its disturbed action, and poets have seized upon and delineated with accuracy some of even the more purely physical phenomena of the extended impulse under strong nervous excitement. Thus the great dramatist, in the Rape of Lucrece:

> "His hand, that yet remains upon her breast
> (Rude ram to batter such an ivory wall l),
> May feel her heart, poor citizen, distressed,
> Wounding itself to death, rise up and fall,
> Beating her bulk, that his hand shakes withal."

But apart from the increase of the beat by mere temporary agitation, a heart may act overfrequently and overstrongly and its action become sensible to the person; in other words, it may palpitate, from some more unremitting excitement dependent upon perverted innervation. This is the main cause, as we shall presently see, of the altered impulse of the heart in the so-called functional disorders.

It has just been stated that the direct symptoms of a cardiac disorder—pain, palpitations, irregular action—are met with when no recognizable structural changes have taken place. Under such circumstances the affection of the heart is termed functional, and its symptoms are those already mentioned, variously combined, sometimes the one, sometimes the other predominating. These functional disorders are very much more frequent than the organic. They are, for the most part, produced by direct excitement of the heart, or by its being sympathetically disturbed by some source of irritation existing remote from it, or in the system at large. The symptoms may be said to constitute the disease. As they have been above examined separately in connection chiefly with organic affections, they may be here examined separately in connection chiefly with functional derangements. And as in the former, so in the latter, one symptom is apt to attend the other.

Disorders characterized by Palpitation, associated or not with change of Rhythm.

We have already briefly alluded to the causes of augmented action which are associated with organic changes, and to those occasioning temporary disturbance of the heart. A more permanent form of palpitation is engendered when the organ is kept more constantly excited by a deranged condition of some viscus remote from it; by the use of stimulating substances; or by some general morbid states. Thus a disordered stomach or liver leads to a reflex disturbance of the heart, which ceases if the disorder of the stomach or liver be remedied. In gouty and rheumatic persons the heart frequently pulsates with increased quickness and violence, and sometimes with marked irregularity. Special articles of diet, especially tea or coffee, produce palpitation; so does the inordinate use of tobacco in any form. Masturbation and excessive sensual indulgence, but particularly the former, are prolific sources of continued palpitation. We also see those affected with it who, addicted to laborious studies, give their minds no rest, and grudge themselves the neces-sary time for food, sleep, and exercise. Women who are hysterical, or whose uterine functions are disordered, suffer continually, or fancy that they suffer continually, from palpi-tation. .So do so-called nervous people invariably complain of the beating at the heart.

In those whose blood is much impoverished, the palpita-tions are often very severe and very constant, and their sen-sitive state of system is apt to be increased by the fear of laboring under an incurable disease of the heart. There is, indeed, from the strong resemblance to an organic affection, apparent cause for alarm. The heart strikes sharply and abruptly against the walls of the chest; its action is very frequent; the breathing becomes hurried on the slightest exertion. Nay, even the physical signs may be those of a structural lesion. The altered blood gives rise to a blowing sound in the heart, which is transmitted into the carotid and subclavian arteries. The difficulty of diagnosis is at times great. The age; the sex; the anemic look; the presence of a continuous humming sound in the veins of the neck; the strict synchronism of the murmur with the impulse; its seat at the base of the heart,—furnish a clue to the nature of the case. Still we have often to judge as much or more by the absence of the signs of cardiac enlargement, and of impediment to the flow of the blood, whether the heart be affected in its valvular apparatus, or whether it be simply functionally disturbed and circulating watery blood. And even with all the assistance which the closest investigation can furnish, the distinction may remain doubtful.

A troublesome kind of palpitation is that attended with marked *irregularity* of the action of the heart, displaying it-self by the beat being now slow, now fast, or occasionally intermitting. Sufferers from gout, or old persons whose stomachs are unable to digest food properly, are particularly liable to it. This form of palpitation is not without its danger. It is very prone to be associated with an alteration in the structure of the heart, such as flabbiness of the walls, which may not be sufficient to yield any distinctive physical signs, but which is nevertheless sufficient to be a source of apprehension.

Some who experience these fits of palpitation faint away during them. But the complete, or almost complete suspension of the movements of the heart which characterizes an attack of syncope, has no definite connection with any form of palpitation, nor, indeed, with any form of cardiac disorder, either organic or functional.

It has been made a question whether, in those who are subject to attacks of palpitation or to irregular action of the heart, the organ may not finally become enlarged. There seems to be no reason why this should not take place, and there is a very decided reason why it should. If the muscles of the arm be placed in constant and very active motion, they increase in size. Why, then, may not the heart, which is composed of the same kind of muscular fibre, also grow, if it be often called upon to act more frequently, and in a different manner from that to which it is accustomed? Hence we ought to be very careful not to neglect any functional disturbance of the heart, but aim at removing the condition which keeps the organ in a state of irritation, lest it should suffer a mishap that no exercise of skill can wholly repair.

We sometimes meet with a singular form of functional disturbance of the heart which leads to textural changes, and to which Graves called particular attention. It consists in a long-continued excitement of the organ, as evinced by its increased force and rapid and irregular action, and is followed by a swelling of the thyroid gland, pulsation of the arteries of the neck, and enlargement of the eyeballs. This strange disease is most commonly observed in females, and connected with hysteria, neuralgia, or uterine disturbance; but is now considered by many as being due to an affection of the cervical sympathetic nerve. All the signs may remit or become aggravated from time to time, and especially during a severe attack of palpitation. The turgescence of the thyroid gland arises quite independently of the usually exciting causes of bronchocele. It is accompanied by a pulsating thrill similar to that of an aneurismal varix, and by a distinct throb. At an advanced period of the complaint, these signs subside, and the gland becomes more solid. Indeed, the whole affection may disappear, and the gland, the eyes, the beat of the carotids, the action of the heart, may all be brought back to a normal condition. On the other hand, hypertrophy and dilatation may result from the cardiac palpitations.

There is another form of functional disorder of the heart, so peculiar as to demand a special notice. It is the curious cardiac malady of which we lately saw so many examples in soldiers. Its main symptoms are habitual frequency of the action of the heart, constantly recurring attacks of palpitations, and pain referred to the lower portion of the precordial region. The palpitations occur chiefly during exercise, but may also take place when the patient is quiet, and in many cases happen most often, or indeed entirely, at night, thus interfering with sleep. It is not unusual to hear soldiers who are subject to the disorder complain much of headache and of dizziness, and especially of being thus affected when suffering from palpitation. The pain is generally dull and constant, but is often also described as shooting, and as taking place only in paroxysms. Its chief seat is near the apex, and it is combined very commonly with excessive cutaneous sensibility. Often there is pain nowhere else in the body; but in some instances the cardiac distress is associated with pain in the back, which itself is not unusually connected with the excretion of oxalate of lime by the kidneys.

The action of the heart is very rapid, and in many instances its rhythm is irregular. The impulse is slightly extended, but not forcible, like that of hypertrophy: it is rather abrupt and jerky. As a rule, to which thus far I have met with but few exceptions, the sounds of the heart are modified as follows: the first sound is short, sometimes sharp like that of the second; at other times extremely deficient and hardly recognizable; the distinctness of the second sound is very much heightened. We hear no murmurs either in the heart or in the neck, or they are inconstant. The area of percussion dulness does not appear to be augmented. The pulse is almost always easily compressible; it may or may not share the character of the impulse. It is usually very much influenced by position, falling rapidly twenty beats or more, when the erect is exchanged for the recumbent posture. The increased frequency of beat is not connected with increased frequency of respiration, for often with a pulse of one hundred, the respirations scarcely exceed twenty in the minute. The disorder is a very obstinate one to manage, and improvement comes but slowly. Keeping the heart quiet by occasional doses of digitaline, or of veratrum viride, or by atropia, and improving its tone as much as possible by tonics, has been the treatment which I found to be the most successful.

What the cause of the morbid cardiac impressibility, is very difficult to ascertain. It seems, in many instances, to have followed fatiguing marches ; in some it occurred after fevers or diarrhœa. As far as I have been able to observe, it was not connected with scurvy, or with the abuse of tobacco. That it was not due to anæmia, was at once proved by the general aspect of the men, which was often that of ruddy health.*

These, then, are the principal varieties of functional disorders of the heart. It is hardly necessary again to state that the physical signs present the most certain, if not the only means of distinguishing the functional from the structural affection. They show us that neither the size of the organ, nor its sounds, with the exceptions above mentioned, are materially different from what they are in health. They enable us, therefore, to decide whether the symptoms which are common to functional or organic diseases are removable, or are associated with conditions which no therapeutic means that have been yet devised can fully remedy.

---

* These statements are not intended to be final. They are but a very short summary of the results of a large number of observations which I had an opportunity of making on these cases of " irritable heart," and which elsewhere, and in a more complete form, will be laid before the profession. Some points bearing on the inquiry have been published in the Medical Memoirs of the U. S. Sanitary Commission.

ORGANIC DISEASES OF THE HEART.

Organic diseases of the heart may be classified as follows:

ORGANIC DISEASES OF THE HEART.

Diseases affecting the walls of the heart, but mostly also changing the size of the cavities.	Hypertrophy. Dilatation. Atrophy.
Diseases affecting chiefly the walls alone. . . .	Fatty degeneration. Malformations. Rupture of the heart. Injuries and wounds. Aneurism of heart.
Inflammations. . . . . { of membranes.	Endocarditis. Pericarditis.
of muscular structure.	Myocarditis (Carditis).
Diseases of the valvular apparatus.	Valvular diseases.
Diseases affecting the pericardium.	Chronic pericarditis. Hydropercardium. Pneumo-hydropericardium.

These are not all the organic diseases of the heart; yet they are all save the rarest. But let us study the cardiac maladies rather according to their symptoms and signs than according to their anatomical classification. And first, of a group of acute affections.

Acute Diseases presenting Pain in the Cardiac Region; the Symptoms of a Disturbed Circulation; and a Change in the Sounds of the Heart, or their Replacement by Murmurs.

All the acute affections of the heart come under this head. In all the sounds are either changed in their character or replaced by murmurs. This is certainly true of the only acute diseases of which we have anything like an accurate knowledge—of endocarditis and pericarditis. All the acute disorders give rise further to more or less pain, and to anxiety of expression; in all there is fever; all are prone to occur in connection with other morbid conditions, and especially with a contaminated state of the blood. In all, moreover, the symptoms of a disturbed circulation are met with: palpitation, irregular action of the heart, deranged flow of blood through the capillaries of different organs, and a tendency to dropsical accumulations. That these symptoms are not so clearly defined as in some of the chronic cardiac maladies, is owing to the shorter time the complaint lasts.

Acute Endocarditis.—Acute endocarditis is acute inflammation of the lining membrane of the heart. It arises, as most other internal inflammations arise, from exposure to cold, or without any cause being discoverable. It sometimes results from violent efforts, or from blows and other injuries to the chest. It is often connected with a vitiated condition of the blood, as in pyæmia or Bright's disease. But more frequently still does it form part of an attack of acute articular rheumatism.

As the anatomical characters illustrate the physical signs and many of the symptoms of the disease, they may be here briefly described. The membrane itself loses its transparency and smoothness, and is injected. On its free surface lymph exudes, and is moulded into patches of various size, which may be torn off by the blood and washed into the circulation: and so may the coagula which form, in severe cases, in the chambers of the heart. The inflammation stops short at the muscular structure. Yet it may implicate this, and result in softening the walls of the heart, or in developing purulent cysts in them. It is not uncommon to find the pericardium involved, and then the serous lining of the heart and its serous covering are both the seat of exudation. But the inflammation inside is not usually so extensive as the inflammation without. Indeed, one of the peculiarities and chief sources of danger in endocarditis is this very tendency it has to limit itself. It confines itself, or is most strikingly developed, at a part which bears least of all any impairment —at the valves—and often leaves behind it some permanent disorganization of their delicate structure. But it does not generally affect the entire valvular apparatus; that of the left side is usually alone the seat of the disease.

What morbid anatomy thus teaches, explains the occurrence and situation of the principal sign by which endocarditis is recognized. The roughness of the surface over which the blood flows, or the lymph deposited on or in the neighborhood of the valves, interfering with their function, occasions a distinct murmur, which, it is scarcely necessary to say, is mostly confined to the mitral and aortic openings.

Independently of the development of this blowing sound, there are other signs worthy of note. It is true, they do not form so leading a feature of the disease; still they aid in its correct appreciation. The excited heart beats with augmented force, and sometimes with great irregularity, as the not unusual doubling of the second sound at the base proves. The size of the organ is not notably increased, excepting in those cases in which its cavities are choked with blood or clots of fibrin. The pulse corresponds to the action of the heart; yet not so closely as might be expected. It is, for the most part, frequent and strong, and rather forcible at first; or sometimes small and frequent. It becomes irregular, one beat being strong, the next weak, if the circulation through the heart be seriously obstructed. But it may be feeble while the heart is thumping with violence against the walls of the chest. Occasionally at the onset of the attack it has been observed to be slower than natural.

The general symptoms are not always uniform. There is usually a sense of uneasiness around the heart, with decided fever, a short cough, difficulty of breathing, and an extreme anxiety depicted in the countenance. To these are not uncommonly added a turgescence of the face, headache, some wandering of the mind, a yellowish hue of the skin, gastric irritability, diarrhœa, and rigors, followed by sensations of heat. Excessive pain in the heart is rare, and is not likely to happen, unless the pericardium or the muscular walls be implicated.

Now, where these symptoms are present; where they manifest themselves in a patient whose system is in a state in which endocarditis is apt to take place; and where, above all, they are accompanied by signs of irritation of the heart, and by a blowing sound recently and rather suddenly developed,—we are certain that inflammation is working its changes in the lining membrane of the heart. Yet some circumspection is requisite before arriving at this conclusion, and before the patient is subjected to bleeding, to mercurials, or some such similar energetic treatment, with the view of saving him from the supposed damage which his heart is about to undergo. A murmur may be attended with febrile signs, and still not be dependent upon acute endocarditis. The sound may be of organic origin; or it may be engendered in the course of an idiopathic fever, and the lining membrane of the heart be unaltered.

In the first instance, the murmur is old, and results from some chronic injury to the valve, the attending fever being an accidental complication. Here is undoubtedly a difficult case for diagnosis. We see the patient for the first time: he has fever; his heart is acting strongly; a distinct, blowing sound is perceived over it. How are we to tell that his complaint is not acute endocarditis? We have no absolute means of deciding that it is not. Yet by careful inquiry we can usually come to a knowledge of the truth. If the patient do not recollect to have suffered previously from dyspnœa, palpitation, or other signs of an affection of the heart; if the cardiac excitement and irritation be well defined; if the face denote distress; if the accompanying symptoms indicate a state which is prone to be complicated with endocardial inflammation,—it is this disease under which he is laboring. I may add another and very important element of distinction deduced from the study of the blowing sound, to wit, that the murmur of endocarditis is not so rough, is not often heard during the distention of the heart, and may be changeable in its seat, which an old-standing murmur never is. Besides, it is not associated with those signs of enlargement which are so invariably found when the valves have been for any length of time affected, unless the acute inflammation occur in a heart the valves of which have been previously spoiled. Under such circumstances, we can only conjecture what is going on within the organ by its increased excitement; and, if I may take my own experience as the general rule, by the character of the blowing sound being altered. It is rendered often less distinct, nay, it is even entirely muffled, by the products of the recent inflammation.

But how are we to distinguish between the soft murmur arising in the course of fevers, and that resulting from effused lymph? It, too, is not rough. It, too, happens with the impulse. It, too, is preceded, as some cases of endocarditis are, by a lengthening of the first sound. Here is assuredly a very strong resemblance, yet by no means an identity. The blowing sound in fevers does not exist until the blood is profoundly altered. In endocarditis it takes place almost as soon as the disease begins,—certainly as soon as we are able to recognize positively its commencement. The heart in fevers may be softened, but it is not so directly disturbed in its action. We do not find those symptoms, local as well as general, which show that the circulation is obstructed. The blowing sound is rarely found at the apex. To the last particular some weight may be attached, since the murmur of endocarditis is very apt to be heard at the apex. But to no fact ought as much weight to be attached as to the one first mentioned, that the murmur takes place early, and not late in the disease.

Throughout this description of inflammation of the interior of the heart, only simple, uncomplicated cases have been kept in view; yet it is not often that the malady is seen in so pure a type. It is more generally accompanied by the friction sounds and other signs of acute pericarditis, and by the swollen joints, the painful movements, the acid perspirations of acute rheumatism.

Nor is what has been said of its manifesting itself by a murmur the invariable rule. If the question be asked, "Can endocarditis occur without a blowing sound?" it must be answered in the affirmative. When the seat of the inflammation is not near the valves, no murmur is generated. There may be also none if no vegetations exist on the valves, and perhaps in states of the exudation with which we are at present unacquainted. We cannot, under such circumstances, detect an attack of endocarditis. Yet it may be even then strongly suspected to be present if great excitement and irritation of the heart manifest themselves in a person who is laboring under a disease which predisposes to endocardial inflammation, such as rheumatism. Cases of this nature are, however, exceptional. They do not happen sufficiently often to invalidate the value of the statement that the development of a murmur is the sign indicative of inflammation of the inner surface of the heart. Yet they happen sufficiently often to impress upon us that our knowledge of endocarditis is not complete.

The clinical study of endocarditis is, in truth, a recent study. There are some points about it which are as yet next to unknown, and others which are now being cleared up, and in a manner that must let in light on many obscure subjects of pathology. To this class belong those interesting researches on the formation of clots in the heart, and the effects produced when they or the vegetations which stud the valves are washed into the circulation. The formation of clots of fibrin in the cardiac cavities, if at all extensive, announces itself by a sudden appearance or a sudden augmentation of the symptoms of obstructed circulation : the skin is cold and the surface may be bluish; there is dyspnœa, the heart's action becomes exceedingly irregular, its sounds indistinct, and the extent of the precordial percussion dulness is somewhat increased. Great anxiety of countenance, nausea, vomiting, excitement of the nervous system and delirium, and fits of fainting are also among the manifestations of the clogged flow of blood through the heart. Now, portions of the clots, or of the vegetations on the valves, are sometimes washed into the current, and occasion symptoms which, before we were aware of the damages to which these detached masses may give rise, appeared inexplicable. At present—thanks to Virchow, Kirkes, and Paget—when we see the circulation speedily diminished or arrested in a limb, and the limb swelling or beginning to mortify; when we find that the flow of the blood through the brain has become suddenly disturbed, and the muscles of one side drop paralyzed; when the difficult breathing becomes rapidly still more difficult, while there are no signs of a superadded affection of the lung, nay, while the power fully to fill the lungs remains unimpaired, or while an effusion of fluid into the air-vesicles follows the dyspnœa,—we know what has happened : we know that a broken off piece of fibrin has been driven into the artery of the limb, or into the brain, or into the branches of the pul-monary artery, and, being too large to go any farther, has stuck fast, and has given rise to all of these sudden and sad consequences. Sad, indeed, they are; for, even if the plugs do not lead to an immediately fatal result, they are apt to lay the groundwork for structural alterations in any organ or tissue in which they become impacted.

With respect to the frequency with which changes remote from the heart are produced by the disintegration of masses of fibrin formed in it, we are not yet in a condition to speak positively. Nor are the signs of either the formation of these clots, or of their dispersion, as well understood as is desirable. We are, indeed, better acquainted with those of the latter than with those of the former; for as great an observer as Dr. Walshe records that the effects of a rupture of a sigmoid valve or of a tendinous cord, during the acute endocardial disease, will give rise to symptoms exactly similar to the ob-struction of the circulation resulting from polypoid concre-tions in the heart. Our knowledge of the whole subject is in truth, still at its commencement.

But let it not be understood that the detachment of vege-tations from the valves, or of fragments of clot formed in the cavities of the heart, happens only in endocarditis. Pieces have been found which were separated from valves that were in a state of chronic induration, or so-called ossification. And the blood in the heart may clot from any interference with the current, or from changes in the vital fluid wholly uncon-nected with inflammation. But when it coagulates, from whatever cause, the symptoms are the same as those just described. A murmur, too, is not uncommonly produced, which is not distinguishable from that due to endocardial inflammation, but which is not of long duration, since death follows the impediment in the heart in a few days at furthest.

Inflammation of the aorta may occasion many of the symp-toms of acute endocarditis; at all events it may do so when the upper part of the aorta is implicated. Nor can it be said that it is a condition which with certainty may be discrim-inated. The most significant signs, though they are by no means constantly present, are a hurried respiration, a sharp,

rapid pulse, tumultuous action of the heart, pain in the precordial region, often severely increased by movements, and
also felt along the course of the spine, and a loud systolic
blowing sound. When the abdominal aorta is affected, there
is a strong local pulsation and a very marked murmur will
be heard with greatest distinctness at or near the seat of the
inflammation. In some cases of aortitis, Bright* noticed an
extremely high degree of morbid sensibility over all parts of
the body, which caused the patient to scream with pain when
his wrists were merely touched. The disorder is most apt
to happen in cachectic persons; and it has been repeatedly
observed in those attacked with erysipelas, or after operations
and injuries.†

Acute Pericarditis.—Acute inflammation of the serous
membrane of the exterior of the heart is very similar to that
of its interior. It is developed under the same circumstances.
It exhibits the same frequent association with rheumatism.
It presents the same symptoms. Nature has not, indeed,
drawn a very strict line of demarcation between the two diseases. When one exists, the other is very apt to attend it.
Yet we do meet with endocarditis without pericarditis, and
more often still, with pericarditis without endocarditis.

The anatomical effects of inflammation of the pericardium
are like those of acute endocarditis, and resemble yet more
closely those which inflammation of the adjoining serous
membrane—the pleura—occasions. The pericardium becomes
injected and dry; plastic lymph accumulates on its surfaces,
and especially on the surface which fits tightly around the
heart. The extent and appearance of the deposited lymph
are very various. It may be limited to part of the covering
of one ventricle, or be distributed in layers all over the inner
face of the membrane. It may give to this the look of having
been besmeared with a sticky substance, or of having been
enveloped with a delicate network resembling lace. More
often it is rough and shaggy, and presents a strong likeness
to the villi of the intestine, to the dorsal surface of a bul-

---

* Guy's Hospital Reports, vol. i.
† Chevers; ib. vol. vi., and 2d Series, vol. i.

lock's tongue, to the mucous membrane of the gall-bladder, and to other objects of uneven outline with which the fancy of different observers has compared it. This stage of the disease corresponds to the dry stage of acute pleurisy. It may have the same termination by the two roughened surfaces adhering. But it is often followed by a stage similar to that of pleural effusion. The bag in which the heart lies is filled with fluid; sometimes with serum in which flocculi of lymph float; at times with a thicker, more highly albuminous liquid; less frequently with a watery blood, or with pus. The effusion may remain stationary or be absorbed, and the rugged portions of the membrane be placed again in apposition.

. Now from a knowledge of these anatomical changes, the physical signs may be foretold. It is obvious that there must be at first a friction sound, just as there is a friction sound at first in pleurisy; that then the fluid which distends the pericardium will increase the area of percussion dulness over the heart, and prevent the sounds and the impulse from being distinctly perceived. But the friction sound is not always the same in extent and character, because the deposited lymph is not always the same either in extent or character. The sound is like the crumpling of parchment, or the creaking of new leather, or it is grazing, or a series of irregular clicks. It is a single or it is a double sound, and is prone to mask the natural sounds of the heart. But these are all points which have been already described; we shall merely add, that when the friction develops itself under our observation, and with signs of excitement of the heart, it is as distinctive of inflammation of the pericardium as a recent blowing sound is, under the same circumstances, distinctive of inflammation of the endocardium. When the effusion takes place, it ceases; but only gradually, and not always completely; and in any case it is not uncommon for the ear still to recognize the murmur at the base of the heart, and around the origin of the great vessels.

The percussion dulness of the effusion is generally considerable. Its contour is peculiar and characteristic. As the fluid gravitates to the lower portion of the sac, this distends,

23

of necessity, more than the part where the pericardium adheres to the vessels. The consequence is, that the dulness,
when the patient is in the erect posture, is pyramidal; when

Fig. 27.

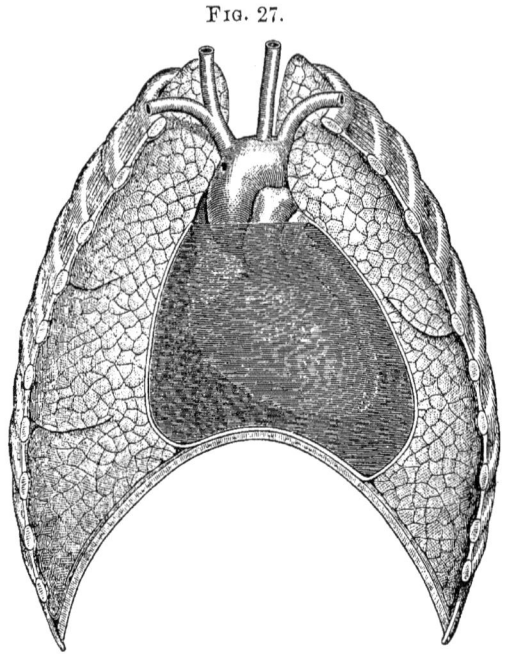

Illustration of the position of the heart in pericarditis, and of the
distention of the pericardium with fluid. The heart sounds are indistinct, excepting above the effusion; the impulse is feeble. The
extent and shape of the percussion dulness may be judged of by the
appearance of the distended sac.

he lies on his back, or changes from side to side, the outline
of the flat sound is somewhat altered. In cases of considerable effusion, the intercostal spaces of the cardiac region
widen, the eye recognizes a distinct bulging, and the dulness on percussion reaches to the second, or even to the first
rib. Within the space of dulness is sometimes seen an irregular, wavy motion; and what the eye detects, the hand feels.
Yet no movements, or only very slight movements, may be
perceptible in the præcordia. The heart, with its point
pushed upward by the accumulating liquid, has to struggle
to reach the walls of the chest. Its contractions are irregular; its impulse is very feeble, or all appreciable impulse has
ceased. The sounds are not clearly heard through the mass

of fluid, but seem distant and muffled. Yet the second sound over the upper part of the sternum and at the base of the heart retains its sharpness.

During the stage of absorption the apex returns to its normal position; the dulness gradually disappears; the sounds and the impulse regain more of their normal character; the friction murmur reappears, and then ceases, leaving frequently the two surfaces of the pericardium glued together—a condition which is not so harmless as the adhesions which terminate an attack of acute pleurisy, since it not unusually leads to dilated hypertrophy, or to dilatation.

There is no saying how long it will take for the disease to run through its different stages. Death may occur in less than thirty hours, the heart being paralyzed by an enormous effusion: on the other hand, the acute attack may last for as many days, and then leave serious traces. But whatever stage the malady be in, it can only be recognized by the physical signs just detailed; by the friction, by the peculiar percussion dulness, by the enfeebled impulse and heart sounds.

There are no general symptoms that prove a pericarditis to exist. There are symptoms by which we may infer that pericarditis is present; but there are none which absolutely belong to it, and would prevent it from being overlooked. The symptoms usually met with are those of inflammation of the endocardium, but with more decided evidence of a local trouble in the chest. We find the same anxious expression; the same fever; the same œdema; the same uncertain or irregular pulse. But there is more pain over the heart—acute, severe pain, shooting to the left shoulder, augmented by movement, increased by pressure; there is more dyspnœa, because the distended sac presses on the lung; and there is sometimes difficulty in swallowing. Yet every one of these symptoms may be absent. The pulse may be regular; the breathing not perceptibly accelerated, nor laborious; and even the symptom regarded as the most important of all—the pain—may be wanting from the beginning to the end of the disease.

When the action of the heart grows weaker and weaker,

the circulation becomes more irregular. The beat of the artery at the wrist is feeble, and intermits; the veins of the neck are prominent; the skin is cold and pale; the extremities are edematous. These are always symptoms of grave import: they tell of the failing power of the heart, and call for agents which will sustain it.

If next we come to inquire with what complaints acute pericarditis is likely to be confounded, inflammation of the endocardium and of the pleura occur at once to the mind. To contrast the signs of the first two maladies, for the slight difference in their symptoms has already been alluded to:

ENDOCARDITIS.	PERICARDITIS.
Blowing sound; excited action of the heart.	Friction sound; excited action of the heart.
Slight, if any increase of percussion dulness.	In stage of effusion, marked and extended percussion dulness.
Impulse strong.	Impulse wavy and feeble.
Sounds normal or more distinct, except at site where murmur is heard.	Sounds feeble and muffled; no blowing sounds.

Such is the distinction of pure cases of each disease. But, as already stated, the affections are often combined. It is not very uncommon to hear with the friction sound a distinct endocardial murmur. But there is sometimes a difficulty of another kind in the way of a precise diagnosis. The murmur produced on the outside of the heart may simulate so closely the murmur produced in its interior that it is next to impossible to discriminate between them. The former may completely possess the blowing characters of the latter. Mostly, however, it is rougher; more prone to be double; and each division is like the other, equally rough, equally superficial sounding, equally lacking in strict correspondence to the systole or to the diastole. And, above all, the sound alters at times both situation and character with amazing rapidity. Perceived now as an ordinary bellows murmur on the left side, it is after the lapse of some hours heard as a rough rasping sound on the right. These changes have a high degree of value. But they are not of constant occurrence; and to say that it is sometimes impossible to tell a pericardial from an endocardial sound, is to say no more than is borne out by every-day experience. Fortunately, in point of treatment, an error, should it be committed, is not fatal to the patient's safety; for, at all events before the stage of effusion in pericarditis, the two diseases require much the same means for their relief; and endocarditis is not likely to be mistaken for pericarditis in its stage of effusion.

Inflammation of the adjoining serous membrane, the *pleura*, gives rise to some of the same symptoms and signs as pericarditis. It develops a friction sound: it occasions dulness on percussion, dyspnœa and cough. But the physical signs are in different situations. In one disorder they are noted in the region of the heart, and are confined there; in the other they are spread over the whole side of the chest, and are most perceptible at the back. This is true of the dulness, and also, for the most part, of the friction sound, which, when of pericardial origin, is very rarely heard posteriorly.

At times, however, we meet with very puzzling cases. A friction sound discerned over the heart may be in reality produced in the adjoining pleura. The patient is directed to suspend his breathing. The friction sound does not stop. Now the inference from this would be that the sound originates in the pericardium; and in the large majority of instances this is a correct inference. But it is not always so. The friction may be engendered in the pleura and be caused by the movements of the heart. To mention an example: a laboring man was attacked with acute articular rheumatism, in the course of which a friction sound was heard over the outer limit of the left ventricle, and also posteriorly over the lower portion of the left lung. Occasionally it ceased entirely when the patient stopped breathing, and during a few beats of the heart. Then it recommenced with unequal intensity while the respiration was still arrested. It is evident that this sound could not have been that of an inflamed pericardium; certainly the one perceived anteriorly was not. I know of no absolute means, besides the intermission of the sound during some of the beats of the heart, of detecting in these rare cases the true seat of the disease.

To confound the dulness on percussion caused by liquid in
the pericardiùm with that due to liquid in the pleura, is a
mistake the more likely to happen, because the two serous
membranes, and indeed the lung, are often implicated in the
same inflammation. But a pericarditis uncomplicated with
pleurisy or with pleuropneumonia, does not change the clear
sound at the back of the chest save in rare, very rare cases
of enormous accumulation of fluid within the sac. Effusion
into the pleura gives rise to a flat sound anteriorly; yet to a
still more perceptible dulness at the inferior portion of the
chest posteriorly; and the sounds of the heart remain unaltered, unless its investing membrane contain fluid also.

These, then, are the diseases with which acute pericarditis
is liable to be confounded. There are several chronic cardiac maladies which will occasion some of the same signs
and symptoms: such are thinning of the ventricles with distention of the cavities, and a dropsy of the pericardium. But
the history of these affections is different, and their signs,
although similar, are not precisely the same. The dropsy
of the pericardium is associated with dropsies elsewhere, and
with some obvious cause accounting for the watery exudation, and at no stage of its existence does it exhibit a friction
sound.

But there is another acute complaint of which pericarditis
sometimes borrows the garb. The thoracic symptoms may
be latent, but the disease may produce the symptoms of extreme *gastric irritation* or inflammation. There are nausea
and vomiting, and tenderness on pressure in the epigastric
region. All the remedies are directed to the stomach; and
at the post-mortem examination, the physician stands amazed
at finding this viscus healthy and the pericardium full of
serum or pus. An inquiry into the state of the heart might
have saved him from a serious blunder, which could have
been avoided and the patient's life been probably preserved.

Another grave error which may be thus obviated is the
mistaking of some cases of acute pericarditis, on account of
the wild delirium they present, for acute *inflammation of the
brain.* Now, both in endocarditis and in pericarditis this
active delirium may throw all the other symptoms into the

background. How it is produced is not easy to understand. It is difficult to see why a pericardial inflammation should give rise to such violent disturbance of the brain. It is not at all unlikely that it has its origin in the contaminated state of the blood which occurs in the affections, such as rheumatism or Bright's disease, with which pericarditis is often associated. At all events, however occasioned, it is necessary to be aware that the cerebral symptoms arising in inflammation of the membranes of the heart may entirely draw off attention from the serious lesions within the chest.

Before dismissing the subject of pericarditis, let us inquire in how far one of its terminations—by adhesion or agglutination of the surfaces—can be recognized. In many of such cases, whether or not there be coexisting dilatation, or hypertrophy, or that rare condition, cardiac atrophy, or even probably when the heart is of normal size, we find changed rhythm and dyspnœa. Yet surely these cannot be considered as special signs of pericardial adhesions. Nor is the "abrupt, jogging, or trembling motion" of the heart, described by Hope, pathognomonic; nor the extinction of the second sound, on which Aran dwells. For the pericardial surfaces may be found most thoroughly glued to each other where neither of these signs was present. But it must be admitted that the double jog is often seen, especially if the enlargement of the heart be at all extensive. The most trustworthy signs of pericardial adhesion are those given by Skoda :[*] a drawing up of the heart's apex during the contraction of the ventricles, with a depression in the intercostal spaces becoming visible at the same time, and sometimes with a simultaneous sinking in at the lower half of the sternum; the limits of the dull percussion sound remaining unaffected during inspiration and expiration; and a confused instead of a distinct and punctuate beat of the impulse against the finger. Gairdner,[†] too, lays stress upon the marked movement of the intercostal spaces over the heart; while Walshe[‡] thinks that the systolic dimpling and the undulatory movements in

---

[*] Zeltsch der K. K. Gesellsch. der Aerzte zu Wien. April, 1852.

[†] Edinburgh Med. Journ., 1851, 1859, etc.

[‡] On Diseases of the Heart. Third edition, p 194, Am. ed.

the præcordia only happen if there be, in addition to the pericardial adhesions, pleuritic adhesions in front of the organ, or if the agglutination of the pericardium be combined with cardiac hypertrophy. When the pericardial surfaces are very extensively and firmly united, the eye is struck by the evident depression of the precordial region.

Carditis.—The substance of the heart itself undergoes at times inflammation. We can recognize such a condition after death, by the changed color, the flabbiness, and the presence of granules of exudation and of pus corpuscles among the fibres of the heart. It is known that the inflammation may also occasion local softening and circumscribed abscesses, and even gangrene and perforation of the ventriele. But though familiar with the post-mortem appearances, we are not enabled to foretell the state of the heart during life, mainly because the muscular structure is rarely affected without the endocardium, or still more frequently the pericardium, being implicated, and thus the manifestations of these disorders occur mixed up with those of true carditis. On analyzing the cases on record, I cannot indeed find either a symptom or sign which can be considered as in the least pathognomonic. Extreme pain in the cardiac region is the most usual and the most prominent of the symptoms. It is sometimes very excruciating and sharp, at other times dull, but most distressing and constant. The breathing is generally much oppressed; delirium is often present; the skin becomes cold; and the patient dies in a state of utter prostration or of apparent suffocation. The pulse is much like that of endocarditis or pericarditis—that is, it exhibits no uniform character. The statement that it is invariably intermittent, feeble, and quick, is not correct. It is so as the disease advances, but it has been reported to be full, and not above eighty, long after the distress in the chest was unbearable.*

---

* Salter, Medico-Chirurg. Transactions, vol. xxii. In several of the cases on record, for instance in the one mentioned by Graves, in his Clinical Lectures, there was coexisting valvular disease, which, of course, invalidates the statements as regards the character of the pulse, and indeed as regards many of the other symptoms.

Chronic Diseases attended with Increased Extent of Percussion Dulness, but with Normal or almost Normal Heart Sounds.

We often meet with a group of affections which present the phenomena of extended dulness on percussion in the cardiac region, associated with sounds like those heard in health: they may be louder or less loud, better defined or less well defined, still they are the natural sounds of the heart, and no cardiac murmur is detected, unless the disorder be no longer uncomplicated.

To this group belong those diseases which affect the walls of the heart or its cavities, without having involved the valvular apparatus, such as hypertrophy and dilatation—types of the two different states of force and of weakness; but both exhibiting an extent of percussion dulness greater than in health, and heart sounds not very materially changed.

Hypertrophy.—Hypertrophy of the heart is an overgrowth of its walls, and most usually also of its cavities; for, although we may have the muscle thickening without the cavity enlarging, nay, even with its diminishing in size, neither this simple, nor the concentric hypertrophy occurs, save in rare instances. It is evident that any one of the chambers of the heart may alone become hypertrophied. But practically, the state we mean, when speaking of hypertrophy of the heart, is an increase of the ventricles, and especially an increase of the left ventricle, in its wall and cavity, with a similar, although much slighter expansion of the right side. Whether the auricles be enlarged or not, is a matter always more of conjecture than susceptible of absolute proof.

The physical and vital manifestations of the heart having outgrown its natural dimensions are these: the pulse is full and strong, and somewhat tense. The face is florid, or else it is pale; but the mucous membranes of the lips and eyelids are injected. The eyes are bright, and apt to be prominent. The carotids pulsate forcibly under the least excitement. Some persons suffer from headache and giddiness; in fact, all the symptoms denote a circulation actively, too actively carried on. Yet the symptons directly referable to the heart are not marked. There is, as a rule, no pain, nor irregular action of the heart, nor do violent fits of palpitation occur. What the patient comes to consult his physician about, are rushes of blood to the head; or a ringing in the ears; or a feeling of weight in the epigastrium which troubles him after a full meal; or on account of shortness of breath; or because the powerful action of the heart, when lying in bed, attracts his attention; or sometimes he is alarmed about a dry cough, and believes himself the victim of pulmonary consumption.

The physical signs are more uniform than the symptoms. We observe a fulness or arching of the precordial region, and an impulse strong, heaving, and extended over several intercostal spaces. The apex does not strike the chest walls between the fifth and sixth ribs, but its beat is perceived lower down, and more inward, toward the median line, in consequence of the enlarged and weighty heart not retaining its normal position. The extent of percussion dulness increases, both longitudinally and transversely; and particularly in the latter direction, if the right ventricle be much enlarged. This peculiarity in the expansion of the dulness on percussion forms, in truth, with the greater dyspnœa, and with an impulse more directly perceived over the right side of the heart, near the pit of the stomach, the sign that hypertrophy with dilatation has principally affected the right side of the heart.

The first sound of a hypertrophied heart is duller than in health, but prolonged and weighty. The second sound is not particularly changed. There are no murmurs, excepting under rare circumstances, which will be alluded to in discussing valvular diseases. Thus the greatest value of auscultation is, that, by showing us that the sounds are but little altered, it enables us positively to exclude a lesion of the valves; just as the chief service of percussion, with reference to an enlarged heart, consists in permitting us to distinguish the excited motions of the simply disturbed organ from the action of a heart the walls of which are thickened; and as the main use in noting the impulse is, that it serves as a

means of discrimination between hypertrophy and those affections in which the beat is weakened, such as dilatation, or
a pericardial effusion, or between the dulness in the precordial region due to hypertrophy and that caused by deposits
in the pleura or lung.

FIG. 28.

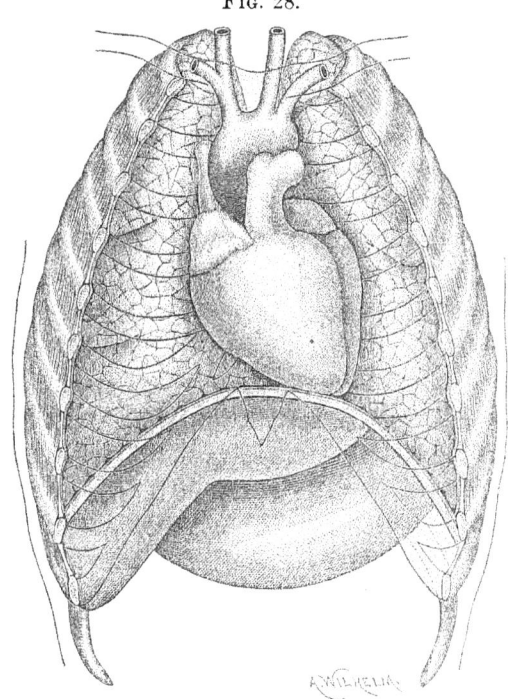

A hypertrophied heart lying in its position in the chest. The cause of the
lowered apex beat, and of the extension of the impulse, as well as of the
somewhat squarer outline of the increased dulness over the enlarged organ,
is obvious from the shape and position of the heart.

Hypertrophy of the heart affects males much more frequently than females. Its causes are various. Continued
functional excitement produces it; so does perhaps excessive
nourishment. But the main cause is an obstruction to the
circulation, either in the heart or in other organs. It is for
this reason that the complaint is so often seen in connection
with diseases of the valves or of the large arteries, and that
the right side of the heart enlarges when the pulmonary air-
vesicles are overdistended. We also meet with hypertrophy
of the heart as a consequence of the obliteration of the pericardial sac by its two surfaces adhering. Of this form of

hypertrophy there are, as we have above seen, no positive and distinctive signs.

Dilatation.—Dilatation of the heart is the reverse of hypertrophy. By this it is not meant that, because the cavities are dilated, the walls may not be increased; for we constantly meet with this form of dilated hypertrophy. But it is meant that the morbid condition in which the cavities have been stretched out of all proportion to the thickness of the muscular walls is the reverse of the condition in which the walls are stronger, firmer, and more powerful than in health; in other words, the latter state is very different from the former, and when it predominates we call the affection hypertrophy; when the former is in excess, we speak of the disease as dilatation, no matter whether the walls be slightly thicker than normal, or of natural thickness, or, as they often are, thinner, and apparently hardly capable of supporting the weight of the blood.

From these almost opposite pathological states, almost opposite physical signs or symptoms might be expected. And so we find it. We look in dilatation in vain for the activity and power with which the blood is forced out of a hypertrophied heart. Everything indicates debility, inaction, and stagnation of the vital current. There is a strong tendency to venous congestions and to dropsies. The portal system is gorged. The liver increases in size. The bowels are constipated. The urinary secretion is interfered with, and sometimes albumen is passed from the kidneys. The hearing may become dull. The patient is languid and feeble, and his intellect obtuse. He suffers from chilly sensations, and from distressing palpitations and uneasiness in the cardiac region. The pulse is small and irregular, and the veins of the surface swollen. The skin around the ankles, and often at other parts of the body, pits on pressure. But since it is the right side of the heart which is usually the most affected, the lungs show most plainly the effects of the venous stagnation. Difficulty in breathing, making itself at times manifest in paroxysms attended with wheezing respiration; a chronic cough; a collection of serum in the pulmonary structure,—all add to the misery which this perilous malady entails. And as it is commonly some obstructive disease in the lungs, such as emphysema, which has given rise to the dilatation of the right side of the heart, so this again aug. ments the morbid state of the lungs, and aggravates the symptoms.

Fig. 29.

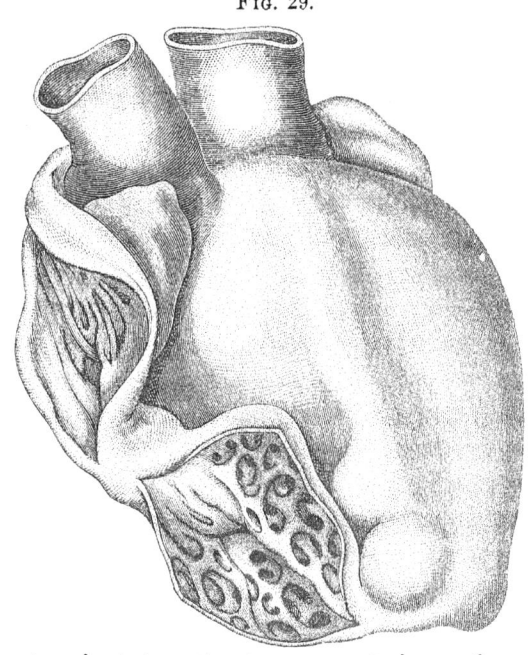

A dilated heart, the right ventricle opened. In this case there was no valvular disease. Hence the characteristic physical signs; the increased dulness on percussion, the extended but weak impulse. The first sound was feeble, for the organ was soft as well as dilated.

The physical signs are very unlike those of hypertrophy. The same extended dulness on percussion exists; but it is associated with a feeble, fluttering, and irregular impulse, which is in strong contrast with the heaving, powerful blow of a hypertrophied left ventricle. The sounds are not always the same. When the walls are thin, they are clearer, sharper, and more ringing than in health; if, however, the muscular structure be at all disorganized, the first sound is faint and very ill defined. But no murmurs are perceived, unless a watery state of the blood produces them, or unless it happens, and it does not unfrequently happen, that the dilatation of the heart is conjoined to valves incompetent, either temporarily or permanently, to prevent regurgitation.

Such is the description of cases of very marked dilatation. All cases are not, however, so distinct, nor are they uncomplicated. Organic affections of the heart are, indeed, indefinitely blended, and dilatation is met with in different combinations and in every possible degree. Accordingly, its symptoms and signs are somewhat dissimilar. But one constant feature it certainly preserves: it always holds up to view both the vital and physical manifestations of a weakened heart. It is thus that it is likely to be confounded with the diseases in which an enfeebled action of the heart is encountered, and these are fatty degeneration and a pericardial effusion.

Fatty Degeneration.—This is one of those disorders with the anatomical characters of which we are far better acquainted than with their clinical history. The microscope has revealed to us that the soft, flabby heart, which appears to the eye but little changed from health, has had its muscular fibres atrophied and transformed into fat granules and oil. It has thus explained to us, what was previously incomprehensible, why a heart seemingly so little altered should rupture, or why death should set in with all the evidences of failing circulation, when nothing in the whole body can be found sufficiently diseased to account for the termination of the vital action. But our power to recognize the fatty change during life has not kept pace with our power to recognize it after death. There is as yet no sign discovered, by which we can say that the dangerous disorganization of the muscular fibres of the heart is in progress. We may, however, suspect it, if the signs of weak action of the heart—feeble impulse and ill-defined sounds—coexist with a pulse permanently slow or permanently frequent and irregular, and be met with in a person who is the subject of a wasting disease, or who has arrived at a time of life at which all the organs are prone to undergo decay. Something more than a suspicion is warranted, if, in addition, there be proof of fatty degeneration elsewhere, such as an *arcus senilis;* or if it be ascertained that the patient suffers from paroxysms of severe pain in the heart; that he sighs frequently; that he is subject to seizures, during which his respiration seems to have come to a stand-still, and that he is liable to be stricken down with repeated attacks having the character of apoplexy, save that they are not followed by paralysis.*

Now, here are certainly a group of phenomena dissimilar to those of a dilated heart. Let us add to them, that the extent of the cardiac percussion dulness remains unaltered, that dropsies and local congestions are not prominent symptoms, or indeed do not happen at all, and the dissimilarity becomes still greater. A differential diagnosis would, under such circumstances, be anything but difficult. But in point of fact, the matter is generally not so easily decided, and there are several reasons why it is not. One is, that all the features described are but rarely combined in the same case; indeed, some of the more marked, such as the peculiar respiration, the seizures like apoplexy, are uncommon rather than common, and the altered breathing occasionally occurs in other cardiac maladies. The second is, because non-fatty softening may, it is believed, present the same vital and physical manifestations. The third, because a fatty heart has a tendency to become dilated, and the symptoms and signs of the former disease are then merged into the symptoms and signs of the latter, throwing us back into the province of conjecture and probability for a diagnosis. With the organ in such a condition, the practical value of a differential diagnosis is, however, not very great; for both affections are benefited by the same treatment : both require that the power of the heart should not be lowered. In both, therefore, the treatment applicable to hypertrophy is to be avoided; instead of weakening the action of the heart, it must be sustained, and the blood enriched. It is hardly necessary to add, that all causes of serious excitement are to be strenuously guarded against.

Persons who have fatty hearts are subject to attacks of faintness, preceded or attended with *sensations of great coldness* or a chill. And sometimes these attacks happen daily, or every

---

* But the exact relation the arcus senilis bears to a fatty heart is not ascertained. See, on its diagnostic value, a paper by Lee. Amer. Medical Monthly, September, 1856.

few days, and in a manner to give rise to the impression that they are due to malaria. A number of instances of the kind have come under my observation, and I have met with them more particularly at the end of fevers or other debilitating diseases happening in those affected with feeble hearts. The seizures, though bearing a certain resemblance to intermittent fever, are unlike it in being associated with signs of great weakness of the circulation, sometimes almost a vanishing pulse and a sense of impending dissolution; in their irregular accession; and in their not being followed by febrile phenomena. In doubtful cases the thermometer, by showing the absence of the great rise of temperature of the malarial disorder, will materially assist us in the diagnosis.

A fatty heart sometimes *ruptures.* Now, in spite of the care with which some authors have detailed the physical signs of this mishap, we know nothing positively about them; for death usually takes place far too rapidly to have permitted of any such observations. The symptoms that are mostly noticed are these: the patient is suddenly attacked with intolerable anguish in the heart; he presses his hand to it; then faints and soon expires. Or else he lives for a short time, suffering from faintness, cramps, and difficulty of breathing, and with death plainly written in his face.

Pericardial Effusion.—Pericardial effusion also presents the signs of a weakened heart with increased dulness on percussion in the cardiac region, and is thus very liable to be mistaken for a dilatation of the organ. Where the effusion forms part of a general dropsy, the detection of the cause of the latter, in connection with the different signs which fluid in the pericardium occasions, will prevent error. Where the liquid has remained after an inflammation of the membrane, both signs and symptoms are like those of the stage of effusion in acute pericarditis, and although there are points of resemblance to a dilated heart, there are also points of contrast, as the subjoined table shows:

DILATATION OF THE HEART.	CHRONIC PERICARDITIS WITH EFFUSION.
Percussion dulness increased in extent, but square in outline.	Percussion dulness increased, but of pyramidal shape.
Heart sounds clear and sharp; sometimes, however, feeble.	Heart sounds feeble and distant sounding at the apex, but distinct near the upper part of the sternum.
No friction sound.	Often friction sound still heard at the base of the heart.
Dropsy; signs of venous stagnation; severe cough, and dyspnœa.	Neither dropsy nor venous stagnation is observed; or, if at all, only in a very limited degree. Cough and dyspnœa are not so prominent symptoms.
History of disease shows it to be gradually developed.	The history frequently points to the acute attack.

These, then, are the marks of similitude and of distinction presented by a chronic pericardial effusion, a fatty heart, and cardiac dilatation; in other words, between the morbid states which occasion the signs and symptoms of a feebly acting heart. Before proceeding to another subject, let us glance at one more condition, fortunately infrequent, which may give rise to some of the same phenomena as those described —*an accumulation of blood in the cavities of the heart.* Like dilatation, this increases the area of percussion dulness; like it, too, it is often associated with perverted rhythm. The chief differences, so far as our very limited clinical knowledge of the subject permits us to say, are these: the impulse is generally much more labored, is more irregular, is sometimes strong, sometimes weak, not so almost uniformly indistinct or tremulous. There is much more venous congestion of the face with greater dyspnœa, and we often find some acute malady, such as endocarditis or pneumonia, giving rise to the cardiac engorgement. But the matter is often a very difficult one to determine; for many of the same states which lead to dilatation may produce an accumulation of blood in the heart; nay, dilatation itself predisposes to it.

24

Diseases of the Heart, exhibiting more or less of the Signs and Symptoms of Enlargement of the Organ, and accompanied by Endocardial Murmurs.

Valvular Affections.—To find the sounds of the heart clearly and well defined, is to know that no disease of the valves exists. No matter whether there be reason to believe that the walls of the heart are hypertrophied to twice their thickness, or the cavities stretched to twice their capacity, if the ear recognize the natural sounds, it is evidence that the valvular apparatus is not affected. When it is disordered, the mischief betrays itself, for the most part, by a blowing sound. If, therefore, a murmur of any permanence be met with in the heart, if especially it be associated with the signs of either hypertrophy or dilatation, the inference that valvular disease exists will in the vast majority of cases be a correct inference.

Yet it will not be always so; for there are other morbid states besides valvular affections which engender a murmur, that may be even accompanied by all the manifestations of enlargement of the heart. Malformations, such as communications between the auricles or between the ventricles, or between the great vessels near their origin, or impoverished blood, or a misdirected blood current, may occasion a murmur.

Now, with reference to *malformations*, their presence in adults, or in children that have passed the days of infancy, is exceedingly rare. The most trustworthy symptom they present is that which indicates the admixture of arterial and venous blood; in other words, the symptom of cyanosis, the bluish discoloration of the skin. In addition, we may perceive the signs of disturbed circulation in the lungs, such as dyspnœa and cough; and of irregular action of the heart; and a blowing sound in the cardiac region. Still, the recognition of these malformations is always more or less a matter of conjecture, and to mistake them for other organic changes in the heart, particularly those of the valves, is a mistake which in the actual state of our knowledge cannot be avoided.

With the aid of more such researches as those of Dr. More-ton Stillé* or of Dr. Peacock,† we shall become accurately acquainted with the pathology of the different lesions, and perhaps ultimately be able to discern them with certainty during life. At present it is in their rarity alone that the safety against errors of diagnosis lies.

As a few points of assistance may be mentioned that com-munication of the ventricles through the septum gives rise to a systolic murmur at or near the base of the heart not propagated into the arteries; that the passage of blood through an open foramen ovale very rarely engenders any sound; and that, whether coexisting with these lesions or not, the majority of instances of cardiac malformation, after the age of twelve, present signs of obstruction at the orifice of the pulmonary artery. In this instance either a systolic or diastolic murmur may be there perceived; in the first case the second sound of the heart is weak or wanting in the second interspace on the left side.

The resemblance borne by cases of *functional disturbance of the heart*, associated with impoverished blood, to valvular affections, has already engaged our attention. The age; the appearance of the patient; the seat of the blowing sound at the base of the heart; the venous hum; the fact that the car-diac murmur is followed by a sharp second sound,—all are points upon which some stress may be laid; yet not so much as upon the absence of the phenomena of an enlarged heart. But, if the question be asked, are the latter absolute demon-strations of the existence of an affection of the valves, cannot a hypertrophied or dilated heart, with sound valves, be com-bined with a condition of blood capable of producing a mur-mur?—we are forced to answer that such is possible. Under these circumstances, the tact of the physician may help him to a well-judged decision; but the only proof of a well-judged decision is afforded by time or the result of the treatment which restores the blood to its normal state.

A murmur caused in violent excitement of the heart by *misdirection of the current*, due chiefly to temporary interference

---

* American Journal of the Medical Sciences, July, 1844.
† Treatise on Malformations of the Heart.

with the closure of the valves, or, perhaps, by altered tension of the valves—causes the exact working of which I have elsewhere fully inquired into*—may become a troublesome source of error in diagnosis, especially when heard over a heart in a state of dilated hypertrophy or of dilatation. Fortunately, a blowing sound of this origin is comparatively rare, and we are generally enabled to discriminate it from an organic valvular murmur by its not being persistent. It is much more likely to be heard at the apex, or rather, according to my own observations, somewhat above the apex, than is a murmur owing to changes in the blood; and it differs from the systolic blowing sound of mitral disease partly by the peculiarity of seat just mentioned, partly by its non-diffusion, its usual absence at the back of the chest, the want of harshness in the inconstant murmur, and the low pitch. Murmurs of this kind are also caused by obstructive diseases of the lungs, without a disease of the heart being present.

These, then, are the causes which impair the value of the cardiac blowing sound as a sign of a valvular lesion. Yet they do not happen often enough to prevent us from regarding a murmur as eminently indicative of an organic affection of the valves.

Let us suppose that we are convinced that the murmur is due to a structural lesion. Can we say what its precise nature is? Can we accurately foretell that the valve is merely roughened; or that it has undergone calcareous transformation; or that it has been bound down; or that it is lacerated; or that vegetations spring from it; or that its muscular attachments are sound or unsound? No, assuredly not. The most we can do is to judge whether the orifices through which the current flows be narrowed, or whether, by the valves not closing, they permit of regurgitation; and to distinguish even this we have to take into account more the time of the occurrence of the sound than its particular character or pitch. Indeed, all distinctions based entirely on either of these are not borne out by clinical experience. Valves incompetent to close the openings at which they are seated may permit a

---

* On Functional Valvular Disorders. Am Journ. Med. Sciences, July, 1869.

murmur to be generated of any character and of any pitch. It is true that a harsh murmur, like that of a saw or of a rasp, is for the most part occasioned by a contracted orifice with rigid valves; but many contracted orifices with rigid valves exist, without producing such a rough noise.

Fig. 30.

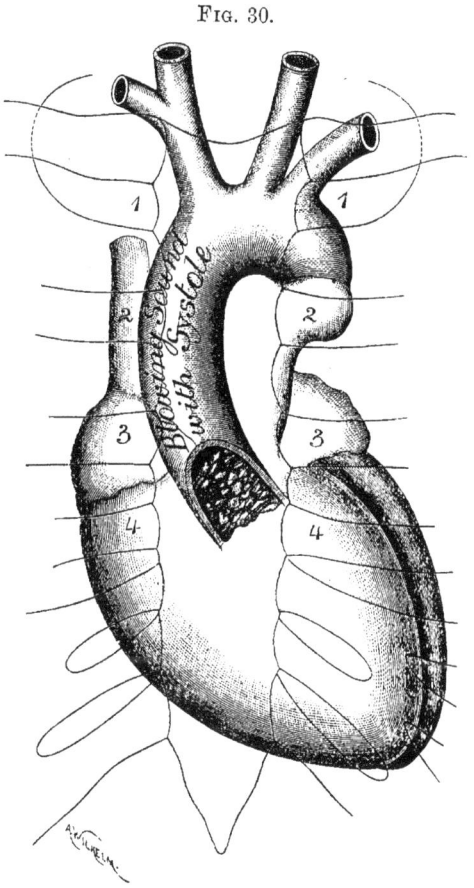

Narrowing of the aortic orifice by vegetations springing from the valves, the structure of which was indeed, to a great extent, destroyed. The engraving illustrates at the same time the physical signs of aortic constriction.

A cardiac sound which is rare, but which, when present, is most uniformly associated with a narrowed orifice, is a distinct musical tone heard at the mitral or aortic valves. It resembles the cooing of a pigeon; or the auscultator listens and listens again, and directs the patient again and again to suspend the respiration before he becomes convinced that the sound is not a sibilant rale in the lung. It is sometimes perceived merely at the end of an ordinary bellows murmur, and disappears and reappears from time to time. Where this rare sound is met with, the valves after death are commonly found to be rigid and unyielding. Yet this is not always the case. Sometimes the musical note is produced by the vibrations of clots which impede the rush of blood through the apertures of the heart, perhaps even by the loose edge of a valve flapping to and fro in the current. Occasionally, too, we hit upon it in chlorosis; but, in truth, only very occasionally, and never unless it be then equally or more marked in the arterial system. We have the authority of Dr. Stokes for the observation, that it may be suddenly developed and precede the signs of structural alteration of the heart.

It has been already stated that, on the whole, we judge best of the state of the orifices and of the valves, by ascertaining the time at which the bellows sound occurs. To do this it is, however, necessary to know in what condition the orifices are during the movements of the healthy heart. Briefly to recapitulate what we have previously discussed: during the contraction of the ventricles, the valves at the auriculo-ventricular openings are closed, since if they were not closed, the blood would regurgitate into the auricles; and the valves of the aorta and pulmonary artery are open, so as to permit the blood to pass along the arterial trunks. During the dilatation of the heart the reverse takes place; the valves at the origin of the great arteries are shut, to prevent the blood which has just been sent forth from regurgitating, and those valves the function of which is to act as gates to the auriculo-ventricular apertures are swung back to allow the stream to flow into the ventricles.

If thus a murmur occur with the contraction of the heart and the first sound, it is either the blood regurgitating from the ventricles into the auricles, or meeting with difficulty in passing into the aorta or pulmonary artery; if, after the contraction of the heart, and corresponding to the second sound, it is the blood passing through a narrowed mitral or tricuspid orifice, or streaming back into the ventricles through incompetent aortic or pulmonary valves. But can we distinguish at which valve the mischief lies? Generally we can. By attending to the site of greatest intensity of the murmur, we become aware of the seat of its production, provided it be

FIG. 31.

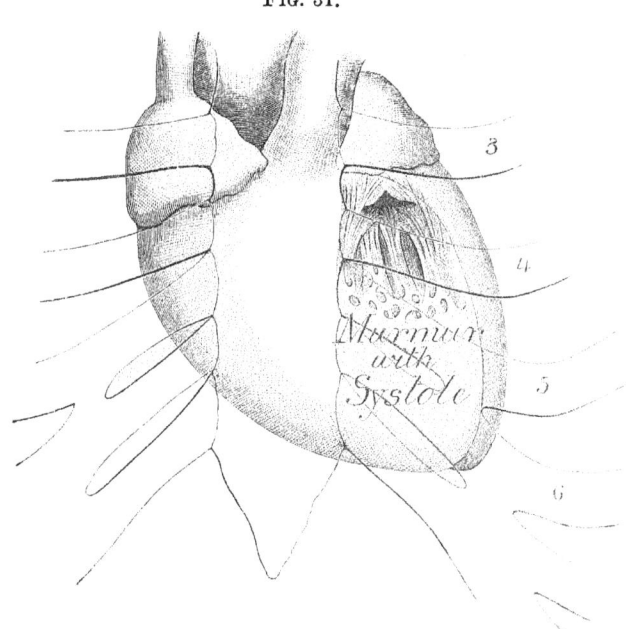

Insufficient mitral valves permitting regurgitation of the blood. The position and time of occurrence of the most significant sign of the affection is indicated in the engraving.

borne in mind what are the points for listening to the different valves. It is, however, also necessary to recollect that, as the whole heart is somewhat lowered, these points are rather below what they are in a natural state of things.

Now, we cannot always say whether more than one valve is affected. A blowing sound in the heart, no matter where generated, is usually transmitted all over the organ. If it mask the natural sounds at other valves, it is very difficult, nay, it is often impossible, to tell positively how many of the valves are injured, unless several spots are detected at which the murmur is intense, and yet not alike in character.

Thus the blowing sound is the most conspicuous and most constant sign of a valvular lesion. The other signs and symptoms vary in individual cases. Where the valves are but slightly affected, let us say slightly roughened, as they sometimes are after an attack of rheumatic endocarditis, the heart does not undergo any decided change in size; the circulation is carried on regularly; and, in spite of the abnormal sound in the heart, the patient's health remains unimpaired, or it is only occasionally that he suffers from slight palpitations. An alteration of the valves of the heart of any extent produces, however, an alteration either in the capacity of its cavities or in the thickness of its walls, and the symptoms of dilatation or hypertrophy make their appearance along with the physical signs of extended percussion dulness and feeble or heaving impulse. Ordinarily it is the latter we meet with, because the valves of the left side are so very much more frequently diseased than those of the right, and their derangements lead to hypertrophy rather than to dilatation.* Affections of the tricuspid valves are very usually connected with dilatation of the organ ; hence dropsy, venous turgescence, and albuminous urine are in them more specially observed. We also find in them, or rather in tricuspid insufficiency, what Mahot has recently more particularly called attention to,—a pulsation of the liver corresponding to each systole of the heart, which can be perceived by gently depressing the abdominal parietes with the hand on the epigastrium.

All valvular lesions may be combined with pain in the præcordia, with palpitations, with restlessness and disturbed dreams. And according as the deranged circulation through the heart interferes with the circulation in other parts, special symptoms show themselves prominently. Thus we find those laboring under a mitral disease suffering most from cough, from dyspnœa, and from attacks of cardiac asthma, since it is the lung which has to bear the brunt of the embarrassed flow of the blood.

---

* But if we may accept Dr. Blakiston's researches as final, affections of the tricuspid valves are both much more common and much more important than is usually supposed. Tricuspid regurgitation, he states, is the most direct and almost constant cause of that engorgement of the vessels of the brain and of the general circulation, with their consequences, which originates within the heart. It is, therefore, the predisposing cause of cerebral apoplexy when in connection with cardiac disease.

If we examine this organ closely, the physical signs afford direct proof of its disordered condition. Here and there are heard plentiful moist sounds from fluid which has leaked into the air-tubes; here and there the respiratory murmur is roughened; here and there percussion elicits impaired clearness. This loss of the natural resonance is at times very manifest at the upper part of the lung, and I have known it to lead to the suspicion of tubercular deposit in cases in which the autopsy showed the pulmonary tissue to be sound, though in a state of extreme congestion.

When the aortic valves permit of regurgitation, this gives rise to effects which are perceptible along the track of the arteries. These all look superficial, and beat with apparent violence, from the force with which the thickened left ventricle is driving the blood through the tubes. Yet when the finger is applied to the artery at the wrist, the strength of the beat is not so great as is expected. A short, abrupt, jerking impulse is indeed communicated to the finger; but then the artery immediately recedes, proving that it was only imperfectly filled. This pulse is the only one which gives us any real information as to the state of the orifices of the heart; otherwise the pulse does not afford any very trustworthy indications. In general terms, it may be stated to be small and rather tense when the openings are narrowed. Still, no stress can be laid on this in a diagnostic point of view. The want of correspondence between its strength and the force with which the heart is acting is often amazing.

Much more information than by merely feeling the pulse can be obtained by studying it with the sphygmograph. But even with this, as thus far developed, we gather in valvular diseases rather corroborative evidence than knowledge which is not attainable by other means of diagnosis. Very probably, with further research, the instrument may be made available to inform us with certainty of the degree of the valvular imperfection, and this would be a great step in advance. As regards the most distinctive graphical signs, we obtain them in aortic regurgitation,—a vertical line of ascent of great amplitude, a sharp and pointed summit, and a sudden descent, with comparatively very little dicrotism. If there be alsò marked aortic obstruction, the line of ascent is oblique, or oftener rather the first part is vertical, and following the sharp point is a gradual curvelike rise; if senile changes in the artery complicate the aortic insufficiency, the sharp-pointed process terminating the line of ascent passes usually into a more or less horizontal plateau. In mitral regurgitation the pulse tracing is usually very irregular; the line of ascent is short, but apt to be very unequal, and the line of descent disposed to be oblique and to present very marked dicrotism.

FIG. 32.

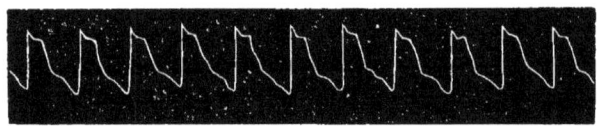

Sphygmogram taken from a patient with aortic insufficiency. The line of ascent does not terminate in as sharp a point, nor is the descent as sudden as we sometimes find it.

FIG. 33.

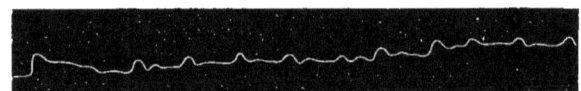

Sphygmogram taken from a patient presenting the signs of mitral regurgitation.

But, instead of entering into a detailed description of the pulse, however studied, or of any separate symptoms of valvular disease, let us group them together with the physical signs, according to the combination in which we are wont to meet with them:

TABLE OF VALVULAR DISEASES.

SEAT OF MURMUR.	SEAT OF DISEASE.	CHARACTER OF DISEASE.	CORRELATIVE PHYSICAL SIGNS AND SYMPTOMS.
Murmur most intense at or near apex of heart.	Mitral orifice.	With impulse, means insufficiency of valves, permitting of *regurgitation;* after impulse, and running into or corresponding to second sound, or preceding first, means *narrowing* of the orifice.	In mitral disease the heart very commonly undergoes dilated hypertrophy, especially the right ventricle. The second sound of the pulmonary artery, heard in the second left interspace, is sharp, accentuated. The cardiac murmur is most often distinctly perceived posteriorly on the left side, near the angle of the scapula. Dyspnœa and dropsy are prominent symptoms, especially dyspnœa. Cough is not unusual, and the pulse is not unfrequently found to be feeble and irregular. In some forms of mitral obstruction, where the curtains are not too rigid, the murmur is always rough.
Murmur most intense at or near the middle of the sternum, or heard with equal distinctness close to the sternum in the second interspace on the right side, and thence propagated into the arterial system.	Aortic orifice.	With impulse, means *narrowing,* or obstruction; with diastole, and taking the place of second sound, means *regurgitation.*	Hypertrophy of left ventricle. The cardiac sounds may all be normal, excepting at the affected valve, although they are often somewhat obscured by the murmur. This is distinct in the carotids, and is sometimes as well heard at the ensiform cartilage as over the sternum, and on a line with the third intercostal space—a fact necessary to be aware of, so as to avoid confounding the aortic lesion with one of the tricuspid valve. When the orifice is constricted, a purring thrill is frequently observed to attend each beat of the heart. The symptoms are often remarkably latent. There is very commonly neither dropsy nor dyspnœa. The pulse is, in constriction, not materially affected, in regurgitation it is abrupt and jerking, and all the superficial arteries pulsate distinctly. It is not unusual to find a double blowing sound attending aortic regurgitation, probably from slight coexisting obstruction of the orifice.
Murmur most intense at or very near to the ensiform cartilage, and over the lower part of right ventricle.	Tricuspid orifice.	With impulse, *regurgitation;* with diastole, and taking therefore the place of second sound, or preceding first, *narrowing?*	Tricuspid regurgitation (for of tricuspid narrowing our knowledge is little else than theoretical) exists very usually in combination with dilatation of the right ventricle, and therefore with the symptoms of this condition: with venous congestions, with dropsies, with difficulty in breathing. On account of the open state of the orifice, the cervical veins may pulsate during the movements of the heart; and in all cases they are distended. The pulsatile motion in the neck becomes especially visible when the breath is held in expiration. The cardiac murmur is ordinarily soft, of low pitch, is not transmitted into the arteries, and not heard above the level of the third rib. In some cases it is so feeble as to be with difficulty discernible.

TABLE OF VALVULAR DISEASES—(*Continued*).

SEAT OF MURMUR.	SEAT OF DISEASE.	CHARACTER OF DISEASE.	CORRELATIVE PHYSICAL SIGNS AND SYMPTOMS.
Murmur most intense at third left costal cartilage near the sternum, or somewhat lower, or in second intercostal space of left side.	Pulmonary orifice.	With impulse, is *narrowing;* taking place of second sound, *regurgitation.*	We have very little actual knowledge, derived from clinical observation, of diseases of the pulmonary valves; of all the valves the ones most rarely affected. Nor does a murmur in the situation indicated, and hardly audible over the left apex or along the sternum, or in the course of the great vessels, having therefore the characteristics of a pulmonic murmur, warrant a diagnosis of disease of the valves: for it may be due to anæmia; be caused by deposits at the upper part of the left lung; or be observed immediately after or during the continuance of hemorrhage from the lungs. But these remarks scarcely hold good with reference to a diastolic murmur, and not at all as regards a double murmur. If this be present, and signs of dilated hypertrophy exist, we are justified in concluding the disease to be a lesion of the pulmonary valves, or at the origin of the artery.

In this manner are the symptoms and signs of valvular affections associated. But I do not pretend to say that this is exactly the combination, and precisely the way in which they happen in every instance. There are too many circumstances which modify them; disorders of several valves are too constantly conjoined; at the same orifice both narrowing and a state permitting of regurgitation are too often found to coexist,—to permit any tabular representation to express either all the symptoms or signs which may occur in individual cases. Apart from this difficulty there is another: even where the affection of a second valve has been correctly fixed upon, the irregularity of the heart's action may be such that it is impossible to say whether the blowing sound which is heard be systolic or diastolic; whether, therefore, the orifice be narrowed or the valves insufficient. Fortunately, this is not a matter of so much consequence; the matter of consequence is, to determine that a disease of the valves of the heart is present.

Presuming that we have been enabled to fix, and to fix accurately, the state of each aperture, there is a point where all our skill invariably comes to a stand-still. We cannot tell how long it is possible for life to continue, or under what circumstances death will happen. It may take place suddenly and most unexpectedly in cases in which the amount of disease in the heart is not found to be very great; and, on the other hand, life, and even a tolerable degree of health, may be maintained with valves so rigid and unyielding that the point of the knife can, at the autopsy, hardly be forced through them. In mitral disease, the patient is liable to be worn out by the dropsy and by the steadily increasing difficulty of breathing; and so, too, in that still more serious lesion—tricuspid regurgitation. In affections of the aortic valves the patient suffers less, but he is more liable to sudden death.

From these remarks, it is apparent that the treatment of valvular disease is very unsatisfactory. In truth, no remedy has any direct action on the valves, and we have to content ourselves with palliating what we cannot cure. The dropsy and the dyspnœa generally demand special attention, and tax the practitioner's efforts to the utmost; for, although they can be greatly benefited by treatment, they cannot be cured so long as their irremediable cause persists.

Before dismissing these valvular affections, there are a few other matters which claim consideration, though the limits set to this work will prevent their full discussion. The blowing sound has been insisted upon as the diagnostic sign of a valvular lesion, and to insist upon this is to do no more than universal experience warrants. But we can rarely thus absolutely connect a disease with a special sign. Undoubtedly there are instances in which no murmur reaches the ear to show that the valves are damaged.

I shall cite, as concisely as possible, two examples. A man, thirty-five years of age, came under my care, complaining of palpitation of the heart, of occasional attacks of bronchitis, and of shortness of breath. His health was otherwise good. A physical examination of the chest showed the action of the heart to be extremely disturbed: the impulse was strong, and the extent of dulness in the precordial region increased. A blowing sound was heard near the apex, but, owing to the great irregularity of the movements of the heart, it was impossible to say whether it corresponded in time to the contraction or relaxation of the organ. The pulse was small, frequent and intermittent. The patient continued in this state for seven months, the beat of the heart becoming more and more tumultuous; but the murmur gradually disappeared. A peculiar clacking sound took its place, which was most distinct near the apex, and was faintly transmitted to other portions of the heart. It occurred with but one sound of the heart,—with which could not be determined. For some time before his death he had considerable cough, with a frothy expectoration and great difficulty in breathing. His face and hands had begun to swell. The immediate cause of death seemed to have been pulmonary apoplexy. The heart was found in a state of dilated hypertrophy, and the mitral valves had been converted into a calcareous mass, which had left but an extremely narrow chink for the blood to pass through.

The next case presents, in several respects, a striking similarity. A gentleman, about fifty years of age, who had led a gay and somewhat dissipated life, noticed that he experienced difficulty in breathing on the slightest exertion. He complained also much of loss of appetite and of distention of the stomach. I could not find any cause beyond flatulency to account for this; the abdomen yielded all over an extremely tympanitic sound. But to the dyspnœa, an inquiry into the state of the heart furnished a clue. The size of the organ was evidently augmented, and its rhythm very irregular. The impulse was strong; but the sounds were normal, excepting near the apex, where, taking the place of one, was heard a dull but very marked clack. When the hand was applied over this point, it felt a vibration of very much the same character as that which the ear could hear, and, like this, it was limited, or certainly only distinctly perceptible, at or near the apex of the organ. The diagnosis of disease of the mitral valves was made, and it proved to be correct. The dyspnœa became greater and greater; the feet, and subsequently the abdomen, were distended with fluid; and the patient died with all the symptoms of an unmistakable valvular lesion.

My note-book would furnish me with many more such

cases; but these two present the main features of all. All the instances I have met with of valvular disease, unaccompanied by blowing sounds, have been instances of disease at the mitral orifice, and of extreme narrowing of that orifice. They were all attended with excessive irregularity of the action of the heart, and with hypertrophy. They all produced difficulty of breathing. They all presented this peculiar clacking sound most marked near the apex. In some, another sound, more like that heard in health, followed it; in others, not. In some, the blowing sound gradually disappeared; in others, none was perceived when first examined; and in others, again, it could be caught occasionally, as a very short whiff, along with the clacking sound. The impulse was in all strong and very variable in its rhythm, and a peculiar movement was felt near the seat of the apex— not the purring tremor which so commonly accompanies the movements of a heart the valves of which are damaged, but a more localized vibration, similar, as far as such similarity can exist, to the sound the ear hears.

These cases are probably of the same nature as those that are every now and then reported as valvular lesions, in which the sounds of the heart were normal. I cannot think that with a disease of the valves they ever are so. There may be no blowing sounds present, but the sounds of the valve affected must be different from what they are in health; and it may again, in all truth, be said, that to hear the natural sounds of the heart well defined, is to be able to exclude a valvular disease.

The other subject to which we may, in conclusion, advert, is the possibility of valves having been insufficient to perform their functions during life, and yet no signs of their incompetence be detected after death, at least none indicated by any structural change in the valves. That such cases occur, is attested by more than one observer. They have generally been found to be connected with dilatation of the ventricles of the heart, and are perhaps due, as suggested by Dr. Pristowe,* to a ventricle becoming dilated without a correspond-

---

* Brit. and Foreign Med.-Chirg. Review, July, 1861; see also cases by Hare, Transact. of London Path. Society, vol. ii., and by Cuming, Dublin Quarterly Journal, May, 1868.

ing elongation of the musculi papillares and chordæ tendineæ. Of course this explanation only holds good with reference to regurgitation through the auriculo-ventricular apertures; but it is to this condition that the instances recorded refer. Yet in explaining them we must not overlook those blowing sounds produced by mere abnormal action of the textures of the heart, to which we have elsewhere alluded, and the existence of which no one can call in question.

Displacements of the Heart.

The heart is a very movable organ. This is proved by the ease with which it is displaced, and with which it returns to its normal position. Its apex is tilted upward by an enlarged liver, by an abdominal tumor, or by a pericardial effusion. It gravitates toward the median line when the walls of the heart have increased in weight and firmness. But these changes are hardly of a nature to attract as much attention as finding a heart beating on the right side of the sternum.

Now, it is nothing very uncommon to meet with it there, and the question immediately arises, what does this strange alteration in its situation signify, and how is it brought about? It is usually produced by pressure exercised on the heart by accumulations of fluid or of air in the left pleural cavity, and therefore denotes, as a rule, a pleuritic effusion or pneumothorax of the left side, and is accompanied by distention of that side. In rarer instances, the heart is pushed across by a highly distended emphysematous lung; in still rarer instances, it is drawn over to the right side by a shrinking of the right lung, attended with dilatation of the bronchial tubes, the so-called pulmonary cirrhosis. It is sometimes found on the right side, because it had been forced there by a pleuritic effusion, and has formed adhesions, so that when the fluid was absorbed it was unable to return to its natural place. In this case the left side will be markedly retracted, and not the right, as it is if cirrhosis be the cause of the abnormal position of the heart.

The displacement may further have been brought about by a cancerous or an aneurismal tumor, or by any of the abdominal viscera having slipped into the chest through a hernial opening in the diaphragm; or it may be congenital. But these are all causes which seldom exist. Practically speaking, transpositions of the heart are met with in connection with diseases of the lungs, as has been explained in a previous chapter. Here we shall merely add, that a congenital displacement cannot be diagnosticated, unless all other causes capable of producing a displacement have been proved to be absent; and that a dislocated heart is able to perform all its functions. It may even be attacked by acute diseases; the recognition of which, under such circumstances,—and they have been recognized,* — belongs most assuredly to the triumphs of physical diagnosis.

SECTION III.

THORACIC ANEURISM.

The heart is not the only part of the circulatory system within the chest which is liable to become diseased. The great vessels which spring from it are subject to the same morbid conditions as the vessels of any other portion of the body. Especially do we find this to be the case with the aorta, the coats of which are frequently roughened by calcareous or atheromatous deposits. These alterations are, however, beyond the discernment of the physician. He may infer that they exist, if a distinct systolic blowing sound be heard in the track of the aorta or its branches, in a person who is not anemic, who is past middle life—and therefore at an age at which these kinds of alterations of tissues happen—and in whom no cardiac murmurs, or only very faint cardiac murmurs, are perceived. But it is not until after death that the practitioner learns the precise nature or extent of the structural lesions. They are thus only interesting to him as a

---

* By Stokes. See Diseases of the Heart, page 463.

pathologist, and important, because he knows that these
changes in the coats of the arteries are often but the first
step toward their laceration or a dilatation of the vessels;
in other words, toward the establishment of an aneurism.

Now, an aneurism of the aorta, whether caused by a disease of the coats of the artery or not, whether true or false,
may affect any part of the vessel. But it is chiefly at the
ascending portion and at the arch that it is met with. Where
it occurs just after the artery has left the heart, it is prone to
elude discovery. Higher up, nearer to, or at the arch, it
more rarely escapes detection. The tumor manifests itself
by a local bulging, varying in extent and situation according
to the extent and situation of the aneurism. A single rib
alone may be raised, or nothing but a fulness be observed.
But some prominent spot is generally detected, and when
this is percussed, it is more resistant, and returns a duller
sound than when there is nothing wrong underneath. Yet
neither the bulging nor the dulness on percussion is of as
much significance as finding a distinct pulsation remote from
the beat of the heart. Every time the latter is perceived, an
impulse is communicated to the finger at the point in the
chest walls which appears to project; that is, usually on the
right side of the sternum in the second intercostal space, or
in the same interspace on the left side, or immediately under
the top of the bone. Occasionally the beat is double, and at
times so violent as to shake the head of the listener.

The impulse may be accompanied by a distinct thrill. Yet
this is not always present, and, when present, not always constant; since it may disappear and reappear. It is thus a
serious mistake to regard the thrill as the requisite sign of
an aneurismal enlargement, and yet there is no mistake more
common, excepting, perhaps, one : to consider that the motion
of the blood in the sac must necessarily engender a murmur.
The ear, applied over the prominence, hears often nothing
that in the least resembles a murmur, but sounds like those
of the heart, sometimes two—the first weighty and prolonged :
sometimes but one, and that one longer and more intense
than the corresponding first sound over the ventricles.

Thus, then, neither thrill nor murmur is essential to the

diagnosis of an aneurism. What is much more so, is to find two points of pulsation in the chest—two hearts, each with its own distinct beat, its own distinct sounds.

The aneurismal tumor in the chest gives rise to symptoms which vary somewhat according to its seat and extent. Prominent among them stand those occasioned by pressure. The sac presses on the adjacent air-tubes, and shortness of breathing, or peculiar cough and signs counterfeiting those of a chronic laryngeal disease, are the result; or it presses on the œsophagus, and the patient suffers from difficulty in swallowing; or it presses on the subclavian artery, and the pulses at the two wrists are noticed to be strikingly different; or on the carotid, and pain in the head, dulness of mind, occasional giddiness, and flashes of light before the eyes, are complained of; or on the venous trunks, and the superficial veins of the neck and thorax are seen to be engorged, and the skin becomes very puffy and swollen ; or on the trunk of the sympathetic nerve or on its ganglia and their communications, and marked contraction, or, in rare instances, dilatation of the pupil of the eye on the side of the aneurismal swelling, is perceived, or profuse sweating becomes a very annoying complication. All these signs, then, denote pressure, and pressure connected with a pulsating tumor in the chest means an aneurism.

I say with a pulsating tumor, because a cancerous or any other *morbid growth* may produce exactly the same signs of compression as an aneurismal tumor,—the same stridor, the same cough, the same feebleness of respiration in one lung from partial obliteration of its bronchial tube. But the solid tumor, large though it be, does not pulsate, or if it does, pulsates but very feebly, and not with the heaving motion of a distending aneurismal sac.* The tumor renders a large surface dull on percussion, and communicates a much greater

---

* This same absence of distinct pulsation was the main point of dissimilarity between an aneurism and an abscess of the mediastinum some time since under my care, and which, after lasting a year, and simulating aneurism most closely in the pain, the dulness on percussion, the difficulty of breathing and of swallowing, and the altered voice, got well by breaking internally and by the discharge, as expectoration, of large amounts of purulent matter.

feeling of resistance to the percussing finger. Yet the ear
listens in vain over the prominence for the weighty sound
with each beat of the heart, or for the hoarse murmur of the
blood streaming through the sac. It is only where a solid
growth weighs on the artery that any murmur is perceived,
and this is different from the superficial, loud sounds or murmurs of an aneurism. Further, a tumor is not confined to
the course of the aorta; it is more commonly connected with
a distended state of the veins of the neck and thorax, and
with œdema of the arm and chest; the pain it occasions is
often more continued, and less neuralgic in its nature. Moreover, as most thoracic tumors are cancerous, the violent constitutional disturbance, the formation of external swellings,
and the peculiar currant-jelly expectoration, aid us in arriving
at a correct conclusion. The obvious inequality of the pupils,
which is found in a certain number of cases among the signs
of an aneurism, is of little aid in a differential diagnosis, for
a thoracic cancer has been noted to occasion the same.* The
rarity of a non-aneurismal tumor in the chest is, however,
very great; and, practically speaking, when the signs of an
intra-thoracic tumor are met with, we are generally correct
in thinking that it is an aneurism we have to treat, even
should the pulsations not be very obvious.

Let us suppose that we are perfectly satisfied, owing to a
marked impulse, that we have not a solid growth to deal
with—does a pulsation uniformly denote an aneurism? Can
we absolutely say, on account of the impulse, that it is an
aneurismal enlargement? If there be also a swelling and
signs of pressure, we can; should these not exist, we cannot
be quite so sure. For a pulsation in the chest not immediately over the region of the heart, although it is nearly
always indicative of an aneurism, may be owing to other
causes:

Where the aortic valves are insufficient, and permit of regurgitation, there may be a pulsation in the aorta; an empyema may pulsate; a dilated auricle may occasion an impulse

---

* MacDonnell, Montreal Medical Chronicle, June, 1858; see, also, the Researches of Gairdner, Clinical Medicine, and of Ogle, Medico-Chirurgical
Transactions, vol. xli.

separate from that of the ventricles ; a pulmonary artery surrounded by consolidated lung may distinctly exhibit its beat.
In all of these the signs of pressure on the surrounding
parts are wanting; and, on the other hand, they show phenomena which an aneurism lacks.

Insufficient aortic valves are accompanied by hypertrophy of
the left ventricle. So is very constantly a thoracic aneurism;
but instead of the throbbing at the upper anterior part of
the chest being attended, as it is in aneurismal swelling,
with a natural, or an unequal and diminished beat at the
wrist, there, as well as in the larger trunks in the neck and
arms, is perceived that strong and peculiar pulsation which
is so characteristic a sign of inadequate aortic valves. Then,
again, a murmur is much more common in this organic
affection of the valves than it is when an aneurism has
formed above the origin of the vessel. And even where a
murmur is heard over the seat of an aneurismal pulsation,
it is better marked there than over the heart, and not unfrequently short, hoarse, and of low pitch ; in truth, it differs in
distinctness as well as in quality from the murmur discerned
at the base of the heart, which may be transmitted from the
aneurism, or depend upon coexisting cardiac disease.

A *pulsating empyema* is very seldom met with; yet it is well
to have a knowledge of the fact that a collection of fluid in
the cavity of the chest may vibrate with the motion of the
heart, and throb with such violence as closely to simulate an
aneurism. To determine the real nature of the pulsation in
these cases, we must attach importance to the situation of
the expanding mass, which is not often that of an aneurism,
and to the signs which point out that liquid has accumulated
within the pleural sac. We also note the circumstance that
over the seat of impulse there are no peculiarly marked
sounds, no murmurs, no thrill.

A *dilated auricle*, the walls of which are at the same time
hypertrophied, may give rise to a movement separate from
that of the beat of the ventricle. Bouillaud cites an example
of this nature, in which a double motion was perceptible in
the second intercostal space of the left side, in a person
whose heart was extensively hypertrophied, and whose mitral

valves were indurated. Such cases are extremely rare. The signs of an accompanying valvular affection and of enlargement of the ventricles, and the probable presence of dropsy would serve to distinguish a dilated auriele from aneurism of the arch. And this is the only form of enlargement of the heart which is at all likely to be mistaken for an aneurism. In cases of hypertrophy or dilatation as we ordinarily meet with them, there is but one motion discernible—that over the ventricles—and not two beats at some distance from each other; the signs of pressure, too, are absent.

A *pulmonary artery* surrounded by consolidated lung tissue may cause—especially if, in addition, the vessel be somewhat widened—a very distinct pulsation. But the seat of the dulness at or near the apex of the left lung; its non-extension over the median line; the limitation of the murmur to the site of the pulmonary artery, or, in some instances, to this vessel and the subclavian; the sharply-defined second sound of the pulmonary artery in the second interspace on the left side; the symptoms and physical signs of phthisis, the most common cause of the consolidation and a morbid condition which of itself would appear to exclude an aneurism; the absence of the phenomena caused by pressure,—all these prove the murmur and the pulsation not to be due to an aortic aneurism.

Another abnormal condition, which may be mistaken for an aneurism, is a *malformation of the chest*, particularly when produced by great prominence of the upper part of the sternum. This error is more specially apt to occur if there be coexisting disturbance of the heart, whether of functional or organic origin. I saw some time since a case where the beating of the arteries of the neck, accompanied by an enlargement of the thyroid gland and by cardiac palpitation, was believed to be an aneurism, mainly because it was combined with very decided prominence of the upper portion of the sternum. But there were neither distinctly localized tumefaction and pulsation, nor altered sounds, nor any signs of pressure.

The signs of pressure play, then, a very important part in the diagnosis of an aneurism. To those morbid states already mentioned, between which they enable us to discriminate, another may be added. Instances have been recorded of constriction of the aorta giving rise to a marked thrill at the upper part of the chest in front, near the sternum, and a murmur much louder there than over the heart. The absence of the signs of pressure, and the throbbing and distention of the vessels of the neck, head, and chest, of the carotid, the subclavian, the temporal, and the mammary arteries may lead to the correct appreciation of such cases.

It is rarely that these signs of pressure are absent, although they do not always manifest themselves in the same manner; sometimes it is bone, sometimes lung, sometimes œsophagus, sometimes nervous fibre which bears the brunt of the distending swelling. They are wanting if the sac be very small, and absent, or not prominent, if the artery be simply dilated, in which case nothing but a constantly pulsating tumor can be detected. Sometimes evidences of compression may be recognized by the attentive physician when no throbbing swelling can be discerned; and from them he infers the true nature of the case, although utterly unable to discover any of the ordinary physical signs of an aneurism. Whenever, indeed, obstinate and anomalous thoracic symptoms, which might be explained by the presence of an aneurismal sac, occur in a person whose lungs and heart appear to be in every respect sound, and whose general health is not very materially affected, we may suspect an aneurism to be the source of the trouble.

So, too, if any laryngeal affection, or if a difficulty in swallowing exhibit rather peculiar symptoms. It is, in 'truth, proper in all cases of chronic disease of the larynx, or where there are indications of a stricture of the œsophagus, to examine the chest carefully, so as to avoid the grave error of overlooking what may be the real and only cause of the whole disturbance.

The symptoms of *chronic laryngitis* especially are at times most astonishingly simulated, and it may happen that the patient, trusting to his feelings, refers obstinately to the chest as the seat of the disorder, while the physician as obstinately sees nothing and treats nothing but the presumed

affection of the larynx.   Even if we cannot discern any pulsation, the following signs may furnish a key to the case.
There is, as in chronic laryngeal disease, alteration of the
voice, with stridor, and peculiar cough ; but the voice is not so
uniformly changed.   Often it retains much of its natural character; and the loss is not so progressive, and the aphonia not
so permanent.   Hoarse the voice may be, but, as the direction of the pressure varies, it alters rapidly both in pitch and
power.   The cough is most commonly loud and paroxysmal, and
has a ringing sound.   Dyspnœa is a very constant symptom,
and is often attended with wheezing or stridulous breathing,
which is not persistent, and is sometimes only produced after
a deep inspiration.   The stridor, however, as Dr. Stokes
points out, differs from that of an obstructive disease of the
larynx by its seeming to issue from the notch at the sternum,
and not from above, from the larynx itself.   If, in addition,
the respiration be found to be markedly unequal in the two
lungs, the diagnosis of aneurism may be ventured upon ; and
it will be confirmed by finding no change in the larynx, when
examined with the laryngoscope, sufficient to account for
the laryngeal symptom, or a change, such as one-sided paralysis of a cord, as can be readily explained by pressure on
one recurrent nerve.*   Of course, the detection of dulness
on percussion, of sounds stronger than or otherwise different
from those in the cardiac region, or the occurrence of a hemorrhage, would place the diagnosis beyond doubt.

In some cases of aneurism, pain is among the earliest
symptoms, and the patient complains much of it before there
is a single physical sign indicative of the presence of a tumor.
I had, several years ago, a case of this kind under my care.
The patient suffered much from fugitive chest pains, very

---

* The aphonia in aneurism is indeed attributable to pressure on the recurrent
laryngeal nerve ; and, as mentioned by Tufnell, a stridulous voice, unaccompanied by aphonia and dysphagia, tends to show that the tumor is on the
right side of the trachea, and does not affect the œsophagus or the recurrent
laryngeal nerve.   When the aneurism presses on the trachea at its bifur-
cation, the voice will be raucous.   In a case of aortic aneurism recorded by
Habershon (Medico-Chirurg. Trans., 1865), the aneurism implicated the left
recurrent laryngeal nerve, and there was atrophy of the muscles of the larynx
as well as left-sided pneumonia.

acute and violent. He had at the same time a cough, but no stridor. The respiration in both lungs was natural, and so likewise was, as far as could be ascertained, every part of the chest. Dyspnœa gradually developed itself, and a cough with a metallic clang and stridulous breathing appeared, while a pulsation became more and more manifest immediately below the notch of the sternum.

The pain is dependent upon pressure on the nervous filaments: it may shoot toward the shoulder or the neck, along the arm, or deep into the centre of the chest. Dull, deep pain, boring and constant, is prone to occur when the pressure of the sac is leading to absorption of the vertebræ. Over the seat of the swelling there is often pain, associated with great tenderness.

The severity of the pain may give rise to emaciation and exhaustion, and become a cause of death; but death does not often take place from exhaustion. More usually the patient's life is cut short by the aneurism bursting, either externally or into internal parts—into the trachea, bronchial tubes, œsophagus, pericardium, pleura, pulmonary artery, or spinal canal. Yet it is not always the first rent which leads to the fatal issue.

Now, can we foretell the course of an aneurism, and the probable mode of death it is likely to occasion? We cannot; for in order to do so, it would be requisite to determine accurately its seat, so as to know what tissues are likely to be encroached upon. And this is very difficult, nay, often impossible. It is true that, when the swelling gives rise to phenomena like those of angina pectoris, we may surmise it to be in the ascending portion of the aorta and near the cardiac plexus of nerves, and look for its breaking into the pericardium or pulmonary artery; when it is accompanied by laryngeal stridor or other laryngeal symptoms, it very probably involves the posterior and lower portions of the arch, and will cause death by strangulation or exhaustion; when it produces much dyspnœa, it is apt to be seated in the descending part of the arch, and death may take place, by the aneurism bursting into a bronchial tube, or by pneumonia. But in regard to all these matters, we can usually do little else than conjecture, because a tumor within the chest leads to such displacements that its relations to the surrounding structures cannot be clearly ascertained during life. The most valuable information we obtain is from a study of the physiological changes, from the symptoms, therefore, of disturbed function ; indeed, the correctness of our conclusions will depend almost entirely on that of our interpretation of these symptoms.

An aneurism of the *descending aorta*, between the arch and the diaphragm, produces, if extensive, dulness on percussion and bulging posteriorly, and may exhibit the same physical signs and symptoms as an aneurism in the neighborhood of the arch. A gnawing sensation in the vertebræ has been especially noticed. Yet, in spite of the most careful scrutiny, an aneurism of the descending aorta often escapes detection, or its physical signs, as a case recorded by Walshe* proves, may exist to the right, instead of to the left of the spinal column, because the vessel has been dragged across the median line by its enlargement, and thus very considerable doubt may be thrown upon the diagnosis.

Let us, in conclusion, glance at the other kinds of aneurism within the thorax—that of the innominate and of the pulmonary artery.

An aneurism of the *innominate artery* is strictly limited to the right side of the body. It differs from that of the arch by the higher situation of the pulsating swelling; by the displacement of the clavicle; the comparative absence of signs of pressure on the larynx and œsophagus; and by the fact that compression of the right subclavian and carotid diminishes the beat of the tumor, while it exerts no effect on an aortic aneurism. Such are, at all events, the marks of distinction which are indicated by the observations in Dr. Holland's† excellent memoir.

An aneurism of the *pulmonary artery* is a very rare disease. Its main phenomena, so far as the few cases which have been placed on record enable us to judge, are: a strongly pulsating swelling, perceptible to the left of the sternum, and limited to the second intercostal space near the costal cartilages; a

---

* Diseases of the Heart.
† Dublin Quarterly Journal, vol. xii.

very marked thrill occurring with each expansion of the aneurism ; and in some instances a rough murmur, which is not discovered at the notch of the sternum or above the clavicles; lividity of face ; dropsy ; and very great difficulty of breathing.* The most significant points of difference between an aneurism of the pulmonary artery and of the aorta consist in the symptoms just alluded to, and in the absence of obvious evidences of pressure. The situation, too, of the physical phenomena is important ; but we must bear in mind that an aneurism of the arch may occasion a pulsating tumor, mainly to the left of the sternum. A mere distinct beating of the pulmonary artery is discriminated from an aneurism by the non-existence of a palpable swelling, of dropsy, or of lividity of the face, and by the usually coexisting signs of consolidation of the lung texture.

---

* In the case detailed by Skoda (Auscultation and Percussion), the dropsy was very great, and the face cyanotic; there was a faint murmur over the base of the heart, but none over the pulmonary artery.

CHAPTER V.

THE diseases of this part of the digestive system need not here be described at any length, because many of them have already been considered in treating of the affections of the larynx, and of the heart and great vessels.

MOUTH.

Soreness of the mouth, pain in masticating, and a fetid breath are usually complained of in diseases of the oral cavity. Let us suppose a patient to present himself with such symptoms; the interior of the mouth is exposed to a strong light, and its different parts inspected.

The gums are noticed to be swollen and injected, and the mucous membrane lining the cheeks reddened.—This is a state of things observed in the different forms of stomatitis. In the common diffused inflammation, be it the result of direct irritation, such as the swallowing of hot liquids or of corrosive substances, or an accompaniment and consequence, as it so often is, of gastric disorder, the redness is very marked; any attempt at chewing is painful; the taste is impaired; and not unfrequently a flow of saliva takes place from the mouth, and superficial ulcerations occur at its various parts. In mercurial stomatitis there are much the same symptoms; but the more copious discharge of saliva; the pain in the jaws; the loosening of the teeth; the enlarged tongue, exhibiting their impress; the painful and swollen state of the salivary glands; and, above all, the peculiar nauseous breath, testify to the specific character of the inflammation. The sore mouth of scurvy may be distinguished from either of the preceding forms by the spongy, purplish, or livid gums, which bleed on the slightest touch; by the eruption on the

(396)

skin, and the other signs which attend a scorbutic state of system.

The gums and the inside of the cheeks and lips are covered with a whitish curd-like exudation.—This is especially noticed in children. It constitutes the form of stomatitis known as "thrush," so frequent in infants at the breast, and so constantly associated with intestinal disorder, with diarrhœa, with colicky pains, and not unusually with a feverish heat of skin and a hot, dry mouth. Very similar to it, regarded indeed by some as identical, is the aphthous ulceration, to which adults as well as children are liable. Here, too, a whitish deposit is perceived in various parts of the mouth; it is apt also to be combined with gastric or intestinal disturbance. The recognized difference consists in the presence of the small ulcers which may be detected when the white crusts that cover them are removed, and in the vesicular nature of the disease during its formative stage. Then the grayish covering of the ulcers in aphthæ is found to be soluble in ether, and to present many oil globules under the microscope. On the other hand, this instrument shows us in thrush a special parasitic formation, the oidium albicans.

Ulcerations are perceived on the gums, tongue, and various parts of the mouth.—We meet with ulcers in the ordinary, in the mercurial, in the scorbutic, and in the aphthous inflammation of the mouth. But ulceration is apt to show its most horrible features in the sore mouth which follows in the train of syphilis, and in that essentially ulcerative disease called canker, cancrum oris, or ulcerative stomatitis. In the former, the fauces as well as the mouth are, as a general rule, chiefly involved, and the ulcers exhibit peculiarities which we shall presently study. The latter is an affection which prevails especially among the poor, and in enfeebled constitutions. It is seen chiefly in hospitals, and not uncommonly in epidemics. It begins with pain in the gums, and these soon swell, redden, and bleed most readily. They are covered with a soft, grayish exudation, which is, however, not limited to them, but often extends to the soft palate. If the layer of exudation be scraped away, a bleeding, ulcerated mucous membrane comes into view, provided the swelling be not so great as to render a careful examination of the mouth impossible. The breath is most offensive; there is usually fever; yet the disease does not progress uniformly with activity. It may last for weeks, or even for months. Owing to the ulceration and to the extreme fetor of the breath, it is often mistaken for gangrene of the mouth. But although it may terminate in gangrene, it does not do so of necessity. It is a far less serious complaint, runs a less speedy course, presents a breath fetid it is true, but not of the peculiar gangrenous odor, and lacks the very symptoms which gangrene within the mouth gives rise to—the rapid extension of the ulceration; the dark-gray tint around it; the extensive swelling of the cheek; its altered color and partial destruction; the constant and profuse flow from the mouth of blood or pus mixed with saliva; and the laying bare of the bones and loosening of the teeth.

The tongue is red and swollen. — Changes in color and in appearance of the tongue are very common, not because the tongue is often diseased, but because it acts as an index to the condition of the system, and especially to the alimentary canal. It is also more or less involved, or at all events its mucous membrane is, in the different forms of stomatitis. An abnormal state of the covering of the tongue is, therefore, far from being a sign that the organ itself is primarily affected.

Occasionally, however, we do meet with diseases of its deeper structures. Its nerves may be the seat of violent neuralgia; its muscles may be paralyzed; it may have become hypertrophied or cancerous; it may undergo progressive muscular atrophy; or it may be in a state of acute inflammation. The latter is, perhaps, the most frequent of its maladies, and is readily recognized by the red, swollen look of the organ, joined to a burning pain in it, and either to great dryness of the mouth or to a constant dribbling of saliva. The swelling usually commences at the anterior portion, and may become so considerable as to threaten suffocation; the inflamed tongue fills up the fauces and protrudes out of the mouth, and the unhappy patient can neither swallow nor utter a word. He has active fever, headache, great restlessness, and intense thirst, which symptoms last for several days, and until the inflammation subsides. But unless properly treated, and sometimes in spite of proper treatment, the inflammation is very likely not to end in resolution, but runs on to suppuration or gangrene. In some instances, it leaves a permanent induration, which may be mistaken for a cancerous nodule. Acute glossitis is always a dangerous complaint; fortunately, it is not a common one. Its most frequent cause, as now seen, is direct injury, either from wounds or the stings of venomous insects, or from the introduction of corrosive substances into the mouth. Its most frequent cause formerly was the abuse of mercury pushed to salivation. It is at times observed as a complication of scarlatina or of erysipelas.

FAUCES.

The fauces—that is, the different parts at the back of the mouth which are brought into view when the lips are widely opened, such as the half arches, the uvula, the tonsils, the posterior wall of the pharynx—may be involved in the same diseases as the parts situated in front. The contiguity of these' structures is in fact such that any morbid action is very apt to spread to them, or, on the other hand, to extend from them either forward or downward into the pharynx, and even into the larynx. Moreover, on this very account a disorder is rarely found limited to any one portion of the fauces, but transfers itself generally from one to the other, from the tonsils to the soft palate, from the soft palate to the tonsils. The most common affections of the fauces are inflammation and ulceration, both of which occasion a feeling of uneasiness in the throat, and also difficulty or pain in deglutition, and both of which are readily enough detected by looking into the mouth when the jaws are widely separated and the tongue depressed.

In the ordinary inflammation of the fauces, the *simple angina*, or sore throat, the parts are of a bright-red color, the uvula is long and swollen, and by dropping on the tongue gives rise to a constant disposition to swallow, although the act of swallowing is attended with pain. Associated with

the angina are coryza and febrile disturbance; and, owing
to the inflammation travelling up the Eustachian tube, the
sense of hearing is impaired.

The same symptoms are observed in the *pseudomembranous
inflammation of the fauces;* but in this dangerous complaint,
instead of the viscid mucus which lines the membrane in
the simple form of sore throat, we find patches of fibrinous
exudation-matter; the discharges from the mouth and nostrils are fetid; there is, as when describing diphtheria we
shall make apparent, a tendency to great prostration, and
not unfrequently to an extension of the affection toward
the windpipe.

Tonsillitis.—When the inflammation penetrates into the
substance of the tonsils, occasioning the disease popularly
known as *quinsy*, much the same general symptoms occur as
in ordinary angina. But the sense of constriction in the
throat is greater, so is the difficulty in swallowing; and
liquids are apt to return through the nose. The voice is
thick, and has often a peculiar sound; it is painful to the
patient to talk, and on looking into the throat, the tonsils
may be seen red and prominent and covered with mucus,
which is not easily detached. Sometimes the swelling is so
considerable that the tumid glands fill up the space between
the half arches, and leave but a small interval for the passage of food or drink. In some instances, we cannot separate the jaws sufficiently to get a view of the throat, and
have to trust to the introduction of the finger to tell us
what is the condition of the affected parts. Occasionally the
inflammation extends from the tonsils to the salivary glands;
the submaxillary and parotid glands swell, and ptyalism takes
place. It is necessary to be aware of this fact, for if a mercurial cathartic has been administered, the profuse flow of
saliva might be incorrectly attributed to it.

There is not much likelihood of confounding this secondary
parotitis with mumps, in which an outward swelling, visible
beneath the ear, is found, but not a swelling within the
throat, and in which no real difficulty in swallowing occurs,
except, perhaps, when the tumefaction is at its height. This
comparative absence of difficulty in deglutition, added to the

tension, fulness, and soreness at the angles of the jaw, the pain felt there, the almost impossible mastication, the purely external character of the tumefaction, and the febrile excitement and disfigured face, are indeed the signs by which parotitis is generally at once distinguished from any of the morbid states which resemble it.

Tonsillitis terminates by resolution or by the formation of pus. There are no positive means of ascertaining that the inflammation is going to end in suppuration, although we may suspect that this will be the case when much pain is felt at the angles of the jaws and shooting to the ear; and when the symptoms have been severe and persistent for more than four or five days. Sometimes the pus may be seen through the covering of the tonsils; but often the vast sense of relief experienced by the patient, and the sudden improvement in deglutition, attended, perhaps, with an unpleasant taste, are the only signs that the collection of pus has been discharged. Attacks of tonsillitis are very prone to be repeated, and may lead to permanent enlargement and induration of the tonsils.

Diphtheria.—There is another kind of inflammation of the fauces which, in obedience to the clinical classification of disease followed in this work, may be fittingly here considered —membranous angina or diphtheria. Not that it is really a purely local malady. On the contrary, it is a general disease, of which the exudative inflammation of the throat is merely the most usual characteristic. Yet the local lesion is so marked, and the symptoms are so nearly related to those of the common forms of acute sore throat, that practically the diphtheritic disorder is best regarded in connection with them.

Diphtheria is an affection of remote antiquity, which had to a great extent disappeared from view, but which in our generation is again extending over all portions of the globe. Let us in a cursory manner view its symptoms.

It begins usually as an ordinary sore throat, with redness and swelling of the arches of the palate, and of the tonsils. There is a slight stiffness of the neck, and the glands at the angles of the jaw are enlarged and tender. Within a period varying from a few hours to a few days, an exudation takes

place on the tonsils, uvula, and the soft palate. This exudation is more or less extensive, generally tough, and of a white
or grayish hue. It may show but little tendency to spread;
or it may extend to the gums and along the walls of the
pharynx, and into the windpipe. In some cases it passes upward into the nares; yet it may commence there simultaneously with its appearance in the throat. The false membrane
once formed, darkens, wastes from the circumference toward
the centre, and gradually disappears. But sometimes the
coat becomes for a time thicker and thicker by the constant
addition of fresh layers. When artificially removed, it is
soon redeveloped. After the first week from its beginning,
however, no further exudation is apt to occur, and the danger
arising from the membrane may be looked upon as over.

The constitutional symptoms vary greatly in different cases.
The pulse may be frequent, the skin hot, there may be much
pain in the head; in fact, the symptoms are those of asthenic
fever. But generally there is little febrile excitement, a sense
of weakness and prostration being prominent from the onset.
In some instances, real typhoid phenomena show themselves;
and the more asthenic the disorder, the more apt is the
exudation to be pulpy and granular.

In diphtheria the danger is twofold: it arises partly from
the depressing effect of the poison, increased as this effect
may be by the absorption of putrid matter from the throat;
partly from the extension of the disease to the larynx and
lungs.* Nor is the termination of the acute disorder always
the termination of the complaint. A chronic irritation of
the throat, lasting weeks or months, and possibly relapsing,
under exposure, into a diphtheritic sore throat, remains; or
albuminuria, which, indeed, shows itself during the height
of the malady, but which also outlasts its acute manifestations; or bronchitis and pneumonia—both of which may be
delayed until after the exudation has disappeared from the
throat—increase the list of the complications of the affection,
and protract or imperil the convalescence. And there are

---

* In some cases death seems to be due to the formation of heart-clots.
John F. Meigs, Am. Journ of Med. Sci., April, 1864.

morbid conditions which may be wholly looked upon as after-symptoms. A paralysis of the velum, palate, and pharyngeal arches, making itself apparent by a peculiar nasal intonation of the voice, and by a proneness to regurgitation of fluids through the nostrils, is among the earliest of them. Later appear impairment of vision, gastrodynia, ulcers in various parts of the body, profound anæmia, and that gradual failing of muscular power, with numbness and increasing weakness, which ordinarily does not take place until after complete convalescence, and which winds up in almost total, although not irremediable loss of muscular force, —in fact, in diphtheritic paralysis.

Now, all these facts go to indicate the malignant character of the disease, and how essential it is, even while the malady is in its acute stage, to counteract, by nourishment and stimulants, the depressing effect of the poison; how essential to continue the treatment long after the throat affection has been removed.

But to look at the differential diagnosis of the disorder. It varies widely from stomatitis, from tonsillitis, from pharyngitis—in truth, from all the ordinary local inflammations of these structures—by the presence of a membrane, by the striking constitutional symptoms, and by the sequelæ.

Yet there are certain sources of error which it is necessary to be on our guard against. In *simple pharyngitis* a mass of mucus, in part derived from the nares, is apt to collect on the inflamed membrane, and looks at first sight like the coating from an exudation; but it may be very easily removed, and a closer inspection proves its true nature. In *tonsillitis*, little yellowish or whitish points form at the opening of the follicles on the surface of the swollen tonsils. But they are very limited, are strictly confined to the gland, exhibit no tendency to spread or to coalesce, are generally small white specks of roundish or oval shape, and when cast off, a superficial ulceration is seen on the gland. I desire particularly to call attention to the possibility of confounding these appearances, which are by no means uncommon in tonsillitis, with diphtheria, for I have known them to have occasioned more than one mistake. Should, in an individual case, the facts mentioned be insufficient to solve the doubt, the microscope can do so readily, for it shows the white masses to be largely composed of epithelium, and not, like the diphtheritic membrane, mainly of fibrillated fibrin, of granular corpuscles, and of pus.

Ulcerative stomatitis, the form of stomatitis most likely to be confounded with diphtheria, and especially with this malady when the exudation lines the gums, is discriminated by the ulceration or sloughing; whereas the mucous membrane in the pseudomembranous disease remains intact, save in the rarest instances. The same feature distinguishes diphtheria from gangrene of the mouth, for which, on account of the extreme fetor of the breath, it is sometimes mistaken, and aids in distinguishing also from other kinds of stomatitis, as from *thrush*. Then here, too, the buccal mucous membrane, and not the throat, is chiefly affected, and the abdominal symptoms, and the other constitutional phenomena, are so different. So are they in *aphthæ*, in which, moreover, the superficial ulcerations, the pustules, and the seat of the disorder—usually on the edge of the tongue, on the internal surface of the lips, and on the gums and inside of the cheek—are points to be taken into account.

Besides these affections, there are others which must be distinguished from diphtheria. We occasionally find cases occurring in epidemics, and where the membrane is limited nearly altogether to the follicles, and chiefly to the tonsils. As the membrane passes away, ulcerations are obvious. Swelling of the glands of the neck, and fever, but not of acute type, attend this *ulcero-membranous angina*, which, moreover, shows a strong disposition to relapses. But though kindred to diphtheria, and in isolated instances perhaps difficult to discriminate, it differs from it in its seat and want of tendency to spread, in the formation of superficial ulcers, its less marked constitutional depression, and its invariably favorable termination.* Whether there are not also other kinds of membranous sore throat to be separated from true diphtheria, is a matter requiring further investigation.

---

* See a paper, in which I have described an epidemic of the kind, in the Am. Journ. of Med. Sciences, July, 1870.

There is an acute disease of the throat to which Dr. Todd, among others, has called attention,* and which presents also some strong points of similitude to diphtheria—*erysipelas of the fauces.* Like diphtheria, it is a most dangerous ailment; as in diphtheria, the morbid process may extend to the larynx; as happens often in diphtheria, the mucous membrane may exhibit a peculiar dusky-red color; as in diphtheria, the poison paralyzes the muscles of the palate and pharynx, and liquids are apt to be rejected through the nostrils and mouth. But the difficulty in deglutition differs from that of diphtheria in being present from the onset; and is not attended with enlargement of the glands of the neck, nor with the formation of a false membrane. In some instances, too, we find vivid redness of the throat, which may be associated with much swelling. If the erysipelatous inflammation extend to the larynx, there is local pain, with urgent dyspnœa and hoarseness; and usually rapid exhaustion supervenes. In cases of this kind, the submucous tissues of the larynx are found extensively infiltrated with pus. They may happen without erysipelas showing itself on any external part of the body; on the other hand, erysipelas beginning in the fauces may spread to the face.†

This erysipelas of the fauces is not a very frequent disease; and it must be stated that there are cases of diphtheria which simulate it very closely. I have seen a number of instances of the malady in which the whole mucous membrane was of a vivid or dusky hue; in which there was much swelling with an effusion of serum, especially in the submucous tissue of the uvula, causing it to look like a small transparent bag; in which immense difficulty or even impossibility in deglutition existed,—yet in which no membrane appeared for days after the violent inflammation of the throat, and was, when it showed itself, very slight in extent, and out of all proportion to the inflammation. But the constitutional symptoms and the sequelæ were the same as those of ordinary diphtheria. In one of the cases of the kind referred to, suppura-

---

* Clinical Lectures on Acute Diseases.
† Cases quoted in Schmidt's Jahrb., 1869, No. 1.

tion of one of the tonsils took place in consequence of the inflammation; a layer of deposit had coated parts of the tonsils and of the half arches and uvula.

How shall we separate diphtheria from *menbranous croup*, a disease with which, indeed, it is by some regarded as identical? Yet this is taking a narrow view of the facts. In the first place, croup is a purely local complaint, and lacks the peculiar constitutional symptoms and sequelæ of diphtheria. Secondly, an affection of the windpipe is not by any means an essential element of diphtheria, for in the majority of cases the disease does not spread to the larynx. Thirdly, when, by the paroxysms of irritative cough, the disturbed breathing, the huskiness or extinction of voice, we may infer that the exudative inflammation has reached the larynx; when, in other words, the symptoms of croup arise, the first manifestations of the membranous affection are perceived in the throat, and not in the larynx. To sum up: pseudo-membranous angina affects primarily the throat, and may extend to the windpipe; pseudomembranous croup affects primarily the windpipe, and may extend to the throat.

Lastly, diphtheria may be confounded with *scarlatina*. When, indeed, we reflect on the similar appearance of the throat, on the occurrence of albuminuria in both maladies, and on the frequency with which both are found at the same time to prevail as epidemics in a community, it is not astonishing that one should be looked upon as but a modified form of the other. Allied they certainly are, but not identical; for the poison of one leads to a thoroughly defined rash, and leaves a protective influence against a second attack, but often also deafness, suppuration of the glands of the neck, and dropsy—phenomena which are not encountered in the other. Moreover, the exudation in the throat is not exactly similar in the two diseases. In scarlatina it is pultaceous, and not coherent, and has no tendency to spread to the respiratory passages. Then the albuminuria happens at a different period. In scarlatina it is a sequel rather than a concomitant; in diphtheria it is a concomitant rather than a sequel. Further, the gravity of the symptom is not the same. In the latter malady, it is an indication of danger; it has not so serious a meaning in the former.

Diphtheria may be intercurrent in various maladies: in typhoid fever, in the exanthemata, in pneumonia. Nor is the exudation always restricted to the throat. It may show itself in a wound or on excoriated skin, on the nasal mucous membrane, the conjunctiva, the nipple, the uvula, or around the anus; it may be found coating the stomach, the intestines, and the ramifications of the bronchial tubes.*

Nasal diphtheria is a serious form of the malady; it may either be present alone, or coexist with a deposit in the fauces and pharynx. In the latter case, particularly, must it be looked upon as very grave. It generally occurs with symptoms of a low type, and we recognize it by carefully inspecting the posterior pharynx, and seeing the membrane extend upward; by noting the irritated, reddened look of the nostril, even where no membrane can be discerned in it, though the membrane may at times be easily seen ; and by the coryza, the sense of obstruction in the nose, and the sanious discharge which comes from it. In cases in which the nasal duct and laryngeal canal are stopped up by the false membranes, tears are constantly rolling down the cheeks.

Chronic Sore Throat.—Attacks of angina are prone to recur, and to lead to chronic inflammation of the structures. Now, an affection of this kind is liable, on any exposure, to be kindled into the acute complaint; and besides, it yields at all times some manifestations of a disorder of the throat. A thickening of the folds of membrane forming the half arches, a tumefaction of the follicles at the upper part of the pharynx, a lengthening of the uvula, are the visible signs of the chronic malady; a constant disposition to clear the throat, and a dry cough are often the attending general symptoms. Owing to

---

* See on this subject, as well as concerning some points which in the above sketch have been but alluded to, Bretonneau's Memoirs ; the writings of Trousseau, Bouchut, and Daviot, which, with those of Bretonneau, were republished by the New Sydenham Society, 1859; Trousseau's Clinique Médicale; W. F. Wade, Observations on Diphtheritis, London, 1858, describing clearly the association of diphtheria with albuminuria ; Greenhow on Diphtheria ; Maingault, Mémoire sur la Paralysie Diphthérique, Paris, 1860; Jenner on Diphtheria, London, 1861; and Slade on Diphtheria.

the habitual coughing, the patient may be suspected to be laboring under' phthisis, and treated accordingly, when the whole trouble lies not in the lungs, but in the throat. Yet an error in the opposite direction is quite as easily, and perhaps more frequently, committed. It is, indeed, the fashion with many to snip off tonsils and uvulas, with the view of curing a cough which really is kept up by a source of irritation in the lungs, forgetting that in scrofula and tuberculosis chronic enlargement of the tonsils and follicular pharyngitis are by no means unusual. A careful examination of the chest ought always to be made, even when inspection of the throat shows disease to be there present.

The *follicular disease of the throat*, or "clergyman's sore throat," is the most frequent of all the morbid conditions which produce a chronic sore throat. As Dr. Green, who so well described the disease, pointed out, the abnormal condition of the follicles of the mucous membrane of the pharynx and fauces often extends to the larynx. There are constant hawking and attempts at clearing the throat, and not unfrequently roughness of voice or decided hoarseness. On inspecting the throat, the enlarged mucous follicles can be readily discerned; those on the pharynx are very prominent. In cases of long standing, the follicles may ulcerate, and very commonly they pour out an acrid secretion. But unless from coexisting enlargement of the uvula or an altered position of the epiglottis, or marked laryngeal disease, or a bronchial complication, there is no decided cough. The follicular disease may occur in consequence of repeated attacks of sore throat, or be an attendant upon gastric disorder, or follow constant exercise and straining of the voice.

Ulcers are not often developed in the fauces during an attack of acute inflammation, except in the specific sore throat of scarlatina; in chronic inflammation, especially if occurring in scrofulous persons, they are more common. The most profound ulcerations are those of constitutional syphilis, implicating, as they do, not only the tissues of the fauces, but the parts in front, and destroying both the fleshy covering of the bones and the bones themselves. With regard to treatment and to prognosis, it is of the utmost im-

portance to distinguish these *syphilitic ulcers* from those produced by other causes. A cutaneous eruption of a syphilitic
character, and enlarged lymphatic glands, or the history of
antecedent syphilis, would lead us to a correct conclusion;
but an accurate history of a syphilitic infection cannot always
be obtained. The ulcers themselves furnish some information by which we may suspect their origin. They are not
superficial and stationary, like those resulting from ordinary
inflammation; on the contrary, they are deep, and have a
strong tendency to spread. They are rounded, or of a ser-
piginous form, with borders well defined and elevated, and
surrounded by a distinct zone of redness; and the inflammation which precedes them is limited to spots, and is not so
diffused, nor attended with so much swelling, as the inflammation which exists prior to simple ulceration.

PHARYNX AND ŒSOPHAGUS.

In describing the affections of the fauces, the affections of
that portion of the pharynx which is most usually the seat
of disease have been at the same time described. Indeed,
when we speak of acute or chronic pharyngitis, we generally
mean acute or chronic inflammation of the fauces, to which
the upper part of the pharynx belongs. Inflammation of
the portion of the pharynx which is out of sight when the
tongue is depressed, is rare. It may be presumed to exist, if
there be pain and an impediment in the act of swallowing
when the food arrives opposite the top of the larynx, while
the respiration remains free, and the voice unaffected. Abscesses sometimes form between the textures composing the
pharynx, and between its posterior wall and the cervical
vertebræ. These *retropharyngeal abscesses* mostly result from
disease of the vertebræ. They occasion very great difficulty
in deglutition and in breathing; an altered voice; dull pain
and stiffness in the neck; external swelling, which may or
may not be edematous; and commonly a tumefaction at the
back of the throat, which can be seen, or which at least can
be felt with the finger pressed against the posterior wall of
the pharynx. On account of the obstructed respiration and

the changed voice, the disease is very liable to be mistaken for laryngeal complaints, especially for croup. Its differences have been enumerated above. I will only add that a safeguard against error is, to bear in mind the possibility of these abscesses simulating. affections of the larynx.*

The œsophagus is not very often the seat of disease. We sometimes meet with acute inflammation of this division of the alimentary canal produced by swallowing boiling water or corrosive poisons, especially nitric or sulphuric acid, or ammonia. The symptoms of acute *œsophagitis* are usually mixed up with, or masked by those of inflammation of the pharynx, or of the stomach. We may, however, infer its presence, if difficulty and pain in deglutition exist, for which nothing in the throat can be found to account, and if these phenomena be associated with hiccough and with a burning sensation between the shoulders, in the course of the tube.

Of the chronic diseases of the œsophagus, *stricture* is beyond doubt the most common. The narrowing may take place at any part of the passage, and a large pouch sometimes forms in front of, or behind it. The constriction results from preceding inflammation or ulceration, from cancerous degeneration of the walls of the tube, or from the pressure of a tumor or an aneurism. The formidable malady manifests itself by an impediment in swallowing—even liquid food cannot pass without great difficulty; and if the stricture goes on increasing, the patient perishes miserably by starvation. In addition to the obstruction to the passage of food, we may find a peculiar pain occurring at a particular part of the tube, and the raising, without cough or vomiting, of clots of blood presenting nearly always the same shape.

The matter ejected in the attempts at deglutition consists simply of masticated food together with more or less mucus. Should there be any doubt as to the seat of the obstruction, a bougie will clear up the doubt, and thus we possess in this instrument the most valuable diagnostic as well as therapeutic agent. But we must not immediately conclude,

---

* See an elaborate paper on the subject of these abscesses by Allin, New York Journ. of Med., Nov. 1851.

because the bougie when introduced meets with resistance, that an organic stricture is present. The narrowing may be simply *spasmodic*, yet give rise to all the symptoms of an organic constriction. But they are not permanent: at times nourishment is readily enough swallowed, and a full-sized bougie passes with the greatest ease. This singular disorder occasionally accompanies ulceration of the larynx; but it is chiefly met with in hypochondriacs and in hysterical women. The latter, indeed, sometimes fancy that they are incapable of swallowing, and reject the food they take without there being the least impediment, or even a temporary spasm, to prevent its passage, just as sometimes they lie in bed and imagine themselves paralyzed and unable to walk, until they are compelled to do so.

The disorders of the pharynx and œsophagus which we have just been considering have as a common symptom difficulty in swallowing. In truth, they are the most usual cause of *dysphagia*. But we must not forget that other causes may produce it, such as paralysis of the muscles of the throat, diseases of the larynx or trachea, particularly ulcerative diseases, and aneurismal tumors within the chest.

CHAPTER VI.

DISEASES OF THE ABDOMEN.

THE abdominal cavity contains viscera of very varied functions ; some form, others break down organic constituents; while others again excrete the broken-down material. They all, however, labor in one cause; they all work together toward preserving a normal state of the blood, either by preparing fit matter for it, and consequently for the healthy nutrition of the frame, or by removing such substances as would be hurtful if they were retained. Any serious derangement of any of these viscera, especially any serious chronic derangement of those which are not simply reservoirs, must therefore inevitably lead to a deterioration of the blood and to a defective nourishment of the body. But, independently of the change of the blood and the falling off in the general nutrition, there are no vital symptoms which characterize abdominal diseases as a group ; and as many other causes may give rise to the same symptoms, they furnish on the whole but little information of real value in diagnosis, and none at all as to the particular organ at fault. This we learn to some extent by examining, where it can be done, the secretions or excretions ; to some extent by noticing the peculiar appearances of the skin which are produced by deterioration of the blood, or by substances, such as bile, circulating in it; and, perhaps, to a still greater extent by the exploration of the organs through the flexible parietes of the abdomen. It is, in truth, by means of the physical method of investigation that we often obtain the most valuable information, not only as to the seat, but even as to the nature of the morbid action; and although physical exploration of the abdomen does not yield as perfect results as when this form

(412)

of diagnosis is applied to the affections of the thorax, the senses of sight and touch still supply us with an amount of knowledge most valuable, and with which it would be difficult to dispense. I speak only of the senses of sight and touch, because the sense of hearing, save in so far as it enables us to judge of the sounds elicited by percussion, is not very applicable to the study of diseases below the diaphragm. But let us pass in review the different methods of physical diagnosis with reference to abdominal disorders.

Methods and General Results of Physical Examination of the Abdomen.

INSPECTION.

By inspection, we learn the size, shape, form, and movements of the abdomen. To inspect the abdomen satisfactorily, the patient should be placed in an easy attitude, either standing or sitting. The recumbent position is less eligible, yet we are often obliged to examine sick persons in this posture. Whenever practicable, ocular inspection must not only be made from the front, but also from the sides, and, under some circumstances, the back ought to be inspected. In appreciating the results thus obtained, it is very necessary to bear in mind, that even in health the appearance of the abdominal walls is modified by certain physiological conditions. The abdomen is much larger, in comparison to the size of the chest, in childhood than in adult age. It is more voluminous in females, especially in such as have given birth to several children. It increases in size with advancing years, particularly when a tendency to obesity exists. Its shape is somewhat altered by the pernicious habit of wearing tight stays. Its upper portion is more distended after a copious meal than when the stomach is in an empty state.

In disease we may observe either a partial or a general abdominal enlargement. The latter is caused by accumulations of air in the intestinal canal; by liquids in the peritoneum; by an edematous condition of the abdominal walls; or by large tumors which fill up the whole cavity. A partial enlargement is mainly produced by the increase in size of particular organs, such as of the liver, or spleen, or ovaries. It may also be brought about by induration and swelling of the mesenteric glands, or by tumors of various kinds—solid or hernial; and it is sometimes due to diseases above the diaphragm. A pleuritic or a pericardial effusion, or emphysema of the lungs, may give rise to a marked fulness below the margin of the ribs.

A retraction of the abdominal parietes is perceived in general emaciation, and very obviously in that dependent upon a narrowing of the cardiac or pyloric orifice of the stomach, or upon chronic diarrhœa and dysentery. It is also noticed in lead colic and in cephalic diseases, especially in tubercular meningitis.

There are some further changes in the appearance of certain external parts which may tend to elucidate the state of the parts within. Thus we learn from the distention of the superficial veins, that an obstruction exists to the flow of blood in the large veins of the abdomen, either in the portal system or in the vena cava. The lessening of the depression at the umbilicus is, unless it be produced by pressure limited to the particular spot where the umbilicus lies, a sign indicative of a general abdominal enlargement.

While inspecting the abdomen, we sometimes see distinct movements of very different kinds. The act of breathing gives rise to a motion which is very slight when a tumor or any other impediment interferes with the free action of the diaphragm, and which is much exaggerated by diseases within the thoracic cavity. The rolling of the intestines is sometimes visible on the exterior; so are at times those shiftings of accumulations of gas which give rise to a series of jerking elevations; so, too, are occasionally the spasmodic contractions and relaxations of the abdominal muscles. But none of these is as often encountered, and none occasions as much alarm as a pulsation, the chief seat of which is the epigastric region, and which, as we shall presently see, is not unfrequently mistaken for an aneurism.

PALPATION.

Palpation teaches us some very important lessons. We learn by the application of the hand to the abdomen many things of which the eye cannot inform us. We can judge of the size, position, and consistence of the viscera which are felt through the abdominal walls. We can determine whether the parts are firmly attached or movable; whether they are smooth or nodulated; and whether or not they possess a motion of their own. We can ascertain whether they are tender or not; and by tapping with the fingers of one hand, while those of the other are applied to another portion of the surface, we can, by the peculiar feeling of fluctuation, detect the presence of fluid in the abdominal cavity. We can satisfy ourselves further, by the sense of touch, of the state of the parietes: whether hot or cold, resistant or elastic, edematous or not.

In order to use palpation with most effect, the abdominal muscles must be relaxed, and to do this the patient should be placed on his back, and his thighs be flexed on the body. Occasionally it is essential to vary this position; to turn him from side to side, or to examine him when erect. The amount of pressure too should not always be the same. When we wish to examine deep parts, the pressure is increased; when it causes pain, the exploration must not be unnecessarily repeated. The character and the intensity of pain which pressure calls forth, often throw considerable light on the disease we are investigating. Thus, if it take deep pressure to produce pain, we are usually right in concluding that the mischief is not superficially seated. The pain of inflammation of the serous membrane is commonly much augmented by pressure, and is of a very severe, cutting character. Pain due to inflammation of any part of the mucous membrane of the intestinal tract is duller. All neuralgic or nervous pain, such as that of colic, is relieved rather than augmented by pressure, and may thus be distinguished from the tenderness caused by inflammation. Yet this is not always the case; it is to be regarded as a rule which has many exceptions.

But we cannòt enter into any fuller particulars as to what palpation teaches us in individual diseases of the abdomen; because, as there is hardly one of any importance in which it is not of some service, we should say here what it would be necessary to dwell upon repeatedly further on.

PERCUSSION.

Percussion is, in the study of abdominal affections, as valuable as, perhaps even more valuable than, palpation. By it we can circumscribe the different organs with great accuracy; we can judge of the position of the stomach and intestines; we can limit the distended bladder; and fix the borders of the liver and spleen. By its aid, further, we tell whether a distention of the abdomen is produced by air, or by a solid tumor, or by liquid. But without entering, for the present, into any particulars as to its use in the recognition of individual abdominal disorders, we may here examine, in a cursory manner, the results it yields when applied to the healthy abdomen.

To render percussion a trustworthy interpreter of the state of the abdominal viscera, the patient should be placed in the same position as for palpation. The sounds are best elicited by mediate percussion, and especially by mediate percussion performed by means of a pleximeter. But to appreciate them fully, something more is requisite than to produce a distinct sound, and be able to tell whether it is dull or tympanitic. We must be acquainted with the relations of the parts concealed from view by the abdominal walls; and more, we must understand the physiology of the organs they cover, and take into account that during the digestive process their contents and position may vary sufficiently to modify the sound.

To commence with the airless viscera. The *liver* is one of the easiest organs to limit. We determine its upper boundary by striking with moderate force in a line from somewhat above the right nipple toward the lower part of the thorax, until marked resistance and dulness tell us that a solid organ has been reached. At this point we draw a line; then we recommence percussing downward from near the median line, and above the dulness just obtained; then we percuss from the axilla downward; then posteriorly from beneath the lower angle of the scapula, and so on, until the line traced out reaches the vertebral column.

The dulness thus elicited marks the upper boundary of the liver; at least of the portion which comes more directly in contact with the abdominal walls. Anteriorly it extends from the lower extremity of the sternum to between the fifth and sixth ribs; at the side, the dulness is generally in the seventh intercostal space; near the vertebral column, it is on a level with the tenth or the eleventh, more rarely with the ninth interspace. The dulness of the left lobe reaches nearly two inches across the median line; but the heart lies here so near to the liver, that we cannot, with any accuracy, distinguish the flat sound of the one from the flat sound of the other; nor indeed is this, for practical purposes, of any very great consequence.

. After the upper border has been fairly traced out anteriorly, laterally, and, should it be thought necessary, posteriorly, we next determine the inferior margin of the organ. This is readily effected by percussing downward from the already ascertained line of dulness, and noting where the large intestine sends forth its distinct tympanitic sound. To determine the lower border correctly, the pleximeter must be pressed firmly on the integuments, and the stroke of the finger be slight; for if it be strong, we obtain the sound of the surrounding hollow viscera through the thin layer of liver which covers them, and before we have arrived at its margin. This mode of procedure is different from the one pursued to determine the height to which the liver rises, because the position of the parts is different. Superiorly, the lung descends between the surface and that portion of the convex surface of the liver which fits into the diaphragm, and it requires very strong percussion to bring out the dulness of the deep-seated solid organ. By forcible percussion, however, we detect a decided loss of the pulmonary resonance at about the fourth intercostal space.

The inferior border of the liver will, anteriorly, be generally found to lie immediately at, or to project below, the last rib; posteriorly, we cannot determine this border positively, for it becomes continuous with the dulness occasioned by the presence of the right kidney. The lower margin of the left lobe is commonly met with at the upper third of a line drawn from the ensiform cartilage to the umbilicus. A much distended gall-bladder may cause a strictly defined dulness lower than the dulness of the surrounding liver.

The *spleen* is a solid organ which is not so easily circumscribed as the liver. Indeed, if the stomach contain much food, or if it or the intestines be distended with gas, it is very difficult to discriminate the dull sound of the spleen. To find its limits, we must place the patient on his right side, with his legs flexed; or let him stand erect, and then begin to strike with some force in a line from the axilla to the crest of the ilium. At the ninth, or sometimes at the tenth rib, the sound becomes dull, and there is much greater resistance to the finger. Here is the upper boundary of the spleen. We mark the spot, and continue to percuss in the same line until, at about the twelfth rib, we arrive at the lower boundary of the organ, as indicated by the distinct tympanitic sound of the intestines.

After the vertical diameter has been thus ascertained, the horizontal is readily determined by percussing from the median line to a point between the lines which trace the superior and inferior margins, and by noticing where the sound of the stomach gives way to the dull sound of the solid viscus. When these three points have been decided upon, we have learned enough for practical purposes. We may then, if we choose, percuss posteriorly; but we cannot circumscribe the spleen with any accuracy behind, because its dulness becomes continuous with that of the left kidney.

The average size of the spleen is four inches in length and three in width; but it may, if in a diseased state, increase to twice or three times that size. Mailliot tells us that when, as occasionally happens, the viscus eludes detection by percussion, we may infer that its dimensions are small. This remark only holds good provided the stomach and intestines be not very much distended with gas.

The information obtained from percussing the *kidneys* is of so little value, that I shall not enter into a description of how these organs are to be percussed; nor, indeed, can they be limited with anything like accuracy, except at their inferior and outer borders, where the dull sound they occasion is surrounded by the intestinal resonance. This dulness extends somewhat lower during a full inspiration.

To set limits to the *stomach* and *intestines*, by means of percussion, requires an ear accustomed to discriminate between shades of sound, since we have to judge more between sounds of different degree, but similar to each other, than between sounds of different character. Nor are the tones elicited always the same over the same spot; on the contrary, they vary according as the contents of the hollow viscera vary. And we can make use of this circumstance for purposes of diagnosis.

The stomach, when not unusually distended with gas or with food, renders a sound which is hollow, ringing, and tympanitic to a certain degree, yet which is not tympanitic as that of the intestine is. It is in fact a sound unlike any other, and experience soon enables us to distinguish it from that of the surrounding viscera. Sometimes the sound is distinctly amphoric.

Now, to determine the boundaries of the stomach, it is necessary to mark out first the lower margin of the liver, for it covers a portion of the stomach; then the heart and the inner border of the spleen. The part which lies between these solid viscera yields the sound of the stomach, mixed at one point, namely, to the left of the apex of the heart, with the resonance of the lung. Near this spot, about opposite to the seventh rib, the cardiac extremity of the stomach is situated; below it is the body of the organ. To ascertain its lower border, we percuss gently in a downward direction, until the alteration in sound shows that we are striking over the colon. The difference is at times very obvious, at times very slight. It is most readily detected if the stomach contain either solid or liquid ingesta. And availing ourselves of this fact, we may sometimes follow, with advantage, Mailliot's advice, and, unless the circumstances of the case forbid it, let the patient swallow a glass of water. By placing him in the erect position, the fluid will gravitate to the greater curvature; and the line of comparative dulness indicates the lower margin of the stomach, which is generally found near the umbilicus.

The *colon* yields, in its ascending and transverse as well as in its descending portion, a sound of a far purer tympanitic character than the stomach, the note of which is, indeed, in many respects, more amphoric than tympanitic. When, however, the tube contains feces, the sound is modified; and as these are prone to accumulate on the left side in the descending colon, and especially where it passes into the iliac fossa,

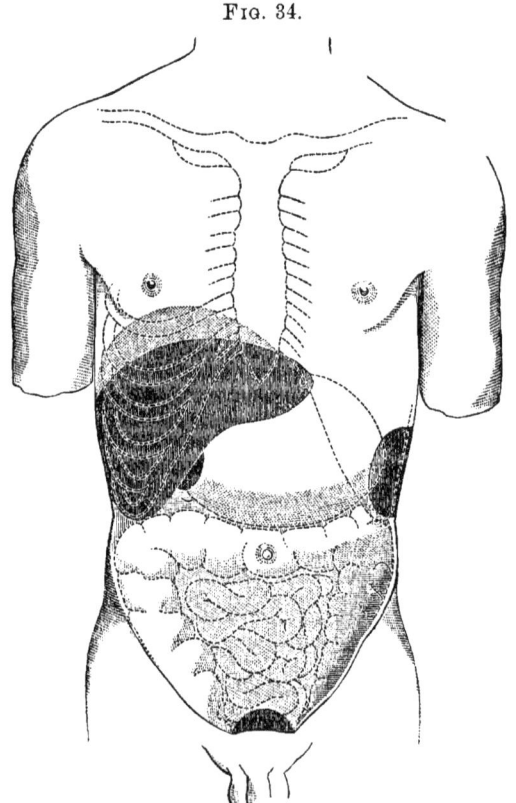

Results of abdominal percussion, as set forth in the text. The dark shades indicate marked dulness; the light shading exhibits a lessening of the clear, or of the tympanitic character of the sound—an approach to dulness.

it is usually not so resonant as the ascending colon. The *small intestines*, unless they are filled with fluid or solids, or distended with gas, render a sound of higher pitch and of smaller volume than the surrounding large intestine, and by this less deep-toned sound their position may be accurately determined.

The position of the viscera in the pelvis cannot be ascertained by means of percussion. It is only when the bladder is much distended, or the uterus augmented in size, that the outline of either can be traced on the walls of the abdomen.

AUSCULTATION.

Auscultation does not stand us in much stead in abdominal diseases. It is serviceable in aiding in the detection of an abdominal aneurism; and sometimes an enlarged spleen gives rise to a distinct blowing murmur; or the rubbing of a roughened peritoneum may occasion a friction sound; but, on the whole, the application of the stethoscope to the abdominal walls is rarely called for. In health, no constant sound is heard save that of the aorta; for the rush of blood through the other arteries, or through the veins, produces no appreciable murmur. When the stomach is distended with air and contains liquid, sounds possessing a metallic character are perceived, which an inexperienced observer is very apt to consider as originating in the lungs; over which, in truth, they are often audible. The passage of gas through the intestines gives rise to those peculiar noises termed "borborygmi." In the pregnant state, auscultation is of value in detecting the pulsations of the fœtal heart and the uteroplacental murmur.

SECTION I.

DISEASES OF THE STOMACH.

As the disorders of the stomach are so common; as we are so constantly called upon to remedy them; as a patient hardly ever gives a history of his ailment without thinking it obligatory to enter into a minute account of the state of his digestion, it would be reasonable to suppose that as a class no affections are so well understood and so susceptible of clear description as those of this viscus. But in point of fact there are none so little understood; and indeed it is only within the last few years that any attempts have been made to penetrate, with the light thrown by modern means of research, the darkness which surrounds the pathology of one of the most important organs in the body. All these attempts have had as their goal to ascertain the exact anatomical changes and modifications in the secretions which give rise to the symptoms commonly referred to perverted function; and to a certain degree they have been successful; but not to that degree which enables us to associate each symptom with some definite alteration in the healthy structure or the normal action of the part.

The symptoms which are very constantly met with in derangements of the stomach, whether organic or functional, are loss of appetite, nausea and vomiting, acidity, flatulency, and pain. Before inquiring into the individual diseases of the viscus, we shall briefly pass these symptoms in review.

Loss of Appetite.—This is one of the most common signs of a disordered stomach. It manifests itself in various ways. It may amount to absolute repugnance to taking any kind of food, or be merely an inability to partake of certain articles. Again, little by little the process of digestion may become more and more difficult and annoying, and the patient in consequence instinctively abstains from eating, excepting in quantities barely sufficient to keep up life. What the loss of appetite depends on, we do not know; nor shall we until the causes of appetite and hunger are definitely settled. That nervous influence has something to do with the anorexia, is seen by the sudden deprivation of all desire to eat when any strong impression is made on the nervous system—such as that caused by the unexpected receipt of unwelcome news. The amount of epithelium on the mucous membrane is also connected with a marked diminution of the appetite; for with a tongue much coated, absolute disgust at the mere thought of taking food often exists, which yields to relish for food as soon as the tongue begins to clean.

Attending the diminished or lost appetite, we meet sometimes with great emaciation and with signs as if even the small quantity of food taken were not absorbed into, or utterly failed to nourish, the system. Moreover, there is apt to be sensitiveness over the abdomen, and spots of particular sensitiveness exist which correspond to the situation of the mesenteric glands. We find, however, no evidence of actual organic disease, either in the abdomen or in the lungs; nor does this *pseudo-tabes mesenterica*, if I may so call it, occur, like the disease it simulates, in scrofulous or tubercular patients. I have met with a number of cases, chiefly in young women with lowered vital force, fond of excitement, and living indolent lives. Some were hysterical, others not. But in all the disorder seemed to be due to deficient nervous power, with impaired function of the stomach, and very possibly of the abdominal glands.

Instead of the appetite being lost, it is at times capricious, or even ravenous. A craving after food is not often combined with a structural lesion. Yet we occasionally meet with it in persons affected with gastric ulcers. It is common to find it in those who suffer from neuralgia of the stomach. And sometimes in cases of mere nervous gastric disturbance, with or without pain, there is an extraordinary exaggeration of the appetite. The patient eats eight or even fifteen times a day largely, digests his food properly, yet is constantly hungry.*

The feeling of *thirst* does not lessen when the desire for food does. On the contrary, it usually increases when the latter diminishes.

Excessive Acidity of the Stomach.—Excessive acidity occurs from various causes. The gastric juice may be secreted in very great quantities, or it may contain an abnormal amount of acid. But excessive acidity is most frequently due to the decomposition of food and to a process of fermentation, dependent rather upon an insufficient amount of the gastric solvent than upon its superfluity. It then manifests itself only after meals. When the mucous membrane is covered with a tenacious mucus or with thick layers of epithelium,

---

* Cases recorded by Guipon, Bulimic and Syncopal Dyspepsia.

slow digestion and acidity from fermentation result; because, although the gastric juice is sufficient, it cannot mix as readily with the aliment.

The acids formed in the stomach are, besides the muriatic acid of the gastric juice, lactic acid, acetic acid, carbonic acid, butyric acid, and oxalic acid. Some articles of food produce these different acids in considerable quantities. Thus sugar generates large amounts of lactic acid. The acids which are created in the stomach may get into the blood, and by vitiating this fluid give rise to various disorders.

When much acid is present in the viscus, it occasions a sensation of heat which extends along the œsophagus. This "heart-burn" is apt to happen in paroxysms, and is attended with a feeling of constriction or with actual pain at the epigastrium. As a symptom it has no special diagnostic value, for it is met with both in functional and organic diseases of the stomach. It simply denotes extreme acidity; and is very common in gouty persons. It probably arises, as Dr. Chambers surmises, from the action of the acid contents of the organ on the oversensitive cardiac and œsophageal nerves.

Flatulency.—The gas in the intestinal canal may be merely air which is swallowed; or may be generated from imperfectly digested food; or it may be a secretion from the blood-vessels of the part. In those who suffer from indigestion, it is produced in the last two ways, and the patient complains greatly of the annoyance it occasions. It causes a disgust for eating, a feeling of distention, and sometimes actual pain. By interfering with the downward movements of the diaphragm, it induces a sensation of constriction in the chest, shortened breathing, and palpitation of the heart; and the sleep is broken by uneasy dreams.

An expulsion of the gaseous contents of the stomach by the mouth gives rise to *eructation*, or belching. The belching which follows the decomposition of food has sometimes the taste and the odor of rotten eggs, owing to the gas evolved consisting of sulphuretted hydrogen. At other times, the eructation is odorless, because the gases formed are carbonic acid, or hydrogen or nitrogen, or some of their compounds. When the gas results from fermentation or decomposition of food, it frequently coexists with acidity occurring only after meals, and we remedy it by administering the mineral acids or agents which promote digestion. When it is a secretion from the blood-vessels, it happens in an empty state of the stomach, and is often relieved by simply regulating the time of taking food, so as to avoid too long intervals between the meals. As a cause of flatulence and eructation which it is important not to overlook may be mentioned thoracic aneurism.*

Nausea and Vomiting.—These are frequently combined. But sometimes there is persistent nausea without vomiting; sometimes vomiting occurs without any or with but slight preceding nausea. Yet they are both occasioned in much the same way: what gives rise to one will give rise to the other.

Vomiting is a very complex act. But its causes, although various, may all be ranged under four heads. It arises either from an irritation of the peripheral extremities of the nerves which supply the parts more directly concerned in the act itself, such as the stomach, the diaphragm, and the œsophagus; or the irritation originates in the centres from which these nerves spring, and is referred to their peripheries; or there is a mechanical obstruction in the stomach or intestines; or the vomiting is purely sympathetic. To illustrate these different forms in full is not necessary. I will merely mention a few examples of each. Under the first head belongs the vomiting observed in acute or chronic inflammation of the stomach, in ulcer, or in cancer; also that following a debauch, or the introduction of irritating substances into the viscus. Under the second head may be ranged the vomiting which occurs in diseases of the brain; perhaps, also, that which arises in morbid states of the blood. Under the third head we may class the vomiting in narrowing of the œsophagus, and of the pyloric or cardiac extremity of the stomach, and in obstructions of the intestine. It may, however, be made a question whether the vomiting in all these cases is not owing to the same ultimate cause as that of the

---

* Walter F. Atlee, Amer. Journ. of Med. Sciences, July, 1869.

first group; whether, in other words, it is not a reflex phenomenon called forth by the irritation at the seat of the
impediment.

The fourth group is exemplified by the vomiting in pregnancy, in wounds of the extremities, by that occurring in
peritonitis, in inflammation of the intestines and of the liver,
and in irritation of the fauces. In the four last instances the
vomiting is due to direct transmission of the irritation, and
must be looked upon as originating through means of that
sympathy called by physiologists continuous. The first two
illustrate the remote sympathy between different parts of the
body, of which disease often furnishes such striking proofs.

Connected thus with so many various conditions, the act
of vomiting, taken by itself, is of very little diagnostic value.
It presupposes a certain amount of irritation existing in the
stomach, or reflected to it; but nothing more. It is of course
a frequent symptom in disorders of the stomach, especially
in those which are organic; yet the error ought to be strenuously guarded against of considering it as having reference
only to derangements of that viscus. As it is allied to morbid states too numerous to be here examined into in detail,
I shall content myself with making a few general statements
regarding the indications to be drawn from it.

When vomiting is observed in a person previously in good
health, we may suspect either the invasion of some acute
malady, or that some poisonous substance has been wilfully
or accidentally taken. Again, it may come on suddenly
from violent mental emotion. When everything that is
swallowed is immediately expelled, the difficulty lies in the
œsophagus, or at the cardiac orifice of the stomach, or in
an extreme irritability of the viscus; and this irritability,
attended as it often is with unceasing nausea, experience
teaches to be far more frequently due to a sympathetic excitement of the organ than to any derangement of its own.

As regards the vomiting which is brought about by gastric disorders, it is of much consequence to note the period
at which it happens, whether before meals or after meals,
and how long afterward. In some diseases, such as ulcer
and cancer, it rarely occurs excepting when food has been

taken. The act of vomiting then affords relief from the pain, and is, as it were, rather physiological than pathological. In narrowing of the pylorus, it takes place some hours after digestion has commenced. But, as vomiting will be described hereafter in its relations to the individual diseases of the stomach, we shall not anticipate what will be more fitly discussed elsewhere. For the same reason we need not dwell on the characteristics of the ejected matter. Yet a few words on the subject can hardly be omitted.

The nature and the quantity of the vomit are of course most various. The following are its most common kinds:

Food or *liquid*, mixed with saliva and some mucus, is expelled when the stomach is very irritable, or if an obstruction exist which renders the entrance into the organ difficult or impossible. Half-digested food, in a state of acetous fermentation and with a strongly acid reaction, is cast out when the proper secretion of the gastric juice or its intimate admixture with the aliment has been interfered with, or when this has been detained for a long time in the stomach. This kind of vomit is usual in chronic inflammation and in cancer of the stomach, especially in the latter. In the ejected matter the particles of food may still be recognized with the unassisted eye; but when the food has been kept for a prolonged period in the stomach, or when it has passed on into the duodenum and is returned, it is changed into an apparently homogeneous mass. Examined, however, under the microscope, the different elementary structures of the animal or vegetable substances partaken of can even then be detected. Mixed with muscular fibre, fibrous tissue, starch corpuscles, and vegetable cells, is usually found a considerable quantity of oil.

Fig. 35.

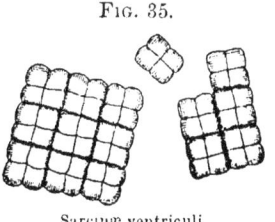

Sarcinæ ventriculi.

Sarcinæ and yeast fungi are sometimes discovered, by means of the microscope, in the vomit. These organisms are the result of a process of fermentation, and are generally associated with most copious vomiting. Of sarcinæ we knew nothing previous to their description by John Goodsir, in 1842. They are small square or slightly oblong bodies, divided into similar smaller portions by cross lines, and each portion thus formed is again subdivided; but the markings of the smaller squares are not so distinct as those of the larger. The accompanying illustration shows a mass of sarcinæ found in the vomit of a patient who suffered from gastric ulcer.

Vomit containing sarcinæ is always indicative of some structural change in the stomach. It is sometimes found in chronic gastritis of long standing; or in connection with ulcer, and yet oftener with cancer, and especially in those cases in which the narrowing at the pyloric extremity has led to distention of the organ. In truth, it is the opinion of several eminent pathologists, and among them Dr. Budd, that the disorder requires that there should be some condition which prevents the stomach from completely or readily emptying itself.

Sarcina vomit has an acid smell and an acid reaction, and often a peculiar brownish appearance. After standing, it becomes covered with a dirty, frothy matter, like yeast; but owing to the amount of half-digested food at times mixed with it, its aspect is not uniform, and it is only by the microscope that the presence of the strange bodies can be recognized with certainty.

The process of fermentation which attends the development of the sarcinæ occasions heart-burn and extreme flatulency, both of which add greatly to the distress of the patient; and the copious vomiting is a source of relief rather than of aggravation of his suffering, since the formation of acid and of wind is, for the time being, almost entirely or wholly arrested. Our aim, in treating cases of this disorder, is of course to remove the cause which incites to the development of sarcinæ; but as this object is not often attainable, we have to rest content in checking the activity of the process of fermentation by the administration of alkalies, and in preventing it as far as possible, by such medicines as creasote, or, better still, by the remedy proposed by Dr. Williams, the sulphite of soda, in doses of from half a drachm to a drachm.

Mucus is occasionally ejected in large quantities, both mixed with food and pure. In chronic gastritis, and in the milder forms of acute gastritis, the mucous membrane is covered with a tenacious secretion, and a considerable amount of a glairy or stringy matter is expelled by the act of vomiting. As a general rule, indeed, it may be stated that, when much mucus is evacuated, an inflammatory state of the mucous membrane, or what is termed a catarrhal state of the stomach, is present.

A thin, watery fluid, looking much like saliva, is discharged in some cases of organic disease of the stomach, and more frequently still in functional derangement of the organ brought on by eating coarse food. Now and then it is met with in pregnancy. This variety of vomiting is popularly known as "water-brash;" technically, as pyrosis. It is not seldom attended with a burning sensation extending to the fauces, and with pain running back to the spine. Generally it is a tractable disorder if proper food be taken. The fluid is commonly alkaline; sometimes, owing to its intimate admixture with the gastric contents, it is acid.

The source whence the fluid is derived is not settled. Frerichs found that it possessed the power of converting starch into sugar. On this account, it has been presumed to be saliva, which, after having accumulated in the stomach, induces vomiting; or saliva which by a spasm at the entrance of the stomach is prevented from entering that organ, and is ejected after collecting in considerable quantities. By others it is regarded as being formed by the glands at the lower part of the œsophagus. It was for a long time looked upon as a secretion from the pancreas; and was considered a sign that the pancreas was diseased, and not performing its function. But these views may be easily proved to be untenable.

Bile may find its way into the stomach, and be expelled by the mouth, imparting to the vomit a greenish or yellowish color, and a very bitter taste. The occurrence of bilious vomiting is commonly held to indicate a disease of the liver, or that the patient is extremely "bilious." It is a proof of neither. It is observed when there is much retching, and when the act of vomiting is protracted and frequently repeated, and is chiefly met with in the various forms of acute gastritis, and at the invasion of some acute malady which gives rise to sympathetic disturbance of the stomach.

Fecal vomiting never depends upon a disease of the stomach. It may possibly be owing to a fistulous opening between the colon and the stomach; but such cases are extremely rare. Generally it is due to a mechanical obstruction to the passage of feces. Occasionally it happens in fevers of a low type, or in peritonitis, and is then, perhaps, the result of paralysis of a portion of the intestinal tube, which acts, to some extent, as a mechanical obstruction. The matter that is ejected has the odor of feces; but it is commonly of less firm consistence, and of lighter color. And this because it is often the contents rather of the small than of the large intestine. Sometimes it is perfectly fluid and quite thin.

It is commonly supposed that fecal vomiting is caused by an inversion of the natural peristaltic action of the bowel. This doctrine has been called in question by Dr. William Brinton. He attributes the reflux of fecal matter to the peristalsis itself, which, acting on an obstructed and distended bowel, occasions, as far as possible, the forward propulsion of the contents of the intestinal tube, but which also gives rise to a current in the opposite direction in the fluid substances occupying the centre of the tube. For the ingenious arguments by which this position is maintained, I must refer to his Gulstonian Lectures.*

Pus in small amount is sometimes found mixed with the vomit in cases of large ulcers in the stomach, simple or cancerous. When in quantities, it is owing to an abscess in the neighborhood of the viscus having poured its contents into it. On the whole, pus is rarely met with in the matters expelled. And the same can be said of other substances which may find their way into the stomach, like echinococcus sacs and worms, and also of masses of false membrane.

Blood, on the other hand, is not infrequently vomited. It is unnecessary that I should describe the appearance of the blood when it comes from the stomach, nor the symptoms which accompany its discharge; this has been done already in treating of the diagnosis of hemorrhage from the lungs. I will merely here, before examining into the circumstances

---

* Lancet for July, August, and September, 1859.

which cause a hemorrhage from the stomach, recall the fact that it is preceded by nausea and followed by black stools, and that the fluid ejected is generally black, and presents an acid reaction.

The quantity of blood lost varies, of course, very greatly; but the amount vomited is by no means a proof of the amount effused. The larger portion may pass off by the bowels, giving rise to peculiar tarry stools. Nay, the whole may be voided with the stools; so that vomiting of blood and hemorrhage from the stomach are not always synonymous.

Hemorrhage occurring from the stomach is differently caused. It may spring from an injury to the organ, or from a disease of its coat; it may be vicarious; it may be the consequence of disorder elsewhere than in the stomach, as of a mechanical obstruction in the portal system; it may depend upon an altered state of the blood. But in all cases, however caused, with the exception of those which arise from a large vessel being eaten into by the process of ulceration, a hemorrhage from the stomach is an illustration of that kind of capillary hemorrhage which modern research has proved to lie at the root of the so-called hemorrhages "by exhalation." The overdistended capillaries burst; yet no traces of their rupture can be discovered with the unassisted eye after death. Nor is this difficult to account for, when the number and the extreme minuteness of the vessels implicated are considered.

In the hemorrhage that follows blows or kicks on the stomach, an *active* hyperæmia of the mucous surface is occasioned, which leads to the extravasation of blood. An active arterial hyperæmia also precedes the hemorrhage that sometimes follows the swallowing of irritant poisons; and it is probably the cause of the hæmatemesis in several of the organic affections of the stomach. Of these, only cancer and ulcer are apt to present hemorrhage as a prominent symptom; and of these two, again, it is much more frequent in the latter than in the former. The blood effused may be so slight in amount as to escape detection; and this is especially likely to happen when it is intimately admixed with food or with bile. Yet, by means of the microscope, the existence of blood corpuscles in the ejected matter can be always demonstrated.

When blood has been detained for some time in the stomach, and has become intimately mingled with the acid contents of the organ, it loses entirely its natural appearance. What is termed " coffee-ground vomit" is blood which has been thoroughly intermixed with other substances. It is the result of a comparatively small or gradual hemorrhage; and as this is the kind which is apt to happen in gastric cancer, it is common in this affection. It has been held to be pathognomonic of it; but it is not. It occurs in other morbid states of the organ. It is also met with in yellow fever, because in this dreadful malady the blood often accumulates little by little in the stomach before it is expelled.

Vicarious hemorrhage from the stomach is not at all unfrequent, and especially frequent is that which takes the place of the natural flow of the menses. It is never dangerous. The blood escapes more or less exactly at the time of the normal discharge, and while the bleeding lasts the stomach is slightly tender, and the digestion impaired. But during the intervals there are no signs of a disturbance of the functions of the organ, and no pain; both of which are points of importance in distinguishing between loss of blood caused by suppressed menstruation and by disease of the stomach.

Gastric hemorrhage, dependent upon a state of *passive* congestion brought on by an obstruction to the flow of venous blood, is occasionally seen in organic affections of the heart. But it is much more common as the result of embarrassment of the portal circulation, from tumors, or from affections of the liver and spleen. It frequently attends, therefore, cirrhosis and enlargement of the spleen, and for obvious reasons it is often joined to intestinal hemorrhage.

The last cause of gastric hemorrhage I have mentioned is that resulting from changes in the blood. The vessels themselves also are toneless, and rupture easily or offer no resistance to their altered contents escaping. This kind of hemorrhage is met with in scurvy, in typhus fever, and in yellow fever.

We see thus that blood is vomited from various causes, and that merely from the occurrence of hæmatemesis, we can determine nothing definite as to its origin. Yet the symptom, for a symptom it always is, is one of serious import, and when taken in connection with other signs is of very great service in diagnosis. We ought, in chronic cases, first to suspect the hemorrhage to be due to some organic disease of the stomach; when there is no other proof of a structural affection of this organ, we turn to the liver, spleen, or heart for its explanation, or examine carefully every part of the abdominal cavity, to see whether or not a tumor is the source of the trouble. If occasioned by none of these conditions, its cause lies probably in altered blood, or in suppressed discharges; of course, the history of the case is indispensable to any induction. Thus, in low fevers there is not often much difficulty in determining what has brought about the hemorrhage. The facts speak for themselves.

There is, however, one difficulty present in all instances; and that is, to tell whether the ejected blood has found its way into the stomach, and has been subsequently expelled, or whether the hemorrhage is really gastric. The only method to avoid being deceived, is to scrutinize closely the history and attending phenomena. Blood may be introduced into the stomach by the bursting of an aneurism, or from an ulcerating pancreas; or it may have been swallowed during an attack of epistaxis or of hæmoptysis, or wilfully, to excite sympathy, or to escape punishment for crime. The records of medicine teem with such instances of deception.

So much for vomiting of blood, and for the different characters presented by the vomit. In describing them we have been led away from the indications they furnish in diseases of the stomach. But it was more convenient here to consider vomiting somewhat connectedly and in detail, than to be obliged to treat of it in various chapters. To return now to the more special symptoms of a deranged stomach.

Pain.—Pain occurs in many of the gastric disorders, and

28

is met with in every conceivable form. It is sometimes very slight; at others, very violent. It is often more a feeling of soreness than actual pain. It may or may not be increased by pressure; and may either be augmented or relieved by the taking of food. If persistent or severe, and accompanied by tenderness at the epigastrium, it is almost always linked to a morbid state of the tissues of the viscus. Mere uneasy sensations, on the other hand, also happen in functional derangement of the organ while the food is being digested; and may even be attended with slight tenderness at the epigastrium.

Now, as both pain and soreness to the touch may be present, as well in functional disturbance as in organic change, how can we tell with which they are associated? Dr. Budd* lays down a law on this point which, on the whole, is borne out by the experience of the profession. The pain and soreness, he affirms, dependent on organic disease may be distinguished from the pain and soreness which result from functional disorder by noticing the time at which they take place. If they are more severe soon after meals, or when the stomach is full, and more severe after a heavy meal of animal food than after a light one of farinaceous substances and milk, they point to a structural affection. If they occur only when the stomach is empty and are relieved by food, they are indicative of a functional derangement. This general rule is as true as most general rules; but no truer. The confidence to be placed in it depends to some extent on the meaning attached to the word pain; for the rule would prove a very fallacious guide, were the uneasiness and sense of weight attendant on the act of digestion, in those whose gastric juice is deficient in quantity or in an unhealthy condition, to be regarded in the same light as pain, and as undeniable evidence of organic disease.

Occasionally the stomach is the seat of violent paroxysms of pain. These are at times linked to a chronic organic affection; at others, they are apparently connected with a perfectly sound state of the viscus, and coexist with a tend-

---

* Diseases of the Stomach.

ency to neuralgic pains all over the body; at others, again, they are brought about by some article of food which the stomach does not tolerate or is unable to digest. This singular disorder is variously described under the name of *gastrodynia* or *gastralgia*, or, by some authors, as a form of *cardialgia*. The pain is supposed to be associated with or be due to a cramp of the stomach; but whether it is so or not, is far from being certain. When the predisposition to it exists, exposure to cold and damp, a draught of cold water drunk when heated, sudden and violent emotions, or a collection of wind in the alimentary canal, will bring it on. And this predisposition is met with in gouty and rheumatic persons, and in those who are debilitated,—in women who are anemic, and in men who have been exposed to exhausting influences.

The pain varies very much in intensity; it is usually severe and agonizing; but it is not permanent: intervals of rest and comfort succeed to the paroxysms of harrowing distress. During a violent attack, the skin is cold, the pulse slow, there are frequently nausea, vomiting, sometimes fainting, and often a feeling of utter prostration and impending dissolution. The seat of the pain is in the epigastrium, immediately beneath the ensiform cartilage. The patient feels as if the coats of the stomach were being violently drawn together, or rent asunder, or rapidly pierced by a sharp instrument. Thence the pain extends toward the umbilicus and the hypochondria. It is sometimes relieved by the recumbent position and by external pressure.

But relief, under these circumstances, depends much on the condition with which the pain is associated. If it be connected with a chronic gastritis or an ulceration, external pressure aggravates rather than alleviates it. This is certainly true as a general rule, yet we cannot always positively announce that the pain which is conjoined with tenderness at the epigastrium is a proof of an organic lesion. There is sometimes sensitiveness to the touch in purely nervous gastralgia; or slight pressure may augment the pain, but firmly compressing the pit of the stomach diminish it.

In a practical point of view, it is very important to discriminate between the cases of gastralgia which may be viewed as pure neuralgia of the stomach and those in which the paroxysms of pain are combined with a chronic lesion. We infer that we have to deal with instances of the former, when the attacks occur in those whose impoverished blood or enfeebled health predisposes to neuralgia, and especially if they happen in women laboring under disorders of the uterus or ovaries, or in persons who suffer from neuralgic pains in other parts of the body. But the broadest line of distinction is drawn from the state of the digestive apparatus during the intervals. The disordered digestion; the pain after eating; the tenderness at the epigastrium; the nausea and vomiting; and the other symptoms common in morbid alterations of the coats of the stomach, are not seen in pure neuralgic gastrodynia. I have already stated that too much stress ought not to be laid on the influence of pressure on the paroxysmal pain during the paroxysm. A sign more trustworthy is the alleviation following the taking of food, for which, in truth, there may be a craving; and occasionally cases of gastralgia are met with, in which the pain occurs only early in the mornings, and is very distressing, but is almost immediately eased by a hearty breakfast.

The form of gastrodynia which is produced by some article of food that disagrees with the individual is readily distinguished from the other varieties, by observing that it is transient and by noting its cause. The indigestible substance undergoes fermentation in the stomach, and acidity, flatulent distention, and nausea attend the pain, which ceases when the offending matter is ejected and the gas expelled.

The remarks just made apply also, in the main, to other manifestations of perverted innervation of the stomach, such as to hyperæsthesia, erethism, with or without persistent vomitings,—forms happening usually in weak or hysterical persons, but which in the present state of our knowledge are still conveniently classed with gastralgia.

The nervous filaments, the irritation of which occasions pain in the stomach whether paroxysmal or not, belong to the vagus; sometimes, perhaps, the distress originates in the branches of the sympathetic that supply the organ. But we must be careful not to ascribe the seat of every pain which is felt between the umbilicus and sternum, or referred there, to the stomach. Diseases of the pleura, of the heart and its covering, affections of the intercostal nerves, abscess of the liver, intestinal disorders, rheumatism of the abdominal muscles, may give rise to a pain in the epigastric region. And again, spasmodic pain, like that of gastralgia, may be caused by colic, by disorganization of the tissue of the kidney and of the pancreas, and by the passage of gall-stones or of renal calculi. The great safeguard against error is to bear in mind that painful complaints of the stomach may be mistaken for those enumerated, and to ascertain carefully, in cases of epigastric distress, that there is no cause beyond the stomach to account for it. The nearer, in many instances, the pain is to the median line, or should it occupy this, and be very fixed and confined to a small spot, the greater is the probability of its being dependent upon gastric disease; and pain of the character alluded to is generally indicative of a serious malady.

Pain is the last of the symptoms directly referable to the derangement of the viscus itself to which we shall allude. But when the great organ of assimilation is disordered, other organs suffer, either through sympathy or because the irritation is transmitted to them, or because a similar state of their mucous surface is induced. The bowels are usually in a very sluggish condition. It is commonly only when the gastric acidity is extreme that they are relaxed. The viscera within the chest are frequently disturbed. The patient is annoyed by palpitation and shortness of breathing after meals; and as he feels the agitation of his heart, and finds that always, after he has eaten, his face is flushed, the palms of his hands hot, and his temporal arteries throbbing, he is apt to overlook the derangement of his stomach, and to fancy himself laboring under an incurable cardiac affection. A dry cough, also, is a not unusual concomitant; but a cough is sometimes the result of coexisting catarrh of the bronchial mucous membrane, or disease of the lung structure; and sometimes the affection of the lungs precedes that of the stomach.

So, too, with the kidneys. They may be irritated by the

crude material which has made its way into the blood, and which they are called upon to excrete. The urine often contains various abnormal constituents; yet not seldom a morbid state of the urine is found previous to the derangement of the stomach, and the indigestion is the secondary, rather than the primary ailment.

Indeed, we must never be too hasty in concluding, when a disordered stomach is associated with diseases of other viscera, that it is their cause; it may exist as their consequence. Diseases of the liver and intestines are especially prone to induce a gastric affection.

One of the worst results of a disordered digestion is the state of mind it produces. It occasions listlessness and sadness, and a disposition to look at all events in a gloomy light, and sometimes brings on the most inveterate hypochondriasis. Aretæus ascribed to the stomach as its primary power, that it acted as the president of pleasure and disgust, "being, from the sympathy of the soul, an important neighbor to the heart for imparting good or bad spirits." Now, although no one at present would agree with the physiology of the learned Cappadocian, who will deny that, mixed up with strange error, there is in the remark a germ of truth ? How few men have not, at one time or another, experienced the depression, the lack of energy which a disturbance in the main organ of digestion brings with it! But here, again, we must be careful not to confound cause with effect; for want of activity or a distressed state of mind may seriously impair the appetite and subvert the normal action of the viscus. The exquisite description of Juvenal, in his Thirteenth satire, of the conscience-stricken perjurer, is hardly drawn with too much poetic license

> Perpetua anxietas, nec mensæ tempore cessat,
> Faucibus ut morbo siccis, interque molares
> Difficili crescente cibo : sed Vina misellus
> Exspuit; Albani veteris pretiosa senectus
> Displicet: ostendas melius densissima ruga
> Cogitur in frontem, velut acri ducta Falerno.

In the rough sketch just finished of the symptoms encountered in gastric disorders, no attempt has been made to separate the signs which belong more particularly to alteration of its coats from those which occur in derangement of its functions; in other words, I have not tried to dissociate the symptoms of "dyspepsia" from those of actual lesions.

And this for two reasons: in the first place, the most palpable indications of organic disease of the stomach are those of disordered function; and secondly, there are no symptoms which belong exclusively to dyspepsia. This complaint consists simply of the phenomena of indigestion, but in such infinitely varied combination as to baffle the pen of any one who attempts to delineate it completely: in some cases we find pain; in others, nausea and disgust for food; in others, again, uneasiness after meals and acid eructations, or flatuleney; in some the gastric symptoms are connected with debility, great depression of spirits, and with wasting; in others a fair amount of health is preserved, the appetite is uncertain or perverted, and the signs of indigestion are only manifest after certain articles of food have been partaken of. Thus it is impossible to present anything like a complete picture of merely functional dyspepsia. Nor is this necessary; for its main features are easily enough recognized. In truth, the liability to error lies in an opposite direction. The faulty performance of the act of digestion is too often regarded as the whole ailment. Too often, if the practitioner has made out the diagnosis of "dyspepsia," he seeks no further, and treats the patient for this, and this alone, by means of some of the innumerable mixtures which enjoy the reputation "of being good for dyspepsia." He does not remember, or choose to remember, that dyspepsia may be bound *as a symptom* to structural alteration of the stomach, just as palpitation and irregular action of the heart may constitute the whole complaint, but may also be joined to a serious valvular lesion. It is true that, in an organ like the stomach, it is particularly difficult to tell where disturbed function ceases and anatomical change begins. Still, that this can be done to a greater extent than it is usually done, cannot be gainsaid. Moreover, there are a great many affections which probably have connected with them definite anatomical lesions and constant modifications of the gastric juice and of the secretions of the mucous follicles of the stomach, which we are as yet obliged to embrace under the name of dyspepsia; and this because we are unacquainted with their clinical expression. But we may fairly hope that, through those admirable physiological and pathological researches which have of late commenced to illuminate the subject, our ignorance will be dispelled, and by their aid we may expect the limits of purely functional dyspepsia to be much reduced; so that what the physician of the present day is compelled to class under the general term dyspepsia will be recognized by the physician of the twentieth century as several distinct affections, each with its characteristic structural change,—much in the same way that the physician of the eighteenth century was obliged to regard and to treat dyspnœa as an individual disease, while now we have learned to separate it into different varieties, in conformity with its prominent anatomical causes, and to treat it in accordance with its source.

Diseases of the Stomach in which Pain and Soreness at the Epigastrium, and Vomiting occur.

After what has been premised, it is obvious that the structural diseases of the stomach, so far as they are known up to this time, present but very few symptoms which can be regarded as at all characteristic. Indeed, the only ones which can lay any claim to be so considered—and we have already seen that this claim is not always valid—are pain and soreness at the epigastrium, and vomiting. We may, then, take these symptoms as a starting-point in diagnosis, and describe the individual organic affections in which they chiefly occur, speaking first of those that are acute.

Acute Gastritis.—This malady is now pronounced by all authors to be exceedingly rare, save as the result of irritant poisons. Yet there was a time, and that not fifty years ago, when acute inflammation of the stomach was held to be very frequent, and when this idea was made the keystone of a wondrous edifice of pathological and therapeutic theory, which counted its admirers by hundreds in every part of the civilized world. The discrepancy of opinion, as regards the frequency of the disease, may, to some extent, be explained by the varying latitude given to the term inflammation. Undoubtedly, inflammation of an intense kind, involving more than the mucous membrane, originating spontaneously, and not from the introduction of any highly acrid or corrosive substance into the stomach, is very seldom met with. But it is no less certain that inflammation of a less active character, limited to the most important part of the stomach, to the mucous membrane, and especially to its surface, is far from being a rare disease; and whether as a concomitant of fevers, or as an idiopathic malady, is a disorder to which the practitioner's attention is constantly drawn.

Thus, then, acute inflammation of all the coats of the stomach, or even of the entire mucous membrane, is uncommon; acute inflammation of its surface is common. Yet it is the doctrine of the day, not to regard any case as acute gastritis, unless serious changes have been wrought by the inflammation in the tissues of the organ, so serious as almost to preclude recovery. To discuss, in a work of this kind, the correctness or incorrectness of this view, would hardly be justifiable. But, before proceeding, I would venture to submit, whether the limits within which acute inflammation is supposed to be confined are not more rigidly marked out for the stomach than for any other viscus; whether it is not very arbitrary and artificial to make severity and consequence the test of acute inflammation; and whether a state of things fully entitled to be called acute idiopathic gastritis is not more frequent than is generally admitted? I am sure that I have seen cases which differed in nothing from the typical and graphically described cases of Andral,* save in the fatal termination and in lacking the symptoms which immediately precede that termination.

To detail one which was very striking: a robust woman, the mother of several children, whom she was obliged to support by hard labor, was suddenly seized with a pain in the epigastric region, and vomiting. There was no apparent

* Clinique Médicale, tome ii.

cause for the attack: she had certainly not swallowed any irritating substance. Although at one time a sufferer from indigestion, her digestive organs had not been markedly disordered for weeks prior to the appearance of the pain and irritability of the stomach. 'The former seemed to come on before the latter. It was of a dull character, increased by swallowing either solids or liquids, and associated with the greatest tenderness. Nausea was constant, and vomiting very frequent. Large quantities of a greenish fluid were ejected, as well as nearly everything she swallowed. The tongue was deeply coated; its edges and tip were red. The bowels were constipated, but not painful on pressure. There was fever, not, however, of an active type; the skin was hot toward evening; the pulse quick and small; the breathing was hurried, and the patient exceedingly restless and prostrated. She complained most of the distress in her head, and of violent thirst. The treatment pursued consisted mainly in opening the bowels by enemata, and in administering ice and repeated doses of calomel, some of which she retained. After the symptoms had lasted for about ten days, they gradually disappeared, and she slowly recovered. The pain on swallowing and the soreness at the epigastrium were the last to leave. Indeed, when she passed from under my care, they had not ceased entirely. I cannot say whether they ever did, for I lost sight of the patient.

Now, here is a case which presented all the symptoms of a severe inflammation of the stomach, similar to that produced when an irritant poison has been received into the organ. In all such instances there are the same nausea and vomiting, and pain; the same restlessness and headache; the same form of fever and small or feeble pulse; the same unquenchable thirst. Sometimes the pain is of a burning kind; and in those cases which prove fatal,—and many do prove fatal, as much perhaps from the destructive effect of the irritant on the tissues as in consequence of the inflammation,—there is hiccough, the skin becomes cold, the features collapse, and the sufferer dies prostrated, yet frequently preserving his mental faculties to the last.

From these severe cases of acute gastritis, however caused,

there exists every grade of inflammation down to an active congestion of the mucous membrane, and to a mere reddening of its surface. Of course, there will not be in the milder forms the same intensity in the symptoms. But the outline is the same, although the filling in be in far less vivid hues. There is in all the same tendency to nausea and to vomiting, with more or less epigastric pain and uneasy sensations, and more or less tenderness at the pit of the stomach, and headache.

A mild gastritis is very commonly brought on by a debauch or by the introduction of irritating articles of diet into the stomach. These cases are popularly known as severe attacks of indigestion; that they are owing to an inflammatory state of the mucous membrane, was proved by the ocular demonstration Dr. Beaumont had of the process in the person of Alexis St. Martin. Dr. Beaumont found that whenever Alexis had been eating plentifully of substances hard of digestion, or drinking freely of ardent spirits, the mucous surface of the stomach exhibited patches of redness of various size, from which now and then small drops of blood exuded. Aphthous spots were also detected, and the secretions were evidently arrested, although occasionally a considerable quantity of ropy mucus collected on the surface of the membrane. The symptoms these changes, when they were marked, produced, were some tenderness at the epigastrium; nausea; vomiting; constipation, or sometimes diarrhœa; a coated tongue, and headache,—in fact, just the symptoms of which patients complain when they are suffering from an acute attack of indigestion.

Another common and kindred kind of mild inflammation of the stomach is that usually called a " bilious attack." The French designate it expressively as *embarras gastrique.* English writers, borrowing a term from the Germans, describe it as a variety of *gastric catarrh.* In truth, it is like a catarrhal affection, and is often associated with catarrh of other mucous membranes. It sometimes occurs in epidemics. The symptoms are those already detailed. There is nausea, and frequently bile is vomited. We do not usually observe much pain in the epigastrium; but rather a feeling of uneasiness, and a slight soreness to the touch. The urine is commonly dark, and deposits urate of ammonia; the tongue is much coated; there is thirst, with generally a slight fever, which exacerbates at night. From the latter circumstance, remittent fever is treated of by some authors as an acute gastric catarrh; but this is giving to one of the phenomena in this disease a prominence to which it is not entitled.

Secondary acute inflammation of the mucous membrane of the stomach is found in association with various disorders. It is met with in remittent fever, in typhus, in the exanthemata, in rheumatism, and oftener in gout, and partakes somewhat of the specific character of the malady with which it happens to be combined. Indeed, instead of being a secondary inflammation, it is oftener, to speak correctly, a local expression of a constitutional state.

Several writers describe a form of gastritis which occurs in very young children, and leads to softening of the mucous lining of the stomach. Jæger, Cruveilhier, and Billard in particular have made this *acute gastric softening* the subject of special study. Yet its nature is not fully understood. There are some who believe the gelatinous softening to be the consequence of inflammation; others who regard it as nothing but the post-mortem result of the solvent powers of the gastric juice; while others again maintain it to be due to a pathological process that is not inflammatory, but which has disorganized the tissues during life. The symptoms which are ascribed to the malady are certainly exactly like those of acute inflammation of the stomach. As I have no experience in this strange disorder, I shall follow closely the delineation given of it by Billard.*

The disease usually commences with the signs of a violent gastritis, with tension of the epigastric region, which is painful to the touch; with vomiting, not only of the milk and the other liquids swallowed, but also of a green or yellow fluid. This vomiting happens either immediately or some time after the child has taken food or drink. There is occasionally diarrhœa; and the discharges from the bowels are frequently

---

* Maladies des Enfants nouveau-nés.

greenish, resembling those from the stomach. The respiration is hurried and jerking; the extremities are cold; the face and cry expressive of suffering; the agitation is great. To this state succeeds one of general prostration and insensibility, and at the end of six, eight, or fifteen days, the patient dies exhausted, from want of sleep and from the constant vomiting and pain. In very young children, there is hardly any fever. The disease sometimes runs a more chronic course. It may be combined with a similar softening of the intestines. Cruveilhier has seen it occur in epidemics. He describes a prodromic period, marked by a rapid loss of strength, and by intense thirst.

Chronic Diseases attended with Pain, Epigastric Tenderness, and Vomiting.

The chronic diseases of the stomach may, like the acute, be considered in accordance with the pain, the soreness at the epigastrium, and the vomiting that attend them. At all events, these are the symptoms common to the chronic diseases which are susceptible of diagnosis. Besides these, there are some chronic disorders with the morbid anatomy of which recent careful researches have made us familiar,—such as destruction of the tubular structures; hypertrophy of the solitary glands; interstitial growths leading to their wasting, and to a gradual fibroid thickening of the entire mucous or submucous coat; fatty degeneration of the atrophied masses,[*] —but which we are as yet utterly unable to distinguish at the bedside, and which, so far as has been ascertained, may even be entirely latent.

Contrasting the chronic diseases with which we are clinically acquainted with the acute, vomiting is found to be a symptom of greater diagnostic value—not the act itself, but the appearances of the ejected matter. And further, the phenomena of dyspepsia stand forth much more conspicuously.

Chronic Gastritis.—In chronic inflammation of the mu-

---

[*] See Handfield Jones, Pathological and Clinical Observations respecting Morbid Conditions of the Stomach.

cous membrane, or chronic catarrh of the stomach, as it is called by some, the symptoms of indigestion are very persistent and very manifold. They vary somewhat according to the extent of the mucous surface involved and the amount of mucus and epithelium which accumulates on it, and probably also according to the healthy or wasted state of the gastric glands. Generally there is a sensation of discomfort, of weight, and of soreness at the pit of the stomach, which is aggravated by food; the part is also tender to the touch. Sometimes, even when the stomach is empty, a burning at the epigastrium and an inward fever are complained of. The appetite is impaired or capricious. Fermentation, heart-burn, and flatulency frequently attend the slow digestion of the food; the tongue is usually heavily coated; it may, however, be clean. The bowels are almost always constipated. The urine contains an excess of phosphates or urates, or exhibits crystals of oxalate of lime. The patient's circulation is languid. He suffers from chilliness. His spirits are depressed. Not unfrequently, when the case has been of long duration, he is annoyed by vomiting, after meals, the half-digested food mixed with strings of mucus. But the vomiting may also take place when the stomach is empty, and the ejected matter be fluid and colorless. Drunkards who suffer from chronic gastritis often throw up a quantity of glairy fluid on rising in the morning. A colorless vomit, joined to symptoms of long-continued indigestion, is always very characteristic of chronic gastritis.

Thus, then, occasionally the character of the vomit, more frequently the coated tongue, the distress after eating, the soreness at the epigastrium, and, especially, the permanence of the symptoms, distinguish the dyspepsia of chronic inflammation of the stomach from that which is purely functional; for, although cases of chronic gastritis may recover, and often do recover, yet the amelioration is very gradual, and months or years elapse before restoration to health takes place.

The causes of the malady are often obscure. It certainly cannot always, nor in truth frequently, be traced to an antecedent acute attack, although those who suffer from the chronic disorder are particularly prone to acute · exacerbations. It is more common in persons over than under forty years of age. It is especially common in gourmands and drunkards, and in those who live on coarse food. It is often found cònjoined with chronic bronchitis, and sometimes with tubercular disease of the lungs. Passive congestion undoubtedly acts as a predisposing element. The inflammation is seen to arise from this cause in the course of chronic affections of the heart, of the liver, and of obstructions to the portal circulation, whether complicated with a lesion of the liver or not.

Chronic gastritis is frequently associated with ulcers in the organ or with cancer, and many of the symptoms of these disorders are clearly attributable to it. Let us inquire whether there are any special symptoms to inform us that something more dangerous than chronic inflammation of the mucous membrane of the stomach exists.

Gastric Ulcer.—Ulcer of the stomach is a disease comparatively rare in this country; but it is not so in some parts of the Continent of Europe and in England. It has, especially of late years, been made the subject of careful study by several eminent pathologists and physicians. The remarks about to be made are based partly on a perusal of the valuable material that has been collected; partly on a number of undoubted cases of the affection which have come under my notice.

The ulcer or ulcers, for there are sometimes several present, are seated most usually in the posterior wall of the stomach, in or near the lesser curvature and toward the pyloric extremity. The great danger arises from perforation of the coats and subsequent peritonitis. But the ulceration may prove fatal by opening a large blood-vessel. Again, the protracted suffering and excessive vomiting may gradually exhaust the vital energies. On the other hand, the ulcers may heal by cicatrization; and this, according to Dr. Brinton, who has written a very able monograph on Gastric Ulcer, takes place in about half the instances. In cases which may be regarded as typical, the malady is announced by symptoms exactly like those witnessed in chronic gastritis—the same uneasiness and pain at the epigastrium, and occasional nausea and vomiting of food, or of a watery fluid. Perforation may at this early stage of the disease most unexpectedly cut short the patient's life. Should perforation not take place, hemorrhage from the stomach, with emaciation and anæmia, next appears. In this way the disease usually continues for several months, or sometimes for a much longer period, the symptoms remitting from time to time, and showing singular variations in their severity.

Of these symptoms, the pain and the vomiting are the most characteristic. Pain is rarely absent; never, perhaps, except in cases which run a rapid course. It is generally a continuous dull feeling; sometimes a burning, at others a gnawing sensation. As a rule, it is rendered more acute within a quarter of an hour after eating, and remains so as long as food occupies the stomach. Its situation is commonly in the middle of the epigastric region, and there it continues strictly limited. At that point, too, there is localized soreness, or even great tenderness to the touch. Sometimes the pain is seated behind the ensiform cartilage, or is referred to the right or to the left hypochondrium. It is often associated with a gnawing pain in the lower dorsal vertebræ, which may shoot between the scapulæ or down the spine; but the dorsal pain, like the epigastric, is, on the whole, very fixed, and radiates but little. Besides this continued feeling of distress occur violent paroxysms of pain, which may last for several hours; nay, with trifling intermissions, even for days. They are aggravated by pressure or by food; and, in fact, they are often thus induced, but not always, for they sometimes come on suddenly when the viscus is empty. The patient refers the suffering chiefly to the pit of the stomach, or to the dorsal vertebræ. He is apt to seek the recumbent posture for its relief. Yet it is a circumstance not a little remarkable in the history of gastric ulcer, that there are sometimes long intervals during which all pain, whether paroxysmal or not, ceases, and during which food can be taken without inconvenience.

The peculiarities the pain exhibits form, on the whole, the

most distinctive symptom of gastric ulceration. The paroxysms just spoken of might be mistaken for a purely nervous gastralgia. And, indeed, when it is considered that both disorders are specially apt to occur in anemic women, and in those whose menstrual functions are deranged, it becomes apparent how easily this mistake may be committed. The soreness at the epigastrium; the persistent symptoms of indigestion; the increase of pain after meals,—constitute, in a diagnostic point of view, the great safeguard against error. To these might be added the vomiting of blood, were it not that vicarious hemorrhages are not at all unlikely to take place in young women who are troubled with amenorrhœa.

This is, in truth, a matter having a very close connection with the diagnosis of gastric ulceration. Persons who suffer from a disturbance of the menstrual function are prone to be hysterical; and it may happen that one of the most marked traits of the hysterical disorder is, that it manifests itself by tenderness in the epigastric region, and by pain in the stomach. We may thus have the most significant signs of gastric ulcer, occurring, as so very many cases of amenorrhœa do, in chlorotic young women; therefore in the very class among whom ulceration of the stomach is most frequently found. Nay, as I had occasion to note in a patient who was under my care, the very history may point to the probability of a gastric ulcer.* Yet generally, by close attention to all of the phenomena of the case, we can arrive at a correct conclusion. The tenderness of the simulated malady, as in all local hysterical affections, is very great on the slightest touch; and there is no severe pain posteriorly corresponding to the spot of soreness in the epigastric region. Pressure upon a spinous process may cause pain; but it is not the peculiar dorsal pain of gastric ulceration. Then, in the hysterical complaint there is often hyperæsthesia of the skin in various portions of the body, and the apparent gastric distress bears no relation to the taking of food or to the circumstance of its being of an irritating character or otherwise. Lastly,

---

* Philadelphia Hospital, Jan. 21st, 1863; reported by Dr. H. C. Wood, in Med. and Surg. Reporter, Feb. 1863.

the cast of the features and other evidences of a hysterical constitution will assist us in the diagnosis.

But to return to the vomiting of blood. When this is not traceable to a suppression of a natural discharge, and when it does not befall a person who suffers from a disease of the heart, or liver, or spleen, or œsophagus, it acquires great significance. It is the only kind of vomit at all distinctive of a gastric ulcer; for the substances ejected present otherwise appearances not different from what they do in chronic gastritis. The blood may be pure and red, but it is more frequently blackened by the gastric juice; and large quantities are sometimes passed by stool. Now, hemorrhage does not take place in chronic inflammation of the mucous membrane of the stomach. In those instances in which erosions exist on the surface, the vomited mucus may be a little streaked with blood; yet anything like a profuse hemorrhage never happens. Hence its occurrence in a case with the symptoms of chronic gastritis renders the presence of an ulcer very probable.

But in concluding this sketch of gastric ulceration, two questions arise which require solution: Does an ulcer always produce the peculiar train of symptoms mentioned? May not the same phenomena be met with in other disorders? The first question must be answered in the negative. Many a case of ulceration of the stomach occasions nothing but the symptoms of chronic gastritis; and even these may not be marked. The second question is to be answered in the affirmative. There is a disorder with symptoms almost identical with gastric ulceration, namely, the corrosive *ulcer of the duodenum.* Now this affection, were it more frequent, would be a constant source of error in diagnosis. It may run an acute, or at least an apparently acute, or a chronic course. In either case, it is scarcely distinguishable from gastric ulceration. Trier,* from an analysis of twenty-six cases, mentions as the most important ground for a differential diagnosis, signs of dilatation of the stomach; a sensitive tumor in the epigastrium,

---

* Quoted in Brit. and Foreign Medico-Chirurg. Review, Feb. 1864; see, also, monograph by Krauss, and remarks on it in Niemeyer's work on Practical Medicine.

proceeding from adhesion with the pancreas; and jaundice or other hepatic phenomena. But these symptoms are far from constant, and in accordance with his own showing, in the acute cases, and in those chronic cases which run a latent course, the diagnosis is, with our present means of research, impossible. It may be added that the perforating ulcer of the duodenum is much more apt than ulcer of the stomach to remain latent, and to lead suddenly to a fatal termination.

There is yet another disorder with symptoms like those of ulcer, a disorder still more serious and destructive—namely, cancer.

Gastric Cancer.—Cancer is found more frequently in the stomach than in any other organ excepting the uterus. Of nine thousand one hundred and eighteen cases of cancer which occurred in Paris from 1837 to 1840, two thousand three hundred and three were in the stomach.* The disease is generally primary. It is most often seated at the pylorus; next in frequency stands the cardiac orifice; most rarely does it involve the whole viscus. We find all the varieties of cancer affecting the stomach; but none is so common as scirrhus. Indeed, what is called cancer of the stomach means, in the large majority of cases, scirrhus; and, moreover, scirrhus at the pyloric extremity, deposited primarily in the textures which intervene between the mucous and the serous coat. It would be out of place to enter here into a minute description of the appearances of a gastric scirrhus. I will only state that I have usually found it to present cell-growths less marked than those of scirrhus of any other part of the body.

The symptoms of cancer of the stomach are the same as of chronic gastritis—pain, tenderness in the epigastrium, disordered digestion, vomiting. In a more advanced state of the cancerous malady they may be those of gastric ulcer, hemorrhage being added to the list above given. There is only one symptom at all distinctive of cancer—namely, the existence of a tumor, and this is so only when it is joined to digestive troubles and to increasing debility and emaciation.

But let us see if there is nothing in the pain and vomiting,

---

* Walshe on Cancer.

or in the accompanying circumstances of the case, by which, even when a tumor cannot be discovered, the presence of a cancer may be suspected. Pain is a very constant symptom; quite as constant as it is in gastric ulcer. But the pain is, as a rule, more continued, much less influenced by the taking of food, and more radiating, being often referred to the right or left hypochondrium. Its character is very varying. It may be dull, gnawing, or it may be lancinating. It may be slight, or it may amount to excruciating agony. It is often of the latter kind. But it is a mistake to suppose that a cancer of the stomach necessarily causes severe or lancinating pain. Again, it should be borne in mind that the part diseased may ulcerate, and then the pain is exactly like that of an ordinary gastric ulcer, and is affected in the same way by food.

Vomiting is not an invariable result of a cancer; yet it is a very frequent one. The seat of the morbid growth determines, to a great extent, the occurrence of vomiting and the period at which it will happen. When the body of the stomach is attacked, but the orifices are not obstructed, it may not take place at all; or if it take place, it is within a brief time after meals. When the disease has narrowed the cardiac extremity, vomiting supervenes almost immediately; the food has hardly been swallowed before it is brought up again. But when, as is so much more common, the pylorus is constricted, the food is not thrown off until it attempts to pass through into the intestine; therefore not until a considerable time after meals.

With respect to the character of the substances ejected, this too depends on the seat of the cancer, and the time at which the vomiting arises. If it ensue several hours after meals, the cast-off matter consists of food partly digested, partly in a state of highly acetous fermentation. An enormous quantity of acid material, the accumulation of several meals, is sometimes brought up during one act of emesis. The ejected matter may be intermingled with blood, and have a blackish or reddish-brown, "coffee-ground" appearance; or the mucus which is thrown up is tinged with black flakes. But it is rare that any considerable amount of unmixed blood is vomited.

Thus a close study of the pain and vomiting may furnish evidence by which the existence of a gastric cancer might be suspected. There are a few other circumstances which would strengthen this suspicion: one of these is the intense acidity of the stomach with the sour eructations; another, the extreme flatulency; another, the fetid breath, for although fetor of the breath may result from putrefactive changes in the food in almost any form of gastric disorder, it is perhaps never so permanent or so much complained of as in cancer. A fourth is the obstinate constipation. A fifth, the progressive loss of flesh and the cachectic appearance of the patient, who is pale and tired looking, or has a complexion slightly jaundiced, or whose face is of a color which seems to have arisen from a combination of the hue of chlorosis and of jaundice. The supposed characteristic straw color of cancer is not often met with; sometimes we observe red spots on the cheek in the afternoon. And there are cases in which irritative fever accompanies the gradual wasting — gradual, because the duration of the malady averages fully a year.

Now, should all these symptoms be met with in a person who is steadily becoming feebler, whose age is above forty, in whose family cancer is hereditary; should cancerous tumors develop themselves in any other part of the body, the suspicion entertained would be converted into almost a certainty. But it is not often that a perfectly typical case, presenting a combination of all the symptoms enumerated, is met with. And I repeat, that the most distinctive sign is a tumor; when this is not detected, considerable uncertainty hangs over any diagnosis of gastric cancer.

To contrast, then, cancer of the stomach, with chronic gastritis and gastric ulcer:

CHRONIC GASTRITIS.	GASTRIC ULCER.	GASTRIC CANCER.
Pain at the epigastrium somewhat augmented by food; also soreness. Both constant, although comparatively slight.	Pain at the epigastrium much augmented by food; subsides when this is digested; paroxysms of pain, but not laucinating; a strictly localized soreness to the touch in the epigastric region, sometimes a painful spot over the lower dorsal vertebræ. Intermissions in the pain of considerable length are frequent.	Pain frequently of a radiating kind, often paroxysmal, not unusually severe and lancinating, but not of necessity associated with soreness. Little or not at all affected by food. Pain rarely remits; never intermits for any considerable time.

CHRONIC GASTRITIS.	GASTRIC ULCER.	GASTRIC CANCER.
Symptoms of indigestion.	Symptoms of indigestion Sometimes very slight.	Symptoms of indigestion. Extreme acidity of stomach.
Sometimes vomiting.	Vomiting may be present or absent.	Vomiting a very frequent symptom.
No hemorrhage, or but trifling hemorrhage; and even a trifling hemorrhage is rare.	Abundant hemorrhage from the stomach common.	Hemorrhage not very abundant; but occasioning frequently coffee-ground looking vomit.
Bowels constipated.	Bowels may or may not be constipated; usually are.	Bowels obstinately constipated.
No fever.	No fever.	Fever not uncommon.
Not much emaciation; no cachectic appearance.	Frequently extreme pallor and debility.	Gradual and progressive loss of flesh, and debility.
Not confined to any age. More common in middle-aged or elderly people.	May occur in middle-aged persons; but is also frequently seen in young adults, especially in young women.	Most common in elderly people; rarely occurs in persons under forty years of age.
Disease may be relieved or cured, or is of very long duration.	Duration uncertain; may get well, may run on rapidly to perforation; on the other hand, may last for years.	Average duration one year; may be shorter, but seldom longer; very rarely reaches two.
No tumor.	No tumor.	Generally a tumor.

The differences laid down in the table are derived from an analysis of well-marked cases. In the early stages of the cancerous malady, a differential diagnosis is impossible. Subsequently, as already stated, the detection of a tumor plays an important part in any induction. But this remark does not apply to cases of cancer of the cardiac orifice, which are rare, and in which a tumor, from its deep situation, almost always eludes discovery. Such cases are, however, discriminated by their presenting the same signs as a stricture of the œsophagus low down; indeed they are very constantly combined with a narrowing of the tube, produced by the cancer spreading to it. Cancer, at other parts of the organ, occasions a perceptible tumor in about three-fourths of all the instances; its situation is of course not always the same. Where no tumor can be discerned, and particularly if, as may happen, portions of the stomach remain healthy and the digestive disturbances are slight, the existence of cancer may not reveal itself by any symptoms, and the case run a latent course.*

A cancer of the anterior wall produces, as a rule, fulness, resistance, and percussion dulness in the epigastric region.

---

* See report of case under my care at the Penna. Hospital, published in Amer. Journ. of Med. Sci., vol. lii. 1866.

A cancer involving the greater curvature gives rise to a swelling near the umbilicus, or to one extending toward either hypochondrium. The tumor formed by cancer of the pylorus is commonly felt plainly a little to the right of the median line, and one to two inches below the cartilages of the ribs. In women its position is apt to be even lower than this; and, indeed, in both sexes the situation of the indurated pylorus is very variable. It may be pushed down to near the umbilicus, nay, it has been discerned near the anterior superior spinous process of the ilium.* It is very rarely found in the left hypochondrium, but not unfrequently in the right. Then it may form adhesions to the liver, which viscus at times so completely covers the tumor as to render it impossible of detection.

The reason why the swelling, in not a few instances, shows itself much lower than the normal seat of the pylorus, is obvious. Meal after meal the organ seeks to overcome the resistance offered by the narrowed pyloric orifice, and does so with great and increasing difficulty. The constantly-repeated and long-continued struggle leads to hypertrophy of the muscular coat and to distention of the hollow viscus.

The tumor may or may not be movable; its surface may be either smooth or nodulated. It may be large and distinct, or small and requiring a careful examination to distinguish it from the surrounding and more yielding textures. It is much more perceptible on some days than it is on others. Its existence, as has been already insisted on, furnishes the most conclusive evidence in favor of a cancer.

But is a swelling in the region of the stomach strictly pathognomonic of gastric cancer? Unfortunately for diagnostic purposes, it is not, even when the swelling has been ascertained to belong to that viscus. A mere fibroid thickening of the pylorus will occasion a tumor, and, moreover, produces symptoms which resemble so closely those of malignant disease at the orifice, that I much doubt the possibility of distinguishing during life, with any certainty, be-

---

* See Lebert's cases in Traité Pratique des Maladies Cancereuses.

tween the two affections. Let us take this case, which I saw
with Dr. Moss,* of this city, as an example.

A woman, aged forty, complained much of pain at the pit
of the stomach, and of a heavy sensation throughout the
abdomen. For some months she had been suffering from
indigestion, and had been steadily losing flesh and strength.
Her countenance had a tired look, and she was very despondent. She had a slight cough; and on percussing the lungs,
impaired resonance was detected at the apices. The bowels
were obstinately constipated, the tongue was smooth and red,
the pulse feeble. She vomited shortly after meals, yet never
anything but the ingesta. There was no pain on pressure
over the pylorus; but a greater resistance to the finger than
usual was detected. The further progress of the complaint
was marked by the most incessant vomiting, only, however,
after meals. Hydrocyanic acid, creasote, opiates were given
in vain to arrest it. Once, and once only, did it cease for
several days; and then without apparent cause. As the
case drew toward its fatal termination, the patient was much
troubled with acid eructations, and had occasionally slight
febrile attacks. The distress in the epigastrium increased in
severity. About three weeks before her death she was seized
with lancinating pains under both patellæ, which were neither
relieved nor aggravated by pressure or motion. They were
accompanied by pricking sensations and numbness in the
legs, and an inability to walk. The pains gradually ceased,
but the loss of motion and numbness increased from day to
day. She died, utterly exhausted by the abdominal pains
and the incessant vomiting, about three months after she began to reject her food. On post-mortem examination, tubercular deposits were found at the apices of the lungs. The
abdominal viscera were healthy, excepting the stomach; and
this, too, was healthy, save at its pyloric orifice, which was so
narrowed that the tip of the little finger could hardly be
forced into it. The mucous lining lay in folds, but on dissection was found to be perfectly normal. At the pylorus,
but only there, the submucous and muscular coat were

---

* Published in full in Proceedings of Path. Society of Phila., vol. i.

uniformly thickened.   Examined microscopically, they contained nothing but fibro-areolar tissue, spindle-shaped fibre-cells, and very distinct organic muscular fibres.

Now, here is a case which evidently was not cancer; and yet it had the symptoms of cancer.   It is true that the absence of blood and of glairy mucus in the matter vomited, and the indistinctness of the swelling, in spite of the great emaciation, were against the supposition of cancer of the pylorus.   Still no inference based on these data alone could be strictly trusted, since every cancer is not associated with the vomit of coffee-ground material, or of glairy mucus, or with a palpable tumor.   The disease was combined with tubercular deposits in the lung.   Nor is this the only example of the combination which has come under my notice. And when a tubercular state of the lung has been fairly made out, and there exist at the same time signs of pyloric obstruction, I should be much inclined to hazard a diagnosis that this is not of a cancerous nature, but consists simply of an increased abnormal development of the submucous coat, with probable subsequent hypertrophy of the muscular tunic.

The *fibroid thickening* may extend throughout the whole stomach.   Such cases differ from cancer by their long duration; the absence of hemorrhage, of vomiting and severe pain; and the more uniform gastric swelling.   They are sometimes observed in spirit drinkers.   Yet their discrimination from cancer is never a certainty, but merely a matter of conjecture.

SECTION II.

DISEASES OF THE INTESTINES AND PERITONEUM.

In considering the diseases of the intestines, we meet again with symptoms into the import of which we have examined in connection with affections of the stomach.   We encounter nausea, vomiting, and derangement of the powers of digestion. These disturbances are to a great extent sympathetic or dependent upon coexisting gastric disorder; they do not serve, therefore, as guides in the detection of intestinal maladies. The signs upon which we rely much more implicitly are pain and the fecal discharges. Now, as regards the former, we draw the most trustworthy inferences, as we shall presently see, from its kind rather than from its mere occurrence. The study of the fecal discharges tells us often in a more direct manner what is going on in the long tract of intestinal membrane.

Alvine Discharges.—To examine briefly into the diversified appearances of the stools:

Watery stools are observed whenever a large quantity of the serum of the blood finds its way through the intestinal coats. They are met with after the administration of saline purgatives, in serous diarrhœa, and in cholera. Their hue varies: they may be almost colorless, or tinged with yellow. Sometimes, although very thin and watery, they are decidedly yellow; again they are rendered turbid by the dissemination of whitish flocculi of cast-off epithelium, or by mucus. Whether they be yellow or colorless depends on the existence or non-existence in them of fecal matter and of bile. In a prognostic point of view, the most colorless evacuations are the most dangerous. Their persistence bespeaks a continued absence of healthy fecal matter and of the proper secretion of bile.

The presence of an excessive quantity of *mucus* renders the discharges less consistent than natural; yet, unless they contain more or less serum, they are not of necessity very liquid. Stools with much mucus are met with in some cases of diarrhœa and in dysentery. The appearance they present is often similar to the white of an egg; or the whitish masses of mucus surround the lumps of feces, or are intermingled with the fluid alvine discharges.

Pus in large amount and unmixed with feces is only discharged when an abscess has ruptured into some part of the intestine. Stools composed of feces and pus are encountered in chronic inflammation and in ulceration of the bowels; and whitish, creamy streaks indicate the presence of the foreign substance. Yet the pus may be so intimately blended with the feces, or with masses of mucus, as to require the microscope for its detection.

Stools consisting entirely of *bile* are very rarely met with. More generally there are other elements joined to the voided secretion of the liver. An excess of bile in the alvine discharges gives rise to evacuations of a yellowish-brown or yellow hue, which darkens on exposure to the air. When the alimentary tube is highly acid, the resulting color is green. Both these kinds of stools are commonly called "bilious;" but the latter is, perhaps, less absolutely so than the former. A deficiency of bile manifests itself by clayey, sometimes even by almost white stools.

Black stools result from the action of certain medicines, as of iron; from a vitiated condition of the bile and intestinal secretions, such as occurs in bilious fever; or from the effusion of blood into the alimentary canal. At all events, when the hemorrhage proceeds from the stomach or upper part of the canal, the stools have a black, tarry appearance; when from the lower section of the tube, pure blood is passed, or, if it be small in quantity, a blood-streaked mucus. Should any doubt exist as to whether the dark discharges be dependent or not upon the presence of blood, let them be diluted with water; they will assume a reddish tinge if this be the cause of the abnormal color.

The *odor* of the evacuations is extremely offensive in fevers of a low type, and when the intestinal secretions are vitiated. So, too, at times in small-pox and in cholera. Acidity of the intestinal canal, as in the diarrhœa of children, or in rheumatism or gout, imparts to the stools a sour smell.

In cases of constipation it may be important to notice the *shape* of the passages, because this may show whether an impediment in the gut has flattened, or otherwise altered them. In fevers, as well as in affections of the intestinal mucous membrane, whether inflammatory or not, we often derive much information from studying the form of the voided matter. Figured stools, succeeding to fluid passages, are always of favorable omen.

Chemical and microscopical examinations of the feces are not often made; yet chemistry and the microscope may be frequently of very great service. They enable us, for instance, to recognize with certainty that the yellowish lumps contained in, or the greasy film which collects upon the surface of the evacuation, consist of fat. The microscope, too, detects pus and blood; and it exhibits, in the fecal discharges of putrid fevers, masses of crystals of the ammonio-phosphates. One drawback to the use of chemical research for clinical purposes, is the uncertain composition of the feces, owing to the number of elements derived from the food. A further objection, both to it and to microscopical investigation, is the repugnance every one feels to the close examination of human excrement.*

So much for the alvine discharges. Their study, it is evident, is of service not merely in intestinal complaints, but equally in the many maladies in which the alimentary tube sympathizes or becomes involved. But to return to the uncomplicated intestinal diseases, grouping them as they may be recognized by pain and peculiarity in the fecal discharges, and describing with them, for convenience sake, the affections of the peritoneum.

Diseases attended with Paroxysms of Pain referred chiefly to the Middle or Lower Part of the Abdomen, and not associated with marked Tenderness or with Fever.

The type of these is colic.

Colic.—This is an intestinal pain, paroxysmal in its character, and usually combined with constipation, but unattended with febrile symptoms. The pain is of a severe griping, or pinching, or twisting kind, and is commonly referred to the neighborhood of the umbilicus. It is generally relieved, or at any rate not aggravated, by pressure. Yet this is not so invariable as it is ordinarily held to be; for sometimes there is some soreness with the pain, and, indeed, a slight soreness not unfrequently remains after the paroxysm has passed off.

---

* See, on the minute examination of the feces, Lehmann's Physiological Chemistry; a paper by Marcet, Proceedings of Royal Society, 1854; and the Inaugural Dissertations of Wehsarg and Ihring, quoted in Brit. and For. Med.-Chirg. Rev., Oct. 1854.

While the pain lasts, the countenance wears an anxious, frightened expression ; the skin is cold, or covered with clammy perspiration ; the pulse is depressed. Occasionally there is vomiting, and in severe cases the abdominal walls are tense or raised in hard knots by the spasmodic contraction of the muscles. A fit may last only a few minutes, or, with trifling remissions, for several hours.

Some persons are very liable to attacks of colic. Those who suffer from indigestion, or are enfeebled by exhausting maladies, are predisposed to them; so also are hysterical, gouty, and rheumatic individuals. As to the exciting causes, they are very various; and somewhat according to its different causes, colic presents different forms. Let us indicate the more prominent.

Colic, simple and unconnected with a disease of the bowel.—Now, in these cases, which are generally called, from the supposed pathological condition, spasmodic colic, the paroxysmal pain may have a threefold origin. It may be the result of direct excitation of the peripheral intestinal nerves by the presence of irritating substances in the intestinal canal, such as indigestible food, acid drinks, hardened feces, gases, morbid secretions, worms, medicines, or poisons. It may proceed from an irritation of the central nervous system reflected to, and manifesting itself in the intestinal nerves. It may be sympathetic, and produced by a morbid state of the adjacent abdominal viscera, at times, perhaps, through the intervention of the central nervous system.

1. Colic, owing to food difficult of digestion, is very common, especially at the time of year when fruit is beginning to ripen. Sometimes it is caused by food which is not in itself injurious, but which is taken in quantities greater than the digestive organs can manage. Hence it is frequent in children at the breast who are overnourished; and in persons in delicate health with enfeebled digestive powers.

The form of colic under discussion is often attended with vomiting and diarrhœa; it may be of only a few hours' duration, or it may last for several days. It is for the most part readily relieved by the administration of a mild cathartic, joined to a small quantity, or, if the pain be very severe, to a full dose, of opium. An emetic is at times of signal service, and so are, as in all forms of colic, warm anodyne fomentations.

Colic arising from distention of the intestines with flatus, or "flatulent colic," is the result of the decomposition of food in the alimentary canal; sometimes, however, the gases are extricated from morbid secretions, or are exhaled directly from the blood-vessels. The abdomen is very tympanitic and greatly distended, and the flatus is from time to time discharged by the mouth or by the anus, with great relief to the patient. Hysterical persons are very subject to this form of colic, which yields, like the preceding variety, to opiates, purgatives, and warm fomentations, and to the administration of carminatives, or of stimulating injections.

Colic from accumulation of hardened feces is preceded by obstinate constipation, and is usually a tedious disorder. The accessions of pain are easily enough remedied by emptying the bowels, but they are constantly recurring.

Colic from the presence of morbid secretions in the intestinal canal is not so often encountered as that from indigestible food or retained fecal masses. Yet it is occasionally met with in cases of diarrhœa attended with a disordered state of the intestinal functions. And it is very probable that even in the so-termed bilious colic, the intestinal pain is not purely sympathetic, but is owing to the irritating character of the bile discharged into the intestine.

This "bilious colic" is often preceded by nausea, loss of appetite, and a coated tongue. The paroxysms of pain frequently go hand in hand with vomiting—first of the contents of the stomach, then of bile. They are in general accompanied or soon followed by a yellowish tinge of the conjunctiva, by tenderness in the region of the liver, and by a desire to go to stool. The bowels are, however, apt to be obstinately constipated. Bilious colic is common in malarious districts; it occurs especially during the summer and autumnal months, and frequently follows exposure. It sometimes begins with a chill, and, unlike the other forms of colic, it has as a companion febrile excitement, and a full, frequent pulse.

2. In the second class of cases to which allusion has been made, colic is dependent upon some abnormal condition affecting primarily the great centres of innervation. The colic arising from fright, from anger; that happening in nervous females and hypochondriac males; perhaps that proceeding from sudden exposure to cold; the form which is sometimes seen coexisting with neuralgic pains in other parts of the body,—in short, all those cases which are spoken of as nervous colic, might here be mentioned.

The attack is sudden, and not commonly of long duration; but it is very apt to be repeated, and requires strict attention to diet, proper exercise, and frequently iron, quinia, wine, or the vegetable tonics for its prevention.

The so-termed "metallic colics" are further instances of colic produced through agents which act primarily on the general nervous system. This is at any rate true of lead colic. Copper colic is not a purely neuralgic colic. It exhibits paroxysms of severe pain like those caused by the poisonous influence of lead; but it is attended with nausea, vomiting, diarrhœa, tenesmus, an abdomen distended and tender to the touch,—in other words, it is rather an inflammation of the intestine with colicky pain, than uncomplicated colic. Lead colic, on the other hand, is, so far as is known, a pure colic; for in the recorded examinations of those who have died of the disorder, no abnormal appearances were found in the intestines. The distinguishing marks of lead colic are the bluish-gray line along the gums; the contracted abdomen; the obstinate constipation; the great relief usually afforded to the pain by pressure; the duration of the pain; its marked and agonizing exacerbations; and the history of the case. The signs of the lead poisoning also manifest themselves in other parts of the body, but I shall not particularize them here, as the poisonous effects of lead will be elsewhere more specially considered.

3. Affections of various organs may give rise to colic, by sympathy, and generally through the intervention of the nervous system to which the irritation is first transferred, and from which it is then reflected. Thus colic is a not uncommon attendant on morbid states of the kidneys, of the

liver, of the bladder, the testicles, the ovaries, and on disordered menstruation. Yet we must not forget that the
pain, although spoken of as colic, is often not strictly intestinal, but is merely a pain radiating from the affected organs
themselves.

Colic arising in consequence of some abnormal state of the bowel.
—In the preceding illustrations of colic, the disorder was
viewed as occurring in a healthy bowel. But colic may have
only the significance of a symptom, and be combined with
an altered structure or a changed position of the intestine.
This is a point to which sufficient attention is not generally
paid in practice. The word colic suggests, to the minds of
most, a paroxysmal pain, constipation, and a spasm of the
bowel. Now, without discussing whether a true spasm be
a necessary attendant on the paroxysmal pain, it would
appear to be certain that there is nothing so absolutely
peculiar about the pain that its association with an involuntary muscular contraction of the intestine can be regarded as
invariable. We meet, indeed, with colicky pains, uudistin-
guishable from those of pure colic, linked to an organic disease of the bowel, and under circumstances some of which
forbid the idea of a spasm. They are encountered in dysentery; enteritis; hernia; ulceration; intussusception; strangulation; twisting; strictures; distention,—in fact, in the most
various morbid states of the intestine. And colic as a symptom can be discriminated, so far as the pain is concerned,
from colic as an idiopathic disorder, only by a careful study
of the history and the concomitant phenomena of the case.
In several of the maladies cited, however, the more transitory
nature of the pain,—or gripings, as they are termed,—in
others, the presence of fever and of tenderness, serve as
guides in diagnosis. Fever and soreness to the touch are
also met with in that form of inflammation of one or several
coats of the bowel which happens after exposure or after the
retrocession of rheumatism from some external part, and
which is commonly known as rheumatic or inflammatory
colic.

Having thus indicated the various forms of colic; having
alluded to the relation they bear to structural diseases of the

intestines, and to affections of adjacent viscera; it is unnecessary to re-examine the field and point out how wide its extent is from a diagnostic point of view.   I shall only here
again insist on the necessity of tracing out in every case, as
far as possible, the cause of the painful malady, so as to know
if any serious mischief lie at the bottom of it; and will but
add a few words with reference to the disorders with which
uncomplicated colic, or that which is held to be purely spasmodic, may be confounded.   They are:

GASTRALGIA;
PERFORATION OF THE INTESTINE;
STRANGULATED HERNIA;
PASSAGE OF GALL-STONES;
NEPHRALGIA;
SPASM OF THE BLADDER;
UTERINE COLIC;
NEURALGIA OF THE DORSAL AND LUMBAR NERVES;
ABDOMINAL ANEURISM AND TUMORS; DISEASES OF THE
   SPINE;
ENTERITIS AND PERITONITIS.

Gastralgia.—In gastralgia or gastrodynia the pain is seated
in the epigastric region; whereas in colic it is either in the
neighborhood of the umbilicus, or rapidly shifts its position
from that point to different parts of the abdomen, and is
often connected with a spasmodic contraction of the abdominal muscles.   Again, the history in cases of gastralgia; the
fact that the attacks happen most frequently after meals;
their association with signs of a diseased stomach,—indicate
the organ in which the paroxysms of pain arise.

Perforation of the Intestine.—When paroxysms of pain have
their origin in perforation of the intestine, the extreme prostration and collapse show that they are not produced by a
harmless disorder like colic.   Further, the abdominal distress is in such cases preceded by symptoms of a diseased
state of the stomach or intestines; and if the patient live
sufficiently long after the accident, the pain is followed by
great distention of the abdomen and extreme tenderness,—
in fact, by the signs of peritonitis.   However, the differential diagnosis is occasionally very difficult.   Especially is it

so in typhoid fever; for in this affection colic is readily induced, or perforation of the intestine may be brought on by
very slight exciting causes, and, moreover, peritonitis, so
several excellent observers think, may occur without perforation.

Strangulated Hernia.—All mechanical obstructions of the
intestine will lead to paroxysms of intestinal pain. They
are met with in cases of intussusception and ileus; they are
equally frequent in cases of strangulated hernia. In all, the
obstinate constipation must arouse suspicion regarding the
true nature of the complaint. But to detect a hernia, a
local examination is required; and a careful search at the
usual seats of this affection ought, therefore, to be made in
every instance of severe or protracted colic. Persons have
lost their lives in consequence of the practitioner neglecting, until too late, this simple precaution against disastrous
error.

Passage of Gall-stones.—The passage of a gall-stone is generally attended with paroxysms of intense pain which might
be readily mistaken for colic. There is, as a rule, the same
absence of fever and of tenderness. Indeed, pressure is often
resorted to in order to mitigate the suffering, and thus the
resemblance to colic is heightened. The points of distinction
from colic are, the position of the pain in the epigastric
region; its sudden commencement and sudden termination;
the severe nausea and vomiting attending the attack; the
jaundice; and the voiding of gall-stones with the stools. The
latter sign, however, though a positive one, assists less in the
discrimination of the disorder than would appear at first sight;
partly because it does not serve as a means of indicating the
nature of the affection until its close, partly because the stone
often escapes detection in the feces. The other circumstances
have, therefore, a more available diagnostic value. Yet even
they do not enable us to distinguish positively between the
transit of a biliary concretion from the gall-bladder to the
intestine, and the bilious colic which is joined to derangement of the function of the liver. The repetition of the attack
is always a strong reason for suspecting it to be owing to a
discharge of calculi from the gall-bladder; and so are severe

retching and vomiting, the sudden supervention of jaundice, and the localized epigastric pain. But these phenomena, too, it may here be mentioned, are produced by hepatic neuralgia, which in very rare cases is believed to happen independently of gall-stones. And there is nothing by which we can discriminate this malady—the very existence of which is indeed denied—except by its recurrence after certain intervals, the alternations with other affections of the nervous system, and by the slightest touching of the part inducing at times the acute pains.*

Where the gall-stones are large and have become impacted in their course toward the intestine, they give rise to inflammation which may lead to ulceration and to the discharge of the concretion—generally then very large—into the intestine or stomach. Subsequently an obliteration of the duct may happen ; or the inflammation and ulceration of the duct may result in perforation into the peritoneum. In some cases the gall-stones are voided through the abdominal walls, in consequence of their having caused inflammation of the gall-bladder and subsequent adhesions to the abdominal parietes. The fistulous passages discharge pus and bile, and occasionally fresh concretions: they may last for years ; but in time they generally heal. As regards the other forms of fistulous communications alluded to, they very rarely present symptoms so peculiar as to warrant anything like a certain diagnosis.†

Nephralgia.—Paroxysms of pain with intervals of comparative ease and unassociated with fever occur in nephralgia, or pain of the kidney, and are, therefore, often mistaken for colic. Now, nephralgia is generally, although not invariably, caused by the passage of a calculus through the ureter. Its symptoms, besides the pain, are numbness of the thigh, nausea and vomiting, a constant desire to make water, and aching and drawing up of the testicle. The patient, as in colic, is restless, and seeks relief by frequently changing his position. The pain comes on suddenly, and is excruciating. It is felt

---

* See the cases of Budd, on Diseases of the Liver; of Andral, Clinique Médicale, tome ii.; and of Frerichs, Diseases of the Liver.

† See a collection of cases by Murchison, Edinb. Med. Journ., July, 1857.

in the loins, usually on one side, and shoots along the track
of the ureter to the corresponding hip and thigh. It sometimes extends to the pelvis or toward the umbilicus, and is
often attended with tenderness in the course of the ureter.
Occasionally it is almost exclusively felt at the hip. When
the stone reaches the bladder, the pain ceases as abruptly as
it began; though sometimes there is still discomfort produced
by the stone interfering with the act of micturition. During
the attack the urine is passed in small quantities at a time.
It is high colored; sometimes it contains a little blood. If it
be collected, and after all pain has disappeared be carefully
examined, a small, hard body or a sandy deposit is generally
detected, and reveals the cause of the past anguish. It is from
the presence of the sandy deposit that the complaint has received popularly the name of a fit of " the gravel."

From the description given it will be seen that, in several
respects, the disorder is exactly like intestinal colic. The
seat of the pain is a point of distinction; yet in neither complaint is the seat entirely characteristic. It is not always
strictly umbilical in colic; it is not always exactly in the
region of the ureter or kidney in nephralgia. Of more importance is the state of the urinary functions, which are comparatively undisturbed in colic. Again, the numbness of the
thigh and the retraction of the testicle are valuable diagnostic
marks; they would be absolutely decisive, were they constantly present in nephralgia.

Spasm of the Bladder.—The bladder is sometimes the site of
paroxysms of violent pain, supposed always to attend upon a
spasm of the viscus. There is an intense desire to urinate,
which the passing of water does not allay. The pain is not
steady; it has its intervals of cessation. It is accompanied
by a sense of constriction at or near the pelvis, and sometimes
by tenesmus, and may extend to the kidneys, to the thighs,
and to the sacrum: or the irritation may be communicated
to the penis, and cause erections. If the sphincters be involved, the urine cannot be voided. The bladder distends;
there is most intense anxiety with restlessness; the pulse is
feeble; the skin cold, and covered with clammy perspiration.

A spasm of the bladder may be caused by the presence of

a stone in it, or of irritating urine. It is also encountered in gout and hysteria, and as the result of stimulating diuretics. Violent fright, too, may occasion it. It sometimes proceeds from a disorder of adjacent structures, such as of the rectum, or of the uterus. Now and then, as Sir Benjamin Brodie pointed out, it is associated with inflammation or suppuration of the kidney, and the vesical pain is so intense that it draws off attention from the organ most affected. To distinguish it from colic is not difficult; the position of the pain and the disturbed condition of the urinary functions serve as guides. It resembles more closely nephralgia, and its treatment is much the same as that of this distressing complaint. It is palliated by hip-baths; by hot fomentations and mustard plasters applied over the seat of pain ; by warm water enemata; by the internal administration of ether and opium, or of Indian hemp; and, if need be, by the inhalation of ether or chloroform. Should symptoms of inflammation supervene, cupping or leeching the parts is, as in nephralgia, proper; and, indeed, if the case be of any duration, this is always, as a matter of precaution, advisable. As in nephralgia, too, after the fit is relieved, the important indication is to prevent its repetition by endeavoring to remove its source.

Uterine Colic.—The painful sensations experienced by some women at their menstrual periods may come on in paroxysms similar to those of colic. In truth, the pain is often spoken of as uterine colic, and at times continues for many days, persisting during the whole menstrual period, or even longer. In some of these cases the trouble is localized in the uterus ; in others more especially in the ovaries, which are then tender to the touch. Similar attacks of pain, also accompanied by congestion, or even by inflammation of the ovaries, are occasionally met with as the result of falls or of blows on the hypogastric region.

Now, with reference to the disorder first alluded to, or ordinary dysmenorrhœa, it may be generally easily discriminated from colic by its concurrence with the setting in of the menstrual flow; by the pain remitting rather than intermitting; by the seat of the pain in the pelvis, or the lower part of the abdomen; by its not uncommon association with sickness, nausea, and vomiting; and by the fact that all the signs of disordered menstruation have happened over and over again at the menstrual periods.

Where the ovaries are very much congested or inflamed, whether or not the affection exist in connection with dysmenorrhœa, or occur in consequence of other causes, among which gonorrhœa may be one, the pain, tenderness, and swelling in the hypogastric region; the not unusual numbness and flexed position of one or both thighs; the febrile irritation, and the hysterical symptoms; the retention of the urine; the violence of the paroxysms of pain, and the duration of the malady form a group of phenomena very dissimilar to those of ordinary cases of colic.

Neuralgia of the Dorsal and Lumbar Nerves; Abdominal Neuralgia.—The dorsal and lumbar nerves are subject to neuralgic affections, which exhibit, like colic, paroxysms of pain unaccompanied by fever. In truth, the resemblance to colic is so great that, until Valleix made abdominal neuralgias a subject of special study, their discrimination from colic was unsatisfactory, perhaps impossible. This distinguished observer has taught us to look for spots painful to the touch in the course of the aching nerves, and has shown that the disturbance of the nerves supplying the abdominal parietes manifests itself only on one side of the body, whereas, as is well known, an irritation of the intestinal nerves obeys no such law.

In neuralgia of the lumbar nerves, or lumbo-abdominal neuralgia, to employ the term sanctioned by Valleix, the pain is commonly felt in the hypogastric region, a little to one side of the median line. In this situation, too, there is localized soreness on pressure; the other tender spots are, generally, one a little to the outside of the first or second lumbar vertebra, and one immediately above the middle of the crest of the ilium. In women, who are by far the greatest sufferers from the disease, there is sometimes also a painful place about the middle of the Fallopian tube, or on the neck of the uterus; in men, a point on the scrotum is here and there found sore to the touch. These spots of tenderness serve as characteristic signs; and they enable us to separate neuralgia not only from colic, but also from lumbago, and from rheumatism of the abdominall walls.

Besides these forms of neuralgia, we find other kinds of abdominal neuralgia, which may be mistaken for colic. They are attacks of pain affecting especially the mesenteric plexus or the solar plexus, happening in paroxysms of great severity, and attended with a sense of faintness and annihilation. The disorder is unconnected with lead poisoning or any of the causes which produce colic, is often excited by exertion, and is associated with debility and relieved by an antineuralgic treatment. In some cases the painful disorder is clearly of malarial origin; and in every case we must lay great stress on the frequent recurrence of the pain and on the history to enable us to discriminate between the neuralgic complaint and colic. The distinction from gastralgia can only be made by the more marked gastric symptoms, and the absence of or the less decided prostration and sense of fainting in this malady.*

Abdominal Aneurism and Tumors; Diseases of the Spine.—In all of these we may find violent pain of a paroxysmal kind referred to various portions of the abdomen, and unaccompanied by fever. We judge that the pain is not colic, by its frequent repetition; by its want of association with intestinal or gastric disturbance; by its being, although liable to exacerbations, so steadily present at some part either of the spine or abdomen; and by the attending symptoms and signs occasioned by an abdominal tumor, or by a disease of the lower dorsal or of the lumbar vertebræ.

Enteritis and Peritonitis.—Inflammations of the intestines and peritoneum also give rise to severe abdominal pain. But it is more constant, linked to great tenderness, and, in acute cases, to symptoms of high febrile excitement. Thus enteritis and peritonitis belong to a different group of diseases—a group of inflammatory affections, which I shall describe somewhat at length, before contrasting the symptoms of inflammation of the intestines or of the peritoneum with those of colic.

---

* A number of cases of abdominal neuralgia are reported by Handfield Jones, in his Treatise on Functional Nervous Disorders; see, also, Porcher's cases in Am. Journ. of Med. Sciences, July, 1869.

Diseases attended with Pain and marked Tenderness in the Umbilical Region or diffused over the Abdomen.

Acute Enteritis.—Enteritis means now, by common consent, inflammation of the small intestine, and especially of the portion that lies between the duodenum and the colon. The morbid process may extend to the colon; if, however, it involve a large portion of the latter, it is colitis or dysentery, and not enteritis, with which we have to deal. There are two forms of enteritis: one in which the mucous membrane of the bowel is alone affected; the muco-enteritis, or the catarrhal inflammation of recent authors, the erythematous enteritis of Cullen. In the second, more than the mucous tunic is implicated; there is also inflammation of the submucous and muscular coats, or even of the serous investment of the bowel. To this variety of the complaint the term enteritis is by several writers restricted; and it is to this form of the malady, occurring acutely, that the description about to be given more particularly applies.

The symptoms of an acute attack of enteritis are those of colic, attended with fever and tenderness. The disorder may begin with the symptoms of colic, and in such cases the inflammation of the bowel is said to have supervened on colic; or it may set in with a chill and fever, and extreme thirst.

When the disease is fully established, the fever runs high; the pulse, tense and full at the onset, becomes small and wiry, although it remains frequent. There are nausea and vomiting, and sometimes most distressing fits of retching, produced either by sympathy, or because the stomach shares in the inflammation. The tongue is clean and of natural appearance, or it is covered with a white coat, or again it may be red and dry. The bowels are constipated; sometimes, however, there is diarrhœa, or constipation alternating with diarrhœa. The stools are, in consequence, of varying consistency and color; they may contain a small quantity of blood, but they very rarely contain pus. The appetite is completely lost; the thirst is unceasing; the pain, as in colic, is paroxysmal. It commences near the umbilicus, and thence may shift to various parts of the abdomen, but not to the epigastrium ; yet it is not so violent, nor does it cease so entirely as in colic, but rather exacerbates, and then changes to a dull feeling of distress. It is greatly increased by pressure, and the patient seeks relief, as in peritonitis, by lying on his back with his thighs flexed, so as to relax the abdominal muscles. Toward the right of the umbilicus, it is not uncommon to find a marked pulsation, as if from throbbing of the abdominal aorta or of its large branches,—a sign to which, if I mistake not, Dr. Stokes* first directed attention. This pulsation may be very annoying. In looking over the notes of cases on which the description of the symptoms of enteritis just given is based, I find one in which neither the thirst, nor the pain, nor the nausea and vomiting occasioned as much distress as the violent throbbing in the abdomen.

In those instances of the malady which advance to a fatal termination, the pulse becomes quick and irregular, and loses its tenseness; hiccough appears; the abdomen swells; the features are haggard, and expressive of great suffering; and the patient's strength becomes gradually exhausted. The worst and most hopeless cases of the disease are those dependent on mechanical obstruction of the bowel, whether it proceed from organized bands in which a loop of intestine is caught, or from invagination, or from accumulation of hardened feces, or from a hernial strangulation.

Among the symptoms and signs of enteritis mentioned, the pain is one of the most important for diagnosis. It is never absent, save in some rare instances in which the inflammation is very intense at the onset.† Still more important is the great tenderness. This enables us to say that the case, in spite of the colicky pains, is not colic. It warns us not to resort to stimulants, and remedies merely to relieve the seemingly spasmodic pain. It tells us, when it succeeds to what began as ordinary colic, that inflammation of the bowel has supervened and requires immediate attention. It ad-

---

* Article " Enteritis," in Cyclop. of Pract. Med.
† Andral, Pathologie Interne, tome i. page 47.

monishes us not to administer strong cathartics to overcome the constipation which appears in consequence of the severe inflammation.

The disease in its violent form just described bears a close resemblance to peritonitis. We shall presently see what are its distinguishing marks. But there is, as above stated, another variety of the disease, a mild variety, or *muco-enteritis*, in which the disturbance is limited to the mucous membrane. The main features of this disorder are the same, but they stand out in less bold relief. There are griping pains, a slight soreness to the touch, general uneasiness, loss of appetite, thirst, nausea, and sometimes vomiting. But we find only slight fever; or rather, the skin is dry and becomes hot toward night, and the febrile excitement remits in the morning. Diarrhœa is always present, and the stools are sometimes very offensive. This form of the disease may terminate, as the severer inflammation generally does, in less than a week; yet it may persist for several weeks, and thus gradually lapse into a chronic complaint. It is common in children, especially during dentition. It is also observed when irritating food or secretions occupy the alimentary canal for any length of time, or after exposure, and as an attendant upon the exanthemata and typhoid fever. Indeed, it is sometimes difficult, particularly in children, to know whether we have to deal with a case of muco-enteritis, or with the intestinal complication of enteric fever. The state of the cerebral functions, and the pain and gurgling in the iliac fossæ may clear up the doubt; yet in some cases nothing but the eruption and the course of the symptoms will do so.

Acute Peritonitis.—As in acute enteritis, so in acute peritonitis, pain and tenderness are the most significant symptoms. To these are joined fever, distention of the abdomen, and frequently cold sweats, nausea, vomiting, and obstinate constipation.

To understand these symptoms, it is necessary to be acquainted with the morbid anatomy of the disease. I shall endeavor to sketch it in a few words. Acute inflammation attacking the peritoneum may be confined to one spot; but it is very apt, even if limited at its onset, to spread over the entire membrane. It commences with injection of the vessels. This is soon followed by an exudation of lymph, or of lymph and serum; or the effused fluid may be hemorrhagic, or purulent, or ichorous. The last-mentioned varieties occur in depraved states of the blood, or in asthenic conditions of the system. The inflammation, even when general, is usually most marked at one or several portions of the membrane. It leads to paralysis of the intestine, and to its distention by gas.

The effects of the exudation are somewhat different according to its kind and amount. If much liquid be effused, the abdomen is swollen; but the fluid, as a rule, is readily taken up again. When the inflammation is followed by the pouring out of coagulable lymph, the two surfaces of the peritoneum are very prone to become either partially or generally agglutinated, and strings of fibrin stretch between the intestinal coils. Nor is the lymph very likely to be re-absorbed. On the contrary, it is often transformed into tissue, and gives rise to induration and roughening of the membrane, or to a permanent attachment of its two layers, or to fibrous bands fastening one portion of intestine to the other. When the serous membrane adheres in spots, it sometimes incloses pus in the sacs thus formed. These abscesses may discharge into the bowel, or, as Rokitansky tells us, they may evacuate their contents through the abdominal parietes. Hence the results of acute peritonitis do not pass off with the attack itself. Indeed, these sequelæ may be as grave as the original malady.

But to return to the symptoms of acute peritonitis, and especially to those characterizing the form in which the inflammation has involved the whole membrane or a very large part of it. The disease begins with chilly sensations or a protracted rigor. To these succeed fever, and abdominal pain and distention. The fever runs high at the onset; it exhibits a dry, burning skin, a pulse frequent, but, as in most of the acute inflammations of the mucous and serous membranes below the diaphragm, small and wiry. However, both the character of the pulse and the temperature of the skin change as the dangerous malady progresses. The pulse

will be less tense and more developed as the inflammation
subsides, or exceedingly feeble and flickering if the disorder
proceed toward a fatal termination.   The skin of the extremities becomes cool, and is frequently covered with cold
sweats.   The features are sharpened and wear the look of
death, even in cases which ultimately recover.

The pain is constant and very severe.   It may exacerbate,
but it never intermits.   At first the pain is confined to a particular point; but as the inflammation extends, so it extends
over the whole abdomen.   It is increased by the slightest
pressure, be that pressure exerted by the hand or by movements of any kind.   To obviate the pressure, the patient lies
on his back with his thighs flexed, and, however tired of retaining the same position, he does not change it.   The descent of the diaphragm augments the pain; instinctively,
therefore, he refrains from drawing long breaths, and his
respiration is short and frequent.   If closely watched, it is
found to be purely thoracic, the abdominal walls neither
rising nor falling during the respiratory acts.

The abdominal distention is in part owing to meteorism,
in part to the liquid effused into the peritoneum.   Percussion
tells us in individual cases how far each acts as a cause of
the enlargement, by the tympanitic or the dull sound elicited.
Palpation, too, reveals the presence of liquid.   Yet neither
percussion nor palpation ought to be employed, save when
really necessary for diagnosis, and then only with the greatest
care, on account of the pain they occasion.   The fluid does
not gravitate as invariably as in ascites to the lower portion
of the belly.   It is often caught in sacs formed by the membrane adhering in spots; and thus circumscribed dulness
may be found at one or several parts of the abdomen.
Sometimes the roughening of the membrane gives rise to a
distinct friction sound.

Independently of the abdominal pain and swelling, we
meet, in acute peritonitis, with constipation, nausea and vomiting, headache, a suppression of the urinary discharge, and
in rare instances with priapism; of these symptoms, constipation is the most constant.   The bowels are never relaxed,
except in the puerperal form of the malady.   The constipa-

tion is caused by the paralyzed state of the intestine, to portions of which the inflammation may spread; or by the lymph gluing together the coils of the bowels, and thus interfering with their peristaltic action.

Death in acute peritonitis is commonly preceded by enormous tumefaction of the belly, by cold sweats, a pinched countenance, a rapid, flickering pulse. When recovery takes place—unfortunately a rarer issue of the malady than its fatal termination—it is commonly very slow and gradual. The symptoms diminish one by one; they do not cease suddenly; and often morbid conditions remain which prolong greatly the patient's illness, and may lead in themselves to a disastrous result. It is, therefore, impossible to foretell the duration either of the acute disease or of its consequences. Andral fixes the average length of an acute attack at between six and nine days, and of a subacute attack at from twenty to thirty days. But the nature of the malady is such, that many cases last a longer, many a much shorter period.

Acute peritonitis arises occasionally from exposure to cold and wet; much oftener in consequence of injuries to the abdomen, such as blows, stabs, or kicks; or from perforation or laceration of some of the abdominal organs, and discharge of their contents into the peritoneal cavity. It also results from some peculiar and poisoned state of the blood, as, for example, that frightful form of peritonitis occurring in childbed fever. It sometimes originates from an inflammation of the abdominal viscera, especially of the spleen, intestines, or uterus and its appendages, spreading to their serous covering, and thence extending more or less rapidly. Again, other morbid states of the abdominal organs, such as cysts of the ovaries, intestinal intussusception, or strangulated hernia, may compress or irritate the membrane, and lead to inflammatory action. Owing to these diverse sources, peritonitis presents varieties which exhibit points of difference sufficient to require special notice.

The inflammation produced by *extravasation* into the peritoneal sac is characterized by its sudden development. The matters extravasated may be blood, or bile, or urine, or the contents of the stomach. Most frequently perforation of the stomach or intestine lies at the bottom of the mischief. Whatever its cause, the perforation is immediately followed by collapse; and tenderness and distention of the abdomen soon make their appearance. Yet peritonitis may set in rapidly in cases in which there has been no rupture; and, on the other hand, in rare, very rare instances, the contents of the alimentary canal may be discharged into the sac without giving rise to inflammation.*

The peritonitis of childbed fever, or *puerperal peritonitis*, is principally distinguished by its occurring during the puerperal state. Its symptoms are, so far as the peritoneal inflammation is concerned, exactly those of any other kind of peritonitis, excepting that diarrhœa, instead of constipation, is commonly present. The uterus or the uterine appendages are generally, but not invariably, first attacked; and it is in these regions that pain and tenderness are first felt. The inflammation begins in those structures and spreads to their serous investment, or it may be primarily seated in that investment; in either case it soon involves the entire membrane.

But, independently of the symptoms of the local disorder, there are phenomena which clearly belong to the general puerperal disease, of which the inflammation of the peritoneum is but a local expression; there are evidences of a poisoned state of the blood and a general disturbance of the system. How else account for the exudations into the pericardium and pleura being like those on the peritoneum? How else account for the black vomit, and for the delirium,— symptoms far from seldom met with in puerperal peritonitis, but not in the purely local disease? How else account for the uniform type exhibited by the malady in some epidemics, and its varied form in others?

What the poison is which determines the terrible disease, we cannot here inquire. It may be, as some think, atmospheric; it may be, as others hold, the absorption of putrid matter from the uterus; it may be an animal virus trans-

---

* Cases reported by Bardeleben and Siebert, quoted in Henoch's Clinic of Abdominal Diseases. Instances of rapid peritonitis without perforation are given by Thirial, l'Union Médicale, 1853.

mitted by the hand of the attendant; the complaint may be, as is now so generally believed, closely analogous to erysipelatous inflammation; it may be eminently contagious; it may not be so at all.   These are not points, however important their solution to the well-being of thousands of lying-in women, which concern us here.   For diagnostic purposes, it is of more consequence to know that the distemper prevails epidemically and endemically, that its features change, and that the puerperal peritonitis of one year is not the puerperal peritonitis of another; in short, that while childbed fever, whatever its cause, occasions peritonitis, peritonitis does not constitute childbed fever.

Taking this view of the disease, it is obvious that those sporadic cases of peritonitis occasionally encountered after delivery, in which the inflammation has either become general or remains limited to the womb and its surroundings, are very different from the pestilential disorder which attacks numbers of parturient females simultaneously, or in rapid succession.   And the inference from these statements is, that under the general name of puerperal peritonitis are grouped together several forms of peritoneal inflammation, having not one, but several causes, accompanying not the same, but diverse constitutional states, and presenting not always identical, but at times most opposite indications for treatment.

Partial or *local peritonitis* is almost invariably owing to a pre-existing morbid condition of some abdominal viscus.   Sometimes the circumscribed inflammation is protective rather than calculated to work mischief.   It arrests a destructive perforation of the membrane, or it limits the matter discharged to a certain spot; it may at least do so for a time, for general peritonitis is very apt ultimately to follow.

Partial peritonitis often pursues a subacute rather than an acute course.   It may end in adhesions or lapse into a chronic state.   Its symptoms are much the same as those of a more general inflammation: the same fever and constipation, the same pain and tenderness.   The fever does not, however, run so high, and the pain and the great tenderness are much more localized.   The abdomen, also, is not so swollen nor so tympanitie.   But perhaps even more frequently than in general peritonitis are found accurately limited spots of dulness on percussion corresponding to circumscribed collections of pus in the peritoneal cavity.

Partial peritonitis is more liable than the general disease to be confounded with other disorders. Yet error can hardly arise, or, should it arise, it is not of much consequence, provided we bear in mind that it is precisely with the morbid states of the viscera which lie below the peritoneum that the circumscribed inflammation of the serous membrane is usually connected, and that local peritonitis, therefore, frequently attends the very disorders from which it is sought to be distinguished. Let us, however, examine into some of the complaints with which peritonitis, whether local or general, may be confounded. They are:

GASTRITIS;

ENTERITIS;

METRITIS;

CYSTITIS AND DISTENTION OF THE BLADDER;

RHEUMATISM OF THE ABDOMINAL WALLS;

ABDOMINAL HYSTERIA;

COLIC.

Gastritis.—Acute inflammation of the stomach can scarcely be mistaken for inflammation of the peritoneum, provided attention be paid to the history of the case and the seat of the pain. The former disorder commences with vomiting, and this continues a prominent symptom throughout; whereas vomiting is neither so constant, nor does it occur so early, in peritonitis. The pain and tenderness are limited to the region of the stomach in gastritis; they are diffused and accompanied by general abdominal enlargement in peritonitis. They may, it is true, be localized when the peritonitis is partial. But acute inflammation of the gastric peritoneum is hardly encountered, save as an attendant on severe inflammation of the stomach, or on a destruction of its coats. And in the first instance it is practically gastritis we are dealing with; in the second, the history of the case, the sudden increase of the pain and tenderness, and the development of fever will go far toward evincing the nature of the disorder. However, if a partial peritonitis occurring in consequence of serious gastric disease be subacute or chronic, it eludes discovery.

Enteritis.—Enteritis differs from general peritonitis by the less extended tenderness; by the seat of the pain near the umbilicus, and its more paroxysmal character; by the comparative absence of tympanites and abdominal tumefaction; and by the greater prominence of nausea and vomiting. It is, moreover, a disease far less violent and dangerous than acute peritonitis; yet it cannot be distinguished with certainty from the partial form of this disorder. In truth, so far as the diagnosis of enteritis is concerned, it is not of much importance that it should be; for inflammation of the intestine is generally associated with a local peritonitis, to which some of its symptoms are clearly owing.

Metritis.—Inflammation of the womb is not likely to be mistaken for general peritonitis; the pain on pressure, which they have in common, is confined in the former disease to the uterus and its annexes, and there is little or no tympanites. It is thus, and thus only, that the acute metritis of childbed fever may be distinguished from the acute general peritonitis of the same malady. For otherwise the resemblance is strong; in both, the disease is ushered in by chills, and the lochial discharge soon diminishes or ceases. When the puerperal malady attacks, as it often does, the uterus as well as the whole peritoneal surface, the signs of inflammation of the serous membrane mask those of inflammation of the womb.

Now, a local inflammation of the peritoneum occurs still more constantly as an attendant on inflammation of the womb and its appendages, whether the disorder of the sexual organs be or be not puerperal. It frequently leads to collections of pus, which can be readily felt through the parietes of the abdomen, or through the rectum and the vagina, and which sometimes discharge into the bowel or vagina after a lingering sickness. The proofs that the uterus is involved in these cases of partial peritonitis, are the signs of its disordered functions and the excessive pain occasioned by pressing on the cervix during an examination per vaginam.

31

Cystitis and Distention of the Bladder.—Both inflammation and distention of the bladder are occasionally mistaken for general acute peritonitis. An acute inflammation of the bladder gives rise to frequent calls to pass urine: yet the act is performed with great difficulty, and in severe cases may become impossible; the bladder distends; a sense of uneasiness is felt in the perineum; the region above the pubis becomes tender to the touch, and sounds dull on percussion; the unhappy sufferer is very restless and distressed; he has the excited pulse and the hot skin of an inflammatory fever; at times vomiting and hiccough supervene; and death is preceded by gradually deepening coma. Such cases resemble in some respects those of peritonitis with suppression of the urinary discharge and with strangury. But the urine which is voided in peritonitis is simply high colored, like that of any febrile state. In cystitis it contains large quantities of mucus and pus, and often blood and crystals of phosphates. Again, the abdominal tenderness is localized, and is frequently accompanied by a smarting in the course of the urethra. Neither of these signs is encountered in peritoneal inflammation. The disturbance of the urinary organs which not unfrequently takes place in the latter disorder has been variously explained; it has been attributed to inflammation of the part of the peritoneum covering the bladder, or its immediate neighborhood. But whether it be so or not, is as uncertain as whether it be an inflammation of the serous investment of the stomach which occasions the nausea and vomiting of the same disease.

An overdistention of the bladder, not the result of inflammation of its coats, may produce a local tenderness spread over a considerable portion of the lower part of the abdomen. But the outline of the dulness coextensive with that of the tenderness; the fact that the patient has generally not passed urine for a considerable time and the sudden cessation of the supposed peritonitis on passing a catheter, show the true nature of the malady.*

---

* A case of this kind, occurring after delivery, is given by Lever, Guy's Hospital Reports, 2d Series, vol. viii. page 41.

Inflammation and Abscess in the Abdominal Muscles.—When the abdominal walls become inflamed, symptoms are occasioned which are not always easily distinguished from those of acute peritonitis.   The disease is attended with some fever, with pain increased by movement, by the act of coughing, and by pressure, and sometimes with excessive tenderness.   The seat of the inflammation is generally the rectus muscle and the surrounding cellular tissue.   The parts on one side of the umbilicus are most commonly attacked, and it is there that a hard swelling is perceived, over which the skin is rather hot and sometimes red.   The tumefaction gradually disappears by resolution, or else fluctuation becomes, from day to day, more distinct, showing that suppuration is taking place; and the pus being discharged, immediate relief follows, and the pain and febrile symptoms instantly cease.

Now, the disorder rarely runs a very acute course; it lasts at least a week or two; and often much longer.   Where much of the muscle is involved, the complaint closely simulates peritonitis; more, however, the partial than the general kind. Where the inflammation of the muscle is not extended, the resemblance to inflammatory affections of the organs lying underneath the point of tenderness is even greater than to inflammation of the peritoneum.   Hepatitis, splenitis, and gastritis have been mistaken for the affection of the abdominal parietes.   These errors can only be avoided by taking into account the absence of disturbed function of the suspected viscus; often, too, the peculiar swelling furnishes a clue to the real nature of the case.

But can we distinguish, with anything like certainty, between these abscesses in the abdominal walls and instances of partial peritonitis leading to collections of pus in the peritoneal cavity?   I believe not: for in both there is a tumefaction; in both the general symptoms are much the same; and, as happens sometimes in peritoneal abscesses, the pus presses its way through the parietes of the abdomen.   How, then, are we to know where was the seat of its formation? Whenever we find a swelling which has come on gradually, or has followed a blow or kick on the abdomen, or a swelling which is very hard before fluctuation appears; whenever the softening of the tumor is immediately preceded by distinct chills, and the skin covering it is tense, and heated, or reddish; whenever there is nothing pointing to the occurrence of partial peritonitis, as an attendant on visceral disease, or as a consequence of an attack of general peritonitis,—we may infer, from the history and the signs, that the affection lies in the abdominal walls. But the skin is not always discolored nor hot; the commencement of the swelling is sometimes veiled in obscurity, and an error in diagnosis is not discreditable, because it is unavoidable.

But it is not every case of abscess in the walls which is attended with symptoms that render it likely to be mistaken for inflammation, or the results of inflammation. Sometimes the preceding tumefaction is so hard, or it is so long before the process of suppuration sets in, that the affection is much more liable to be confounded with abdominal tumors. The most trustworthy points of difference are furnished by a study of the history of the case, and of the mode of invasion; by the slow growth of the tumor on the one hand, its far more rapid growth on the other; and by the absence, or at all events the comparative absence, of signs denoting serious disturbance in one or several of the abdominal viscera. Then, in doubtful cases, the exploring needle may be of use. The fluid thus obtained shows, under the microscope, shreds of broken-down muscle and of areolar tissue, mixed, if suppuration have commenced, with pus. Again, stress may be laid on the occurrence of chills preceding the softening of the mass. In some patients the inflammation is unaccompanied by any appreciable signs; it leads to gradual changes in the muscular fibres, which do not reveal themselves until the disorganized muscle gives way. The fibres undergo softening or a true fatty metamorphosis, and the slightest force suffices to produce a rupture. Not a few cases have been reported in which one of the recti muscles has been torn asunder during a fit of coughing. The seat of laceration is generally about midway between the umbilicus and the pubis, a little to one side of the median line; the rent fills with blood, occasioning a circumscribed swelling and rigidity of the abdomen. There is sometimes pain, with nausea, vomiting, and obstinate constipation.   Nay, the symptoms have mimicked so closely a strangulated ventral hernia as to have led to the performance of an operation.*

Rheumatism of the Abdominal Walls.—Occasionally rheumatism attacks the abdominal muscles, and gives rise to local symptoms similar to those of peritonitis. But the pain is not so constant, nor is it spontaneous, as in this disorder. It is also less affected by movements or by pressure. Not that these diminish it; on the contrary, they aggravate it. But deep pressure causes little or no more pain than slight pressure; and it is only during certain motions—when the muscles are placed on the stretch—that the pain is severe, or sometimes, indeed, at all produced.

The pain is often one-sided, or, at any rate, much more marked on one side, and we find no meteorism and but slight fever, and not the anxious expression of countenance of peritonitis. So strong a degree of similarity may, however, exist between the two diseases, as to keep judgment in suspense. In such cases it is better to treat the disorder as if it were inflammation of the peritoneum. In point of fact, it may happen that such inflammation does succeed to the rheumatic affection of the abdominal muscles, and this occurs chiefly when the disturbance in the muscles forms part of an attack of acute rheumatism having a decided tendency to shift its seat.

Abdominal Hysteria.—No disease simulates peritonitis so closely as hysteria. The abdomen may be extremely painful to the touch, swollen and distended with gas, fever may set in, and yet the whole disorder be purely hysterical. To illustrate which I quote the following instance of this remarkable affection :

An unmarried woman, twenty years of age, placed herself under my care, on account of extreme tenderness of the abdo-

---

* Richardson's case, Amer. Journ. of the Med. Sciences, January, 1857. Further instances of this accident are given by Virchow, in the "Würzburg. Verhandl.," Band vii.   The description of abscesses in the abdominal parietes I have drawn from cases coming under my own notice, from manuscript notes taken by Dr. J. K. Kane, at the Philadelphia Hospital, and from the cases collected in the Dictionnaire des Dictionnaires de Médecine, art. "Abdomen."

men and febrile irritation, both of which had become developed in a few days. The abdomen was swollen and tympanitic, and so sensitive that it would not bear the pressure of
her clothes; the pulse was frequent; the skin dry and hot;
the tongue was slightly coated; the bowels constipated; the
countenance expressive of distress. Here was certainly a
group of symptoms like those of acute peritonitis. But the
absence of the wiry pulse, the comparatively slight fever,—
slighter, at any rate, than was to be expected from such general and great tenderness,—and the expression of countenance,
which was not that of acute inflammation of the peritoneum,
arrested my attention. I inquired more closely into the case,
and found that the patient had had similar attacks previously;
that they had come on sometimes shortly before, sometimes
shortly after, her menstrual period; but that for several months
her menses had ceased to flow. The abdominal tenderness
was in reality, as she represented it to be, very great; yet
strong pressure produced no more pain than the lightest
touch. Nor was the pain increased by deep inspiration, or
by coughing, or by extending the thighs. Taking all these
circumstances into account, as well as her age and sex, instead of treating her for acute peritonitis, cold water injections, mild purgatives, and a mixture of assafetida and vale-
rian were employed. Under these remedies, all the symptoms
of the apparent peritonitis speedily vanished.

Yet all cases of abdominal hysteria do not pass off so
quickly; sometimes they are much more persistent. Then,
however, they are from the onset unattended with fever, or
the fever soon ceases, which fact would in itself clear up any
doubt as to the non-inflammatory nature of the complaint.
The absence of febrile excitement, too, especially if taken in
connection with the several localized and more or less distinctly circumscribed spots of tenderness, enables us to
distinguish between peritonitis and those instances of neuralgia of nerves supplying the abdominal parietes, to which
women who are laboring under disorders of the uterus are so
liable.

  Colic.—As already stated, the pain of colic is paroxysmal,
and not attended with fever, or with much, if any, tender-

ness; while it is hardly necessary to repeat that the pain of an inflamed peritoneum is constant, and associated with the greatest tenderness and with fever. Cases of colic do indeed occur in which we find fever and some tenderness; but these signs then are out of proportion to the amount of pain. The pulse is not wiry, nor the tenderness so exquisite or so diffused. Further, it is not at all unlikely that in such cases the peritoneum is really in parts injected and slightly inflamed. We know that even a more severe form of peritonitis may follow colic; why should not an injection of the membrane frequently coexist?

The same remarks are applicable to those severe paroxysmal pains which accompany the passage of gall-stones or of urinary concretions, or which occur at the menstrual periods. They are frequently spoken of as varieties of colic, and, so far as their discrimination from peritonitis goes, there is no difference—it rests on the same grounds precisely; for when there is fever or tenderness on pressure, it is likely that inflammation has been set up in those parts in which, or in the neighborhood of which, the pain is felt. In the so-called uterine colic, an injection of the peritoneum has positively been demonstrated.

Chronic Peritonitis.—An acute attack of peritonitis may imperceptibly assume a chronic form. The fever gradually disappears, or at all events lessens; but the exudations into the peritoneal cavity, whether organized or not, remain, and so do some abdominal pain and tenderness. In this condition the patient may continue for many months; now and then a fresh inflammation starting up in the peritoneum and giving rise to acute symptoms, or an intercurrent severe diarrhœa leading to rapid loss of strength. In all such cases, indeed, if they last for any length of time, debility and emaciation become marked symptoms; then hectic fever is observed; the legs become edematous; and the patient may die, worn out and presenting the symptoms of pyemic poisoning. When recovery takes place, the exudation into the peritoneal cavity is either discharged through adjacent viscera; or it may be gradually reabsorbed; or it may be transformed, more or less quickly, into tissue. When the disease terminates in this way, it is apt to leave traces of its action in a chronic thickening and roughening of the peritoneum.

But chronic peritonitis now and then comes on, and ends in a different fashion. It is insidious in its approach, and its fatal termination is preceded by evident signs of tubercular or cancerous deposits in the abdominal cavity or in the lungs. The disease is not then simply chronic peritonitis, but chronic peritonitis in connection with a cachexia. Cases of the kind are commonly of long duration. They are attended with ascites, and often with very considerable abdominal distention. I shall, therefore, postpone most of what I have to say about their diagnosis until I come to abdominal enlargements, and shall then consider what differences there are between these various forms of chronic peritoneal affections and other disorders leading to ascites, and to consequent abdominal distention.

Diseases attended with Pain and Tenderness in the Right Iliac Fossa.

Affections of the Cæcum and its Appendix.—Standing clinically in close connection with inflammatory affections of the peritoneum, are the disorders of the cæcum and its appendix. They frequently give rise to a partial peritoneal inflammation; they sometimes lead to fatal general peritonitis. Their chief manifestations are localized pain and tenderness, and a tumefaction in the right iliac fossa. In truth, they are the disorders which pre-eminently occasion signs of disturbance in this region.

Inflammation is the most common of the morbid processes affecting the cæcum and its appendix. This inflammation may be limited to the cæcum; it may have its seat entirely in the appendix. It may be equally violent in both; it may cause ulceration in one and not in the other. It may originate in the loose areolar tissue around the cæcum; it may begin in the cæcum, and spread from its peritoneal covering to the areolar tissue of the iliac fossa. Here are certainly conditions which are different, and between which it would be very desirable, in a prognostic point of view, to be able to discriminate. But such discrimination is clinically, for the most part, impossible. If an inflammatory affection of this out-of-the-way corner of the alimentary tube has been detected, we cannot, with any certainty, go further. The history and progress of the disease may determine the exact diagnosis; but we cannot always rely upon their aid.

Inflammation of the cæcum or of its appendix is, in the majority of instances, caused by accumulation of hardened feces, or by hardened bodies which have there become impacted. Both structures are also at times found highly inflamed in cases of dysentery. But here the inflammation forms part of a more general inflammation of the bowel; and as it is not my present object to consider the disorders in which the cæcum may participate, but rather those in which it is chiefly concerned, and without any other part of the tube being implicated, such accidental inflammation need not be further alluded to.

Now, the morbid phenomena which attend inflammation of the cæcum or its appendix will vary materially according to the acuteness of the disorder, its course, its termination in ulceration, the presence or absence of peritonitis, and the extent and rapidity of appearance of this dangerous complication. Sometimes the cæcal disease sets in suddenly with all the symptoms and signs of a severe local peritonitis in the right iliac fossa. There is pain, with tenderness, a chill, and fever; and the pain and tenderness soon spread, as the peritoneal inflammation becomes more general. But usually the complaint is of more gradual formation, and presents the following history and symptoms: the patient has been suffering for some time from constipation, or alternately from diarrhœa and constipation. He has a dull pain referred principally to the iliac fossa, and sometimes radiating to the hips. When this region is examined, it is tender to the touch, full and hard, and sounds dull on percussion, while around the dulness there is a very tympanitic sound, if the gut, as it often is, be much distended with gas. Colicky pains occur from time to time, but are mainly confined to the lower portion of the abdomen. In such cases there has been, in all likelihood, a distention of the cæcum, which favors an accumulation of feces, and these again have acted as exciting causes to an inflammation; or foreign bodies, such as cherry-stones or concretions of various kinds, have become impacted in the cæcum or the vermiform appendix, and have gradually provoked the morbid action.

In its further progress the case exhibits varied features: it may end in resolution; or the tenderness in the iliac fossa may become greater, and vomiting, fever, and the marked signs of a local peritonitis appear; or ulceration of the bowel, and more frequently still of the appendix, may allow a discharge of extraneous matter into the peritoneal cavity, which produces violent general peritonitis; or, again, the bowel may become so paralyzed that it can no longer contract to propel its contents, and the patient dies with all the distressing signs of intestinal obstruction. In more fortunate instances the constipation at length yields to remedies; large quantities of hardened fecal matter are passed; and the distended and irritated intestine gradually regains its tone.

Inflammation of the loose areolar tissue around the cæcum presents much the same symptoms and signs. This *perityphlitis* is, in truth, frequently combined with inflammation of the cæcum or its appendix. Even where perforation has taken place, the matters may be detained in the neighborhood of the lesion, giving rise to circumscribed inflammation around the cæcum, and to an abscess. Subsequently, the collection of pus may find its way into neighboring viscera, or be discharged externally, when the ruptured intestine may heal; although sometimes the perforation remains open, and fecal matter is found oozing through the abdominal parietes. The tumefaction which the abscess occasions, whether it be or be not connected with disease of the intestine, is generally very evident. When, however, the pus burrows under the iliac fascia, the swelling may be slight. But under such circumstances there appears a characteristic sign: the pain, on moving the right foot, is intense, because the iliac muscles become involved in the disorder. If the swelling be great, there may be œdema of the foot and numbness of the thigh, from pressure on the vein and nerves.

When these abscesses in the right iliac fossa are not combined with disease of the adjoining bowel, they give rise to but slight fever and pain; the action of the intestine is not very materially interfered with; there is no nausea; and, as the abscesses frequently have a favorable termination by discharging into the intestine, or through the abdominal parietes, we do not observe acute peritonitis supervening on them, as it does so often on ulcerative disease of the intestine or its appendix. Yet there are cases in which judgment is held in suspense; in which it cannot be said whether the swelling does or does not communicate with the gut. Fortunately, this makes little difference in respect to treatment. Inflammation of the tissue around the cæcum requires chiefly leeching, warm fomentations, and opiates; and, in case of suppuration, surgical aid to produce an early exit for the pus. Inflammation of the cæcum or its appendix is remedied, when it can be remedied, by the same agents.

Independently of the difficulty of distinguishing between the inflammatory disorders of this portion of the alimentary tube and its surroundings, there are sources of perplexity introduced by the circumstance that other diseases of the cæcum and affections of adjacent structures may simulate typhlitis and perityphlitis. Thus distention and cancer of the cæcum; inflammation and ulceration of the ilium; suppuration of the kidney or its envelopes; psoas abscess; abscesses of the abdominal walls; intussusception of the intestine; and inflammation of the ovary,—occasion some of them pain and tenderness in the right iliac fossa, some of them a fulness in this region: therefore all of them have signs which they share with an inflammation of the cæcum. But although they all offer points of similitude, they also offer points of contrast.

A *distention of the cæcum* gives rise to fulness in the right iliac fossa, and to pain; but, unless associated with inflammation, not to tenderness or to fever; copious enemata too, or purgatives, clear out the feces which accumulate from want of power of the bowel to propel them, and the dulness on percussion vanishes after the free evacuations. Another element of distinction is furnished by the circumstance that those who suffer from atony of this portion of the alimentary tube labor under it for a long time; they are generally highly nervous persons, of sallow complexion and with impaired digestion, whose bowels are habitually constipated, and who complain of attacks of spasmodic pain and fulness in the iliac region. Yet, although there is fulness, there is no dulness on percussion, and no hard swelling is detected, unless the cæcum be loaded with feces. On the contrary, the cæcum and ascending colon generally show, by the excessive tympanitic resonance when they are percussed, that they are distended with flatus.

In that rare disease—*cancer of the cæcum*—there is a fixed, firm swelling; but it is of very gradual growth, and the disorder generally produces a stricture of the gut, and is associated with malignant disease in other parts of the body. Ulceration of the ilium produces pain and tenderness in the iliac fossa. But combined as it generally is with phthisis or with typhoid fever, the history of the case gives a clue to the probable nature of the disorder. Moreover, there is not present a tumefaction which sounds dull on percussion. Should, however, perforation of the bowel take place before the patient is seen, and general peritonitis come on, the diagnosis is not so readily made, because we are deprived of the decisive proof furnished by the hard swelling.

As regards *tumors of the kidney and abscesses in it, or connected with its envelopes*, the situation of the swelling is not exactly in the ilio-cæcal region, or at all events it is not confined to this spot. The mass of the tumor lies in the loin, or above the anterior termination of the crest of the ilium; and the urine contains ingredients, such as pus, or blood, or heavy deposits of urates or phosphates, which show that the secretion of the kidney is abnormal.

An *inflammation in or about the right ovary* gives rise to pain and tenderness in the right iliac region, and to fever. But it is attended with disturbance of the uterine functions, and occasions no very perceptible swelling. A tumor of the ovary or of the uterus may produce a visible tumefaction; but springing as it does out of the pelvis, its exact seat, its bulk, its shape, the absence of marked intestinal symptoms, and a per vaginam examination will, under ordinary circumstances, permit its cause to be discovered.

An *invagination of the intestine* has a different history, and makes its appearance suddenly with such peculiar signs that, although it may be likewise the occasion of a tumor in the right iliac region, it can generally be distinguished from cæcal disease. Yet, where the latter leads to intestinal obstruction, the diagnosis is not always obvious. In truth, as I shall further on attempt to enforce, to determine the precise character of an intestinal impediment may baffle the skill of the most experienced diagnostician.

So, too, it is with abscesses in or near the region in which those connected with the cæcum occur. Their discrimination is far from being invariably an easy matter. *An abscess in the abdominal walls* furnishes very many of the signs of abscess around the cæcum. The most trustworthy source of distinction is, that the former is unassociated with intestinal irritation, while the latter, from its being often connected with a disorder of the cæcum, is not uncommonly so combined. Then the pus discharged is, for the same reason, in some cases very offensive, and of fecal odor.

Now, this character of the pus, were it more generally observed, would serve equally as a most valuable differential mark between the matter which finds its way to the surface from a cæcal and from a *psoas abscess*. But as it is not constant, we have to apply other tests to the recognition of a psoas abscess. A psoas abscess is associated with caries of the vertebræ; an excurvation of the spine, dorsal pain and tenderness testify to this connection. It occurs in scrofulous persons, and, although gradual in its formation, is often sudden in its manifestation; for not unusually a fluctuating, painless tumor appears below Poupart's ligament as the first positive sign of this formidable disorder. Yet, preceding the pointing of the abscess at this spot, there are often indications of irritation in those muscles in the sheath of which the pus travels; there is difficulty in extending the leg; an inability to stand upright; and a dull, uneasy sensation in the loins, which the patient persists in regarding as rheumatic. Of all these signs, there are none more important, as sources of distinction, than the seat of the visible abscess and its painless nature. The interference with the movements of the right leg is not so valuable as it appears at first sight; since when the iliac muscle is involved, the same difficulty in moving the limb may exist; and the iliac muscle may be implicated in an inflammation of the loose areolar tissue around the cæcum by the inflammation extending to the iliac fascia and causing pus to collect under it; what surgeons term iliac abscesses are, indeed, collections of pus under this fascia. And, in point of fact, they not unfrequently originate near the cæcum, or spread to the tissues surrounding this portion of the gut, break into the cavity of the peritoneum, and therefore practically constitute perityphlitic abscesses.*

Disorders attended with Constipation, and of which it is a Prominent Symptom.

To enumerate all the complaints in which constipation may occur, would require me to pass in review the majority of all the affections of the body. Nor would this serve any useful purpose; for the inactive state of the bowels is often but a concomitant of some disorder which presents phenomena much more striking than the imperfect voidance or the prolonged retention of the feces. But there are cases in which the constipation is a very prominent symptom, in which it constitutes the ailment for which we are consulted, and in which it furnishes the most decisive proof of a serious morbid condition of the intestine. Now, these cases are either those in which the constipation arises, as it were, suddenly, or at any rate becomes suddenly aggravated, is attended with severe symptoms, and is often insuperable; or cases in which it is a habitual state, and not associated with any signs of urgent distress.

---

* See, for collection of cases, and for observations on these abscesses and on diseases of the cæcum, J. Burne, Med.-Chirurg. Transact., vol. xx.; Copland, Dictionary of Practical Medicine, article "Cæcum;" Dunglison, Practice of Medicine; Jackson, Letters to a Young Physician; Oppolzer on "Perityphlitis," Allg. Wien. Med. Zeit., Nos. 20 and 21, 1858; and Bartbolow, Amer. Journ. of Med. Sciences, Oct. 1866.

I shall describe the former set of cases first, because they bear a close relation to affections we have just been considering—to acute enteritis and peritonitis. Not that I mean here to dwell upon the constipation which occurs in these maladies,—it forms only one of the symptoms, and that not the most distinctive,—but I wish to discuss at some length the constipation, frequently insurmountable, produced by an obstruction to the passage of the intestinal contents, and which often brings with it acute inflammation of the bowel and of its serous investment.

Intestinal Obstruction. — Intestinal obstruction, when coming on suddenly, manifests itself generally in the following manner: a person, previously in good health, or perhaps of costive habit, notices that his bowels have not been moved for several days, and that he has an uneasy feeling in the abdomen in consequence. He takes the purgative he is wont to employ, but without the usual effect. Something more active is tried, and still the bowels remain obstinately bound. Colicky pains have in the mean time made their appearance, or, if present from the onset of the disorder, have become aggravated. He becomes alarmed, and sends for his physician. On his arrival, the medical attendant sees that there is indeed cause for alarm. He finds the abdomen somewhat distended, but not painful, or perhaps only slightly painful on pressure. But through its parietes may be noticed the violent, rolling motion of the excited intestine. Vomiting sets in—first, of the substances contained in the stomach or of a bilious fluid, and, as the case progresses, of stercoraceous matter. In this way, unless nature or art comes to the rescue, the disease continues; and signs of inflammation of the bowels, and with them fever, appear as preludes to the fatal termination. Sometimes, however, the patient becomes gradually exhusted; there are no tenderness and fever, but a cool skin, a quick, small pulse, a countenance ghastly and panic-stricken. Severe paroxysms of pain, alternating with intervals of ease, may occur to the last moment. But in spite of the utter prostration, the mind generally retains its clearness until death comes to put a merciful end to the prolonged and irremediable suffering. Should recovery take place, large quantities of fecal matter are discharged, and all the symptoms of the impediment speedily disappear.

Such are the phenomena presented by an intestinal obstruction. They are too striking to permit of errors in diagnosis. And yet errors have been committed, and are still of frequent occurrence, because the history of the attack and the sequence of the symptoms are not taken into account. Many a person laboring under enteritis or peritonitis has been violently purged to remove the stubborn constipation, believed to be due to a mechanical hinderance in the bowels; and, on the other hand, many a case of intestinal obstruction has been treated solely with reference to the inflammation which may attend it, and without regard to the source of this inflammation. Yet it is not ordinarily difficult to distinguish which is cause and which effect. A case that commences with colicky pains and obstinate constipation, in which, at first, in spite of the pain, there is little or no tenderness or fever; in which vomiting soon occurs; in which fecal matter is ejected by the mouth after a stoppage of the bowels of a few days' duration,—is not primarily, whatever may be the ultimate complications, enteritis or peritonitis. A case presenting almost from the onset fever and great tenderness, in which vomiting of fecal matter, if it happen at all, does not happen until late; in which diarrhœa is sometimes found to supersede the enduring constipation,—is inflammation of the intestine or of the peritoneum, but not a mechanical obstruction.

Only in rare, very rare instances, and especially when the bowel is invaginated, is this formidable malady so quickly succeeded by inflammation as seemingly to make its appearance with the signs of peritonitis. Should the disease then run a rapid course, and stercoraceous vomiting not occur, an error in diagnosis is unavoidable. Should it be, however, of some duration, the unyielding constipation and the character of the vomit come to our aid; and casting, as they do, the signs of inflammation more and more into the background, force the conviction on the mind that they are not simply the result of a paralysis of the tube, the consequence of the inflammation, but are dependent on an impassable barrier to the passage of the intestinal contents.

The symptoms upon which I have been dwelling as pointing toward an intestinal obstruction bear a close resemblance to those of external strangulated hernia. In truth, they not only resemble, but are identical with those of this affection. Hence, in every case of obstinate constipation, each point which may be the seat of a hernia must be explored by the eye and the hand. No motives of false delicacy, no reluctance on the part of the patient, should prevent the practitioner from insisting on a search, the neglect of which will cost a life entrusted to his care, should he fail to discover, until too late, the real cause of the alarming symptoms he has been endeavoring to alleviate.

It would be foreign to the object of this work were I to attempt to discuss the external signs by which a strangulation of the intestine at a hernial opening manifests itself. This belongs to surgical, and not to medical diagnosis. Nor shall I, for the same reasons, do more than indicate that it is at the groin, at the umbilicus, at the side of the anus, or through the ischiatic notch that the gut descends and forms a tumor, and that these are, therefore, the regions to be scrutinized.

But there is one part of the subject, alike of importance to the physician and to the surgeon, which I cannot pass by without a few words, since it may be a cause of much perplexity, namely, the possibility of intestinal obstruction taking place in a person laboring under an irreducible hernia and simulating strangulation without any strangulation having occurred. Of this the following case furnishes an example:

In October, 1857, I was requested by a physician in this city to see with him a person, the mother of thirteen children, who had been for several days laboring under obstinate constipation. Large doses of mercurials, croton oil, and turpentine enemata had failed to procure a passage, and the patient was becoming very much frightened about herself. Nor was her situation one free from danger. She had considerable pain in the abdomen; she had been vomiting stercoraceous matter profusely; the rolling of the intestines could be plainly perceived. On her right side was a small irreducible femoral hernia, which, on inquiry, was found to have existed for many years. It was not painful on pressure, nor was the skin covering it discolored ; neither did the mass itself communicate an impulse during the act of coughing. Now, here were signs of a serious impediment to the onward passage of the intestinal contents, as the fecal vomiting and the rolling of the intestines showed plainly. But what was its nature? Was it due to strangulation at the hernial opening ? Was it an internal intestinal obstruction ?

An accurate examination of the abdomen did not throw much light on these all-important questions. The belly was moderately tympanitic, and not painful to the touch, excepting when the pressure was considerable. The rolling of the intestines was perhaps more obvious on the left side; but nowhere could a tumor be felt. Taking all the circumstances of the case into account : the fact that the patient was of very costive habit ; that she was subject to attacks of colic and of obstinate constipation ; that there was nothing to prove that the hernia had recently increased, or was in any way inflamed,—I was led to the conclusion that the case was not one of hernial strangulation, but of internal intestinal obstruction ; and she was treated for this. Copious warm water injections were thrown into the colon through a flexible tube ; her abdomen was rubbed with mercurial ointment. But all in vain : she continued vomiting fecal matter.

Her situation now appeared desperate. She had not had a passage for six days—remedies had failed to procure her one; she was steadily sinking. Knowing that sometimes the gut may be strangulated at a hernial opening without much pain or tenderness, the counsel of an eminent surgeon was sought, to aid in determining whether this was not the cause of the impediment. He thought it probable that it was, and proposed an operation, to which consent was reluctantly obtained. The patient was etherized, and the hernial section rapidly and skilfully performed ; but no constriction was found. The wound was closed, and large doses of opium administered to the unhappy sufferer, so as to mitigate, as far as practicable, the torturing distress of the only termination to the case which seemed possible. On the day after the operation, the intestines had ceased to roll; there was no vomiting. But stercoraceous vomiting reappeared two days afterward, and the rolling of the intestines was occasionally, although faintly, perceptible.

The patient's exhaustion was now extreme; her pulse was very quick and small; her skin cold, of a dirty look; the odor of the breath and of the whole body offensive; and the eyes sunken and surrounded by a broad leaden ring. There was slight pain on pressure between the umbilicus and the sigmoid flexure. The vomiting had ceased, or occurred only very occasionally. Although there was little hope, we had, as soon as admissible after the operation, recommenced rubbing mercurial ointment over the abdomen, and giving injections in the manner before described. This was continued until, to our great gratification, one morning, after a tube had been passed a distance of several feet into the colon, the patient had a copious discharge of tarry fecal matter from her bowels,—seventeen days after the symptoms of complete intestinal obstruction had declared themselves by the occurrence of stercoraceous vomiting.

This case is instructive in several respects. It teaches that recovery may take place most unexpectedly after the patient has been kept at death's door for many days. It shows the beneficial results of filling the colon with fluid in instances of intestinal obstruction; and, in a diagnostic point of view, it illustrates a difficulty which any practitioner may have to encounter in attending a patient who is the subject of a long-standing hernia.

Supposing, however, that we have sufficient grounds for the opinion that no hernia exists, and that the symptoms are altogether owing to an obstacle seated at some portion of the intestine within the abdomen,—can we go any further, can we determine the exact position of the impediment, and what its nature is? We know, from dissection, how varied are the conditions which lead to sudden and invincible constipation. We know that intussusceptions, twists, displacements, strictures of the gut, bands and adhesions, or gaps in the omentum, foreign bodies, impacted feces, gall-stones, and spasmodic contraction of the intestine,*—may all occasion intestinal obstruction, and some of these states even an internal strangulation. Can we distinguish these different lesions from each other at the bedside? In certain cases we can,—we can determine exactly both the position and character of the lesion; in others there is no clue to an accurate discernment of either.

Of the causes of intestinal obstruction, *intussusception* or *invagination* is the most frequent and at the same time the most susceptible of being recognized during life. Part of the gut becomes inverted, slipping for a variable distance into the cavity of the adjoining upper or lower portion. Inflammation is generally soon set up, and produces infiltration of the tissues and their tumefaction, and often leads to adhesions between the opposed serous surfaces, and to effusions of blood and mucus into the canal. The swelling entirely blocks up the tube; yet it does not of necessity do so. The congestion and inflammation which have caused the tumefaction may spread rapidly over the serous membrane, and the patient may die from general peritonitis. But sometimes in this inflammation that is lighted up at the seat of the ileus lies the safety of the patient. It may give rise to a sloughing off of the invaginated part and its discharge into the bowel, and thus pave the way to a favorable issue by restoring the calibre of the tube—sufficiently at any rate to permit of the transit of its contents.

Now, these pathological peculiarities develop special symptoms which not unfrequently enable us to determine the nature of the obstruction. When the intussusception takes place rapidly, a sudden local pain is produced, recurring in paroxysms, and likely to be referred to the seat of the disturbance. The pain is quickly followed by vomiting, by constipation, and by peritonitis. But the constipation is not so absolute as in other cases of intestinal impediment. Sometimes, in fact, owing to the invaginated bowel remaining open, the liquid contents of the intestine may pass through the intussuscepted part and produce a deceptive diarrhœa;

---

* Archives Génér., Aug. 1868.

yet oftener will occur tenesmus, and discharges of the bloody serum which has accumulated in the intestine. Both of the latter signs are eminently diagnostic of the lesion. Still more so would be feeling the end of the invaginated gut by an exploration of the rectum, or finding the loosened segment of the bowel in the stools. But of course it is only in a certain class of cases, those in which the lower portion of the canal is affected, or which have been sufficiently protracted to allow of the curative efforts of nature being accomplished, that signs so strictly pathognomonic are met with.

The casting off of the sloughed portion of the intestine is, we are informed by several observers, always attended with hemorrhage. Whether this be the cause of the hemorrhage or not, it is undoubted that purging, nay, sometimes vomiting of blood, are among the most important differential signs of intussusception. But a sign yet more valuable, because so much more common, is the presence of a tumor. Its seat varies, of course, with the seat of the lesion. And as the most frequent of all invaginations are those of the ilium and cæcum into the colon, or those at the inferior portion of the ilium, it is at the lower part of the belly, and generally passing in direction from left to right, and in the right iliac fossa, that the swelling is detected. The malady occurs at all ages. It is often preceded by diarrhœa.

The course invagination pursues is very rapid. The acute inflammation it occasions soon leads to a fatal termination, or the patient dies generally in less than a week after the occurrence of the accident, utterly prostrated. Yet the records of medicine furnish us with instances in which life has been prolonged for several months. The cases which get well, recover either gradually after the invaginated bowel has been discharged, or, in very rare instances, more quickly by the inverted bowel righting itself.

As regards other forms of intestinal obstruction, they are, with our present knowledge, undistinguishable from each other. However desirable it might be on therapeutic grounds to be able to diagnosticate a twist of the intestine, or its blocking up by hardened feces or gall-stones, or its strangulation by bands; however desirable to know whether, if medical means do not bring relief, the hazardous operation of laying open the belly may be attempted with some hope of success, or whether the impediment is not even to be removed by such a mode of succor,—it must be confessed that there are no positive signs which enable us to decide on the nature of the obstacle.

Yet there are sometimes circumstances in the case which may help us to a correct decision. For example, if the complaint occur in one who has previously suffered from the passage of gall-stones, it is likely that a large concretion of this kind has been arrested in its passage through the intestine, and is the cause of the mischief. Should the disorder be encountered in a person who has before had attacks of constipation almost invincible; who at all times has difficulty in voiding the contents of the tube; whose feces present peculiarities in shape and size, and are sometimes mixed with blood; whose health has been gradually breaking down; whose abdomen is much distended and yields a ringing tympanitic resonance on percussion; in whom a bougie passed into the rectum has detected a marked resistance,—should such a person have an attack of constipation more than usually protracted, attended with enormous distention of the bowel, and in wlich the remedies, whether mechanical or medicinal, that hitherto barely procured a passage, now fail utterly, it would not require much sagacity to discern that a stricture of the intestine, and probably of a cancerous kind, is the source of the cruel and irremediable suffering. If, in addition to the symptoms enumerated, a bougie passed into the rectum meet in its course with a decided obstacle, an error in diagnosis is hardly possible. When, however, the stricture is not accessible to instrumental examination, although we can commonly recognize its presence, we cannot fix its site. The distention above the narrowed part is often so extreme as to lead to displacement of the colon and to an almost uniform swelling of the whole abdomen, thus baffling all attempts at determining the point of constriction. For instance, in a case reported by Dr. Albert H. Smith, the enormously dilated colon had broken loose from its attachments and concealed the rest of the viscera. It was in several places eighteen, in none' less than fifteen inches in circumference; and fully two-gallons of liquid feces were found in the bowels.*

In the other kinds of obstruction the same difficulty—although not of necessity arising from the same cause—may exist in determining with certainty the location of the lesion. There are, however, a few circumstances which may aid us in arriving at such a determination : one is the interesting fact pointed out by Dr. Barlow,† that the higher up the obstruction is in the canal, the nearer therefore to the stomach, the smaller is the quantity of urine passed; another is the early occurrence of the vomiting and the want of stercoraceous character of the matters ejected—both of which render it likely that the impediment is in the small intestine and remote from the cæcum.   Yet another is the speedy presence and the greater severity of hiccough when the mischief is in the small intestine.   Sometimes the patient is himself aware of the exact seat of the cause of his suffering ; he notices that the injecting tube or the enemata seem to reach a certain point and go no farther; so, also, with the rumbling of the wind.   Again, these borborygmi are especially apt to occur in obstructions of the large intestine, and, if joined to tenesmus, are signs of some importance.

The position of the pain, too, may furnish a clue to the position of the impediment.   If this be in the small intestine, the pain is apt to be chiefly, if not entirely, in the neighborhood of the umbilicus.   Another circumstance on which some stress may be laid, is the distention of the intestine above the point of interception.   Indeed, this distention may occasion a visible fulness, sounding extremely tympanitic on percussion ; at times, too, a slight dulness is found, attended with some resistance at or immediately above the seat of the obstruction.   But with reference to the swelling and the tympanitic dilatation of the bowel, there are—as Dr. Brinton‡ sets forth in his extended researches on the subject—several reasons which render these signs uncertain guides in a diag-

---

* Proceed. of Path. Society of Philadelphia, Dec. 1858, vol. i.
† Guy's Hospital Reports, 2d Series, vol. ii.
‡ Cronian Lectures ; see London Lancet, vol. i. 1859.

nosis of the situation of the affection. The distended intestine may not be capable of being traced by the eye or by
percussion, owing to its occupying a large portion of the
abdominal cavity. Moreover, a stoppage at the descending
part of the large intestine, for instance at the sigmoid flexure,
may lead to most palpable distention of the cæcum, and to
pain in that region; while pain and swelling are also observed
in the same locality in obstructions which affect the small
intestine. Thus, then, there are several modifying circumstances which prevent too much importance being attached
to any of the signs mentioned as proofs of the seat of the
obstacle; for, with the exception of a tumor dull on percussion and resistant to the touch, there is nothing absolutely
indicative of the lesion being at a particular spot. And it
is hardly necessary to say that a swelling of this kind cannot
always be found.

Internal strangulation—as by a band acting as the con-
stricting agent, or a diverticulum, or the pedicle of an
ovarian tumor—has it seat almost constantly in the small
intestine. Dr. Hilton Fagge,* who has recently very ably
investigated the subject, considers these symptoms as significant, and warranting a diagnosis of internal constriction:
the sudden and definite onset of the illness; the occurrence
of collapse at its commencement; the comparatively early
age ; the severity of the pain, which is generally referred to
the umbilicus; the absence of external or of discoverable
obturator hernia; the absence of precursory symptoms and
of visible peristole—such as happen in stricture and contractions—of tumor, hemorrhage, and dysenteric symptoms
—as seen in intussusception—and of that extreme intensity
and rapidity of the disorder which characterize the more
acute forms of volvulus.

In referring to the usual seat of pain and swelling in the
right iliac fossa, and to the difficulties which on this account
beset the recognition of the precise site of the hinderance, one
source of error deserving of special notice was not mentioned.
The pain and the fulness in this region may be caused by a

---

* Guy's Hospital Reports, 3d Series, vol. xiv.

disease of the cæcum or of its appendix. Moreover, affections of this part of the alimentary tract, like intestinal occlusion, give rise to constipation which is most obstinate and in some instances incurable. Therefore they in reality enter at times into the category of intestinal obstructions, from the other varieties of which they are, under such circumstances, undistinguishable save by the history of the case and the different sequence of the phenomena. The tumor and the other local signs do not follow the insuperable constipation, but they precede it. Yet if the patient be seen for the first time when he is laboring under an irremovable intestinal impediment, it may be impossible rightly to determine its character.

Habitual Constipation.—We are often called upon to remedy a sort of constipation which is very different from that of an intestinal obstruction. It is a chronic state unattended with fever, or, under ordinary circumstances, with urgent symptoms of any kind. Still it is a very annoying disorder, and so prevalent that there is hardly a person, among the thousands who lead sedentary lives, who does not or has not suffered from it. The symptoms encountered, independently of the rare and difficult fecal evacuations, are headache, giddiness, sluggishness of the mind, a want of the natural appetite, and, joined as the complaint not unfrequently is to derangement of the stomach and of the biliary secretion, digestive disturbances and a sallow complexion. In women there are also often added to the list of evils to which costiveness gives rise, neuralgic pains, palpitation of the heart, cold feet and hands. Not that infrequent evacuation of the bowels always produces such unpleasant consequences. It may indeed in individual cases be compatible with perfect health; for what is costiveness in one person may be a natural state in another. But when the bowels are acting less frequently than is their wont, the disagreeable symptoms mentioned are apt to arise.

Habitual constipation is produced by various causes. It may be brought about by the peculiar nature of the diet. It may depend upon a deficiency or a faulty composition of the intestinal secretions, or upon disorders of those neighboring

glands which pour their secretions into the intestines.   It may
result from impaired power of the bowel to propel its contents,
the consequence either of some mechanical interference with
its action, or of nervous influences, or of exposure to the
poisonous effects of certain substances, as of lead.   To particularize the numerous conditions which furnish illustrations
of each of these different causes would be tedious, and serve
no useful purpose.   I shall select only a few for special notice.

We have often to treat constipation in those who are dyspeptic and suffer from piles.   In them there is, in all probability, some congestion of the portal system, and not unfrequently a constant derangement of the flow of blood through
the liver.   The normal secretion of intestinal juices is interfered with, healthy bile is not supplied, and thus costiveness
results.   A similar congestion of the intestinal mucous membrane has its share in producing the constipation which is
encountered in diseases of the heart.   Sometimes, however,
enough healthy fluid is poured out within the intestine ; yet
there is practically a deficiency, because the inclination to go
to stool is resisted, and the liquid that has been mixed with
the matter to be voided is reabsorbed.   In women who neglect
the calls of nature from carelessness, or because circumstances
prevent their being obeyed at the proper time, this is a very
common cause of constipation.

The influence of the nervous system on the alimentary tube
is shown by the confined state of the bowels which attends
excessive intellectual exertion and violent emotions.   And
when these states are protracted, they lead to a permanent
and annoying debility of the intestine.   The colon especially
becomes torpid in its action, and all the evil results of constipation show themselves in their most marked degree.   Not
that an atony of the bowel is always due to psychical agencies.
Any disorder which induces loss of power in the muscular
fibres may give rise to it.   We find it where the blood is
watery and deficient in red corpuscles, and in those who lead,
so far as bodily exertion is concerned, a sluggish life.   In
some cases—fortunately rare—the weak intestine distends
greatly, and becoming, as above explained, unable to propel
the accumulated feces, insuperable constipation occurs.

The same complete paralysis of the tube, attended with the same unfortunate consequences, may be brought about by chronic lesions of the brain or spinal cord. Perhaps, however, the inveterate constipation which is so constant an accompaniment of these states is partly owing to the powerless condition of the abdominal muscles.

Among the different organic changes in the intestine which, by interfering *mechanically* with the peristaltic wave and the onward transmission of the feces, set up constipation, we find distention of the tube, with atrophy of the muscular fibres; various infiltrations into the walls, producing a narrowing of the calibre; and adhesions between the serous coats of the intestines, or between these viscera and the parietes. Of the first, it need only be said that the symptoms are due to the same paralyzed condition of the intestine, whether complete or incomplete, which has been just considered, and which has been dwelt upon more at length when discussing diseases of the cæcum, and intestinal obstruction. The second group embraces those infiltrations which result from inflammations, and new growths of different kinds which lead to strictures.

The former of these are recognized, as far as they can be with certainty, by the history of the case. The latter present peculiarities in the form and size of the feces, distention of the bowels above the seat of the narrowing, vomiting, attacks of colic, gradual wasting and exhaustion; besides which, extreme costiveness, deepening gradually into invincible constipation, furnishes a key to the grievous nature of the disorder.

When the constipation arises as the result of peritoneal adhesions, there are sometimes signs in the case—such as tenderness at a particular spot from still existing inflammation, or partial distention or retraction of the abdomen—which point out its nature. In the absence of these, the history is our only guide, excepting in those instances in which, as Dr. Bright* first informed us, a peculiar sensation is com-

---

* Cases illustrative of the diagnosis of adhesions and other morbid changes of the peritoneum, Med.-Chirg. Trans., vol. xix.

municated to the touch, varying between the crepitation produced by emphysema and the feel derived from bending new
leather in the hand.

Thus a protracted state of constipation may be due to
several causes, some of which are of very serious character.
And this only proves how important it is to look further
than the mere constipation; how necessary in every case to
endeavor, as nearly as possible, to arrive at the determining
cause of the imperfect or difficult alvine evacuations.   Still it
is often impossible to assign any one cause, because the complaint is, in fact, dependent upon the union of several of
those which have been mentioned.   Moreover, we must not
forget that a constipated state is often joined to affections of
the stomach or liver, and our treatment for the habitual constipation should merge into that of the disorder of which the
constipation is a symptom.

Disorders in which Morbid Discharges from the Bowels occur.

Matters, very unlike the healthy alvine evacuations, are
often voided from the intestinal canal; loose watery stools,
large quantities of mucus, pus, or blood may be discharged.
I shall here describe the disorders which occasion these discharges.

Diarrhœa.—The remark made of constipation is equally
applicable to diarrhœa.   Both occur as an accompaniment
in a vast number of diseases which present symptoms more
characteristic than the confined or loose state of the bowels.
At this place, therefore, diarrhœa will be merely treated of
as we meet with it constituting, so far as can be ascertained,
the entire ailment, or at all events by far its most prominent
symptom.   There are several varieties of diarrhœa.   Difference in time gives rise to marked varieties—to an acute and
a chronic form.

Acute Diarrhœa.—Now, acute diarrhœa proceeds from more
than one cause: it may be excited by the irritating character
of the food taken; it may be brought about by the morbid
nature of the secretions poured into the intestines; it may
be owing to atmospheric influences—to heat, to moisture, to

contaminated air; it may be due to mental emotions, and especially to fear. Its symptoms are thirst; a griping pain in the bowel, of all grades of severity; pallor; a slight debility, and frequent fluid alvine evacuations.

In the diarrhœa caused by a debauch or by indigestible food, nausea and a furred tongue are added to the list of symptoms mentioned. This kind of diarrhœa is generally of very short duration. It is an effort of nature to get rid of obnoxious matter; and when this is effected, the looseness of the bowels ceases of itself. The discharges from the intestines are therefore rather to be favored than suppressed. And we can greatly aid the recovery by enjoining abstinence from food, and by administering diluent drinks and a purgative, to which a small quantity of some opiate is added, sufficient to soothe, but not sufficiently to interfere with the aperient action.

The variety of diarrhœa under consideration sometimes goes hand in hand with a disturbance of the biliary functions, and the stools discharged are fetid, and present the appearance generally described as bilious. This "bilious diarrhœa," too, is not uncommon in persons whose livers are habitually sluggish. It is also frequently encountered during the hot months of summer and early in the autumn, and has a tendency to run on.

Owing to the extreme rarity with which an opportunity offers to examine it, the state of the mucous membrane during an attack of acute diarrhœa is not accurately determined. In some instances redness, swelling, and other evidences of acute inflammation have been found. But these were cases in which during life the symptoms had been severe; in fact, more or less those of an inflammation—pain, some soreness to the touch, and, what is not ordinarily met with in diarrhœa, heat of skin and excited pulse. These graver kinds of acute diarrhœa, or rather of muco-enteritis with diarrhœa as a symptom, are often the result of irritant poisoning. They are still more usually observed as secondary disorders in typhoid fever and in the exanthemata.

Chronic Diarrhœa.—In chronic diarrhœa the lesions encountered are much more marked than they ever are in the acute form. The mucous membrane is tumid and discolored; its follicles are not unfrequently ulcerated. Chronic looseness of the bowels originates in a diarrhœa which is permitted to continue, either from neglect or because the patient remains for a long time exposed to the original cause. But the disorder, no matter under what circumstances it originated, is apt to prove rebellious, and to end by breaking down the constitution. When of long standing, the patient becomes gradually weaker and weaker, and more and more emaciated. The abdomen is sunken; the expression of the face despondent; the complexion pale; the eyes are surrounded by a dark ring. The character of the discharge is very various. They are often dark colored and very offensive. Sometimes the looseness of the bowels alternates with an opposite condition, but the irritability of the intestines never intermits.

This morbid excitability of the intestinal tube is more especially brought about in persons of nervous temperament and of dissipated habits. The abuse of purgatives, too, induces it, and in consequence chronic diarrhœa is not an uncommon result of the cathartic pills which many of the patrons of quack medicines so habitually swallow.

But perhaps the most persistent irritability of the intestines is found in the diarrhœa to which soldiers are so liable, and which, as the result of hardships, exposure, and defective diet, is so apt to pass, no matter what its beginning, into the chronic form of the disease. And this complaint, which is generally associated with a morbid state of the large intestine as well as of the small, which combines therefore some of the features of chronic dysentery with those of chronic diarrhœa, is one that often clings to its victim through life; many a soldier, in truth, escapes the bullet and the sword, only to die of the intestinal affection long after his return to his home.

The causes of the diarrhœa of soldiers are the ordinary causes of chronic diarrhœa already mentioned, favored in their development by fatiguing marches, by want of personal cleanliness, by the exposure and drawbacks of life in camp or in the field, by hot weather, by malaria, and in many instances by a specific epidemic poison in the atmosphere. To this origin are chiefly referred the numerous instances of atonic diarrhœa which happened among the British troops in the Crimea.* During the late war on this continent, we did not escape the scourge of all armies. Irrespective of the causes always acting whenever large numbers of men are collected together for warlike operations, scurvy is stated to have been a prolific source of the thousands of cases of diarrhœa which occurred in the army during the past conflict.†

The chronic diarrhœa among soldiers is not materially different in its symptoms from chronic diarrhœa of civil life, excepting that perhaps we find more frequently thickening and ulceration of the colon; more frequently, therefore, stools containing pus and more of the evidences of chronic dysentery than usually coexist with what is known as chronic diarrhœa. Then, the affection is very often witnessed as a complication of other disorders. Two-thirds of the fever patients received in the hospitals at Constantinople during a long period of the Crimean war were affected with diarrhœa or with dysentery. Diarrhœa was so very general that nearly all disorders were preceded by acute diarrhœa, and terminated in chronic diarrhœa.‡ To any one who had opportunities of observing cases of the Chickahominy fever and diarrhœa so prevalent during General McClellan's peninsular campaign, a parallel will at once occur.

But chronic diarrhœa, as the practitioner of medicine commonly sees it, is not always so strictly an idiopathic ailment as are for the most part the forms of the malady just discussed. It is often attendant on general constitutional affections, or on abdominal diseases which have led to a secondary disorder of the secretions, or even of the coats of the intestine. Thus we find chronic looseness of the bowels in scurvy, in pyæmia, in Bright's disease, in scrofula of the mesenteric glands, and in tuberculosis. In the last of these complaints, the diarrhœa may be occasioned by changes in the secretions of the intestinal glands. But it is not seldom dependent

---

* Blue Book, Medical and Surgical History of the War against Russia, vol. ii. page 101.

† Woodward, Outlines of the Chief Camp Diseases, page 253.

‡ Baudens, La Guerre de Crimée.

upon a true tubercular disease of the intestines, which leads, like phthisis, to softening and ulceration. The discharges are generally copious and very offensive. They contain frequently undigested food. The abdomen is retracted, and presents spots very tender to the touch. Yet, after all, the signs of tubercle, or scrofula elsewhere, furnish alone any positive indications by which the true nature of the wasting malady may be discerned.

In the chronic diarrhœa of strumous children there is sometimes a scrofulous infiltration into the intestinal walls, sometimes scrofula of the mesenteric glands, sometimes both, but in some cases neither. Improper nourishment may be the exciting cause of the continued purging; for do we not see even healthy infants, surrounded by every comfort and every care that wealth can procure, when unsuitably fed, or weaned too soon, suffer from continued irritation of the alimentary tube?

These facts teach us that, in the treatment of the chronic diarrhœa of children, the regulation of the diet is of the utmost importance; and the same is true of the chronic diarrhœa of adults.

Sometimes chronic diarrhœa assumes an *intermittent type*, and its malarial nature is clearly proved by the readiness with which the disorder yields to quinine.* In this respect this malarial diarrhœa differs from cases of diarrhœa we sometimes encounter, in which the pain and discharges come on at an early hour of the day, and cease toward evening and during the night.

Another form of looseness of the bowels is the *membranous*. Here the discharges show shreds of membrane, either in connection with the loose stools, or sometimes in such quantities that the whole mass voided seems to consist of them. Griping pains and tenderness usually precede this form of diarrhœa, which may happen in attacks of a subacute form, or as a persistent and very obstinate disorder. The fecal discharges are usually loose, but occasionally for a time there is constipation.

---

* See contribution by Dr. Sanford B. Hunt on *Diarrhœa*, in Medical Memoirs of U. S. Sanitary Commission, p. 306.

Dysentery.—Frequent and painful passages of mucus mixed with blood, accompanied with straining and bearing down, are the characteristic symptoms of dysentery. In its acute form we find thirst, restlessness, and heat of skin super-added; and sometimes, in severe cases, especially when the disease prevails epidemically, those symptoms of prostration which, grouped together, are commonly designated as typhoid.

Acute Dysentery.—The acute disorder is at times ushered in by a chill; at times it is preceded by diarrhœa. The fever which attends it is not generally intense. It is the exception to find a hard, rapid pulse, and a very hot, dry skin; and in slight cases the pulse is but little excited, and the skin remains cool. More or less pain is always present. It has its seat mostly, but not invariably, at some part of the colon, and this is tender on pressure. It is not constant, but intermitting and shifting, and is often accompanied by a disagreeable, weighty feeling near the anus, which causes a continual desire to go to stool. Yet no relief follows the frequent attempts at defecation; the violent straining only adds to the discomfort of the patient.

The matters voided are small in quantity. They consist of blood mixed with mucus; but, like nearly all of the so-termed mucous discharges, they are composed not simply of mucus, but also of pus corpuscles, exudation globules, granules, and large quantities of cast-off epithelium. They are in some cases highly offensive, and resemble the washings of meat; in others, they are like jelly, or greenish in color. They do not contain feces, or only here and there small, firm lumps of fecal matter; hence we may justly say that, for the most part, dysentery is in reality attended with constipation. When the dysenteric inflammation subsides, the bowels are unloaded of their contents; in consequence, the passage of quantities of small, hard masses of feces is generally a sign that the acute malady is inclining to a favorable termination.

But how long it will take for the disorder to run its course, or whether the acute disease will pass into chronic dysentery, cannot be foretold. Generally this is not its termination; it very often ends, within a week from its commencement, in

33

recovery. But severe cases occur which are of much shorter duration, and in which the symptoms hasten on to complete prostration, and death takes place early in the malady. In these frightful cases—most frequently encountered in epidemics and where the distemper prevails among large bodies of men—collapse may happen with almost the same rapidity as it does in malignant cholera.

Dysentery is essentially a disease of hot climates. It is very common in this country in summer and in autumn, Eating green fruits, exposure to a chilly night after a hot day, or sleeping on damp ground, are prolific exciting causes. It is occasionally found in combination with malarial fevers, adding greatly to their danger. The immediate cause of most of the symptoms is the inflammation of the large intestine, and especially of the portion which commonly bears the brunt of the disorder—the descending colon. Yet in many cases of dysentery we see phenomena manifested which are clearly not to be accounted for solely by the local morbid appearances detected after death, and which show that dysentery is often something more than mere inflammation of the colon. In truth, inflammation of the colon may give rise to the symptoms of acute diarrhœa; for it is a great mistake to suppose that the cause of diarrhœa is only to be sought in some abnormal change in the small intestines. Thus colitis is not always dysentery; and dysentery, to repeat, is often something more than mere colitis.

But whether we believe dysentery to be simply inflammation of the colon; or an inflammation of the colon arising from a diseased state of the blood, and forming, therefore, only part of a general malady; or believe it to be sometimes one, sometimes the other,—we have to admit that it presents peculiarities which render it easy of recognition at the bedside.

Yet we should take good care to ascertain that the supposed characteristic tenesmus and bloody discharges are not really owing to piles or to morbid growths in the rectum. There is less danger of confounding enteritis or diarrhœa with dysentery, for symptoms exist in the latter which do not belong to either of the former. Enteritis has fever; so has dysentery, though, as already stated, the febrile disturbance is not often of a very high grade. And, independently of the differences arising from the absence of the peculiar discharges of dysentery, the pulse of enteritis is small, tense, and quick; that of dysentery, if the febrile action be marked, full and rapid. Diarrhœa differs from dysentery by the liquid fecal evacuations, and by the fact that neither tenesmus, nor bloody stools, nor discharges of mucus occur. Yet in practice we meet with cases which commence with diarrhœa and end with dysentery, or begin with dysenteric symptoms and terminate in diarrhœa, and in which it becomes, therefore, puzzling to say whether we are dealing with the former or with the latter disorder.

Chronic Dysentery.—In chronic dysentery this mingling of the two complaints is especially apt to happen. We rarely see chronic dysentery without chronic diarrhœa. At all events, we seldom find instances of the former, in which the tenesmus and the discharge of blood and mucus mixed with pus are not accompanied by frequent loose alvine evacuations, by griping, by the same gradual wasting and the same irritability of the bowels as are encountered in chronic diarrhœa; nay, the symptoms of the latter, and the difficulty of determining the presence of pus when mixed with fluid feces, may so obscure the true nature of the malady, that what has been regarded as chronic diarrhœa turns out, at the autopsy, to be chronic dysentery. The mucous membrane of the colon is found to be extensively inflamed; its texture altered and irregularly thickened; its surface riddled with ulcers. In such cases the patient goes on steadily losing flesh; but no pain on pressure or localized distress exists to denote the ravages the disease is making in the alimentary tube.

The prognosis is never very favorable. To say, indeed, that it is wholly unfavorable, would hardly be to overrate the serious character of the disease. Many die exhausted; others, in consequence of abscess of the liver, which chronic as well as acute dysentery may induce.

Intestinal Hemorrhage or Melæna.—The discharge of blood in large quantities from the bowels is not apt to occur in dysentery. It is much more common as the result of a mechanical hinderance to its flow through the liver, or of a depraved state of the circulating fluid—such as exists in typhus fever, in yellow fever, and in scurvy. Occasionally the bleeding proceeds from a fungoid growth in the intestine, or an ulcer in the duodenum, or from the bursting of an aneurism. Rokitansky informs us that intestinal hemorrhages sometimes follow extensive burns of the abdominal parietes. And in very young infants, a discharge of blood, both by the mouth and rectum, is not of unusual occurrence.

The blood passed by stool is generally of dark color, like tar. When it is not, we may fairly infer that it flows from the lower part of the intestine and has not had much chance to become admixed with other matters. In all such cases, however, we must make sure, before arriving at any conclusion as to the source of the bleeding, that it does not proceed from hemorrhoids. The exact seat of the hemorrhage cannot be determined; nay, blood may be evacuated by the bowel, and not be poured out at all from the intestine, but from the stomach. In some instances the blood accumulates in the bowel, and before the clots moulded to its shape are discharged, death results.*

Fatty Diarrhœa.—The occurrence of cases in which large quantities of fat, mixed or pure, are voided by the rectum, is attested by many observers. In some of these cases oil was at the same time passed with the urine; in others the urinary secretion was healthy; some cases ended fatally, others in recovery; some were found to be connected with a disease of the pancreas, others were not; in some the disorder was not of long continuance, while in others it lasted, with occasioual intervals, for years. Thus the morbid state with which fatty diarrhœa is associated is far from being always the same.

As a rule, the occurrence of fatty stools is a matter of serious concern. The recognition of the malady is easy. The white, fatty masses, or the oily matter which collects on the

---

* See observations of Cheyne, Dublin Hospital Reports, vol. i.; and of Belcombe, Medical Gazette, vol. iv.

discharges, are soluble in ether, and are readily proved to be fat by the microscope; they burn, too, like fat, with a flame. In some instances the bowels are very constipated, and lumps of hard feces are discharged along with the fatty substance. This happened in a marked example of the disorder that came under my observation. The patient, a man twenty-six years of age, passed a considerable amount of fat both by the rectum and with the urine. He suffered much from digestive disturbance, from constipation, and from weakness. He had a good appetite, but a dislike to fats of any kind. In his case there was, so far as the physical signs indicated, no tumor in the region of the pancreas. The man's condition was much improved by the administration of cinchona and rhubarb; but whether permanently or not I cannot say, as I lost sight of him.

Diseases attended with Vomiting and Purging.

There is a group of diseases in which vomiting and purging are very prominent symptoms. It embraces those disorders in which the intestine and stomach are equally involved. To this group belong some affections which have already been considered, which begin in one viscus and then spread to the other. But those in which both are primarily affected, still remain to be described. The most important of them are the various forms of cholera. Now, there are several very different complaints classed together under the head of cholera. Let us proceed to consider them one by one.

Cholera Infantum.—And first, of the so-called cholera of infants. It is an endemic in the larger cities of the United States during the hot months, and one fraught with danger to all young children. Hundreds die of this summer complaint every year in our densely populated towns.

It commences generally with diarrhœa. Vomiting soon follows; and for a time the two go hand in hand; but unless the case be of very short duration, the spontaneous vomiting ceases, or at all events gives way to occasional exacerbations of irritability of the stomach, while the looseness of the bowels remains, or even augments. The discharges are colorless, or yellowish, or greenish. There is thirst; sometimes fever. The abdomen may be sunken or swollen; and it may be tender. Sometimes the disease runs its course within three or four days; at the end of which time the child dies, worn out by the constant vomiting and purging. More generally the disorder is of longer duration; for weeks or for months it continues; the diarrhœa improving and then returning with redoubled severity. The irritability of the intestinal canal, and the utter impossibility of retaining enough food to nourish the wasting body, gradually wear out the system. The child before death is wan and distressingly emaciated; sometimes restlessness, plaintive cries, rolling of the head, strabismus, coma,—the symptoms of hydrocephalus, —precede the fatal termination.

Such is a sketch of grave and intractable cases. Yet many cases are far from being so desperate. Under judicious treatment a large number are annually saved. Recoveries would bear a still higher proportion to the deaths, were it not that the greatest sufferers from the disease (the children of the poor) are unable to obtain the means most certain to restore them to health—change of air. Cooped up in crowded neighborhoods, surrounded on all sides by filth rapidly decomposing under the burning rays of the sun, they are compelled to breathe the hot, noxious atmosphere which has been the chief agent in generating the complaint. And by bearing this fact in mind we may do much to alleviate the disorder. Even when circumstances render exchanging the city for the country impossible, much good may be effected by directing the child to be carried daily into situations where the air is pure. In all cases, irrespective of the medicinal means employed, the diet must be regulated, and the gums carefully examined to see that the irritation of teething does not keep up or increase the gastro-intestinal excitability.

Cholera Morbus.—Like the cholera of infants, cholera morbus is a disease of the hot season; yet it is also observed at other times of the year. But, although the chief predisposing cause is undoubtedly heat, there is generally an exciting cause which develops the disorder: such as exposure, checked perspiration, drinking large quantities of ice-water, or imprudence in eating. The attack is characterized by spasmodic pains in the abdomen, by cramps in the legs, by rapid loss of strength, and by repeated vomiting and purging. The matter ejected both from the stomach and intestines is liquid, and contains a large quantity of bile. In truth, the affection is in reality a cholera, a flow of bile, which its more formidable namesake, Asiatic cholera, is not.

The disease is sometimes preceded by colicky pains, nausea, and rumbling in the intestines. More generally it comes on suddenly. When at its height, the cramps in the calves of the legs cause the muscles to rise up in hard, knotty masses; the stools are fetid; the vomiting is constant; the thirst is very great, and the skin is cool or cold. But the patient does not long remain in this condition. In the course generally of a few hours, or at the utmost of a day, the symptoms mitigate. or yield entirely to treatment; and pale and visibly emaciated though he be, he speedily regains his previous health. Only in some cases the disease proves intractable, and, after running on for several days, passes into a state of hopeless collapse.

There are not many morbid states with which cholera morbus is likely to be confounded. It may be mistaken, as we shall presently see, for epidemic cholera. We find many points of similarity between it and irritant poisoning, and some between it and acute gastritis. But there are also strong points of difference: the vomiting and purging produced by an irritant poison do not come on at the same time; the vomiting precedes the purging. The pain is first in the epigastrium, thence it may spread. Moreover, we detect often signs in the mouth or fauces which prove the irritating character of the substance swallowed. The vomiting of acute gastritis is accompanied by a hot skin, a small, tense pulse; whereas the skin of cholera morbus patients is commonly cool, and the pulse very compressible and feeble.

Cholera.—The formidable complaint known as epidemic cholera, Asiatic cholera, malignant cholera, or by the simple name of cholera, has some striking features of resemblance to the disorder just considered. It shares with cholera morbus the vomiting and purging, the cramps, the sudden depression; but it is an affection of different origin, and of much more serious import, and presents symptoms not encountered in the cholera that occurs yearly during the hot weather. And, although I am describing it, on account of the gastric and intestinal disturbances which form so prominent a part of its manifestations, in the same group with cholera morbus and among the disorders of the alimentary tube, I am doing so for the sake of clinical convenience, and contrary to sound pathology; for cholera is not an affection either of the stomach or intestines; it is an epidemic constitutional disorder of the most formidable character, generated by a poison transmitted to us from the East. The poison leads to a casting off of the epithelium of the mucous membrane of the alimentary tube; perhaps to changes in the membrane. But the engorged veins all over the body; the ready exosmose of the watery parts of the blood; the frightfully rapid prostration; the sudden blight which befalls the nervous powers,—are elements even more characteristic, and which throw more light on the nature of the fearful malady, than the comparatively uncertain and far from uniform appearances of irritation in the intestinal canal.

The access of cholera is at times sudden and most unexpected; the patient, previously in good health, is stricken down without warning by the force of the poison. More generally there is a premonitory stage: a stage of languor, low spirits, uneasiness, headache, and diarrhœa. The effects of the tainting of the atmosphere with the morbific matter are indeed visible in hundreds of individuals who, during the prevalence of cholera, suffer from these premonitory symptoms without any of greater danger arising. Nay, the same influences which give rise to a *choleraic diarrhœa* in healthy persons have the effect of rendering the bowels of those habitually constipated regular, and sometimes even loose.

When the malignant disease is fairly developed, there is vomiting as well as purging. The contents of the stomach and intestines are first voided, and then large quantities of a rather turbid fluid resembling rice-water, and with whitish particles like rice floating in it. They are the epithelial cells of the alimentary tube, which have been thrown off from the mucous membrane. Simultaneously with the vomiting and purging, or very shortly after, come on severe spasmodic pains in the abdomen and cramps of the muscles of the belly and extremities. With all this there are a burning sensation in the epigastric region; an unquenchable desire for cold drinks; a cool skin; a pulse slightly more frequent than normal; a hurried and oppressed breathing; and a rapidly progressing exhaustion. The case now stands on the very verge of collapse. Should this succeed,—and unfortunately it does succeed in a fearfully large number of instances,—a state of things is witnessed which, once seen, remains indelibly engraved on the memory. The pulse is quick, but hardly perceptible. The discharges cease, and so do often the cramps. The skin is cold, covered with a clammy sweat, and has a bluish look. The nails and the lips have the same unnatural appearance. The whole body shrinks, and seems at times almost to wither visibly even while under inspection. The countenance assumes the aspect of death; the eyes are sunken and have a glassy look. The intellect is commonly clear; but when the patient talks, the words fall strangely on the ear. It seems as if a corpse had spoken, and the voice is husky and faint. The tongue and the expired air are cold. No symptom, indeed, has struck me more forcibly than the icy breath.

But the symptoms do not always take place in the order described, nor are all uniformly present. The vomiting and purging may be wanting from the onset, and so too may the cramps. Only one symptom is never absent—the tendency to early sinking. And sometimes a stage of perfect collapse is reached with frightful rapidity. Instead, as is commonly the case, of several hours elapsing before complete prostration comes on, the vital powers are at once laid low by the assault of the dreadful malady. When cholera prevailed in Philadelphia some years since, I attended a woman who at six o'clock in the morning was in perfect health, and in a little more than half an hour afterward was a lifeless body.

There was neither vomiting nor purging; nothing but cramps, stupor, and speedy collapse. Such cases are not uncommon in the home of cholera—India. Post-mortem inspection shows the thin rice-water fluid locked up in the alimentary canal. Nature may have made an effort to eliminate the poison; but before she completes her task, life is palsied.

In those cases that recover, the vomiting and purging gradually subside, the skin becomes warm, the pulse fuller, the urine—which, while the disease was at its height, was not passed, perhaps not secreted—is again voided, the patient falls into a refreshing sleep, and, the symptom most favorable of all, bile reappears in the stools. Even in apparently hopeless cases of collapse may we be fortunate enough to witness these favorable changes. But where the prostration has been great, the reaction is apt to be violent. A decided fever of low type, with rapid pulse and heat of skin, and attended very often by alarming cerebral symptoms, succeeds; and the urinary secretion, even if it have been restored, becomes again very scanty. Thus the period of reaction brings with it new dangers, and of a kind which are sometimes insurmountable. And this low form of fever, very similar to typhoid, though readily enough distinguished by the preceding symptoms, may last for upwards of a week before death takes place or the signs of danger gradually yield. Now this cholera typhoid may be preceded by scanty urine and marked uræmia, but it may also exist independently of this morbid state, though probably due equally to the blood being loaded with broken-down material. In cases in which uræmia sets in, whether it be followed or not by a fever of low type, there is at first but little, if any, heat of skin and a slow pulse; the patient is wild, restless or drowsy, the kidneys act very imperfectly, the urine is greatly deficient in urea, and usually contains albumen. These are very dangerous cases, and if the secretion is seriously retarded for more than twenty-four hours they are likely to perish.

In any case of cholera convalescence is apt to be slow. For weeks or months irritability of the intestinal canal remains;

and I have met with instances in which it has never disappeared.

It would be needless to go into any minute description of the differences between cholera and other affections; its features are not to be mistaken. Cholera morbus is the only disorder which really resembles it. The dividing line is drawn by the absence of bile in the discharges, the rice-water evacuations, the greater severity and more rapid progress of the symptoms, the bluish color of the surface in the stage of collapse, and the epidemic character of the more fatal disease. In the truly epidemic nature of the distemper, and in the speedy collapse, which shows but too plainly that some highly deleterious matter has poisoned the system, lie even in doubtful cases the proofs that we are dealing with malignant cholera; for sometimes rice-water discharges occur in bad cases of cholera morbus; occasionally, too, this disorder appears to be epidemic; but it is only so on a very small scale. To speak more accurately, it is an endemic on a large scale. We find no proofs of a virulent poison wafted about in the atmosphere, or directly conveyed by human intercourse and traffic, and so noxious as to smite animals as well as man.

The mortality of cholera is very various. In many epidemies one-half, or more than one-half, die. In some the havoc is far less. The first cases that occur almost invariably perish; and, taken altogether, the disorder ranks among the most destructive to life. Its epidemic visitations are what the plague was to the Europeans of the seventeenth century, and what yellow fever still is to the inhabitants of this continent. It is at least as dangerous; its nature is as hidden; its management quite as unsatisfactory.

But although science has not as yet taught us how, with any certainty, to cure the pestilent disorder, she has taught us how we may do much toward averting it. Cleanliness; free ventilation; avoiding indigestible food; separating the sick from the well; and immediately checking the copious watery diarrhœa,—will reduce greatly the number of cases in every epidemic.

SECTION III.

DISEASES OF THE LIVER.

We have already inquired into the clinical methods of examining the liver, so as to form a judgment of its position, size, and other physical characteristics. Let us now look at some of the symptoms which a disease of the viscus generally manifests.

Pain is one of these. It is generally dull, and radiates from the seat of the liver to the upper portion of the thorax, to the scapula, to the shoulder, to the umbilicus. Commonly it is persistent and increased by strong pressure, but the exceptional cases are numerous.

Digestive troubles are very usual accompaniments of hepatic affections. They are of all grades: from mere indigestion to the signs announcing chronic gastritis.

Disturbance of the portal circulation is another very frequent consequence of disease of the liver. The flow of blood is interfered with, and the result is seen in the occurrence of dropsy, of piles, of partial peritoneal inflammation, of hemorrhages from the engorged stomach and intestines, or of enlargement of the spleen and of the veins on the surface of the abdomen.

Jaundice.—But the most frequent, and certainly the most significant manifestation of hepatic disorder, is jaundice. This marked sign shows itself by the yellow tinge imparted to the skin and to the conjunctiva; yet the yellowness is not confined to these structures. It may often be found in internal organs. Besides the peculiar aspect of the surface, icterus is usually attended with depression of the circulation; with pruritus; with high-colored urine, in which the main ingredients of bile can be detected; with constipation, the feces passed being hard and knotty, and often of bad odor, and almost devoid of color, or sometimes of a leaden hue.

Jaundice, there can be no doubt, is due to the presence of biliary constituents in the blood; but it is as yet not satisfactorily solved how they get there. It was the opinion of Haller and of Boerhaave, and it is still the opinion of many, that the bile, in consequence of some impediment to its outward passage after it is formed in the liver, is reabsorbed and conveyed into the circulation. Others hold that the liver is at fault by not performing its function and clearing the blood of the ingredients which form the bile ; these, whether they be bile pigment, or the biliary acids, or cholesterin,* accumulate in the blood, and give rise to the characteristic discoloration of jaundice. Now, neither of these theories will explain all cases : many instances of jaundice are at once interpreted by the former supposition ; but in others it does not suffice, and the view of jaundice from suppression appears more probable. Yet other theories have been advanced to account for some obscure forms of jaundice ; such as the view of Frerichs, that the metamorphosis of the colorless bile acids which enter the blood and are there changed into urinary pigment, is arrested by the action of some poison, and that the acids are converted into bile pigment, which, circulating with the blood, changes the hue of the surface and of the secretions.

The diagnosis of jaundice is easy. The only two morbid states with which it is liable to be confounded are the slightly yellowish hue of chlorosis, and the yellow appearance of the conjunctiva which is natural to some persons. The changed color of the countenance due to alteration of the blood is discriminated by its association with a bluish-white or pearly-tinted eye. The yellow look of the eye sometimes found in health is known by the unequal distribution of the color and the absence of a yellow hue of the complexion. But in negroes, and it is in them especially that we meet with the discolored conjunctiva, we have to judge by the character of the coloration alone. In doubtful cases, the chemical tests by which we recognize bile in the urine would solve the doubt.

When once jaundice has been recognized, the difficulty in diagnosis may be said to begin. Of the very many distinct

---

* Austin Flint, Jr., Amer. Journ. of the Med. Sciences, Oct. 1862.

sources of icterus, which one is before us? Now, clinically speaking, the causes may be thus grouped: 1. Diseases of the liver. 2. Diseases of the bile ducts. 3. Diseases of parts remote from the liver, or general diseases leading to a disorder of the viscus. 4. Certain poisons acting upon the blood. In the first two of these causes there is, as it were, a mechanical difficulty impeding or arresting the excretion of bile; in the third and fourth, no obvious impediment exists, and the origin of the jaundice is usually very obscure. Cases belonging to the third group, however, may be at times explained on the supposition of a derangement of the hepatic circulation. Let us now look at some of the peculiarities of these groups.

1. The jaundice connected with diseases of the liver is, as a rule, recognized by its association with changed dimensions of the organ, and with pain or other palpable signs referred to the hepatic region. It is met with in all disorders of the liver; but does not exist in all in the same degree of intensity. It reaches a high development and is combined with cephalic symptoms in acute yellow atrophy. In fatty liver, in waxy liver, in cancer, in cirrhosis, and in acute hepatitis it is not very marked, and may be, indeed, absent; in truth, it can hardly be looked upon as belonging to the first-mentioned morbid states.

2. Jaundice arising from disease of the larger biliary ducts, or, what is more common, in consequence of their obstruction by pressure exercised by a morbid enlargement of adjacent parts, such as of the pyloric extremity of the stomach or the pancreas; or by their stoppage by inspissated bile or a biliary calculus,—is a form of the malady in which the icterus is commonly very intense. It occasions no head symptoms: and when these are absent in a case of very deep jaundice; when, further, the stools are completely discolored,—we are generally correct in attributing the morbid phenomena to an impediment to the flow of bile through the common bile duct or the hepatic duct. If this impediment be due to the impaction of a gall-stone, severe colicky pains are encountered in addition to the signs just mentioned.

As a further means of discriminating the jaundice due to

obstruction, no matter what the immediate cause, we may avail ourselves of the researches of Dr. Harley.* This physician found that in the jaundice due to reabsorption of the bile into the blood,—precisely the form of jaundice, therefore, that happens if any serious obstacle in the biliary passages exists,—the biliary acids which have been formed in the liver pass into the blood, and thence into the urine. This does not occur if the jaundice be due to suppression. Hence, if we may accept these researches as conclusive, an examination of the urine will throw much light on the cause of jaundice, and especially on the circumstance whether or not it be due to obstruction of the bile ducts.†

3. Illustrations of jaundice following some local lesion of other parts of the body, or appearing in the course of a general constitutional affection, are furnished by the jaundice which happens in some cases of pneumonia, or which is encountered in remittent, in typhus, or in yellow fever. In these fevers, the jaundice is generally found to be connected with an acute enlargement and with structural changes in the organ; and in the latter malady, with disordered hepatic circulation and a fatty degeneration of the secreting cells.

To recognize the form of jaundice under discussion, we must examine all the viscera of the body with care, laying at the same time stress upon the history of the case and the phenomena attending the jaundice. Otherwise, too much importance will be attached to this symptom, and the disturbance of the liver be regarded as forming the whole complaint, when in reality it is but a very small part of it.

4. Poisons acting upon the blood sometimes give rise to jaundice very rapidly; for instance, the jaundice from snake-bites or from pyemic infection is very apt to be suddenly developed and to become quickly intense. In the history of the accident and the signs of alteration of the blood, we possess the means of distinguishing this form of jaundice at the bedside.

---

* Jaundice, its Pathology and Treatment. London, 1863.

† The accuracy of the conclusions as well as the availability of the modification of Pettenkofer's test, by which the biliary acids are tested for, is denied by Murchison in his recent work on Diseases of the Liver.

Thus, then, we can bring, clinically speaking, most of the varieties of jaundice under one or the other of the four heads mentioned. But there are a few kinds of jaundice which it is far from easy to classify; one of these is the jaundice from mental emotion; the other, the jaundice of newly-born children.

As regards the former, it is very difficult to explain its cause; nor, indeed, has any satisfactory explanation been given. All we know is, that violent anger or fright may lead, within a very brief space of time, to the development of jaundice, and that the quickly-occurring discoloration of the skin is not generally dangerous, nor, in fact, of long duration.

The jaundice of newly-born children—*icterus neonatorum*—is ordinarily a very mild complaint which appears soon after birth, and which rarely lasts over two weeks. The yellow hue of the skin is often very deep; yet the child does not suffer, and has no febrile excitement. The bowels are constipated, but the stools are not necessarily altered in their color, nor do they usually present the clayey look which might be expected from the aspect of the skin and conjunctiva. The origin of the jaundice is very obscure. It was attributed by Frank to a stoppage of the choledoch duct by meconium. Dr. West states that it is most frequently observed in children prematurely born.

The prognosis of jaundice depends upon its cause. In general terms, we may say that, if the icterus last upwards of two months, it is always a matter of some danger, as showing, in all likelihood, an organic lesion of the liver or biliary passages. If the discoloration of the skin be attended with cerebral symptoms, the patient's state is precarious. Icterus accompanying affections of the blood, peritonitis, or pneumonia is an unfavorable sign; so is a very dark color of the skin. Indeed, cases of "green" or "black" jaundice generally prove fatal.

The treatment of jaundice turns upon the condition of the liver to which it may be owing. Still, although in accordance with this view the indications for treatment are drawn rather from our recognition of the source of the icterus, and although we ought to be on our guard against treating a symptom instead of the primary cause of that symptom, yet there are certain general indications which are constantly recurring, and of which we must not in any case lose sight.

One of these is to increase the action of the skin; another to keep up the action of the kidneys; a third indication is to stimulate the bowels to free action.

Before examining the hepatic maladies according to their clinical features, let us look at their pathological classification:

DISEASES OF THE LIVER.

Diseases of hepatic parenchyma.	Hyperæmia	{ Acute congestion. Chronic congestion.
	Inflammation and its consequences.	{ Acute hepatitis. Chronic hepatitis. Interstitial inflammation, or cirrhosis. Abscess. Softening. Syphilitic hepatitis.
	Atrophy	{ Acute or yellow, with suppression of function of liver. Simple chronic atrophy.
	Hypertrophy	{ Partial. General.
	Degeneration and new formations	{ Fatty liver. Waxy liver. Pigment liver. Cancer. Hydatids. Tubercle, etc.
Diseases of biliary passages.	Inflammation of gall-bladder and gall-ducts	{ Catarrhal. Exudative. Suppurative.
	Occlusion of biliary passages.	
	Dilatation of gall-bladder.	
	Morbid growths.	
	Foreign bodies; concretions, such as gall-stones.	
Diseases of blood-vessels.	Of hepatic artery.	
	Of hepatic vein.	
	Of portal vein	{ Suppurative inflammation. Coagulation of blood.

Acute Diseases of the Liver attended generally with slight Enlargement of the Organ, and with more or less, though rarely very much, Jaundice.

Acute Congestion.—This arises, like chronic hyperæmia, from organic disease of the heart, from obstructed portal circulation, from disturbed digestion, or from malarial poison; sometimes it is caused by a high temperature, by a blow on the hepatic region, or by arrest of the menstrual flow. The acute congestion is characterized by pain in the right shoulder and loin, by an unpleasant sensation of weight and of tension in the right hypochondrium, and by nausea and vomiting. At the same time the action of the bowels is deranged, being generally too frequent; the tongue is coated; there is depression of spirits, with loss of appetite and of strength; and the liver is enlarged. But we find ordinarily only slight jaundice, and there is no fever. Gradually these signs disappear; the increased hepatic dulness, however, remaining for some time after the gastric and intestinal disturbances have abated. Not unfrequently the acute disorder passes by imperceptible degrees into a chronic state.

Acute Hepatitis.—The symptoms of this affection are much the same as those of acute congestion, excepting that we observe more thirst, greater gastric irritability, a more embarrassed respiration, heat of surface, dry cough, and in some cases an accelerated pulse, enlargement of the spleen, and albumen in the urine. The pain is dull, and associated with a feeling of tension in the hypochondrium. It is somewhat increased on pressure, but not much so, unless the peritoneal covering of the liver be involved. Jaundice is not generally very marked; indeed, at the commencement of the disease it is often absent.

Acute hepatitis is very common in hot countries, and many of the cases are found to be connected with dysentery. It may end in resolution; but the inflammation often terminates in suppuration, and pus collects in the substance of the liver. The occurrence of this untoward event is indicated by recurring rigors, by cold and clammy perspirations, by prostration, and loss of flesh. Not unfrequently, too, a decided fulness of the side may be noticed, and occasionally careful palpation detects deep-seated fluctuation. After an abscess has formed, the danger is very great. The patient is apt to perish from peritonitis or from blood-poisoning; delirium, singultus, and meteorism preceding the fatal issue. Yet recovery may take place. The matter may be discharged through the abdominal walls, or burst into the intestine, or find its way through the diaphragm into the pleural cavity, to be discharged through the lung. But as the phenomena of abscess of the liver following acute inflammation are the same as when the collection of pus is consequent upon other morbid states, we shall not here indicate what we shall have presently more fully to consider.

Let us now examine the maladies with which acute inflammation of the liver may be confounded, premising the statement that, making allowance for the febrile phenomena and the other slight signs of difference just indicated between hepatic inflammation and hepatic congestion, the same remarks will apply to the distinction between this morbid condition and the affections about to be mentioned. The complaints resembling acute hepatitis are:

PERIHEPATITIS;

INFLAMMATION OF THE PORTAL VEINS;

PIGMENT LIVER;

CHRONIC HEPATIC DISEASES WITH ACUTE SYMPTOMS;

ACUTE NON-HEPATIC DISEASES WITH JAUNDICE;

DIAPHRAGMATIC PLEURISY;

INFLAMMATION OF THE BILIARY PASSAGES;

ACUTE YELLOW ATROPHY.

Perihepatitis.—Inflammation of the serous covering of the liver, limited to this covering, or spreading perhaps here and there to the most superficial portions of the structure of the gland, is not a very frequent disease. It is generally caused by the extension of inflammation from organs adjacent to the liver,—as for instance from the stomach, intestines, diaphragm, or pleura,—and may therefore be looked upon as a local peritonitis; or it is an attendant upon disease of the liver itself. In the latter case, it presents no peculiar

symptoms, excepting, perhaps, that it adds tenderness to the
signs of the hepatic malady it complicates.   In the former
case it is more likely to be confounded with acute inflammation of the liver texture, yet the far greater tenderness, the
pain upon motion or deep inspiration, the perfectly normal
size of the gland, the evidences of a disease in the neighborhood of the liver which is likely to have caused the malady,
the absence of jaundice and of splenic enlargement, and the
slight fever, distinguish the perihepatic inflammation from
true hepatitis.

Inflammation of the Portal Veins.—An inflammation of the
portal veins, terminating in suppuration, is very liable to be
mistaken for acute inflammation of the liver.   Nor are there
in truth any positive symptoms by which we can discriminate
between the two maladies.   Still, we may sometimes suspect
that the veins are the seat of inflammation, rather than the
structure of the liver, if, with the signs of acute and painful
enlargement of the organ, we find jaundice, thin and copious
stools, recurring chills and profuse sweats, emaciation, increase in size of the spleen, without any apparent fluctuation
or other signs of a hepatic abscess ; if there exist pains between
the ensiform cartilage and umbilicus, or in the epigastrium
or right hypochondrium, or shooting to the lumbar and sacral
regions; if following these symptoms appear striking evidences of hectic fever, or peritonitis; and if these phenomena
are encountered in a person who, on account of a previous
affection of the intestines or spleen, or any other organ
having a direct venous connection with the portal circulation,
is liable to disease of the portal system.   Enlargement of the
spleen is a very constant feature of impediment in the portal
vein, whether from inflammation or thrombosis.

Pigment Liver.—" In individuals who die from the effects
of marsh poison, under symptoms of severe intermittent,
remittent, or continued fevers, we frequently find peculiar
changes of the liver associated with functional derangements
of the organ, and of the parts pertaining to the portal system.
The liver presents a steel-gray, or blackish, or not unfrequently a chocolate color; brown insulated figures are observed upon a dark ground.   This change of color is pro-

duced by pigment matter which is accumulated in the vascular apparatus of the gland." So says Frerichs, the observer who has most carefully described the pigment liver.*

But the liver is not the only organ implicated in the morbid process: the spleen is commonly affected; the blood becomes watery, its corpuscles are broken down, and it contains large quantities of pigment; and pigment accumulates in the kidneys or brain. Now, the effect of all this is to occasion marked symptoms, besides those referable to the derangement of the liver; for it is not unusual to find grave cerebral disturbance, albuminuria, hemorrhage from the intestines, profuse diarrhœa, and enlargement of the spleen. Irrespective of these manifestations, we must note the singular ash, or grayish-yellow color of the skin, the evident hydræmia, and the very great amount of pigment which is readily detected in even a few drops of the blood. The fever that accompanies the morbid condition is of an intermittent type; the pulse is not, as a rule, much accelerated, and the jaundice is generally slight. In India pigmentary degeneration of the liver tends to suppurative hepatitis.†

When we contrast the phenomena described with those of acute hepatitis, we see at once the difference. The fever, the aspect of the patient, the blood full of dark pigment, and the frequency of cerebral symptoms are entirely unlike the indications of acute hepatic inflammation.

Chronic Hepatic Diseases with Acute Symptoms.—We occasionally meet patients who, when they first present themselves to us, seem to be laboring under an acute affection of the liver, either some form of acute inflammation of the liver structure or the biliary passages, or acute congestion of the liver; but in whom the acute symptoms have merely supervened upon a chronic complaint. Such cases are very puzzling; it may be indeed impossible to arrive immediately at their solution, and we have to wait until the acute symptoms subside, before the diagnosis is determined. Sometimes,

---

* Treatise on Diseases of the Liver, vol. i.
† Aitken's Pract. of Medicine, vol. ii.

however, an accurate inquiry into the history of the affection will lead to a knowledge of the real condition—still, far from always; for the malady may have been latent and scarcely attracted the patient's attention. In hepatic cancer, as an example presently to be mentioned will show, the sudden and rapid development of the malady amid the signs of acute congestion is not very uncommon. Occasionally the peculiar physical phenomena of individual hepatic diseases, such as the nodular tumors of a malignant growth, or the fluctuation of a hydatid cyst, will assist materially in the diagnosis.

Acute Non-hepatic Diseases with Jaundice.—As we have already observed, while treating of jaundice, there are many acute affections, such as pneumonia, pyæmia, puerperal fever, and some forms of poisoning, in which jaundice may coincide with febrile symptoms, and excite suspicions of acute hepatitis, or, at all events, of an extreme degree of acute hepatic congestion. But the yellowness of the skin which may attend the non-hepatic disorders mentioned is accompanied by symptoms so different from those connected with the jaundice of acute inflammation of the liver, that a mistake is not likely to arise if the history of the case be taken into account, and other viscera besides the liver be explored. A careful examination will therefore prevent a serious error.

Diaphragmatic Pleurisy.—The manifestations of inflammation of the pleural covering of the diaphragm are in several respects similar to those of inflammation of the liver. We find, for instance, pain in the right hypochondrium, nausea and vomiting, cough and embarrassed respiration, occasionally jaundice—much the same symptoms which we observe in hepatitis, especially if the serous envelope of the liver be at the same time implicated. But the pain in diaphragmatic pleurisy is greater, more suddenly developed, and is much more aggravated by movements and by full inspiration; the difficulty in breathing amounts to orthopnœa; we frequently encounter hiccough and great anxiety, sometimes a sardonic grin on the features, and the cough comes on in paroxysms. And although, as a case recorded by Andral* proves, there

* Clinique Médicale, tome ii.

may be jaundice; yet this is in reality so very generally wanting, as scarcely to belong to the symptoms of diaphragmatic
pleurisy. Then in this complaint we may find friction sounds,
—though the physical signs will not always aid us, being, as
the febrile excitement is, often but slight and uncertain.*

   Inflammation of the Biliary Passages; Acute Yellow Atrophy.—
Both of these maladies may be readily confounded with hepatitis. But the former, although presenting more jaundice
than the other maladies of the group now under discussion,
is otherwise so similar that it may be classed with them, and
will be described as one of the main affections of this group;
the other belongs clinically to a different section—namely,
among diseases characterized by decrease in size of the liver,
and it is there that we shall point out its differences from
acute hepatitis.

Inflammation of the Gall-bladder and Gall Ducts.—
Inflammation, when it attacks the biliary passages, is most
apt to affect the gall-bladder and the ductus choledochus.
Very frequently the morbid process is propagated from the
stomach or intestines to the common duct, and nausea, furred
tongue, a feeling of weight in the epigastrium, and diarrhœa
occur previously to the discoloration of the feces, the jaundice, the increased hepatic dulness, and the very slight tenderness on pressure in the right hypochondrium; in other
words, the symptoms of gastric or gastro-intestinal catarrh
precede those of "icterus catarrhalis,"—by far the most
common form of inflammation of the gall-bladder; for suppurative inflammation is very rare.

   Now, this icterus catarrhalis is generally a very tractable
disorder; and after continuing for two or three weeks, it
usually subsides. But it may last for as many months; and
in rare instances the inflammation leads to an occlusion of
the bile ducts, and to a fatal issue. I had such a case in 1863
under my charge at the Philadelphia Hospital. The patient,
a man upwards of sixty years of age, died deeply jaundiced
and comatose. He had presented, during life, the signs of
enlargement of the liver; little or no tenderness in the

---

* Cases by Habershon, Guy's Hospital Reports, 1869.

hepatic region; no fever; but much gastric irritability and obstinate constipation, both of which had existed for three weeks prior to a noticeable discoloration of the skin. The whole disease was, so far as could be ascertained, of only two months' duration ; and the jaundice steadily deepened from the time of its first appearance. At the autopsy, the gall-bladder was found enormously distended, its coats thin, yet otherwise scarcely abnormal ; but the common duct was obliterated by inflammation. The stomach and upper bowel were congested, while the coats of the stomach toward the pylorus were thickened.

Now, in point of diagnosis, it is not generally difficult to distinguish the catarrhal inflammation of the gall-bladder, excepting in those rare instances in which the common duct or the hepatic duct is obliterated. It differs from hepatic inflammation chiefly by the absence of fever and of grave constitutional disturbance ; from the ordinary congestion of the liver, by the different etiological elements in the history of the case,—the one disorder occurring most commonly in connection with disease of the heart or an obstruction of the portal circulation, or a miasmatic poison ; the other following most usually exposure to cold and damp. Then, inflammation of the gall ducts gives rise to very much more jaundice. Further, we must not forget that what is called congestion is often really the disease we are discussing.

From the jaundice of chronic hepatic maladies—such as cancer or cirrhosis—we separate catarrhal icterus by the non-existence of the significant physical signs of these maladies, by its acute course, and by the dissimilar progress of the symptoms. Inflammation of the biliary passages, and the jaundice arising in consequence of biliary calculi, are distinguished by the severe pain, the sudden appearance of the icterus subsequent to the paroxysms of pain, its increase after such paroxysms, and its often rapid fading after the gall-stone is voided. The symptoms of the early stages of acute atrophy of the liver, as well as those of some cases of acute inflammation, may be so like the phenomena of inflammation of the gall-bladder and gall ducts, that their discrimination is for a time impossible.

Acute Diseases characterized by a Decrease in the Size of the Liver and by Deep Jaundice.

Acute Yellow Atrophy.—This dangerous affection consists in a rapid diminution in size of the liver, with changes in its secreting cells, amounting often to their complete disintegration. The functions of the liver are, in consequence, almost wholly suspended, and the evil effects of the accumulation of the elements of the bile in the blood show themselves plainly in the deep jaundice, and the profound disturbance of the nervous system. To this disease belong most of those cases of malignant jaundice which terminate rapidly in death after violent cerebral symptoms. The malady scarcely ever lasts a week; generally a few days only elapse before the patient becomes comatose and dies.

The complaint is sometimes ushered in by nausea, a coated tongue, irregular action of the bowels, a frequent pulse; at other times it begins abruptly with pain in the head, and vomiting, at first of the contents of the stomach, but soon of coffee-ground material, which is evidently altered blood. The skin is of a deep yellow, and becomes from hour to hour more intensely discolored. Jaundice is, indeed, never absent: it may not make its appearance before the other urgent symptoms; but sometimes it precedes the signs of serious trouble for several days, or even for longer— perhaps for upwards of two weeks.* There are not uncommouly pain in the hepatic region, meteorism, enlargement of the spleen, and hemorrhage from the bowels. The pulse exhibits extraordinary changes: it is generally very rapid, but sinks at times, without any assignable reason, to a normal frequency; during the deep coma of the last stages of the malady, the beat of the artery is apt to become slow and full, but it may be very quick and very small. There is fever, generally, however, not very active or presenting a marked rise in the temperature; and the surface may be covered with petechiæ, on account of the progressing dis-

---

* As in Observation No. XVII. of Frerichs' Treatise on Diseases of the Liver, vol. i. p. 214, Sydenham Society's Transl.

solution of the blood. But if we except perhaps the deep jaundice, the most significant symptoms are those referable to the nervous system. Severe headache, delirium, tremors, spasms, or a constantly-increasing stupor and sluggish pupils are the phenomena which show clearly what disturbance the poisoned blood is creating in the nervous centres.

Now, how does this fatal malady differ from acute inflammation of the liver? By the marked jaundice, the cerebral symptoms, the rapid diminution in the volume of the liver, the frequent pulse, and the occurrence of hemorrhages. Then, the circumstances under which acute atrophy makes its appearance are very dissimilar: we find it not unusually following violent mental emotions or excesses; or it occurs during pregnancy, and is then accompanied by renal disorder.

Indeed, the diagnosis is not generally a difficult one ; not nearly so difficult as between acute atrophy and typhoid fever, or between the former affection and yellow fever or certain local diseases, such as peritonitis, pneumonia, and meningitis, when accompanied by jaundice and delirium. The character of the eruption, the presence of diarrhœa instead of constipation, the milder nature of the mental wandering, and the slower progress of the disease are of much value in enabling us to distinguish between enteric fever and acute yellow atrophy of the liver. From yellow fever, acute atrophy differs by the epidemic character of the former and the different circumstances under which it arises, by the intense pain in the back, limbs, and forehead, the stages the febrile malady presents, the high fever temperature, the comparative absence of cerebral symptoms, and the enlargement rather than the atrophy of the liver.

From the other affections named, the hepatic disorder may be discriminated by a thorough examination of the various organs of the body, and by a careful weighing of all the symptoms. In truth, it is thus only that we can avoid error in diagnosis, since, unless we can establish satisfactorily the most positive sign of acute atrophy—the diminution of the percussion dulness corresponding to the wasting of the liver—there is hardly a manifestation of the hepatic malady so exclusive that it may not occur in the diseases mentioned, when these are complicated by jaundice. It is true that vomiting of blood is scarcely among their symptoms; but this does not invariably happen in acute atrophy. In many cases of doubt we may turn to account the researches of Frerichs on the character of the urine in this complaint, and seek in the urinary secretion for the deposition of sediments of tyrosine or for leucin; and test for the urea, which is greatly deficient or absent. We may in this connection remark that leucin and tyrosine have also been found in the blood and in many tissues of the body. This happened in a case which I saw with Dr. H. C. Wood, and which he has fully and carefully reported.*

The occurrence of the fatal malady in pregnant women has already been alluded to. Now, jaundice from mental emotion, or produced by the pressure of the gravid womb, is in them not unusual; and we may be called upon to distinguish this simple and harmless form of icterus from that of yellow atrophy. In the serious derangement of the nervous system, and the graver character of all the symptoms, lie the marks of separation.

Chronic Diseases attended with Enlargement of the Liver, and with slight or no Jaundice.

Chronic Congestion.—This morbid condition is observed chiefly in persons of sedentary habits, who indulge too freely in the pleasures of the table, in those who use large quantities of alcoholic drinks or fermented liquors, and is very frequently met with in hot climates and in malarial districts. It may also occur in scurvy, and in connection with abdominal affections which interfere with the portal circulation, and thus produce a fulness of the blood-vessels of the liver; or it may happen in consequence of a disturbance of the flow of blood through the liver, dependent upon disease of the heart.

Whatever the source of the hyperæmia, the symptoms are very similar. They are usually an impaired appetite, a coated tongue, a feeling of tension and weight in the right hypo-

---

* Amer. Journ. of Med. Sciences, April, 1867.

chondrium, depression of spirits, loss of strength, and occasional nausea and diarrhœa, or looseness of the bowels alternating with constipation. The conjunctiva has constantly a more or less jaundiced tinge; the dulness on percussion in the hepatic region is increased in extent. In some cases, the habitual congestion leads to an altered condition of the bile ducts and of the secreting cells of the liver; but ordinarily, unless the hyperæmia be kept up by some exciting cause which it is impossible to remedy—such as an abdominal tumor, or an organic affection of the heart—we can, by a carefully regulated diet and by active exercise in the open air, together with the use of laxatives, restrain the congestion, and, indeed, in time remove it. A very troublesome feature, however, of the malady is its disposition to return.

By attention to the signs mentioned, there is usually little difficulty in recognizing chronic hepatic congestion. How it may be discriminated from other forms of enlargement of the liver, we shall presently inquire. It is sometimes confounded with, or rather there is sometimes mistaken for it, a liver which has been pushed downward by the habit of tight lacing. But the absence of any signs of hepatic derangement, and the lowered outline of the upper border of the displaced right lobe, will generally enable us to distinguish this state from chronic congestion of the liver.

Chronic hepatic congestion, as indeed any disease of the liver which leads to its enlargement, may be confounded with chronic gastritis; and on account mainly of the fulness in the epigastric region which may happen in the hepatic malady, and which is so constant in the gastric affection. The error is particularly likely to occur in those cases of enlarged liver in which there is pain on pressure. But the outline of the dulness when the liver is increased in size, the jaundiced hue of the conjunctiva, the altered character of the stools, and, on the other hand, the more marked indigestion and the fulness and tenderness being equally perceived in positions to which the liver, unless very greatly augmented, does not extend, will ordinarily enable us to arrive at a correct diagnosis. Yet in attempting to do so we must not forget that the two morbid states may be conjoined.

Hypertrophy of the liver, it is believed, may present at times the manifestations of congestion. The little we know of an increased formation of the liver-cells, teaches us that this may happen as a partial hypertrophy, to compensate for loss of substance, in instances in which a portion of the gland has been destroyed; or as a more general increased growth in diabetes, in leucocythæmia, and as a consequence of malaria. Perhaps the history of the case may enable us to arrive at the discrimination of the rare disease. Yet there is never any certainty in the diagnosis: in truth, we cannot be said to possess the means which would enable us at the bedside to distinguish hypertrophy of the liver from other forms of hepatic enlargement.

Chronic Hepatitis.—The symptoms of this malady are very obscure; indeed, it is difficult to say what are its symptoms, because of the extreme latitude which has been given to the term chronic hepatitis, under which have been ranged most of the chronic affections of the organ—especially, however, the waxy, the fatty, the congested, and the cirrhotic liver. If, following Andral, we call only that state chronic inflammation in which the liver is augmented in size, harder than natural, yet easily torn, of deep-red color, and in which the exudation is very apt to become purulent, we find these manifestations: dull, heavy pain in the hepatic region, somewhat augmented by pressure; dry, heated skin, of sallow hue, and often the seat of distressing itching; a yellowish conjunctiva; indigestion; whitish stools, generally hard; a short cough; and the physical signs on palpation and percussion of an enlarged liver, the border of which is uniformly thickened and hardened.

The inflammation may be chronic in its course almost from its onset, and be developed under much the same circumstances as chronic congestion; or it may succeed to an attack of acute hepatitis. But chronic hepatitis is not a common disease, excepting in hot climates, and is scarcely to be distinguished, with any certainty, from persistent hyperæmia of the organ, unless when the inflammation leads to the formation of abscesses.

Abscess of the Liver.—Hepatic abscesses, as we have

already seen, may form as the result of either acute or chronic inflammation of the liver. In the tropics this is not at all an unusual termination of the inflammation; in temperate climates we seldom encounter the affection, save as the consequence of metastatic or pyemic inflammation of the liver, or in connection with some disease of the intestines.

The symptoms of hepatic abscess are very obscure. In pyæmia the collection of pus may take place in the liver without causing scarcely any phenomena which direct attention to the viscus. In the other forms of inflammation of the liver which produce abscesses, we are likely to have the same symptoms as in acute hepatitis, excepting that the formation of pus is apt to give rise to rigors, to quicken the pulse very much, to lead to night-sweats, and not unfrequently to the development of a fever simulating that of a quotidian or tertian intermittent.

The local signs, too, are far from being always very obvious, or indeed uniform. In some instances the hepatic region is more prominent than natural, and we can detect fluctuations over portions of the enlarged gland; but neither sign is constant, and the latter depends greatly upon whether or not the abscess be deeply seated in the hepatic parenchyma. Tenderness, either general or limited to a particular spot, is found only in a certain proportion of cases. It is frequently associated with a throbbing or a dull pain, which may be transmitted to the right shoulder. According to Annesley,* this sympathetic pain in the right shoulder indicates that the convex part of the right lobe of the viscus is affected. Conjoined to the feeling of weight, and to the throbbing in the hepatic region, is at times a tension occasioned by palpation of the abdominal muscles, especially of the rectus. Twining† regards this circumstance as a very significant manifestation of deep-seated abscess.

But a positive diagnosis of abscess of the liver is often a very difficult matter; for there are a number of other affections with which it may be readily confounded. Prom-

---

* Researches into the Diseases of India.

† Diseases of Bengal.

incut among these are hydatids, cancer of the liver, diseases of the gall-bladder, and a pleuritic effusion on the right side.

From *hydatids* of the liver, the febrile symptoms, the disturbed nutrition, and the pain distinguish a hepatic abscess, excepting in those cases in which the cyst becomes the seat of suppuration. Under these circumstances error can scarcely be avoided, unless we are fully cognizant of the history of the patient, and are in possession of facts furnishing clear evidence as to the state of the liver prior to the formation of pus.

Cancer of the liver differs from an abscess by its dissimilar history, by the hard nodular masses, and by the absence of fluctuation. It is only in rapidly growing medullary cancer that we can discern a sense of fluctuation; but even here we can generally distinguish some nodules which do not fluctuate; and should the soft cancerous matter impart to the finger a feeling of fluctuation, it is very rarely as distinct as that of an abscess. Further, the marked febrile phenomena and the other constitutional symptoms are not like what occur in hepatic cancer.

Of the *diseases of the gall-bladder*, the one which is most liable to be confounded with hepatic abscess is distention of the bladder. This occurs either from a closure of the cystic or common duct, especially from the former, or from an inflammation of the gall-bladder itself, and perhaps a subsequent closure of the ducts. In such a case the gall-bladder may become enormously distended with irritating and decomposing bile and puriform matter, and thus may be occasioned a fluctuating tumor, tender on pressure, and readily mistaken for an abscess.

Now, we are sometimes able to distinguish the soft swelling caused by a diseased gall-bladder by its situation, its pear-shaped form, its mobility and absence of adhesions to the abdominal walls, its distinct and persistent fluctuations; by its never having been hard; by the normal appearance of the parietes of the abdomen; by the non-existence of local œdema and redness; and by the fact that affections of the gall-bladder are frequently preceded by repeated attacks of violent pain due to the passage of biliary calculi, or by bilious

fever. Then we find very little jaundice, or none at all; and
no hectic fever. But to neither of these circumstances can
we trust implicitly. For there is apt to be very intense jaundice in an affection of the gall-bladder, if the common duct
also be implicated; and jaundice is, in abscess of the liver,
a symptom much more frequently absent than present. And
with reference to hectic fever, the continued suppuration in
the distending sac may produce it, and lead, indeed, as in a
case reported by the late Dr. Pepper,* to very great constitutional disturbance. As regards the shape of the swelling,
due to an enlarged gall-bladder being diagnostic, we must
bear in mind that it may be changed by contraction of the
muscular coat.

A *pleuritic* effusion on the right side of the chest is distinguished from a hepatic abscess by the same phenomena which
we found, in discussing pleurisy, to separate this affection
from all forms of enlargement of the liver. But abscesses
may open into the right pleural cavity. Then we observe
the physical signs of a pleuritic effusion subsequent to
those of hepatic abscess. Generally, too, the pus which has
made its way through the diaphragm destroys the lung
texture, until it reaches the bronchial tubes, when large
quantities of purulent sputa are expectorated; or, in rarer
instances, it is discharged through the walls of the chest. In
the former case, the disturbance in the pleura, and the accumulation of pus there, may be very limited: the inflammation of the pleural membrane may be circumscribed, while
the signs of an inflammation at the lower portion of the right
lung, dulness on percussion, tubular breathing, rusty-colored
sputa are very evident. These phenomena may subside, and
the respiration in parts become inaudible, when a discharge
of a large quantity of a reddish or whitish pus takes place,
in which the elements of bile, and the microscopical appearances of the hepatic tissue may be detected. Gradually this
expectoration ceases, and the affected textures heal. But in
some instances the discharge never stops, and the patient
dies worn out by the constant drain upon his strength.

---

* American Journal of the Medical Sciences, Jan. 1857.

When the abscess forces its way *externally*, it may, prior to its discharge through the thoracic or abdominal walls, occasion difficulty in diagnosis as regards abscesses originating in these walls. Nothing but a careful consideration of the attending symptoms and of the history of the case will lead to a differential distinction. Nor does the difficulty wholly cease when the slowly developed tumor, which a hepatic abscess forms, has opened, since it is far from always that we find in the pus the evidences of the broken-down liver tissue; and it is only occasionally that the fluid is of yellow or greenish color and yields the reactions of bile. The means of discrimination most to be relied upon is a probe, for by the depth to which it can be passed, the direction it takes, and the feel of the structures it encounters, we are placed in possession of many important facts bearing on the diagnosis. It was only thus that in a case under my charge at the Pennsylvania Hospital, and in which the symptoms were very conflicting, a positive diagnosis could be reached.

Fatty Liver.—A fatty liver occurs in drunkards; in persons who lead indolent lives and are large eaters; in wasting diseases, especially in phthisis; in the course of a protracted diarrhœa; and sometimes in children after exanthematous fevers. But of all these causes, pulmonary consumption is the most common.

Now, a knowledge of the sources of fatty liver is the most important element in the diagnosis; for neither the physical signs nor the symptoms present anything which is really characteristic. The physical signs are simply those of an enlarged liver. The symptoms are much the same as of hepatic congestion, excepting that there is perhaps greater tendency to diarrhœa, and that we find, in some instances, a pale, smooth, greasy-feeling skin. The amount of jaundice is always very slight; in truth, this symptom is frequently wanting. And partly in consequence of the absence of this important symptom of hepatic affections, and partly because of the little appreciable disturbance a fatty liver may occasion, this morbid state, especially if it be slight, at times escapes our observation entirely.

Waxy Liver.—A peculiar infiltration into the structure

of the liver, or its degeneration into a substance rendering it firmer and more glistening, gives rise to that appearance of the liver which is variously designated as waxy, lardaceous, amyloid, albuminous, or scrofulous liver.

The symptoms of a waxy liver are those of a hepatic derangement which manifests itself rather by the signs of disturbances of other organs than by the direct proof of altered function of the viscus really affected. Thus disordered digestion, nausea, vomiting, tympanites, discolored stools, and diarrhœa are very much more frequent than jaundice, which, indeed, is infinitely oftener absent than present. There is a feeling of fulness in the hepatic region, but little or no pain; while physical exploration exhibits an increased percussion dulness, and shows the organ to have a well-defined though somewhat rounded margin.

Enlargement of the spleen very commonly coexists with the enlargement of the liver, and in many cases the urine is albuminous from waxy disease of the kidneys. Dropsy, as a rule, is not encountered; but in this respect much depends upon the state of the kidneys and of the blood.

The etiology of a waxy liver teaches us that it is more common in males than in females; that the malady is most usually caused by constitutional syphilis; that in rarer instances it is produced by the tubercular diathesis; also that it coexists with scrofulous diseases of the bones, with collections of pus in various parts of the body, with repeated attacks of intermittent fever, or results, perhaps, from the abuse of mercury. In some cases we cannot trace the pathological process to any known cause; yet even in these cases we find it attended with signs of impaired nutrition, and occurring in persons evidently cachectic.

Now, when we contrast a waxy liver with other hepatic complaints in which the liver is enlarged, we find it resembling most closely the fatty and the syphilitic affections. But in the former although there is enlargement, there is not often so much increase in volume as in the waxy liver. Besides, the organ has a softer feel on palpation, and the disorder is not associated with a diseased spleen or kidney, and is far less likely than a waxy liver to give rise to dropsy. A syphilitic

hepatitis, with which indeed the waxy liver is at times combined, is mainly distinguished by the prominent nodules felt
on the surface of the liver, and which result from syphilitic
inflammation of the organ.

From congestion of the liver, waxy liver is readily discriminated. A comparatively slight affection in which jaundice
is frequent is very different from a grave malady in which the
hepatic disease forms but part of a general cachexia, and in
which jaundice is very infrequent.

Cancer of the Liver.—In cancer of the liver the size of
the organ is almost invariably increased, and sometimes it
reaches an enormous volume. The form of the gland, too,
is generally altered. It is irregular and uneven, nodules of
various size being developed in its substance and projecting
from its border and surfaces. These prominences are usually
harder than the surrounding hepatic tissue; but there are
exceptions to this rule, for sometimes, especially in the en-
cephaloid variety of the malady, the elastic tumors impart,
when pressed, a very deceptive sense of fluctuation. The
cancerous masses generally increase, and in some cases with
great rapidity.

The malignant disease is rarely confined to the liver; it
frequently supervenes upon cancer of the mammary gland or
of the uterus. It is an affection pre-eminently of middle life
or of old age; yet it occasionally occurs in young persons. I
have seen two cases of primary cancer of the liver in women
not twenty-five years of age.

Now, many of the pathological facts just mentioned have
a strong bearing on the diagnosis of hepatic cancer. They
especially throw light on the most important signs of the
malady—to wit, the increased percussion dulness in the hepatic region, and the uneven surface detected on palpation.
The enlarged liver is found extending across the epigastrium
far into the left hypochondrium; it reaches at times lower
than the umbilicus, and presses the diaphragm upward. The
nodules can often be felt distinctly through the abdominal
walls. The diseased organ is painful, and usually tender to
the touch. In cases in which the peritoneal covering is
affected, the tenderness is greatest. And, although any of

these three phenomena—the enlargement, the uneven surface, and the tenderness—may be absent, they are tolerably constant attendants on cancer of the liver. The tenderness is, I think, the sign least frequently wanting.

Among the symptoms of hepatic cancer, we find gastric and intestinal disturbances, pain in the right shoulder, rigidity of the abdominal muscles, a disordered nutrition of the whole body, a cachectic look, occasional febrile attacks, and, in the latter stages of the disease, sometimes hemorrhages from the stomach or bowels, and diarrhœa. Ascites, too, is observed among the symptoms of the malignant malady, and is generally dependent either upon chronic peritonitis attending the development of the cancer, or upon the pressure this exerts upon the larger branches of the portal vein. Jaundice may or may not be present; it is, on the whole, most frequently wanting. There are cases in which all these symptoms are perceived; while in others only some, in others, again, even these few may not be well defined. Indeed, when we consider the amount of deposit which is generally present; when we regard its character; when we take into account the necessarily impaired function of one of the most important glands in the body; when we reflect upon the pressure which the enlarged organ must occasion,—it is truly astonishing that often so little dropsy, so little jaundice, so little pain, so little constitutional disturbance should be produced by the disease.

Yet, in point of diagnosis we can generally discern the malady by the combination of the symptoms and signs indicated. It is only at an early stage of the disease, or when the liver is not enlarged, that we are apt to be in doubt. Under the former circumstance, a swelling in the hepatic region, pain upon pressure associated with nausea and vomiting and with failing health, occurring in a person above thirty-five years of age, may well excite our suspicion. But unless there be a cancer in some other part of the body, we cannot be certain that the commencing swelling in the right hypochondrium is malignant. When the liver is the seat of cancer, but is not increased in size, the recognition of the malady is next to impossible. In these obscure cases, the persistent tenderness in the hepatic region, accompanying the evidences of disturbed function of the liver, ascites, and a cachectic appearance, are the signs most trustworthy and most likely to lead to a correct conclusion.

But let us pass in review the affections with which well-marked cancer of the liver is likely to be confounded. Omitting here hydatids, abscess of the liver and cirrhosis, they are:

WAXY LIVER; FATTY LIVER; CHRONIC CONGESTION;

ACUTE CONGESTION AND ACUTE HEPATITIS;

SYPHILITIC LIVER;

DISEASES OF THE GALL-BLADDER;

CANCER OF THE STOMACH;

CANCER OF THE OMENTUM;

ENLARGEMENT OF THE RIGHT KIDNEY.

Waxy Liver; Fatty Liver; Chronic Congestion.—A waxy liver presents often as much increase in size as cancer; moreover, like cancer, it is associated with evident signs of cachexia. The main points of distinction are the combination of the former morbid condition with enlargement of the spleen and albuminous urine, and the history of the case pointing to constitutional syphilis or to diseases of the bones, or long-continued suppuration,—in fact, to the causes which generally lie at the root of the development of a waxy or lardaceous state of organs. When distinct nodules are perceived in examining the liver, of course the difficulty in diagnosis ceases.

A fatty liver is much easier to discriminate from hepatic cancer. The occurrence of the non-malignant malady in consumptives or in drunkards, the absence of pain,—in truth, of any decided indications of hepatic disease, excepting increased size of the organ,—enable us to distinguish between the two affections with certainty. The slighter signs of disturbance, both constitutional and local, the dissimilar history, and the uniform enlargement of the liver separate chronic congestion from cancer. As a mark of distinction, too, of the cancerous from all of these non-malignant disorders, Virchow lays stress on the existence of swollen jugular glands.

Acute Congestion and Acute Hepatitis.—It is very rarely, indeed, that either of these ailments is confounded with cancer of the liver, because the history in this malady and the course it takes are so dissimilar to an acute hepatic disorder. Yet there are cases in which the malignant disease is either developed with great rapidity, thus simulating acute congestion or acute inflammation, or in which it has lain dormant and passed unnoticed until it begins suddenly to increase. Under such circumstances even, we may be able to recognize the malignant complaint, if its physical phenomena be well defined; but if these be not clearly marked, the diagnosis becomes one of very great difficulty.

To cite a case in illustration:

A married woman, twenty-five years of age, was admitted into the Philadelphia Hospital on January 14th, 1862, with jaundice and slight fever. She stated that she had been in excellent health until about two weeks before, when she caught cold by sleeping in a damp apartment. Her appetite and digestion had been good previous to her present illness, and she had been fully able to perform her household work. Since she was taken sick she had noticed a feeling of weight in the region of the stomach and liver. When examined, rales indicative of bronchitis were found in the chest, and the impulse of the heart was feeble. The hepatic percussion dulness was observed to be increased in extent, especially that of the left lobe; but the outline of the organ appeared regular and even. Tenderness at the lower portion of the abdomen, but more particularly in the epigastrium and right hypochondrium, was also noted. There was nausea, but no vomiting; the tongue was clean; the evacuations were discolored.

Now, here was certainly a patient presenting none of the signs of hepatic cancer, excepting, perhaps, the tenderness over the enlarged gland. Yet at the autopsy, which was made within a week after her reception into the hospital, and therefore not three weeks from the apparent beginning of the complaint, whitish nodular spots, evidently cancerous, and many of them soft, were found in the substance of the liver, but not at its edges, nor forming anywhere distinct protuberances which could have been detected during life, and which, had they existed and been discerned, might, notwithstanding the history of the case, have furnished a clue to the cause of the tenderness and of the hepatic enlargement.

Syphilitic Liver.—As a consequence of constitutional syphilis, the liver may at times exhibit cicatrices on its surface, and scattered nodules, consisting of connective tissue, and extending into the parenchyma. This condition is styled syphilitic inflammation of the liver, or the syphilitic liver. The organ becomes uneven from the contraction of the cicatrized parts, and is very apt to be somewhat increased in size, from coexisting waxy degeneration. The patient has a pale, cachectic look, but is not jaundiced;* nor is dropsy present, unless there be at the same time an affection of the kidneys or enlargement of the spleen. But the most important elements in the diagnosis are the history of the case and the detection of syphilitic cicatrices in the throat. When contrasted with cancer, we find, besides these points, the chief distinctive marks to be: the much more usual absence of jaundice and of dropsy, the not uncommon increase of the spleen, the want of local hepatic tenderness, and the smaller size and softer feel of the nodules.

Diseases of the Gall-bladder.—Dilatation and cancer of the gall-bladder are both very liable to be mistaken for cancer of the liver. The former affection may result from occlusion of the hepatic and common bile ducts, produced by pressure of surrounding tumors or by an impaction of gall-stones; or it may be owing to the distention of the bladder with an albuminous fluid—the so-called dropsy of the gall-bladder. Now, in either instance the bladder may attain an enormous volume, and give rise to a marked tumor at the lower margin of the liver. The prominence is very apt to be rounded or pear-shaped, and, excepting in those cases in which the occlusion is in the cystic duct or at the neck of the gall-bladder, the impediment to the flow of bile is accompanied by intense

---

* No jaundice is mentioned in the cases of Dittrich, Prag. Vierteljahrschr., Bd. vi. and vii.; of Gubler, Mém. de la Société de Biologie, tome iv.; or of Bamberger, Krankheiten der Leber, in Virchow, Pathologie, etc.; of Moxon, in Guy's Hospital Reports, 1867.

jaundice and by decided hepatic swelling. Hence, in the deep hue of the skin, the uniform enlargement of the liver, the peculiar contour of the prominence, and the history of the case, which not unfrequently points to repeated attacks of colic from the passage of gall-stones,—we find the clue which permits us to determine that we have not to deal with hepatic cancer.

Cancer of the gall-bladder is scarcely ever met with in young persons, and is, as a rule, associated with cancerous formations in the liver or in other organs. It is very diffi-cult to make out a certain diagnosis of the affection, for it presents a strong likeness both to cancer of the pyloric extremity of the stomach and to cancer of the liver. From the latter it is undistinguishable, unless the situation and form of the tumor be such that we can clearly recognize it as belonging to the gall-bladder. Jaundice, as in cancer of the liver, may be absent or present: in five cases reported by Bamberger* it was found in all, and was even very intense. Frerichs, on the other hand, states that in most instances it is wanting. The signs of the cancerous cachexia are always very strongly marked; perhaps, as a rule, more strongly than in hepatic cancer.

Cancer of the Stomach.—This is discriminated from cancer of the liver by the far more constant vomiting, by the dark appearance of the ejected matter, by the more obvious symp-toms of indigestion, the persistent pain in the stomach, or the pain radiating from there to either hypochondrium. Moreover, the seat of the tumor is different; it is epigastric, or extending downward, but not often passing into the right hypochondrium, and it shows on percussion a very different contour from an enlarged liver. Yet there are cases in which we are kept in doubt; especially those in which the left lobe of the liver is chiefly affected with the cancerous malady and presses upon the stomach, inducing perhaps—and thus making the likeness still closer—obstinate vomiting. The only traits of distinction are then found in the presence or absence of the signs of marked derangement of the functions of the liver.

---

* Krankheiten des Digestions-Apparates.

Cancer of the Omentum.—The absence of jaundice, and the unaltered appearance of the stools are here, too, of great value in indicating that a tumor near, or joining the left lobe of the liver, is not due to cancer of that viscus. Moreover, the boundaries of the morbid mass are very different from those of a diseased liver. But we cannot always trust to this. Cancerous tumors of the lesser omentum may so surround the liver, and correspond so closely to the irregular form produced by hepatic cancer, that the two maladies cannot be distinguished; at least not by the local signs. Again, a loop of intestine may be thrust across the enlarged liver at a point corresponding to the usual limit of the percussion dulness of its left lobe, thus dividing the most prominent nodules from the greater portion of the viscus, and making it appear as if the tumor were to the left of, and below the stomach, and belonged, therefore, probably to the omentum.* Such cases, unless the history and the attending symptoms throw light upon them, are beyond the reach of diagnosis.

Enlargement of the Right Kidney.—A tumor formed by an enlargement of the kidney does not present the same outline of percussion dulness as a cancerous liver. The dulness is, moreover, bounded by the tympanitic sound of the intestine, and is not lowered by a deep inspiration; and the signs of disturbed function of the kidney, and an examination of the urine, will generally materially assist the diagnosis. Still, cases may occasionally happen in which, owing to a peculiar shape of the diseased kidney and to the obscurity of the symptoms, an error in diagnosis can scarcely be avoided. The difficulty in discrimination is heightened by the circumstance that most cases of morbid growth of the kidney, at least of one-sided growth sufficient to give rise to a palpable tumor, are cancerous; and are therefore, so far as the manifestations of a cachexia go, similar to cancer of the liver.

Hydatids of the Liver.—The development of one or of several cysts in the liver, containing within them echinococci, is not as a rule a disorder which occasions any serious dis-

---

* This happened in a case seen with Dr. S. Weir Mitchell, and published by him, Proceedings of Path. Society of Philadelphia, vol. i. p. 275.

turbance of the general health. Nor do the hydatids usually give rise to either jaundice, dropsy, or any marked signs of gastric or intestinal irritation, or to fever, or local pain. Their most constant manifestations are a decided increase of the size of the liver, and the presence of elastic tumors discernible in the hepatic region.

The growth of the hydatid is generally very slow, but in most cases it attains considerable dimensions, and the liver may be found to encroach upon the lung as far as the second intercostal space, or to extend far down into the abdominal cavity. On percussion, the line of dulness either of the upper or the lower boundary of the viscus, or of both, is perceived to be very irregular, and occasionally on striking a series of abrupt blows on the pleximeter, or the fingers of the left hand used as such, we discern a peculiar vibration (similar to the sensation perceived on striking a mass of jelly), to which Piorry was the first to call attention, and which is very significant of the existence of the cyst. Owing to the pressure the increasing tumor may exert on adjacent structures, we observe in some cases dry cough; palpitation and displacement of the heart; vomiting,—possibly jaundice and ascites.

Hydatids ordinarily last for years. The echinococci may die, the sac become much reduced in size, or obliterated, and recovery take place; or the cyst may discharge its contents through the stomach and intestines, through the bronchial tubes, or through the walls of the abdomen, and the patient then gets well. But so favorable a termination cannot be counted upon. A fatal issue may at any time ensue by the hydatid tumor bursting into the pleura or peritoneum, and leading to violent inflammation, or by inflammation and suppuration occurring in the sac, or in the tissues immediately surrounding it. Even when the hydatids are discharged through the stomach, intestines, or bronchial tubes, recovery is apt to be very slow; nor is it, indeed, very uncommon to find the patient's strength giving way before the contents of the sac have been entirely voided and it has closed.

In some countries hydatids are much more frequent than in others. In Iceland these growths developed from the eggs of a tapeworm are so common that they cause one-seventh of the human mortality.

Now, in point of diagnosis, it is not generally very difficult to detect the presence of hydatids. It is true that when these are small or deep seated, it may be impossible to discern them. But a large and superficially seated hydatid tumor can usually be distinguished, and can be separated in most cases from the maladies to which it bears a resemblance.

It differs from an abscess of the liver by the want of that febrile action, pain, and great constitutional disturbance to which the formation of an abscess is so prone to give rise; from cancer of the liver, by the absence of evident cachexia; of local tenderness and of the unevenness of the surface which the small, hard tumors projecting from it occasion. A distended gall-bladder may, like a hydatid tumor, be free from pain on pressure, but unlike this, it is preceded by attacks of colic, is generally accompanied by deep jaundice, and its situation corresponds to the normal seat of the gall-bladder.

An aneurism of the aorta differs from hydatids in the pulsation and the severe pain the patient suffers, so utterly dissimilar to the absence of pain or to the mere feeling of tension and weight of a hydatid swelling.

Pleuritic effusions have many features in common with those cases of hydatids of the liver in which the growing tumor extends upward into the chest. All the physical signs of a large effusion may be present, even the dilatation of the thorax and a sense of fluctuation in the intercostal spaces. But the irregular outline of the dulness on percussion of the hydatid cyst, the great displacement of the heart, and the lowering of the upper margin of dulness upon deep inspiration enable us commonly to detect the real nature of the disease. When the cyst has opened into the lung and the hydatids are being expectorated through the air-passages, the harassing cough, the copious sputum, and the inflammation of the pulmonary tissue which is apt to be occasioned, may cause the affection to be mistaken for pulmonary abscess or phthisis. The surest marks of distinction are furnished by the changed form of the lower part of the thorax, and by finding bile and the hooks of the echinococci in the sputum.

But though we may thus generally distinguish hydatids of the liver from the maladies which have similar symptoms, there are unquestionably cases in which it is extremely difficult to arrive at a satisfactory conclusion. Under these circumstances, an exploratory examination with a grooved needle or a very fine trocar has been recommended; but this proceeding is not wholly free from danger unless the swelling be prominent and superficial. The character of the fluid drawn off will assist us materially in diagnosis. It is as clear and colorless as water, has a specific gravity of 1007 or 1009, and contains not a trace of albumen, but large quantities of chloride of sodium. No other fluid in the human body, whether in health or in disease, presents these peculiarities.*

Occasionally portions of the liver are transformed into a mass, consisting of connective tissue stroma, and numerous large and small cells filled with a gelatinous substance. The disorder looks like alveolar carcinoma, but it is really multilocular hydatids or echinococcous tumors. The centre of the mass suppurates, but even this does not diminish the great resistance of the hepatic tumor, nor is fluctuation, save in the rarest instances, perceptible. The liver may retain its normal shape, or elevations may be perceptible, such as we observe in carcinoma and syphiloma of the organ. No jaundice usually attends the hard hepatic swelling; but in cases in which the bile ducts are obstructed we meet with jaundice without dyspeptic symptoms or previous paroxysms of pain, and usually without enlargement of the gall-bladder. In cases with icterus, unlike what we find in syphilis or in cancer, there is complete discoloration of the feces.†

Let us now, in concluding the review of the hepatic maladies which are attended with decided increase of the size of the organ, briefly contrast their most important manifestations. We have found that, as regards the enlargement, they

---

* Murchison, Lancet, Nov. 1865; also Lectures on Diseases of the Liver, 1868.

† See the cases of Friedrich and of Niemeyer, referred to in his Practice of Medicine.

differ materially. Simple congestion, chronic inflammation, a fatty liver, do not attain nearly the volume of cancer, of hydatids, of abscess, nor even of waxy disease of the liver. The three affections first mentioned differ, moreover, from all of the others, excepting the waxy liver, by presenting a uniform, and not an irregularly-shaped swelling nor uneven outline of the percussion dulness.

Concerning the symptoms, we observe that, although these hepatic disorders all agree in not being in any way characterized by jaundice, yet that this sign is more commonly present and more distinct in some than in others. In hydatids, and in the syphilitic liver, there is no yellow hue of the skin or conjunctiva; so, too, as a rule, in waxy liver. In fatty liver and in abscess it is, on the whole, most frequently wanting. The same may, perhaps, be said of cancer, though sometimes there is decided icterus in this malady. In chronic congestion and in chronic inflammation we ordinarily find jaundice, though it may be but a slight yellow tinge of the skin and eye. With reference to dropsy, we are not apt to encounter it in any of the hepatic affections under consideration, excepting in cancer and in waxy disease. It is in these two, also, that the most obvious signs of a cachexia are met with; while in abscess we find fever, and perhaps the greatest and most evident constitutional disturbance.

Viewed with regard to their *prognosis*, none of these diseases, unless it be congestion and fatty liver, can be stated to be devoid of danger. Abscess, waxy infiltration, and cancer have the most unfavorable prognosis.

In point of *treatment*, the different maladies present very dissimilar indications; indeed, the treatment must be guided chiefly by our knowledge of the particular condition of the liver, and by the constitutional state of the patient.

Chronic Diseases attended with Decreased Size of the Liver, and with Abdominal Dropsy.

Cirrhosis.—A liver reduced in bulk, very dense and hard, exhibiting granulations of various size separated by bands of fibrous tissue, and surrounded by a thickened serous en-

velope, presents the morbid state known as cirrhosis, or by
the familiar name of hob-nail liver. The change in the organ
is produced by a new formation of areolar tissue, due to inflammation of the fibrous texture, called Glisson's capsule,
which accompanies the vessels and biliary ducts in their ramifications through the hepatic parenchyma. The bands that
result from the thickening of the areolar structure compress
the parenchyma and destroy some of its secreting cells. The
inflammation which leads to these alterations in the tissue of
the liver is generally developed from a chronic congestion
consequent upon the abuse of spirituous liquors. But this
cause does not explain all cases : in some, the malady is connected with disease of the heart; in others, with constitutional syphilis ; in others, again, it cannot be attributed to
any known agency. Sometimes it is combined with fatty or
waxy degeneration.

In the first stage of cirrhosis, the organ is somewhat increased in size; then, as Glisson's capsule thickens more
and more, the bulk becomes lessened. It is, however, very
doubtful whether the stage of enlargement invariably precedes that of shrinking; probably the process of reduction
constitutes at times the first morbid change.

But without entering into this question, we may state that
there are no symptoms by which we can recognize the disease at an early period, whether or not the liver be augmented in volume; for the symptoms at first are the same
as those of chronic congestion or chronic inflammation of
the organ — namely, dull pain, perhaps tenderness at the
hypochondrium, disordered digestion, and a sallow or a
jaundiced hue of the skin. Nor can we say, even after the
stage of contraction is fairly developed, that the diagnosis
of the affection is easy, or indeed always possible. It may
rest on no stronger grounds than finding in a person who is
known to be a spirit drinker an intractable ascites, without
any obvious cause to account for the dropsy.

Besides the dropsy, the other clinical features of the malady are not very marked. The most significant signs consist
in the diminution of the percussion dulness in the hepatic
region, and the detection, by the touch, of firm, irregular

granulations on the margin and under surface of the liver. But both these signs are very difficult to discern, on account of the distention of the abdomen by the fluid effused within it, and the displacement of the liver this may occasion. In fact, it is often only after the performance of paracentesis that the abdominal walls, then no longer tense, will permit us to judge of the altered state and volume of the organ. This is more especially true with reference to palpation; as regards percussion, it is sometimes possible, even when the abdomen is still full of dropsical effusion, to detect, by repeated and careful examination, the lessened extent of the hepatic dulness.

Irrespective of these phenomena, we find at times other manifestations which will assist us in the diagnosis of cirrhosis. They are enlargement of the spleen; dilatation of the veins of the abdomen; gastric and intestinal derangements; loss of flesh and strength; jaundice; a decidedly cachectic appearance; and hemorrhages from the nose and mouth, or stomach, or into internal cavities. The increase in size of the spleen is, however, far from constant, and rarely reaches a very considerable extent. The dilatation of the abdominal veins is not perceived until an advanced stage of the disease, and is sometimes connected with a peculiar vascular network, stretching from the umbilicus upward and downward, and, as Sappey* was the first to describe, with a decided enlargement of the epigastric and mammary veins, the blood flowing through the former in a reversed direction from what it does in health—namely, not toward the liver, but from it to the veins of the abdominal wall, and thence to the vena cava.

The gastric and intestinal derangements are rarely wanting; they manifest themselves by failing appetite, impaired digestion, both gastric and intestinal, flatulency and constipation, or the frequent voiding of pale-colored stools. The jaundice does not often attain a very high degree. It shows itself usually in a yellowish tinge of the skin and conjunctiva; but in some cases even this hue is absent, and we find the pale skin and pearly eye of anæmia.

---

* Bulletin de l'Académie de Médecine, tome xxiv.

Yet not one of these symptoms is really characteristic; they only become so when viewed in connection with the dropsy, with the local signs in the hepatic region, with the history of the case, and with the absence of any organic disease of the stomach or intestine, which might account for them.

Let us now look at the marks of distinction between cirrhosis and some of the maladies which resemble it; and first let us compare its traits with those of other hepatic affections. From diseases of the liver attended with enlargement, such as waxy liver, fatty liver, chronic congestion, fully developed cirrhosis is discriminated by the presence of ascites and the other signs of seriously obstructed portal circulation, by the diminished, certainly not augmented, size of the organ, and the different history of the disorder. From hydatids of the liver, we diagnosticate cirrhosis by the irregularity of outline of the enlarged liver in the former complaint, by the sense of fluctuation and the comparatively unimpaired general nutrition of the body. Cancer of the liver is unlike cirrhosis in the distinctness and size of the protuberances, in the obvious hepatic enlargement, in the less marked or entirely absent dropsy, and in the normal size of the spleen. But when a cirrhosed liver is associated with syphilitic nodules, or when its volume is augmented by waxy infiltration, the discrimination from cancer becomes a matter of extreme difficulty; indeed, it may be impossible to avoid erroneous conclusions.

An inflammation of the portal vein, with coagula forming in it, may occasion the same manifestations of deranged abdominal circulation, the same tumefaction of the spleen, and decrease of the liver as cirrhosis. And what complicates the diagnosis very much is, that cirrhosis is one of the chief diseases which lead to obstruction of the portal vein. Indeed we cannot, under any circumstances, positively discriminate this affection from cirrhosis. Still, we are sometimes enabled to distinguish the former disorder by laying stress on the much quicker development of the symptoms, and by noting the rapidity with which the dropsy returns after the performance of the operation of paracentesis. Compression of the portal vein and of the biliary ducts in the fissure of the liver, in consequence of the inflammation of the areolar tissues surrounding them, may be separated from cirrhosis chiefly by the intense icterus and the complete discoloration of the stools.

Of non-hepatic affections, cirrhosis is most liable to be confounded with *chronic peritonitis;* a mistake rendered the more likely, because chronic congestion, or even chronic inflammation of the peritoneum, may exist as a complication of cirrhosis. But even when no such complication is present, the diagnosis may be difficult. It rests chiefly upon the greater tenderness of the abdomen in peritonitis, the absence of splenic enlargement, the usually unchanged, or certainly not jaundiced, hue of the skin, the association with signs of disease in other viscera, especially of the lungs, and the dissimilar history of the case.

Under rare circumstances, *cancer of the stomach* may simulate cirrhosis. I had some years since a case under my charge at the Pennsylvania Hospital, in which, with very slight digestive symptoms, and without discernible epigastric tumor, considerable ascites and effusion into the left pleural cavity existed. Owing to this effusion, the state of the spleen could not be very accurately ascertained. There was some fulness of the abdominal veins, and the hepatic percussion dulness did not extend entirely to the margin of the ribs. Bile pigment was present in the urine, and the bowels were loose, and progressive emaciation ensued. The man had been very intemperate, and his case might certainly have been selected as an illustration of cirrhosis; yet at the autopsy, the liver, though small, rather hard, and deeply congested, was not cirrhotic, and a cancer, involving nearly the whole stomach, excepting the pylorus, was found.*

Chronic Atrophy of the Liver.—Although cirrhosis is the most frequent, it is not the sole cause of dwindling of the liver. We have just alluded to its diminution in consequence of obstruction of the trunk of the portal vein; but, besides this cause, we find others, such as a decrease of the organ from long-continued closure of the common duct, or

---

* See, for a fuller report of the phenomena in this singular case, Proceedings of Pathol. Society, Amer. Journ. of Med. Sciences, vol. lii., 1866.

its atrophy in old age, or as an accompaniment of chronic disease of the intestine. The first of these morbid states is mainly discriminated by the deep jaundice; the second by the absence of any important symptoms referable to the liver and associated with the diminished hepatic dulness; the other form presents the phenomena of cirrhosis, and cannot be distinguished from this unless the surface of the liver can be distinctly felt through the abdominal walls, and be ascertained not to be irregular. We may sometimes suspect the cause of the shrinking of the organ from the persistent and intractable diarrhœa and disturbance of the stomach. But, on the whole, this decrease in size of the liver following gastroenteric inflammation is not frequent; in truth, there is no cause of simple atrophy of the liver so common as coagulation of blood in the portal vein.

———•———

SECTION IV.

ABDOMINAL ENLARGEMENT.

In describing the causes of abdominal enlargement, I shall view them as they occasion a general and uniform, or a more circumscribed and partial swelling.

General Abdominal Enlargement.

Ascites.—The collection of serous fluid in the peritoneal sac gives rise to dropsy of the belly, or ascites. This may form part of a general dropsy, and be dependent upon an organic disease of the kidneys or the thoracic viscera, or the accumulation of liquid may be confined to, or at all events occupy principally the abdomen. In either case the local signs are much the same. They are: enlargement of the belly; a dull sound on percussion, due to the presence of liquid; and the sense of fluctuation imparted to the hand on one side of the abdomen by a wave of fluid put into motion by a tap on the other side.

As regards the former of these signs, it is uniform and progressive, and is usually very evident—so evident as frequently to attract the patient's attention; although, of course, when the quantity of liquid is small, enlargement of the abdomen may escape detection. The percussion dulness is most readily perceived at the lower portion of the abdomen, where the fluid gravitates, unless when prevented from so doing by being circumscribed by peritoneal adhesions. The bowels float usually to the upper part of the liquid, and at that spot their tympanitic resonance may be distinctly discerned. When the patient is in the erect position, the intestinal percussion note is commonly discoverable in the epigastric and umbilical regions. If he be placed upon his back, the tympanitic sound. is, for the most part, found to extend lower than the umbilical region, while dulness will be elicited in the hypogastric region and the flanks. If the person affected with ascites be placed upon his side, the flank which is uppermost becomes resonant. This alteration of the level of the fluid with the change of position is thus a very significant sign, and always happens except when the effusion is encysted; it is also, as a rule, detected without difficulty, save where very great flatulent distention of the bowels accompanies the accumulation of liquid.

Ordinarily the fluctuation wave felt by the hand is easily discerned. It is, however, obscured by thickening of the abdominal walls from œdema, or from the accumulation of fat in the subcutaneous tissues; it is, moreover, indistinct if adhesions circumscribe the fluid in the peritoneum.

The other symptoms often found in ascites, such as a pushing upward of the liver, spleen, and stomach, embarrassed breathing, perhaps compression of the lungs, and digestive disturbances, need not be specially described, as they present nothing characteristic. Nor is it necessary to insist upon the self-evident fact that a diagnosis of ascites is only half the diagnosis of a case, and that we should in every instance endeavor to ascertain the cause of the collection of fluid in the peritoneal sac. And we may at once proceed to consider the morbid states with which dropsy in the peritoneum is liable to be confounded.   They are chiefly:

OVARIAN DROPSY;

CHRONIC PERITONITIS;

DISTENTION OF THE BLADDER;

GRAVID UTERUS;

CHRONIC TYMPANITES.

Ovarian Dropsy.—It is not until an ovarian cyst rises above the brim of the pelvis that it occasions a swelling marked enough to be mistaken for abdominal dropsy.   Supposing that it has led to considerable enlargement of the belly, we are yet able to discriminate between the two disorders by attention to the physical signs and the history of the case.

As regards the former, we perceive these differences: the sound on percussion over an ovarian cyst is dull in the umbilical and hypogastric regions, while at the sides the tympanitic resonance of the intestines may be obtained.   Moreover, when the patient assumes different postures the dulness in ovarian dropsy does not change its position; and, like all ovarian tumors, it causes a projection in the centre of the abdomen, not a flattening there and a bulging of the flanks, as is not uncommon in ascites.   Lastly, the fluctuation from an ovarian cyst is rarely as perfect as from a collection of fluid in the peritoneum, and is apt to be very unequal at different parts of the distended abdomen.   Thus the physical phenomena of the two maladies are very dissimilar.

When, however, there is ascites complicating an ovarian tumor, the diagnosis is very difficult.   Finding the fluctuation unequal, and an irregular outline of the ovarian growth, may aid us; but a preliminary tapping may be necessary to settle the diagnosis.   The microscope often shows lymph and pus in the fluid from an ovarian disease; yet we cannot trust exclusively to the character of the fluid voided.

In uncomplicated cases, the history assists us greatly in arriving at a correct diagnosis.   In ovarian dropsy, we can, as a rule, make out that the distention of the abdomen has commenced at its lower portion, and has gradually spread upward, one side being very much more prominent than the other, until the abdominal enlargement has become considerable. Again, the constitutional disturbance is less,—often, indeed, the general health is scarcely disturbed; and we do not find those signs of disease of the liver, heart, or kidneys which are so apt to coexist with ascites.

Attention to the history and progress of the complaint is especially valuable in the class of cases in which the physical signs are modified by the intestines not being able to float to the surface of the fluid in the peritoneal cavity, in consequence of adhesions to each other, or of a diseased omentum, or in which the fluid has been limited in sacs by inflammatory adhesions. These cases are those in which a peritoneal inflammation has led to the effusion of liquid; and the history of antecedent peritonitis, or of peritonitis in connection with tubercular disease, the pain and tenderness, the signs sometimes of a tubercular affection of the peritoneum and mesenteric glands, and the evidences of serious impairment of the whole system, will go far toward elucidating the diagnosis.

Chronic Peritonitis.—The effusion which forms in consequence of inflammation of the peritoneum is very commonly spoken of as one of the forms of ascites. Excluding the kind of chronic inflammation which is due to an attack of acute peritonitis passing into a chronic state, let us inquire how cases of chronic peritonitis, in which the disease was gradual in its development, can be distinguished from pure dropsical effusion.

Now, these cases of chronic peritonitis are almost invariably associated with tubercle or with cancer. In the former instance, by far the most common, the malady generally occurs in those who have at the same time tubercles in the lungs; and when we find such a patient complaining of abdominal pain and uneasiness, of soreness to the touch, of nausea, of an irregular state of the bowels, of having more or less fever, and of losing flesh and strength; when we discover the abdomen to be very tense and much distended, in part with liquid, but especially with wind, and sometimes very resistant to the touch, and exhibiting clearly on its exterior the tracings of the convolutions of the intestines,—we can hardly be wrong in presuming the signs of chronic peritoneal inflammation to be owing to the presence of tubercular granulations or of tuberculous disease of the mesenteric glands. Even when the signs of disease of the lungs are wanting, or are not well defined, we shall generally be correct, if the abdominal symptoms mentioned exist, in determining the peritoneal affection to be tubercular.

In some instances the tubercular abdominal disorder develops with rapidity, and the disease has not so much the aspect of a chronic as of an acute complaint. The tumefaction and tension of the belly produced may be so great as to simulate an abdominal tumor.*

A cancer of the peritoneum gives rise to many of the same phenomena as tuberculous disease. But there is this difference: the malady usually happens consecutively to an external or an internal cancer, and scarcely ever, save in persons advanced in years; there is less fever; no diarrhœa, or but little diarrhœa, and no profuse sweats occur; and as the omentum is the most common seat of the cancerous growth, we can generally detect a tumor stretching across the upper portion of the abdomen, and extending perhaps from the epigastrium nearly to the pelvis. The morbid mass is unequal and usually detected readily, excepting where separated by fluid from the abdominal parietes.

Now, it is not necessary to point out at any length the differences between these forms of chronic peritonitis and the ordinary kind of dropsy of the peritoneum. Both the local and general symptoms are very dissimilar, as will be seen at once by contrasting the description just given with that of ascites.

Distention of the Bladder.—This may give rise to a sense of fluctuation and to very marked abdominal enlargement; so marked, indeed, that patients have been tapped, under the supposition that they were laboring under dropsy of the abdomen. But when the bladder is so much distended as to simulate ascites, there is usually more or less tenderness on pressure over the seat of the obvious swelling: which, moreover, presents a rounded outline of dulness on percussion.

---

* See case in Liverpool Hospital Reports, 1868.

Again, we either have the history of retention or of apparent incontinence of urine.* But, so as to avoid all possible chance of error, in any case of doubt a catheter should be introduced into the bladder. This mode of procedure, it may here be mentioned, is the one which leads most speedily and decisively to a true appreciation of the abnormal phenomena in those rare cases of anasarca which are produced by distention of the bladder, and of which Trousseau has recorded several.

The Gravid Uterus.—A gravid womb is readily distinguished from abdominal dropsy by the peculiar form of the dulness on percussion, its steady and uniform increase corresponding to the enlargement of the womb, the absence of fluctuation, the detection of the sounds of the fœtal heart, and the production of movements in the womb on making an examination per vaginam. Very much the same signs, too, enable us to discriminate between pregnancy and ovarian dropsy.

Chronic Tympanites.—A great prominence of the abdomen, due to flatulent distention of the bowels, is, if at all a persistent state, very apt to be mistaken for dropsy of the belly. But the large abdomen yields not a dull, but everywhere a tympanitic sound, and there is no fluctuation. Then, as we shall presently discuss, the history of the case and the attending symptoms throw light upon the nature of the ailment.

Besides the complaints just reviewed, which are those most commonly confounded with ascites, there are a few very rare disorders which might be mistaken for collections of fluid in the peritoneal sac. They are: dropsy of the womb; dropsy of the Fallopian tubes; dropsy of the omentum; very large serous cysts in the kidney; hydatids of the liver, of size so great as to lead to general abdominal distention; and a dilatation of the stomach so extensive that the viscus occupies almost the whole abdomen. With reference to the latter affection, which has been encountered in cases

---

* In a case recorded by Dr. Watson, in his Lectures on the Practice of Physic, although the bladder was enormously distended, large quantities of urine were constantly passing from the patient.

of boulimia, and in cancer of the pylorus, or stricture of the duodenum, we may distinguish it from ascites by the history of the case, by the gurgling discerned on sudden pressure, by the indistinct fluctuation, which is not noticed except over the most dependent part of the organ, and the metallic or amphoric sounds which are perceived when its contents are agitated.* The other maladies mentioned can only be separated by taking into account their history and progress, by laying stress upon the absence of those morbid states which generally cause ascites, and upon the occurrence of special phenomena which point to the structures implicated. Yet it may not always, even with the utmost care, be possible to form a correct diagnosis.

Chronic Tympanites.—A collection of gas in the cavity of the peritoneum is of rare occurrence; but is frequent in the intestinal tube, and the accumulation become sometimes a chronic condition, and leads to very great and uniform enlargement of the abdomen. We find this form of tympanites in some cases of hysteria; in instances of constriction of portions of the intestinal canal, either in consequence of cicatrization, or of cancer of the bowels, or of their compression by a morbid growth; as a sequel of enteritis or peritonitis, or of a spinal lesion, under which circumstances it is evidently due to atony of the muscular fibres; we also observe it in persons whose digestive powers are not strong, and who partake much of food—such as cabbages, beans, and peas—which is apt to occasion flatulency.

Among soldiers this chronic tympanites—owing, perhaps, in many cases to the character of their diet and consequent digestive disturbances—is far from being an uncommon disorder, and may be a very obstinate one. It gives rise to abdominal enlargement, which is constantly mistaken for dropsy, but which does not yield a sense of fluctuation, nor return, on percussion, any other than a well-marked tympanitic sound. The distention produces, moreover, an inability to take active exercise, sensations of cutting pain under

---

* See cases of enlargement of stomach, by Oppolzer, quoted in Ranking's Abstract, July, 1868, p. 65; also Am. Journ. of Med. Sciences, Jan. 1869.

the ribs, and palpitation of the heart; pressure on the abdomen occasions much discomfort; the soldiers, therefore,
walk with their clothes unbuttoned, and find it very irksome
to wear their belts.   They are sometimes troubled by indigestion, and feel particularly uncomfortable after meals; or
the symptoms of indigestion, although they may have been
present at the beginning of the complaint, disappear, but
the swelling of the abdomen persists for many months.
According to my experience, the ailment is always gradual
in its development.

Partial Abdominal Enlargement.

Abdominal Tumors.—I propose here to offer a few observations on abdominal tumors, even at the risk of repeating
much that has been already said while discussing affections
of individual abdominal viscera.   But for clinical purposes,
it is a matter not only of convenience, but of importance, to
point out connectedly the relations an abdominal swelling
is likely to bear to the normal structures of the abdominal
cavity, and to consider, moreover, the fact of the swelling as
constituting, what in truth at the bedside it so constantly
becomes, the starting-point of our diagnosis.

Let us first examine the meaning of an abdominal tumefaction occupying solely or principally one region of the
abdomen.

Right Hypochondrium.—The most usual cause of a tumor
in this region is an enlargement of the liver, whether that
enlargement be due to congestion, to fatty or waxy degeneration, to chronic hepatitis, to cancer, or to an abscess.   The
mere fact of the swelling teaches us nothing as to its cause ;
to discern this, we have to trace the outline of the morbid
increase, to ascertain its feel, and to inquire into similar
points that we have already discussed when reviewing the
hepatic diseases attended with enlargement of the organ.

Sometimes a tumor which seems to be principally in the
right hypochondrium, or to proceed from the termination of
this region, is simply a displaced liver, or an affection of the
gall-bladder.   In the first instance, the recognition of the

disorder—such as a pleuritic effusion—which has given rise to the displacement; in the second, the history of the case, the shape of the swelling, and the symptoms attending it,— will give us, as has been elsewhere indicated, an insight into its cause. Again, a tumor in the parts mentioned may be due to an enlarged kidney,—enlarged either by cancerous trans- formation or cystic degeneration. Careful examinations of the urine and the history of the case furnish the most certain means of discrimination. Then we must also bear in mind that all enlarged kidneys displace the bowel in a particular manner; they press it forward, and the dulness over the tumor is largely mixed with a tympanitic sound, or the dul- ness is, indeed, not very appreciable.

Left Hypochondrium.—The most usual tumors in this region are those produced by enlargement of the spleen. Now, an increase in size of this viscus, if acute, is either owing to in- flammation or to those alterations in its structure which take place during typhoid or the malarial fevers. Under the latter circumstances, the cause of the swelling is disclosed by the history of the case and the symptoms accompanying the fever.

Inflammation of the spleen is an affection very difficult to recognize. The most trustworthy symptoms are: pain in the left hypochondrium, radiating thence in various directions, as far as the left shoulder, and augmented by pressure, by coughing, and by a deep inspiration; nausea; vomiting; fever having irregular fits of exacerbation; sometimes de- lirium, dry cough, and a sense of suffocation. The extent of the splenic percussion dulness is decidedly increased, and when we are sure that the spleen is not displaced, the widened area of dulness always forms a most important element in the diagnosis.

Chronic enlargement of the spleen may be caused by hyper- trophy, by waxy disease, by fibrinous infiltration, by malig- nant growth, and by congestion with subsequent structural changes, such as occur, for instance, in miasmatic affections. There are scarcely any symptoms which are characteristic of these states, excepting it be the alteration the blood under- goes, as evinced by a diminution of the red globules and an increase of the white, and the waxy hue of the face. Dropsy, bleeding from the nose, stomach, or intestinal canal, and digestive disturbances, though far from infrequent, are less constant, and have thus a less available diagnostic value. And in truth, all of the phenomena mentioned, unless, perhaps, the microscopical evidences of deteriorated blood, are, in the recognition of a splenic tumor, of secondary importance as compared with the extended percussion dulness in the splenic region. There is said to be a constant relation between the variations of the volume of the spleen and of the temperature.* In some cases the symptoms are very ill defined, and death may result from rupture of varices of the enlarged viscus, without any signs of a lesion than those of increased size of the organ.† When enlargement of the spleen has reached a certain point, the organ curves into the hypogastric and right iliac regions, and a notch or notches may be felt on its anterior and inner surfaces.‡

Having determined the persistent swelling to be due to the abnormal size of the spleen, we must next endeavor to ascertain the cause of it. The history of the case forms, in this inquiry, the main element in diagnosis.

A fulness projecting from the left hypochondrium toward the umbilical or lumbar region may be owing to *fecal accumulations* in the colon, as well as to an enlarged spleen. Now, although these fecal accumulations do not occur so often in, or near either hypochondrium as they do in the iliac regions, yet they are not very uncommon, and we should be on our guard against confounding them with organic disease. Their irregular outline, and close attention to the history of the case and to the accompanying disorder of the digestive functions, will generally enable us to detect the true nature of the swelling. But we must not lay stress on the non-existence of constipation, for sometimes great irritability of the bowels or persistent diarrhœa is kept up by a large collection of fecal matter in the colon. Repeated attacks of colicky pains and

---

* Am. Journ. of Med. Sciences, July, 1867.

† Traube, Virchow's Archiv, and Brit. and For. Medico-Chirurg. Rev., October, 1869.

‡ Fagge, Guy's Hospital Reports, 1868.

some soreness to the touch are not unusual in cases of extensive fecal accumulation.

As regards swellings of any kind situated in either hypochondrium, or in fact at any portion of the upper third of the abdomen, it is always to be inquired into whether they are affected by the act of respiration. This, as Dr. Kennedy* has pointed out, is a very valuable sign, for if the morbid mass move in consequence of the depression of the diaphragm, it is because structures are involved, such as the stomach and transverse colon, the liver or spleen, which admit of some mobility; whereas a tumor that is uninfluenced must appertain to a fixed part,—for instance, to the aorta.

Epigastrium.—The most common cause of an epigastric tumor is cancer of the stomach. The swelling is then associated with extreme gastric acidity, with frequent vomiting, with pain, and with gradual and progressive loss of flesh, and debility.

But a tumor in this region may be also produced by a *disease of the pancreas.* Now, practically speaking, there is but one affection of the pancreas which we can recognize with anything like certainty—cancer; for neither acute nor chronic pancreatitis, nor fatty degeneration, nor uniform simple hardening of the gland, can, as a rule, be discerned at the bedside. With reference to the two forms of inflammation, we suspect their presence if a large quantity of matter like saliva be passed by stool, or if profuse salivation happen; but though these symptoms have been observed in individual cases, they are far from being constant. As regards cancer, the most trustworthy symptoms are: a tumor in the epigastric region; pain there or in the back, not increased by the taking of food, but usually augmented by the erect posture; progressive emaciation and debility; an appetite capricious rather than diminished, and in some instances, indeed, a ravenous desire for food; constipation, and, at times, but far from invariably, fatty stools.† Besides these indications, we

---

* Dublin Quarterly Journ., Aug. 1864.

† In analyzing forty cases that have been placed on record by different authors, and some that have come under my own notice, I do not find this symptom mentioned in one-third.

not uncommonly find, as the disease advances, obstinate jaundice and occasional vomiting. Very many of these phenomena belong also to cancer of the stomach ; in truth, we never can be certain of the existence of the pancreatic malady until we have excluded the gastric affection. In a differential diagnosis of this kind, the early presence and habitual occurrence of vomiting after meals, the sour eructations, the hæmatemesis, the absence of jaundice, assist us very materially in locating the seat of the disease in the stomach.

An epigastric tumor is sometimes simulated by a contraction of the upper portion of the rectus muscle on palpation ; but the swelling in the latter case generally soon subsides, especially if rubbed. Occasionally, however, a tumefaction due to contraction of an abdominal muscle may be of some duration.* And I have known a contraction of the rectus muscle in a case of gastric cancer occasion so obvious a resistance and swelling, that it was looked upon as due to malignant disease of the intestine, or peritoneum. Moreover, the rigid muscle gave rise to dulness on percussion. But though the phenomena lasted for some time, and were indeed for a lengthened period a marked feature of the case, it was observable that the muscle was raised and rigid to a decided degree only in certain positions; at all events, that certain positions gave a distinct outline to the swelling, and that this then, like the line of dulness, was regular and straight, evidently corresponding to the contour of the muscle.

The muscular contractions are not always confined to one muscle, or to the whole of one muscle, and when irregular, and particularly when associated with tympanitic distention of the intestine, give rise to most of the so-called " phantom" tumors of the abdomen. These swellings are often very perplexing, and are constantly mistaken for serious abdominal tumors. The history of the case, the absence generally of grave constitutional symptoms, the most frequent occurrence of the tumefaction in females, especially in hysterical females, and the usually existing constipation furnish us with valuable

---

* Greenhow's cases, London Lancet, 1857.

signs of distinction.   But I believe the use of anæsthetics to
be the most important means of diagnosis.   I was first led to
employ them, a number of years ago, in a case which had
baffled the skill of several eminent surgeons, one of whom
had proposed to the patient an operation as the only means
of relief from what was considered an ovarian disease.   The
patient was thirty-one years of age, a widow, and evidently
of highly hysterical temperament.   She was very subject to
constipation ; and the swelling of which she complained was
of irregular outline and occupied the centre of the abdomen,
extending some distance on each side of the median line.   It
was hard and resisting to the touch, but, on strong percussion,
yielded a tympanitic sound.   Whenever it was touched she
shrank.   Thorough relaxation was produced by the administration of ether; the hand could be pressed almost against
the vertebral column, and all signs of the tumor had disappeared.   A complete recovery took place; and thus terminated a case which had lasted for fully one year, and in which,
it is highly probable, from the fact that the patient was fond
of having her urine drawn off by the catheter, and had shown
other manifestations of a similar type of hysteria, that
the swelling was in part at least artificially produced.   But
in any of the phantom tumors I would recommend the use
of anæsthetics for purposes of diagnosis; nay, they may be
most advantageously employed for similar reasons in all cases
of abdominal swelling in which the rigid state of the abdominal walls interferes with accuracy of investigation.

In soldiers we at times observe one or several small movable tumors, yielding a tympanitic sound on percussion in the
epigastric or at the upper part of the umbilical region.   Their
nature is very obscure : they are, probably, small portions of
intestine which have been pushed between the fasciculi of a
ruptured rectus muscle.

Umbilical Region.—Tumors which are found in this region
form, as a rule, merely portions of a swelling that is principally seated in the epigastrium or the hypochondria, such as
cancer of the stomach, of the liver, of the pancreas, or of the
omentum, and dilatation of the gall-bladder.   The only two
affections which are apt to occasion a swelling solely, or at

least principally, limited to and perceptible in the umbilical region, are tuberculous disease of the mesenteric glands and a movable kidney.

The symptoms of the former malady, or *tabes mesenterica*, are much the same as those which we have already described as characterizing tubercular peritonitis. Indeed, unless the enlarged mesenteric glands can be felt through the abdominal parietes, the discrimination is very uncertain. The abdomen is prematurely large, is slightly tender on pressure, and has often a doughy feel; the child—for it is almost exclusively in children that the disease is seen—loses flesh, its digestion is impaired, its evacuations frequent and unhealthy. It often presents signs of scrofulous disease elsewhere; and under such circumstances, we cannot be at a loss in determining the nature of the tumefaction in the umbilical region. The simulation of the disease in adults, especially in young women, from mere ataxia and probable functional disorder of the glands, has been described in reviewing the affections of the stomach.

When the *kidneys* are not firmly held by their attachments, they become displaced, and are then apt to give rise to serious errors in diagnosis. The dislocated organ is generally perceived under the margin of the ribs on the right flank, or in the umbilical region, and sometimes extends across the median line. The apparently morbid mass is very easily moved, may be, by careful and methodical pressure, returned to the renal region, and presents, on percussion, the outline of the kidney. The lumbar region yields a tympanitic sound on percussion, and we find less resistance and a slight depression over the usual seat of the organ, which depression is effaced by pressing the tumor into the lumbar region. There is in some instances sensitiveness over the displaced organ, especially after fatigue, or a blow, or strong pressure; and pressure in examining the part is very apt to give rise to the same sensation as when the renal region of the non-affected side is pressed; but we never find any disturbance of the urinary functions, nor, in fact, excepting a disagreeable feeling in walking, does any real inconvenience result from the accident, save in those cases in which the movable kidney has become painful, or, by compressing the vena cava or portal veins, occasions dropsy. The disorder is most apt to occur after violent exertion, or after many pregnancies, or may be due to attacks of congestion of the organ. The right kidney is more frequently movable than the left; and women are more liable to displacements of the organ than men.*

The affection may of course be mistaken for any form of abdominal tumor; but can be distinguished by the absence of signs of constitutional disturbance; by the history of the case; and by the physical phenomena already alluded to. To these may be added the comparatively slight dulness, or the rather tympanitic character of sound elicited, excepting on very strong percussion, over the seat of the tumor. This is an important fact as regards the discrimination of a movable and *displaced spleen,* in which, as the organ is generally enlarged, there is considerable and extended dulness on percussion. Moreover, the history of the splenic disorder, which not uncommonly can be traced to a malarial affection, the usually great tenderness, and the nausea and dyspeptic symptoms and hemorrhagic tendencies which attend the displacement of the spleen, will assist us in our diagnosis.†

Yet another of the abdominal organs is occasionally displaced and movable—the liver. Now, a *movable liver* would be often mistaken for a movable spleen, were it a more common affection. But only very few well-authenticated cases are on record.‡ In these the peritoneal attachment of the organ had become lax, usually in consequence of pregnancy; in the hepatic region there was a tympanitic sound on percussion; and in the umbilical region and toward the right flank a solid body was discerned, the upper border of which presented a convex outline, the lower border was in

---

* See the cases of Henoch, Klinik der Unterleibs-Krankheiten; and of Fritz, Arch. Gén. de Médecine, 1859; Becquet, ib., Jan. 1865; Hare, Med. Times and Gazette, 1860; Oppolzer, quoted in Canst. Jahrb., vol. iii. p. 212; Durham, Guy's Hosp. Reports, vol. ix., 3d Series; Trousseau, Clinique Médicale.

† Cases of displaced spleen are quoted in Archives Générales, 1858, tome ii.; Brit. and For. Med.-Chir. Rev., Oct. 1860; see also Clarke, Dubl. Hosp. Gazette, Aug. 1860; and Med. Times and Gazette, Nov. 1869.

‡ See Cantani, Ann. univers. di Medicina, 1866; and Meissner's article in Schmidt's Jahrb., 1869, No. 1.

the inguinal region. The displaced organ was very easily pushed about, and could be replaced in its proper situation. The spleen was found in its usual seat; the symptoms were merely those of weight and uneasiness in the abdomen.

Lumbar Region.—Tumors in this region, or on either flank, are apt to be occasioned by some morbid growth of the kidney, or by an abscess in it or its surroundings, or in the psoas muscles. Again, they may be due to fecal accumulations; or, if on the right side, to very considerable increase of the liver; if on the left, to a greatly enlarged spleen. To discriminate between these different conditions, we have to determine whether the swelling fluctuates or not; we must also analyze the urine, and inquire minutely into the circumstances preceding and attending the tumefaction. It is thus only that we can hope to attain the necessary data for a diagnosis, which has, indeed, often to be reached by the process of exclusion.

Tumors behind the peritoneum may give rise to a visible prominence in either lumbar region, extending to the upper part of the iliac region. The most common cause of these tumors is cancer of the lymphatic glands lying by the sides or in front of the vertebral column. The disease is very difficult of detection. Still, we may suspect its existence if, in a patient who is evidently cachectic, and who is steadily losing flesh and strength, we discover, on deep palpation on one side of the linea alba or in the flank, a tumor which, owing to its being surrounded by intestine, returns a tympanitic percussion sound. In some cases the swelling communicates the beat of the aorta and simulates an aneurism, or it presses on the vena cava and gives rise to enlargement of the abdominal veins and of those of the lower extremities, and to œdema of the legs. The disease may involve the iliac glands and the tumor extend into the pelvis, or it may reach upward to the diaphragm; and by the cancer spreading to the posterior mediastinum and softening, it may finally open into the aorta, producing hemorrhages precisely like those coming from an aneurismal sac.*

---

* Case reported by Haldane, Edinb. Med. Journal, Aug. 1868.

Iliac Regions.—Tumors in either of these regions may be due to many different causes. They are, as we have elsewhere discussed, principally owing to ovarian affections; to fecal accumulations; to diseases of the large intestine, such as intussusception or cancer; and to pelvic abscess. Sometimes they are caused by displacement of the kidney, by enlargement of the spleen, and in women by periuterine hæmatocele, or by extra-uterine pregnancy.

The ovarian tumors are, as a rule, distinguished from the other disorders mentioned by their more or less globular form, by their movability from side to side or in an upward direction, by their seeming to spring out of the pelvis, and their evident attachment below, by the displacement of the womb, by the comparatively unimpaired general health, and by their indolent and generally painless nature. These remarks do not apply to the very slight swelling occasioned by ovarian inflammation, for here the tumid spot is often the seat of severe pain. The healthy ovary is not sensitive to the touch. To examine the ovary with exactness, the abdominal muscles must be as completely as possible relaxed; the patient is best placed in the attitude recommended by Dr. Marion Sims: on her back, with the shoulders supported, the legs drawn up so that the heels are a few inches asunder, and that the thighs fall easily apart.

But to return to ovarian tumors. As these grow and spread upward they give rise to difficulties in diagnosis, which we have already examined into, so far at least as is possible in a work of this kind. We may here again allude to the manner in which ovarian may simulate renal growths,—a similarity so close that even as accomplished an expert as Mr. Spencer Wells has been deceived. This distinguished authority dwells particularly* on the absence of fluctuation in the vast majority of instances of enlarged kidney; on the renal tumor being first detected between the false ribs and the ilium; on the signs in the urine, and on the absence of those changes in the quantity and regularity of the menstrual discharges which are common in ovarian disorders. More-

---

* Dublin Quarterly Journal, Feb. 1867.

over, the ovarian growth usually displaces the intestine back-ward; in the renal growth it is pressed forward; and large tumors of the right kidney ordinarily have the ascending colon on their inner border, while tumors of the left kidney are generally crossed from above downward by the descending colon.

Among the causes of a tumor in either iliac fossa *periuterine hæmatocele* has been mentioned. The tumor rising above the brim of the pelvis is traceable into it, and the quick manner in which the swelling has formed, the faintness and prostration which the effusion of blood occasioned, and the swelling, commonly of rounded shape, either hard or soft, discernible by an examination through the vagina, render the meaning of the tumor generally a clear one. Much the same physical phenomena are presented by the swelling due to *pelvic cellulitis*. But the slow way in which the tumor forms, the presence of that hot, puffy, thickened, brawnlike condition of the vaginal wall, so especially dwelt upon by Simpson, the usually greater tenderness of the swelling felt through the walls of the vagina, and the feverishness and constitutional symptoms attending the gradual formation of the abscess, are distinguishing marks, excepting where the contents of the hæmatocele suppurate; when for a differential diagnosis we may have to rely on the history of the case.

Hypogastric Region.—Distention of the bladder and enlargement of the uterus, whether produced by air, by liquid, by a morbid growth, or by pregnancy, are the most usual sources of a swelling in this region. If due to either of these causes, the outline of the tumor is regular and rounded; and by the aid of the catheter, of explorations through the vagina and the rectum, and of the history of the case and the attending symptoms, we are generally enabled to arrive at a correct diagnosis.

A tumor in the hypogastrium may also have its origin in splenic enlargement, in disease of the peritoneum, or in hæmatocele. In the latter case, it is apt to be uniform, and to extend to the iliac fossæ.

In concluding this sketch of abdominal tumors, we shall briefly glance at those which are likely to occupy more than one region, and sometimes even the whole or the greater part of the abdomen. In rare instances, a cancer of the liver, or hydatids of that organ, or a fibrous tumor of the uterus, or a solid ovarian growth, or an enlarged spleen, or a kidney the pelvis of which has become enormously distended in cousequence of obstruction of the ureter, may lead to the formation of a swelling which occupies nearly the entire abdomen. But the most usual cause of so extensive a tumor is malignant disease of the peritoneum.

This affection may give rise to a uniform swelling stretching across the abdomen, and equally extensive on both sides of the median line, or, as is not at all unusual, to several small tumors, which are evidently unconnected with any organ beneath. It is, moreover, apt to occasion a peritoneal friction sound, to exhibit a varying resistance to pressure at different points, to lead to ascites, to loss of flesh and appetite, and to the occurrence of irritative fever. Much the same symptoms may be produced by hydatid disease of the peritoneum, though here there is usually less fever, the swelling is even more irregular, the abdominal enlargement greater, and—the test which alone is certain—we may be able to detect the hydatid fremitus.* Peritoneal abscesses inclosed by adhesions will also, if large, give rise to several of the signs of a cancer; but the history of an antecedent local or general peritonitis, the swelling not being influenced by changes in the posture of the patient or by the acts of respiration, the indistinct fluctuation of the tumefaction, and its acute course, will ordinarily enable us to distinguish the non-malignant from the malignant affection.

In some cases, too, the malignant disease is closely simulated by dilatation of the colon. This, though it may present but a single swelling, generally occasions several, which are commonly seated at the middle third of the abdomen, are apt to appear on both sides, be movable, change their position slightly at intervals, and become occasionally less in size. Then, after the case has been for some time under observa-

---

* See the cases of Bright, in Clinical Memoirs on Abdominal Tumors, republished from Guy's Hospital Reports by the New Sydenham Society.

tion, we may be able to notice large and characteristic dis. charges; though we must not forget that a mere sluggish state of the bowels, or even diarrhœa, may exist while the colon is dilated and perhaps filled with fecal accumulations.*

————•——

SECTION V.

ABDOMINAL PULSATION.

Aortic Pulsation.—By far the most frequent cause of a pulsation visible in the abdomen, and especially at the epigastric region, is a throbbing of the abdominal aorta. It is not at all uncommon in hysterical persons. Some women are liable to it immediately before their menstrual periods or during the earlier months of pregnancy. In men it is most often seen in those who suffer from inveterate dyspepsia; and is apt to come on in severe paroxysms, which are very alarming to the patient, but which generally disappear under brisk purging. In hypochondriacs whose abdominal walls are thin, the beating at the epigastrium, from which they may suffer, becomes a source of continued study and distress.

The increased action of the aorta, or, as happens in emaciated persons, the greater distinctness with which the beat of the artery is perceived, without there being really much, if any, abnormal throbbing, may be distinguished from an enlarged and somewhat displaced heart by the circumstances of the case and the absence of any physical signs of cardiac disease; and from an aneurism, by the mode of invasion, and by the want of those signs which, as will be presently described, characterize an aneurism.

Abdominal Aneurism. — Aneurism of the abdominal aorta is a disease of middle life, and of males. Its most frequent cause is excessive muscular exercise; sometimes it is produced by a blow on the abdomen. Its duration is very

---

* For several interesting cases of the disorder, see Kennedy, *loc. cit.*

uncertain: occasionally six or seven years elapse from its earliest indications until the fatal termination; and not unusually the patient lives twenty to thirty months after the outbreak of the manifestations of the complaint.

The chief *symptoms* of the aneurismal disorder are pain, and an absence of dropsy, of fever, or of any considerable constitutional disturbance. The pain is generally felt in the back, or in the right hypochondrium, or shooting down the sciatic nerves to the lower limbs. It may be constant and dull, or occur in protracted and violent paroxysms; ordinarily there is a persistent pain which has periods of fierce exacerbation. The disproportion between its violence and the otherwise almost unimpaired health is a striking and common feature of the disease, and is apt to continue until the aneurism becomes very large and occasions displacement of important organs.

The *physical signs* of an abdominal aneurism are: an impulse communicated to the hand when placed over the swelling; a systolic blowing sound; a thrill; and in some instances a distinct prominence and alteration in the form of the abdomen. The impulse corresponds, with very rare exceptions, to the beat of the heart, is single, and ordinarily very forcible. Generally it cannot be felt from behind; it is a beat discerned only anteriorly and on either side of the pulsating sac. Corresponding to the throbbing of the tumor, we often hear a short blowing sound, sometimes perceived in the recumbent posture only, or a dull, muffled sound; but rarely are there two sounds. A thrill felt at the same time as the pulsation is not unfrequently noticed; still, it may be absent, even in large-sized aneurisms.

Aneurism of the abdominal aorta may be confounded with—

RHEUMATISM; NEURALGIA; COLIC;
DISEASE OF THE SPINE;
AORTIC PULSATION;
LUMBAR AND PSOAS ABSCESS;
NON-ANEURISMAL PULSATING TUMOR.

The first four of these affections are likely to be mistaken for an abdominal aneurism, on account merely of the pain;

the others, because of the presence of pulsation, or of a swelling, or of both pulsation and swelling.

Rheumatism; Neuralgia; Colic.—The pain caused by an aneurism may closely simulate rheumatism of the lumbar muscles, or sciatica, or abdominal neuralgia, or colic. There is nothing in the pain itself which would lead to the detection of its origin; this can only be effected by a recognition of the physical signs of the aneurism. When these are not well defined, the diagnosis is doubtful. Yet, even when they are slightly marked or absent, if the pain be very obstinate, and we have excluded the affections named or cannot trace them to their usual causes, we shall often be right in attributing the pain to an aneurism. This is especially true as regards abdominal neuralgia occurring in males,—a disorder which ought always to make us examine for an aneurism, and which is not unfrequently found to be due to it.

Disease of the Spine.—Patients who are suffering from aneurism often complain of pain in the spine, and present sometimes an obvious spinal curvature. But a careful examination, by detecting the physical signs of an aneurism, will generally enable us to distinguish the source of the trouble. The constant boring pain so much complained of in cases of aneurism, is usually thought to be due to absorption of the vertebræ; but, as the observations of Stokes have proved, it has no necessary connection with this lesion.

Aortic Pulsation.—Simple abdominal pulsation, such as we observe in hysteria, in dyspepsia, and in pregnancy; or excessive pulsation in the abdomen due to an enlarged right ventricle, or to insufficient aortic valves,—may be readily mistaken for an aneurism. But in the former case the history will generally lead us to a correct conclusion, especially if taken in connection with the facts, that the pulsation is not heavy and slow, as in an aneurism, but jerking and sudden; that there is no thrill; no tumor with corresponding dulness on percussion, if we except pregnancy; no systolic murmur audible in front of the abdomen or along the spine; and no pain.

The pulsation due to disease of the heart is discriminated

by the physical signs in the thorax. Regurgitation at the aortic orifice, which is the cardiac affection most liable to be confounded with an aneurism, on account of the marked pulsation it may occasion in the left hypochondrium or at the scrobiculus cordis, is distinguished by the single or double blowing sounds, which are heard not only over the thorax, but over so many arteries of the body.

Lumbar and Psoas Abscess.—In some cases, soft, fluctuating, deep-seated tumors, which are really produced by an aneurism, may arise in the lumbar region ; nay, they may seem to point, as happens in psoas abscess, at Poupart's ligament. But, unlike an abscess, the effusions of blood give rise, with rare exceptions, to impulse and to murmur.

Non-aneurismal Pulsating Tumors.—When a tumor of any kind presses upon the aorta, a distinct pulsation is communicated, which is very apt to be mistaken for an aneurism ; and the similarity to this is heightened by the circumstance that the morbid growth may produce a murmur. The tumors which most usually occasion the phenomena mentioned, are enlargement of the left lobe of the liver, cancer of the pylorus, disease of the pancreas, or in the omentum or mesentery; and, in rarer instances, enlargement and distention of the kidney, fecal accumulation, and cancer of the lumbar glands.

Now, to avoid error, we must pay close attention to the history of the disorder; we must trace, by percussion, the outline of the solid mass, and see if it correspond with any viscus; we must lay stress on the presence of digestive disorders, and on the amount of constitutional disturbance—both of which are so slight in abdominal aneurism ; we must examine the urine carefully, and find out whether there are renal symptoms in the case. Then, in non-aneurismal tumor the patient has almost always been in bad health before the tumor is detected, and the swelling rarely causes pain of such severity as is observed in an aneurism: moreover, the transmitted aortic impulse is, as a rule, lessened by placing the patient on his hands and knees, thus taking away the pressure from the artery. A varicose state of the epigastric veins and the existence of ascites will also decide against the diagnosis of an aneurism; while, on the other hand, the lateral as well as the forward direction of the impulse, violent neuralgic pains in the loins or shooting down the back, and an immovable tumor are in its favor. Still, there are cases in which a morbid growth lying across the aorta may occasion symptoms so nearly like those of an aneurism, that the most skilful diagnostician finds himself at a loss to determine their real meaning.

In these remarks on abdominal aneurism, it has been assumed that certain well-defined physical signs are always present. But it is very necessary to be aware that there are cases in which the physical signs are obscure or absent, and in which an aneurism affords no indication of its existence, beyond, perhaps, pain. Under these circumstances we may suspect the occurrence of the affection, but we cannot be certain of it.

But supposing that, from the combination of the physical signs and symptoms, we are certain that we are dealing with an abdominal aneurism, can we be sure that it is aortic? We cannot; for, although this is generally its seat, an aneurism of the splenic or the cœliac artery, of the superior mesenteric artery, or of the renal artery, may, so far as the collected cases enable us to judge, produce the same phenomena.*

When an aneurism bursts, it gives rise to symptoms which vary much with the seat of the rent. The blood is often effused behind the peritoneum or into it. Death may not follow for several days; but usually very great tenderness of the abdomen, not due to inflammation, and changes in the physical signs are at once produced by the accident.

---

* See Ballard, Physical Diagnosis of Diseases of the Abdomen, page 217.

CHAPTER VII.

ON THE URINE, AND ON DISEASES OF THE URINARY ORGANS.

THE diseases of the urinary organs with which the praetitioner of medicine has to deal are mainly those of the kidney. In the delineation about to be attempted, they chiefly will be discussed; and along with, or rather for the most part preceding their consideration, I shall briefly notice the urine in its pathological and clinical aspects.

URINE.

Physiology teaches us that the main function of the kidneys is to remove water and nitrogen from the system, at the same time that it takes from the blood many of its salts. The excreted liquid contains, therefore, a variety of elements, and by its study we are fortunately enabled to arrive not only at the condition of the organ which prepares it, but also at the state of the circulating fluid, and often indirectly at that of several viscera, the disorders of which give rise to impurities in the blood, which the kidneys endeavor to eliminate. Hence the urine, besides being the most accurate index of the condition of the urinary organs, also becomes a fair indication of that of many of the more important secreting glands in the body; and furthermore, though to a less extent, throws some light on the workings of the nervous system.

But to glean the full benefit from an analysis of the urine, we must be acquainted with its complex composition; be able to explore it not merely qualitatively, but quantitatively, and be accustomed to examine its deposits with the microscope. An immense field of useful research is thus thrown open, the

(586)

limits of which are indeed, in our time, almost daily widening by the active exertions of many devoted laborers. Modern chemistry especially is endeavoring to find means which will bring it within the power of the busy practitioner to determine, by apt volumetric processes, the exact proportion of the ingredients as accurately and as easily as hitherto we have detected their presence. But this is a subject which cannot be more than indicated in these pages; in this brief inquiry, only such of these ingenious investigations will be noticed as have furnished results that may be made readily available for the exigencies of professional life. A few remarks, however, as to the mode of procedure: we must have at hand accurate test solutions, the strength of which is exactly known; be provided with graduated pipettes, for sucking up and measuring the fluid to be examined prior to its transfer to a convenient vessel; and with graduated glass instruments, or *burettes*, from which exact quantities of the test solutions may be dropped. Graduated flasks, also, for the preparation of the solutions of the reagents are very useful, and beaker glasses to hold the urine. It is further customary, in the quantitative analyses, to use the French system of measures, and to employ instruments on which cubic centimetres are marked. One thousand cubic centimetres are equal to one litre, or 61·028 English cubic inches, or to a thousand grammes of water; and one gramme is equal to 15·434 troy grains.

The urine, in its healthy state, is a fluid of acid reaction, of an amber-yellow color, and of a specific gravity of about 1018 to 1020 as compared with distilled water at 1000. On standing from eight to twelve hours, a slight cloudy deposit takes place, consisting mainly of epithelial cells from the urinary passages, and of a few crystals.

The manner of obtaining a specimen of urine is not unimportant. We should always instruct our patient, as is so strongly recommended by Sir Henry Thompson,* to pass the first two ounces into one vessel, and the remainder into another. We thus procure a specimen of the renal secretion,

---

* Clinical Lectures on Diseases of the Urinary Organs.

in addition to anything in the bladder, separate from any urethral products, and avoid the error of confounding prostatic or urethral with vesical or renal disease. When it is essential, for a positive diagnosis, to obtain a specimen of urine absolutely pure, and unmixed with products of the bladder, the same authority recommends the drawing off of the urine by means of a soft gum catheter, of medium size, while the patient is standing. The bladder should then be carefully washed out by repeated small (one ounce) injections of warm water. The urine is now to be permitted to pass, as it will do, drop by drop, into a small glass vessel. The bladder contracts around the catheter, and the urine percolates direct from the ureters, through their virtual prolongation,—the catheter,—into the receptacle. The urine passed in the morning, immediately after rising, will be found to represent with sufficient accuracy the general process of disassimilation; but if greater accuracy be desirable, a specimen of the mixed urine of the twenty-four hours should be used.

The *quantity* of urine daily voided is, at a low estimate, from thirty-five to forty ounces; Vogel places it at fifty-seven ounces, and some observers even higher. Becquerel states the diurnal average to be in men forty-four, and in women forty-seven ounces. In summer, when the skin is acting freely, less fluid passes off by the kidneys than in winter. The more liquid that is taken into the system, the greater is the secretion of urine, unless the other organs which eliminate water, as the skin, lungs, and intestines, are excreting with unwonted activity.

The quantity is diminished in all cases of increased specific gravity, with the exception of diabetes, in which it is largely increased; it is diminished in acute diseases, in fevers, and in the early stage of dropsies; in some forms of Bright's disease through their entire course; and in the last stage of all forms. It is, on the other hand, augmented in all cases of diminished specific gravity; in hysteria; in the atrophic, nodular kidney, in the contracted kidney, and in waxy disease. In almost all vesical and kidney affections frequent micturition is a marked symptom; not always, however, associated with increased quantity of urine.

The *ingredients* of urine are very various. The principal are: urea, the alkaline sulphates, phosphates, uric acid and urates, chloride of sodium, mucus, coloring matter, and a large proportion of water. Small quantities of lime, silica, alumina; of iron, hippuric acid, and carbonic acid have also been detected by careful analysis.

Yet it is not only requisite to be aware of the ingredients, but, so as to have a basis for comparison, it is necessary to know the quantity of each ingredient commonly present in healthy urine. Here is Lehmann's analysis of 1000 parts, and side by side with it Thudichum's estimate of the average composition of the urine passed within twenty-four hours:

LEHMANN		THUDICHUM	
Water	932·019	Water . .	1345 to 1534 grammes.
Solid matter	67·981	Solids . .	850 to 1020 grains.
Urea	32·909	Urea . .	463 to 617 "
Uric acid	1·098	Uric acid . . .	7·5 "
Lactic acid	1 513	Creatine	4·5 ..
Lactates	1·732	Creatinine . . .	7 0 "
Water extract	·632	Sarkine . . .	
Spirit and alcohol extract	10·872	Uræmatine . .	} Undetermined.
Chloride of sodium, } Chloride of ammonium, }	3·712	Uroxanthine .	
		Hippuric acid . .	7·5 grains.
Alkaline sulphates . . .	7·321	Chlorine . . .	92 to 123 "
Phosphate of soda . . .	3 989	(or chloride of	
Phosphates of lime } and magnesia, }	1·108	sodium) .	154 to 200 "
		Sulphuric acid	23 to 38 "
Mucus	·110	Phosphoric acid . .	56 "
		Potassa and soda, } Lime and magnesia, }	Undeter- mined.
		Earthy phosphates .	19 grains.
		Iron	Undetermined.
		Ammonia	10 grains.
		Trimethylamine, } Carbonic acid, } Phenylic acid, } Damaluric acid, }	Undetermined.

Some of these constituents are derived entirely from the food; others from the metamorphosis of the tissues. Hence we find them in increased or diminished quantities in the urine, as a greater or smaller supply enters the body, or according to the activity of the process of nutrition. Their amount is furthermore influenced by the power of elimination of the kidneys and the proportion excreted, and sometimes vicariously excreted, by the skin, lungs, and intestines.

Besides the elements mentioned, the quantities of which it is evident must fluctuate much when the system is deranged, we meet, in morbid states, with substances that do not exist at all in healthy urine, or the presence of which is, to say the least, doubtful, such as albumen, sugar, blood, bile, fats, oxalate of lime, and certain pigments. Some of these are dissolved in the urine, and are not detected, except by chemical tests; others soon form in sediments after the urine has been discharged, and may be at once recognized by the microscope.

Having thus, in a general manner, mentioned the constituents of the urine, habitual and accidental, let us, in the same general manner, look at the points of clinical interest to be decided by an analysis of the urine ; in other words, let us endeavor to ascertain what the physician, not the professed chemist, is commonly in quest of in his explorations. And here it may be stated that, in a search of the kind, we are always somewhat guided by our knowledge of the nature of the case. We would, for instance, be most likely to look for albumen in dropsical affections ; or for sugar where a large quantity of urine was habitually passed.

Usually, we endeavor to fix all, or very nearly all, of these waymarks: the specific gravity, the color, the quantity, the reaction, the presence or absence of such important abnormal ingredients as albumen and sugar, and the character of the deposits. Frequently, too, we extend our examination until we have determined approximately, if not accurately, the increase or diminution of the main constituents of the urine, especially of the urea, uric acid, chlorides, phosphates and sulphates, and the distribution or non-distribution of bile and other unusual constituents through the fluid. To examine these points more in detail:

Color.—As is well known, the color of the urine varies considerably. Its hue is very much affected by food and medicine, as well as by various morbid processes; so readily, indeed, affected, that we must be very chary of drawing conelusions from the appearance of the secretion alone. Yet we may sometimes suspect the presence of certain substances, or be nearly positive of their absence, by the look of the fluid. Thus a smoky or a red aspect is apt to be owing to the admixture of blood ; a very light color denotes generally an increase of water, and is commonly found in diabetes, in hysteria, and in nervous affections of a similar character. It is never met with in diseases attended with fever, for the urine of persons suffering from fever is always of a dark hue. A greenish-yellow or brownish tint of the discharge is indicative of bile; but a similar tinge may be present when rhubarb has been taken. Strong coffee darkens the urine ; turpentine darkens and imparts a violet odor to it; senna gives it a yellowish color ; tar and creasote render it black; so does disintegrated blood.

In most of these instances the altered appearance is due to the respective coloring matter of these articles being excreted with the urine. But sometimes the unnatural hue cannot be thus accounted for, and is rather owing to a change in the normal coloring matter. Now, this pigment, on which the complexion of the urine depends, has been subjected by several chemists to careful examination, and consists, accord- ing to some, of a substance called urophæin, or urohæmatin, bearing a close relation to the pigment of the blood, and, like it, containing iron. Its presence may be demonstrated by adding about double the quantity of strong sulphuric acid to urine, which then assumes a decidedly brown tint. If it become very dark, we may infer that the quantity of the uro- hæmatin is increased, which is the case in pyrexias and in affections of the liver. But according to Schunck,* the color of normal urine is not due to one substance, but to two dis- tinct and peculiar pigments; one urian, soluble in alcohol and ether, the other, urianine, soluble in alcohol, but insoluble in ether.

A method for estimating the quantity of the pigment with accuracy has been proposed by Vogel.† It consists in com-

* Proceedings of the Royal Society, vol. xvi. p. 73 et seq.
† Vogel and Neubauer, "Anleitung," etc., Guide to the Analysis of Urine. Translated for the New Sydenham Society by Dr. Markham.

paring the hue of the urine with a table of fixed colors which serve as starting-points, and each shade of which represents a definite proportion of pigment.

There are besides pigments developed in the urine, owing to the decomposition of substances pre-existing in that fluid. Thus, for instance, indican does not itself impart any color to the urine, but·by its decomposition, to which it is very prone, it yields indigo-blue, indigo-red, and glucose. Schuuck* finds it as a normal constituent of the urine, and Carter† gives the following test for its detection: into a test-tube pour urine to the depth of half an inch; to this add one-third of its volume of commercial sulphuric acid of the sp. gr. 1830, by allowing it to trickle down the side of the tube so as to form the lower stratum. The fluids should then be intimately mixed by agitating them together. There is produced, according to the amount of indican present, a color varying from the faintest tinge of pink or lilac, to the deepest indigo-blue. Unless due regard be paid to these minutiæ, the reactions mentioned will not be observed. A tolerably correct estimate of the share taken by the different coloring matters in the production of a given tint may be made by neutralizing the sulphuric acid, added as above, with caustic ammonia, then agitating the mixture with one-third of its volume of ether, and allowing it to remain at rest for a few minutes. The ether rises to the surface, holding the indigo-red in solution, and the blue in suspension— if any have been generated—leaving the ordinary urine pigment dissolved in the aqueous fluid below. ,

There can be little doubt that a considerable number of the coloring matters mentioned as present in the urine are produced by spontaneous decomposition, or by the action of agents on substances, either colored or colorless, existing in the urine. Schunck has already proved the identity of indican and the products of its oxidation, indigo-blue and indigo-red, with the uroxanthine of Heller, and the products of its decomposition, uroglaucine and urorhodine.

---

* Philosophical Magazine, Aug. 1857.
† Edinburgh Med. Journ., Aug. 1859.

Uroxanthine, or indican, as Heller describes it, is detected by dropping twenty to thirty drops of urine on at least five or six times as much strong hydrochloric or nitric acid. After the fluid has been agitated for some time, it becomes red or faintly violet; and if it contain more than a very small quantity of the uroxanthine, it assumes a very decidedly violet or blue color. Exposure to air, too, evolves this pigment, which in composition is closely allied to hæmatin and to the coloring matter of the bile. It is noticed in considerable excess in very concentrated urine, and in affections of the nervous system, of the serous membranes, and of the kidneys.

Of the pathological coloring matters peculiar to the urine, the purple or pinkish, the uroerythrine of Heller, the purpurine of Bird, is the most common. It has a strong affinity for uric acid and the urates, and stains their deposit deep-red or pink. It abounds in the urine of febrile or inflammatory diseases, and is common in acute rheumatism, in gout, and in diseases of the liver. Its test is a solution of acetate of lead, which produces a pinkish precipitate.

Specific Gravity.—We take the specific gravity of urine to judge of the solid matter it contains. The readiest, although not the most exact, means of proceeding, is by the use of an instrument—the "urinometer"—now in the hands of nearly every physician. But for the implement to yield trustworthy results, the fluid should be brought to the temperature at which the urinometer has been graduated—generally 60° F. A difference of temperature of 7° F. corresponds with about 1 degree of the urinometer.*

From the specific gravity we may calculate the quantity of solid matter passed by multiplying the number above 1000 by 2 for the specific gravities below 1018, and by 2·33 for those above. For instance: in urine of specific gravity of 1010 there would, according to this formula, be 20 grains of solid matter in each 1000 grains of urine; in urine of 1030, 69·90 grains. This information obtained, it is easy to find the whole amount of solids contained in the urine of twenty-four hours, by ascertaining first the quantity passed in that time,

---

* Simon, quoted by Neubauer, *op. cit.*

and then working the problem out by a very simple calcula-
tion. To take the first illustration: if 1000 gr. yield 20 of
solid matter, how much would 20,000 yield? (the quantity
passed, we will say, in twenty-four hours).

$$1000 : 20 : : 20,000 : x. \quad x = 400 \text{ grains.}$$

This method is not, however, very precise; indeed, where
exactness is required, the urine must be evaporated until
nothing but a dry residue is left, which should then be carefully weighed.

The amount of solids in healthy urine is variously estimated.
Golding Bird rates it at about 650 grains in the twenty-four
hours; Beale and other recent observers place it approximatively at from 800 to 1000. As a general rule, the proportion
is greatest in persons of heavy weight; if, therefore, we wish
to make nice comparisons, the weight of the body must
always be stated. To ascertain how much of the solid matter
consists of the salts, the organic substances must be driven
off at a red heat. The following process, recommended by
Neubauer, insures accuracy: a measured quantity of urine,
20 to 30 c. c., is evaporated in a porcelain crucible of ascertained weight by means of the water-bath. When the residue
has become nearly dry, from one to two grammes of finely
powdered and carefully weighed spongy platinum are mixed
with it by the aid of a small platinum wire, and the whole is
then evaporated to dryness. The residue, with the platina, is
then heated over a spirit-lamp, at first very gently, and then
more strongly, until the whole of the carbon in it is con-
sumed, and the residue has assumed a light-gray color. By
subtracting the weight of the crucible and of the spongy
platinum, we obtain the amount of the incombustible salts
in the urine.

In disease, the solids, and with them of course the specific
gravity, fluctuate very much. We find the specific gravity
decidedly increased, rising to 1030 or higher, when sugar or
an excess of urea is present, and when the urine is concentrated and of deep color. A low specific gravity is met with
in certain forms of Bright's disease, in many cases of hysteria,
and in all pale urines excepting that of diabetes. But to be
accurate,—and indeed accuracy in regard to the other physi-

cal and chemical properties is unattainable without attending to the same rule,—we must not lay stress on the specific gravity without taking into account the measure of urine passed in the twenty-four hours, as well as the quantity of drink and of food swallowed; all of which of necessity influences the specific gravity. So, too, does the activity of the tissue metamorphosis.

Reaction.—Healthy urine reddens blue litmus-paper—a proof of its acid reaction. The *acidity* depends, in all probability, upon acid salts, especially upon the acid phosphate of soda.* The degree of acidity is, even in health, not always equal, and is much influenced by digestion, as Bence Jones has pointed out. If no food have been taken for hours, the discharge is highly acid; that passed after a meal, and while the process of digestion is going on, is but faintly so, or neutral, or even alkaline. In about three or four hours after meals the alkaline tide turns, and the acidity of the urine slowly increases until food is again taken. There seems, however, to be a limit to the increase of acidity, for Bence Jones found that continuing to fast for twelve hours beyond the usual meal time did not intensify the acidity of the urine. The alkalinity of the urine after meals is rarely detected at the bedside. For, although it may be alkaline when secreted by the kidneys, it is generally mixed in the bladder with urine which collected before or after the alkaline tide, and the mixed urine when passed may have an acid reaction.†

The acidity of the urine is augmented by the administration of the vegetable or mineral acids; yet they do not cause, even in large doses, as great variations as does digestion.

---

* Dr. Thudichum announces that he has just discovered a normal free acid in the healthy urine, which he designates as kryptophanic acid.—(Med. Times and Gazette, June, 1870.)

† Dr. Roberts (Urinary and Renal Diseases) attributes the occurrence of the alkaline tide after meals to the entrance of the newly-digested food into the blood. "If, as is believed, the normal alkalescence of the blood is due to the preponderance of alkaline bases in all our ordinary articles of food, a meal is, pro tanto, a dose of alkali, and must necessarily, for a time, add to the alkalescence of the blood; and as the kidneys have delegated to them the function of regulating the reaction of the blood, the urine immediately reflects any undue addition to, or subtraction from, the blood's proper alkalescence."

We find, too, this condition of the urine strongly marked if any acid be present in it which sets the uric acid free from the ammonia with which it is combined, or if the former be in decided excess.

We estimate the amount of free acid in the urine by a solution of caustic soda, or by a solution of carbonate of soda, containing 53 grammes to the litre or 530 grains to 10,000 grains. Some of this solution is added drop by drop to 100 c. c. of urine, which has been measured off in a beaker glass. After the addition of each half cubic centimetre, a drop of the mixture is placed, by means of a glass rod, on well-pre-pared litmus-paper. When the paper is no longer reddened, the analysis is finished; and by noting how much of the standard solution has been used, we can determine the acidity of the urine, which it is customary to express as equal to so many grains of oxalic acid, that being the sub-stance used to determine the activity of the soda solution.

Urine, when voided, remains ordinarily acid for at least a day; but it may lose its acidity much sooner. This is always a significant fact, having much the same meaning as if the fluid had been discharged in a neutral or alkaline state.

Now, an *alkaline* reaction may result from several causes: from the effect of digestion, as already mentioned; from the presence of a fixed alkali, as the carbonate of soda or potassa; or from a volatile alkali, due to the decomposition of the urea into carbonate of ammonia. In the former case, heat does not restore the color of the red litmus-paper—it re-mains blue; in the latter, a gentle heat soon brings back the original red tint. Moreover, in alkalescence from either cause, the earthy phosphates are precipitated, the fixed alkali causing the precipitation of the amorphous phosphate of lime; while by the volatile alkali, the phosphates of ammo-nia and magnesia, in conjunction with the phosphate of lime, are thrown down and the triple phosphate is abundantly formed, and can be easily recognized under the microscope by its beautiful prismatic crystals.

Alkalinity of the urine from a fixed alkali is not incon-sistent with health. We have already alluded to the effects of digestion; and alkaline urine also results from the use of certain articles of vegetable food, or of the salts of soda and potassa administered as medicine. Urine owing its alkalinity to a volatile alkali, like carbonate of ammonia, is always to be viewed as pathological. The disturbance is generally long continued, and the urine loses its acidity in the bladder, in consequence of a disease of the mucous coat of the viscus; or from being very long retained there, as in cases of paraplegia; or from admixture with pus, which acts as a kind of ferment, and leads to decomposition of the urea.

Changes in the Quantity of the more Important Constituents of Urine.—Here we shall have mainly to investigate the excess or deficiency of urea, of uric acid, the urates, phosphates, sulphates, and chlorides.

Urea.—The amount of urea excreted by adult males in the twenty-four hours is differently estimated. Becquerel places it, in round numbers, at 286;* Bischoff, at 542 grains; and Roberts estimates it in a healthy adult man at 3½ grains per pound weight of the body. Thus the amount is very variable; yet it is not so variable that a study of the quantity may not answer useful practical purposes. Urea is the principal product of the change of nitrogenized substances. Its proportion fluctuates, therefore, with the food partaken of, as well as with the activity of the transformation of the structures of the system; and hence it becomes the most important index of the waste and repair of tissues. Exertion of body and of mind leads to the discharge of a larger quantity of urea. If this be replaced by a nourishing diet, nothing is lost; the body retains its health. But when the requisite amount of nitrogenized aliment is not taken, or, if taken, cannot be assimilated, owing to a disturbance in digestion, the person wastes. We notice, too, in acute febrile states, hand in hand with the emaciation, an increase of this significant urinary constituent† — a proof, then, of the rapid

---

* Traité de Chemic Pathol.   Paris, 1854.

† Rosenstein, in his researches on the excretion of urea in exanthematous typhus, found that, in the commencement, the quantity eliminated with the urine is remarkably increased, and then, according to the previous mode of living of the individual, sooner or later sinks, with simultaneous increase of the fever, to far beneath the normal standard, to rise again with the augmented ingestion of food.—(Med. Times and Gaz., 1869, vol. i. p. 90.)

and unsupplied disintegration of the tissues. We see the same in inflammations, and in some cases of nervousness; also in certain forms of indigestion, in which the food is speedily passed off in the shape of urea instead of acting its part in the nutrition of the economy.

A lessened quantity of urea is excreted in many long-continued organic diseases which slowly and gradually undermine the general health; but the diminished amount in the urine may also be due to a want of secreting power of the kidneys. The urea then acts as a poison in the blood; and headache, nausea, convulsions,—in fact, the train of symptoms classed as uræmic poisoning is encountered. Many affirm that the morbid phenomena are not so much owing to the retention of the ingredient as to its decomposition into carbonate of ammonia; but this view of the subject is controverted by the experiments of Bernard and of Hammond.

Urea is sometimes not found in the urine at all, or only in traces, having been replaced, as Frerichs tells us, by leucine and tyrosine.

There are several tests for urea; for Liebig, Bunsen, and other distinguished chemists have proposed ingenious methods of determining both its presence and its quantity. Liebig's process is based on the fact that if bichloride of mercury in solution, and bicarbonate of potassa in excess, be added to a solution of urea, we obtain a compound of urea and mercury which is perfectly insoluble in water. The method of procedure is thus given: first separate the phosphoric acid. This is accomplished by measuring off with a pipette 40 c. c. of urine, and adding 20 c. c. of a baryta solution, obtained by mixing one volume of a solution of nitrate of baryta with two volumes of a caustic baryta solution, both prepared by cold saturation. The precipitate is separated by filtration; and 15 c. c. (corresponding with 10 c. c. of the urine) of the filtered fluid are placed in small beakers for each analysis. To this quantity of urine a solution of nitrate of mercury of known strength (and the strength recommended is that 20 c. c. of the solution exactly suffice for the precipitation of the urea in 10 c. c. of a standard solution of urea, in which this quantity contains precisely 200 milligrammes of urea) is added by a pipette or from the burette in very small quantities, the mixture being constantly stirred. When no further precipitation or turbidity is observed, a few drops of the mixture are placed by means of a glass rod on a watch-glass, and some drops of a solution of carbonate of soda are brought in contact with them. So long as the fluid in the watch-glass retains, even for some seconds, its white color, it still contains free urea; and more of the test solution of the mercury must be dropped into the beaker, until, on a renewal of test in the watch-glass, a distinct yellow color becomes instantly apparent. The amount of urea is now calculated from the quantity of the mercurial solution employed; first we find how much the 10 c. c. of urine contained, and then the total discharge in the urine passed in twenty-four hours is readily determined. When albumen is present, it has first to be coagulated by exposure to heat, and the fluid carefully filtered before the amount of the urea can be ascertained.

An easier method, and one which gives results corresponding closely with Liebig's, is Davy's, with the hypochlorite of soda or Labarraque's solution. With the imported French solution this method, Dr. Austin Flint, Jr., states,* is all that can be desired, but with the American article it is very uncertain. The process is as follows: a strong glass tube, with a bore not larger than the thumb can conveniently cover, twelve or fourteen inches in length, closed at one end and ground smooth at the other extremity, capable of holding from two to three cubic inches, and graduated into tenths and hundredths of a cubic inch, is filled more than a third full of mercury, to which afterward a measured quantity (from a quarter of a drachm to a drachm) of the urine to be examined is added. The tube is then to be exactly filled with a solution of hypochlorite of soda (Labarraque's solution). The mouth of the tube is then instantly tightly covered with the thumb, inverted once or twice to mix the urine with the hypochlorite, and finally placed beneath a saturated solution of salt in water contained in a cup. The mercury then flows out, and the solution of common salt takes its place; the mix-

* Chemical Examination of the Urine, p. 46.

ture of urine and hypochlorite, being lighter than the solution of salt, remains in the upper part of the tube. Decomposition of the urine soon takes place, bubbles of nitrogen escape and collect in the upper part of the tube. When decomposition is complete, which is known by the cessation of the evolution of bubbles of gas, the quantity collected is read off the scale on the tube. When great accuracy is required, corrections must be made for temperature and atmospheric pressure, if these vary from the standard of comparison. Each cubic inch of gas represents 0·645 of a grain of urea. Several of the substances found in urine during disease, as, for example, sugar, albumen, biliary and excess of urinary coloring matter, produce scarcely any effect on the results obtained by this method.* Another method for fixing the quantity of urea approximately is proposed by Prof. Samuel Haughton.† It consists in the use of tables showing how many grains of urea are excreted in the urine, of which the amount daily passed and the specific gravity are predetermined. On the opposite page is the table, as abridged by Roberts. It explains itself, and can, for practical purposes, be depended on, excepting when sugar or albumen is present.

A rough way of estimating the urea is to drop nitric acid into a porcelain capsule holding urine which has been evaporated to a mucilaginous consistence. Crystals of a pearly lustre, which the microscope at once shows to be nitrate of urea, are developed; and by always evaporating the same quantity and using a capsule of equal size, we may judge of the amount of the important ingredient as compared with that contained in other specimens of both normal and abnormal urine. If crystals form without the urine being concentrated by evaporation, simply on the addition of about an equal bulk of nitric acid, urea is always in considerable excess. But we may often, even without subjecting the fluid to this test, guess that the urea is increased by observing the

---

* Vide Thudichum on the Pathology of the Urine, p. 68, or Dublin Hosp. Gaz., June, 1854, p. 134, quoted in Braithwaite's Retrospect, 1854, vol. xxx. p. 109.

† Medical Times, Oct. 1864.

Prof. Haughton's Table for the Estimation of the Daily Excretion of Urea from the Specific Gravity.

Fluid Ounces.	Specific Gravity.																									
	1003	1004	1005	1006	1007	1008	1009	1010	1011	1012	1013	1014	1015	1016	1017	1018	1019	1020	1021	1022	1023	1024	1025	1026	1027	1028
20	35	36	43	57	71	85	100	103	106	118	130	136	142	151	160	196	233	241	249	257	265	274	276	278	279	280
22	38	40	47	63	78	94	110	113	117	130	143	150	156	166	176	216	256	265	274	283	292	301	304	305	307	308
24	42	43	51	68	85	102	120	124	128	142	156	163	170	181	192	236	279	289	299	308	318	329	331	333	335	336
26	45	47	55	74	92	111	130	134	138	154	169	177	185	196	208	255	302	313	324	334	345	356	359	361	363	364
28	49	50	60	80	99	119	140	144	149	166	182	190	199	211	224	275	326	337	349	360	371	384	386	389	391	392
30	52	54	64	86	107	128	150	155	159	177	195	204	213	227	240	294	349	362	374	386	398	411	414	416	419	420
32	56	58	68	91	114	136	160	165	170	189	208	218	227	242	256	314	372	386	398	411	424	438	442	444	446	448
34	59	61	72	97	121	145	170	175	181	201	221	231	241	257	272	334	395	410	423	437	451	466	469	472	474	476
36	63	65	77	103	128	153	180	185	191	213	234	245	256	272	288	353	419	434	448	463	477	493	497	500	502	504
38	66	68	81	108	135	162	190	196	202	225	247	258	270	287	304	373	442	458	473	488	504	521	524	527	530	532
40	70	72	85	114	142	170	200	206	213	237	261	272	284	302	320	393	465	482	498	514	530	548	552	555	558	560
42	73	76	89	120	149	179	210	216	223	248	274	286	298	317	336	412	488	506	523	540	557	575	580	583	586	588
44	76	79	94	125	156	187	220	227	234	260	287	299	312	332	352	432	512	530	548	565	583	603	607	611	614	616
46	80	83	98	131	163	196	230	237	244	272	300	313	327	347	368	451	535	554	573	591	610	630	635	638	642	644
48	83	86	102	137	170	204	240	247	255	284	313	326	341	362	384	471	558	578	598	617	636	658	662	666	670	672
50	87	90	106	143	178	213	250	258	266	296	326	340	355	378	400	491	581	603	623	643	663	685	690	694	698	700
52	90	94	111	148	185	221	260	268	276	307	339	354	369	393	416	510	605	627	647	668	689	712	718	722	725	728
54	94	97	115	154	192	230	270	278	287	319	352	367	383	408	432	530	628	651	672	694	716	740	745	749	753	756
56	97	101	119	160	199	238	280	288	298	331	365	381	398	423	448	550	651	675	697	720	742	767	773	777	781	784
58	101	104	123	165	206	247	290	299	308	343	378	394	412	438	464	569	674	699	722	745	769	795	800	805	809	812
60	104	108	128	171	213	255	300	309	319	355	391	408	426	453	480	589	698	723	747	771	795	822	828	833	837	840
62	108	112	132	177	220	264	310	319	329	367	404	422	440	468	496	608	721	747	772	797	822	849	856	860	865	868
64	111	115	136	182	227	272	320	330	340	378	417	435	454	483	512	628	744	771	797	822	848	877	883	888	893	896
66	115	119	140	188	234	281	330	340	351	390	430	449	469	498	528	648	767	795	822	848	875	904	911	916	921	924
68	118	122	145	194	241	289	340	350	361	402	443	462	483	513	544	667	791	819	847	874	901	932	938	944	949	952
70	122	126	149	200	249	298	350	361	372	414	456	476	497	529	560	687	814	844	872	900	928	959	966	971	977	980
72	125	130	153	205	256	306	360	371	383	426	469	490	511	544	576	707	837	868	896	925	954	986	994	999	1004	1008
74	129	133	157	211	263	315	370	381	393	438	482	503	525	559	592	726	860	892	921	951	981	1014	1021	1027	1032	1036
76	132	137	162	217	270	323	380	391	404	449	495	517	540	574	608	746	884	916	946	977	1007	1041	1049	1055	1060	1064
78	136	140	166	222	277	332	390	402	414	461	508	530	554	589	624	765	907	940	971	1002	1034	1069	1076	1082	1088	1092
80	139	144	170	228	284	340	400	412	425	473	521	544	568	604	640	785	930	964	996	1028	1060	1096	1104	1110	1116	1120

deep-yellow color, the strong urinous smell, and high specific gravity of the discharge.

Uric Acid.—Uric acid, like urea, is a product of the metamorphosis of tissue. It is, indeed, supposed by Liebig that the acid is an early stage of the transformation of urea; but this view has not been generally adopted. Hoffman* teaches that uric acid is deposited owing to the decomposition of the urates by the acid phosphate of soda. Under ordinary circumstances the deposition of uric acid occurs subsequent to the expulsion of the urine; but should the acid phosphate of soda be in excess, the uric acid may then be precipitated before the secretion is voided, and may thus give rise to gravel and calculi. This may also occur through too great coneentration of the urine.

In healthy urine the presence of uric acid cannot be detected without the addition of a strong acid, since it exists in the form of soluble urates, which must be decomposed before the uric acid separates. It is gradually thrown down in small red grains, which, should it be desirable to determine the quantity of the acid, are washed, dried, and then carefully weighed. And where accuracy is called for, it is best to allow the acid to separate at a low temperature, by keeping the fluid in a cool place for about four days, after acidulating it with nitric acid about one ounce to fifty.† It is also advisable to use always the same quantity of urine. Neubauer recommends 200 c. c. of urine and 5 c. c. of hydrochloric acid.

The characteristic reaction of uric acid is furnished by the murexide test. A few drops of nitric acid are mingled with the suspected deposit in a capsule, and the mixture is slowly evaporated nearly to dryness over a lamp; a drop of ammonia is then added, which produces instantly a rich purple— Dr. Prout's purpurate of ammonia.

But both uric acid and the urates can be much more easily and quickly discriminated by the microscope. The crystals of uric acid are very readily discerned, notwithstanding that

---

* Med. Times and Gaz., 1868, vol. i. p. 346, or Medical News, vol. xxvi. p. 77.

† Lee and Atlee on Under-estimation of Uric Acid, Amer. Journ. of Med. Sciences, April, 1869, p. 355.

they vary both in size and form. Rhombic plates with rounded angles are very frequent. To obtain the crystals rapidly, where they are not passed as uric acid, a portion of the suspected deposit is dissolved in a drop of potassa, and the alkaline solution then treated with an excess of acetic acid; after the lapse of a few hours crystals of uric acid will be formed.

FIG. 36.

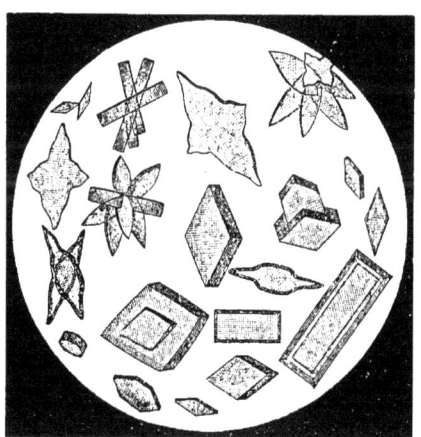

Crystals of uric acid, magnified about 200 diameters ; most of these forms are seen in the urine of acute rheumatism.

In disease, the fluctuations in the quantity of uric acid are very great; as a general rule, they correspond to the rise and fall of urea. We find the acid diminished in affections in which the eliminating power of the kidneys is interfered with, as in the more advanced stages of Bright's disease; an increase is encountered in acute inflammations, in fevers, and in acute rheumatism. In the latter malady this increase is very decided, and little red granules, visible to the naked eye, form a deposit in the urine soon after it is voided.

We must, however, be very careful not to suppose the uric acid to be in excess because it is readily precipitated. It may or may not be in larger amount; the sediment merely proves an augmentation of acidity in the urine sufficient to take away the base from the uric acid. Very frequently urates are separated along with the uric acid; we find then generally a dark urine of high specific gravity and very acid reaction.

Persons who habitually pass urine of the character described are subject to gastric disorders or are affected with a chronic hepatic malady. They are also, for the most part, intemperate or indolent in their habits. Hence it is not uncommonly perceived that exercise in the open air, attention to the action of the skin,. and mild aperients, by tending to eliminate the acid and by keeping the blood from becoming vitiated, afford more real and permanent benefit than the exhibition of alkalies to neutralize the acidity of the urine.

Occasionally precipitates of uric acid or urates occur in the urinary passages. Now, these sediments may concrete and form the nuclei of calculi; or they may be passed in small particles, commonly spoken of as "gravel." If they are formed in the kidney or ureter, their onward passage, presuming the concretions to be of sufficient size, is attended with severe pain, with nausea, and retraction of the testicle,—with the symptoms, indeed, attributed to an attack of nephralgia.

Urates.—The pathological conditions in which the urates are found to be changed are much the same as those in which alterations in uric acid occur. It only remains, therefore, to indicate how the salts may be chemically and microscopically distinguished. The urates consist principally of urate of soda and of ammonia, and of small quantities of urate of lime and magnesia. The deposits formed by their precipitation are of a pink color, yet sometimes brown, or even white. They are dissolved with great readiness by heating the urine. Acids decompose them and separate uric acid.   `

Under the microscope, the urates are seen to be either irregular amorphous particles, needle-like crystals, or round globules of varying size, from some of which fine needles project. The latter are commonly supposed to be urate of soda; the globules and crystals, urate of soda and of ammonia; the fine powder, urate of lime and soda.

But these are not facts which are established beyond doubt; it is only certain that the granular amorphous deposit, until lately called urate of ammonia, really consists of the mixed urates, more especially of the urate of soda and ammonia. These amorphous urates may, under the microscope, be mistaken for phosphate of lime. The differential test consists in their behavior with acids; the phosphate is dissolved by acetic or hydrochloric acids; the urates are gradually transformed into crystals of uric acid. Then, a deposit of phosphate of lime is often more cloudy and less defined than the

FIG. 37.

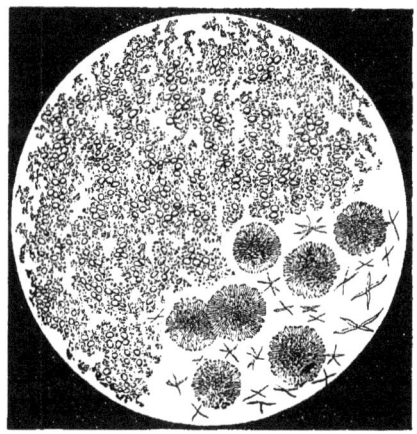

Mixed urates.

urates, and, unlike them, not soluble in liquor potassæ. From carbonate of lime, which also occurs in a granular form, both urates and phosphate of lime are distinguished by the effervescence of the carbonic acid which happens on the addition of a strong acid.

Urine containing a sediment of urates is generally very acid, or soon becomes so, either from an absolute increase of the uric acid, or in consequence of changes in some of the constituents of the fluid—as of the pigment—which take place either before or shortly after emission. Not unfrequently, too, it is scanty, and the urates are deposited as soon as the urine cools to the temperature of the atmosphere. Their precipitation may be, and indeed often is, owing to there not being water enough to hold them in solution. We may judge of this being the case, by ascertaining the amount of urine passed in twenty-four hours. If the quantity be about normal, the deposit is in all likelihood due to an excess of urates. In cold weather these deposits occur more quickly and more extensively than in warm.

But sediments of urates are encountered irrespective of these conditions. They are met with in pale urine, and without either diminution of water or excess of acidity to account for their presence. The urine yields but a faintly acid or a neutral reaction, and under these circumstances phosphate of lime, or even triple phosphates, may be observed to accompany the urates.

Phosphates.—The phosphates are derived in part from the food, in part from the disintegration of, or rather the oxidation of the disintegrated, albuminous substances, and especially of the nerve structures. They occur as the combination of phosphoric acid with soda, lime, and magnesia. In health they are kept in solution by the acidity of the urine; but as soon as the secretion ceases to be acid, they come into view,

FIG. 38.

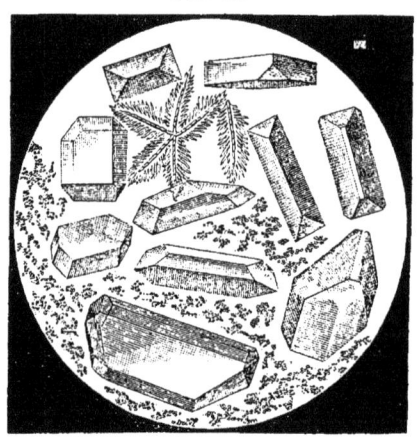

Earthy phosphates; the granules are phosphate of lime, the rest triple phosphates.

and are very quickly deposited. We may hence lay down the general law, that the appearance of phosphates goes hand in hand with a neutral or alkaline condition of the urine. Very often the fluid, as we have already seen, becomes alkaline from the decomposition of the urea into carbonate of ammonia. The ammonia unites with the phosphate, forming triple salts, ammonio-magnesian phosphates, which crystallize commonly in transparent prisms or in feathery-looking bodies, easily distinguished from the amorphous powder, or round, small globules of phosphate of lime. Yet we must remember that there is, as Dr. Roberts has pointed out, a crystalline form of phosphate of lime, which may be mistaken for one of the stellar forms of crystallization of uric acid, from which it may be distinguished by being invariably colorless. These earthy phosphates are all readily soluble in acids, even in weak acids like acetic acid. In many specimens of urine they are precipitated by heat; but the addition of an acid soon dissolves them, and thus prevents the turbidity from being mistaken for that due to albumen.

The triple phosphates are often met with in heavy deposits mixed with pus; in the alkaline purulent urine resulting from chronic vesical catarrh they are very common. They are also seen in cases of retention of urine in the bladder due to its temporary or permanent paralysis, as in low fevers, in hemiplegia, or in paraplegia. They are found, too, in many affections in which the vital powers have been seriously lowered and the acidity of the urine diminished, as during convalescence from acute disease. Under the latter circumstances, and in fact whenever the urine has become alkaline from the presence of a fixed alkali, the phosphatic deposit is apt to show a large excess of the amorphous phosphates, if, indeed, it does not altogether consist of them.

Urine alkaline from fixed alkali, and depositing phosphates, is, unless this condition have been brought about temporarily by fruit or other food, a matter of serious import. We encounter it in persons laboring under great general debility and indigestion associated with an impaired tone of the nervous system,—in fact, in those of whom it is the fashion, or has been the fashion, to speak as exhibiting the "phosphatic diathesis." Such a morbid state is not at all uncommon in men depressed by mental toil or intense anxiety, and is mostly benefited by rest, change of scene, tonic medicines, and generous diet. Opiates, too, have an excellent effect in restoring the acid character of the urine, by their quieting influence on the nervous system.

In these cases, in spite of the distinct sediment of the phosphates, it is very doubtful if they are really increased in quantity. The want of the acidity of the urine permits their precipitation, and causes them to become readily apparent. On the other hand, they may be actually in excess, and yet this excess be concealed from view until a careful analysis has been performed. This happens especially with the alkaline phosphates, the phosphate of soda and the ammonio-phosphate of soda, the proportions of which change in disease much more than do the earthy phosphates, and indicate much more clearly the variations of the phosphoric acid. And, paradoxical as it may appear, the acidity of the urine may be so much augmented by the increase of the phosphoric acid, that a very large excess of alkaline phosphates may be present in solution in a highly acid urine.

Now, a real, not merely an apparent increase of the phosphates, occurs, according to Dr. Bence Jones, in acute inflammatory diseases of the nervous structure during the existence of the most marked febrile symptoms, and in fractures of the skull when an inflammatory action takes place in the brain. We find the phosphates also augmented by the abundant use of animal food, by very active exercise, and in acute rheumatism ; while the phosphoric acid, as well as the sulphuric acid, the urea, and the chloride of sodium, is excreted during the course of a maniacal paroxysm, in epilepsy and in melancholia in less amount than in health.*

To determine the proportion of the *earthy* phosphates, a few drops of ammonia are added to the urine; soon a whitish precipitate is produced, which is not dispersed by heat. From the quantity of the deposit we may form a rough estimate of that of the earthy phosphates. But if the amount is to be accurately ascertained, we must employ a graduated glass, separate the precipitated phosphates by filtration, ignite them in a platinum capsule, and weigh the ashes. The *alkaline* phosphates are not thrown down by alkalies, and, unlike the earthy phosphates, are very soluble in water. They are procured by taking the fluid from which the earthy phosphates have been carefully removed by filtration, and adding to it a saturated solution of sulphate of magnesia.

---

* Adam Addison, Brit. and Foreign Med.-Chirg. Rev., April, 1865. As regards the excess of phosphates being a sign of wear and tear of nervous tissue, this is not universally admitted. Beale, for instance, does not so regard it.

From the deposit obtained in testing for the phosphates, some idea may also be formed of the quantity of *phosphoric acid* in the urine. The average quantity passed by an adult male in twenty-four hours is, according to Vogel, about 3·5 grammes, or nearly 53 grains. But for more minute information respecting this point, as well as for the several admirable volumetric processes by which the amount of the acid may be not only approximately, but precisely determined, I must refer to special treatises on the chemistry of the urine, especially to such works as those of Neubauer,* of Beale,† and of Thudichum.‡

Chlorides.—Unlike the phosphates, the chlorides in the urine are exclusively derived from the food; they correspond closely with the amount of salt ingested. In consequence, the chloride of sodium—the main chloride in the urine, for it does not contain much more than a trace of chloride of potassium—is, even in health, liable to great fluctuations; in twenty-four hours the mean is estimated by Vogel and Parkes at 11·5 grammes, or about 177 grains. Bischoff states the average at 14·73 grammes. In disease, very various amounts are eliminated with the urine. In typhus fever and in acute inflammatory affections, the chlorides sink to a very low level, and rise again in convalescence; an increase after a diminution is thus always a very favorable sign. We may study these changes to advantage in pleurisy and pericarditis, but especially in pneumonia. At the period of hepatization, the chlorides are absent from the urine, and appear in increased quantity in the sputum; during resolution they reappear in the urine; between these stages there is, probably, a determination of the salt to the inflamed organ.

Chloride of sodium is detected with great ease. The urine is strongly acidulated with nitric acid, and a solution of nitrate of silver is added; a dense white precipitate of chloride of silver quickly takes place, insoluble in nitric acid, but soluble in ammonia. The amount of the chloride is estimated by comparison with healthy urine; but to determine its quantity,

---

* Op. cit.   † On Urine, Urinary Deposits, and Calculi.
‡ Treatise on the Pathology of the Urine.

or that of the chlorine, with accuracy, Liebig's volumetric process, by means of the nitrate of protoxide of mercury, should be employed. It consists in first removing the phosphates by the standard baryta solution, of which 20 c. c. are mixed with 40 c. c. of urine. The mixture is poured upon a dry filter, and the filtered liquid is rendered very slightly acid by the addition of a few drops of nitric acid; 15 c. c. of the fluid thus prepared, and which correspond to 10 c. c. of urine, are measured off into a beaker glass, and the test solution of mercury is then dropped from a burette into it until a distinct cloudiness, or a precipitate which does not disappear by stirring, is produced. The amount of the mercurial test solution used is now read off from the burette, and we calculate the amount of chloride of sodium or of chlorine, by estimating that each cubic centimetre corresponds with 10 milligrammes of chloride of sodium, or 6·065 milligrammes of chlorine.

Sulphates.—The sulphates are found in the urine in large quantities. They consist of sulphate of potassa and sulphate of soda; the former in excess. Like the alkaline phosphates, they are dissolved in the urine, and must be precipitated by chemical reagents. To effect this, a few drops of nitric acid are added to urine, and subsequently from fifteen to twenty drops of a saturated solution of chloride of barium, when a white precipitate insoluble in acids is thrown down.

The sulphates are obtained in part from the food, in part from the oxidation of the sulphur entering into the constitution of the albuminous substances of the body and the subsequent union with a base of the sulphuric acid which is formed. They are enhanced by an exclusively animal diet, and after violent exercise; in truth, their increase is apt to go hand in hand with that of urea. An exception to this is noticed by Dr. Parkes* to occur in rheumatic fever. Here the sulphuric acid in the urine is greatly augmented, but the urea not correspondingly so. The administration of potassa raises, in a very striking degree, the proportion of the sulphates.

---

* Brit. and For. Med.-Chir. Rev., vol. xiii.

The average daily quantity of sulphuric acid passed in the urine is about 2 grammes. Vogel gives an easy method of determining approximately whether it is increased or diminished. After ascertaining the whole amount of urine in twenty-four hours—say it is 2000 c., and then each 100 c. c. would contain 0·10 gramme of sulphuric acid—100 c. c. are rendered acid, and as much of a test solution of chloride of barium* is added as corresponds with 0·05 gramme of the acid. The mixture is now filtered, and if the filtered liquid is not made turbid by the chloride of barium, we may infer that the patient has secreted less than 1 gramme of sulphuric acid in the twenty-four hours. If the liquid, however, is rendered turbid by chloride of barium, then a further quantity of this agent corresponding with 0·5 gramme of sulphuric acid is added; and if the filtrate is still rendered turbid, it is evident that the quantity of sulphuric acid is greater than normal.

Creatine and Creatinine.—These substances found in the urine are purely excrementitious, and are derived from a disintegration of the muscular tissue. Creatinine exists in larger quantities than creatine, and is the product of its decomposition.

But few observations have as yet been made on their increase, or on their significance in showing the activity of nutrition in the muscles in health or in disease. Active muscular exercise augments their quantity; and the same effect is probably produced by all spasmodic affections.

Both are generally included, in analyses, under the head of extractives. Their separation is effected by a process proposed by Liebig, consisting of the addition to the urine of lime-water and chloride of calcium, and subsequently of chloride of zinc. But for the chemical particulars I must refer to special works on the chemistry of the urine. Under the microscope, the crystals of creatine are colorless and beautifully transparent. Their appearance, as well as that

---

* Made generally by dissolving 30·5 grammes of crystallized chloride of barium, powdered and air dried, and diluting the solution up to 1 litre; 1 c. c. of it then equals 10 milligrammes of anhydrous sulphuric acid.

of creatinine, is faithfully represented in Robin and Verdeil's plates.*

Presence of Abnormal Substances in the Urine.—Here may be mentioned the ingredients which are observed in the urine in disease only, as bile and blood; and along with them, I shall notice those constituents the occurrence of which in healthy urine is so occasional that it is still undetermined whether they belong to health or disease, but of which it is certain that their presence in any marked degree is abnormal.

Oxalate of Lime.—This appertains to the class just alluded to. There can be no doubt that the salt may be detected in the urine of persons who enjoy good health; but there can be equally no doubt that the crystals are not found in large numbers, excepting in a morbid condition. Some pass habitually a considerable quantity of oxalic acid in the form of oxalate of lime. They are generally persons weighed down by care and anxiety, or who overtask their brains by incessant application to study, or weaken their nervous power by excessive sexual indulgence or by masturbation. Sometimes they are troubled with frequent seminal emissions and irritation of the bladder, or they are dyspeptic, and suffer from uneasiness after meals; but not uncommonly the appetite is good, and the digestion unimpaired. They are always languid, and either very irritable or very dejected. Frequently they complain of loss of memory, and of a sensation of weight, or a dull pain across the loins. They are very liable to boils and carbuncles, grow thin, and evidently are generally out of health. The urine voided is of high specific gravity, shows an increase of urea, and ordinarily a cloudy deposit consisting of mucus and the crystallized oxalates.

This is the disorder called by Dr. Golding Bird " oxaluria," and which is very generally combined with tissue changes and increased excretion of urea. Its existence as a separate affection has been denied; but that the formation of oxalate of lime in any considerable quantity is associated with the symptoms described, can be satisfactorily ascertained by any one who will take the trouble to examine the urine with care,

---

* Traité de Chemie Anatomique.   Paris, 1853.

in cases like those referred to. The origin of the oxalic acid, however, is not certain ; Golding Bird attributed it to a secondary or destructive assimilation of tissue. The evidence is certainly in favor of its being formed in the system, for it has been found in the blood. Still it is not improbable that it may at times be the product of a species of fermentation occurring in the urinary passages, and therefore after the

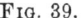

Fig. 39.

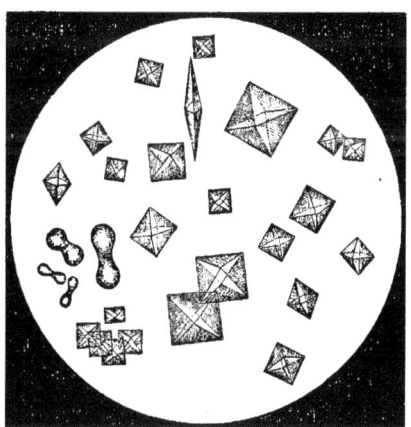

Crystals of oxalate of lime.

urine is secreted. Probably in the former class of cases alone are the constitutional symptoms described present. In the latter we may at times detect evidence of the irritation of a calculus, or of disease of the bladder or kidneys.*

---

* As regards the origin of oxalic acid, Dr. Owen Rees, in his Croonian Lectures in 1856, stated that it was formed after the urine had been secreted by the kidneys, and was derived directly from the decomposition of uric acid and the urates. In a recent valuable contribution to the chemistry of the subject, Schunck* establishes the presence in the urine of oxaluric acid, which he thinks presents an easy and satisfactory solution of the formation of oxalate of lime. The conversion of oxaluric acid into oxalic acid may take place after the urine is voided, or commence in the bladder, or even in more remote parts of the urinary apparatus, and thus lead to the formation of calculi of oxalate of lime. The oxaluric acid is derived from the oxidation of uric acid.

---

* Proceedings of the Royal Society, vol. xvi. p. 140, On Oxalurate of Ammonia as a Constituent of the Human Urine.

Oxalate of lime may be detected in the urine when articles which contain it, such as the rhubarb plant, have been eaten. It may be also found in the urine of patients recovering from severe acute maladies; and is encountered, but only in very small quantities, in the urine of healthy persons. But in neither instance is it at all permanent, nor can the presence of a few crystals be looked upon as of the least practical importance.

The microscope is incomparably the readiest means of detecting the salt. This appears in the urine in well-defined octahedra of most varying size, and in dumb-bell bodies. The former are much the more common and characteristic, for the dumb-bells are not frequent, nor is this formation peculiar to oxalate of lime; occasionally, long or pointed octahedra or prismatic crystals are observed.

The oxalates are often mixed with deposits of urates or uric acid. Sometimes—Beneke says constantly—the earthy phosphates coexist in large amount with the oxalates. Occasionally the irritation the passage of the crystals produces gives rise to tube-casts. A case came under my observation, in which a patient suffering from a protracted and severe attack of oxaluria voided for weeks, along with the oxalates, casts of the character known as hyaline, exudative, or small waxy casts. Neither heat nor nitric acid detected albumen. Under treatment, the crystals disappeared from the urine, and with them the casts. The gentleman recovered perfectly, and is now in excellent health. He has not to this day had the slightest signs of degeneration of the kidneys.

Leucine and Tyrosine.—Both these substances are the result of the decomposition of highly nitrogenous animal matter, are very similar, and usually associated. They have been found in the urine only in disease, as in yellow atrophy of the liver, in typhus fever, and in small-pox. Tyrosine is most readily detected by the microscope. It crystallizes in long, very fine, shining needles, which may congregate in globular bodies.

Hoffman has proposed the following delicate chemical test for tyrosine: a solution of mercuric nitrate, nearly neutral, is to be treated with the solution suspected to contain tyrosine; if it is present, a reddish precipitate is produced, and the supernatant fluid is of a very dark rose color. Leucine crystallizes in granular masses, consisting of roundish globules, sometimes of concentric form, and for the most part of yellowish color, and resembling oil-drops. The chemical test for leucine is to place the suspected deposit on platina foil, and then to evaporate it with nitric acid. The residue that is left is moistened with caustic soda, and this mixture carefully heated over a spirit-lamp. It is gradually condensed into oily-looking drops; a property which Scherer has pointed out as characteristic of leucine.

Bile.—The occurrence of bile in the urine imparts to it a very dark color. Its presence is a proof that the bile passes into the blood, and that the kidneys are performing a function forced on them by the deranged action of the liver, or by an impediment in the biliary passages. All the constituents of the bile may appear in the urine, or only the pigment, without the acids or their salts. The pigment is sometimes found transiently, and in small quantities, without yellowness of the skin; its more permanent and marked occurrence is, however, always attended with jaundice. It may be discerned both before the discoloration of the skin is noticeable, and after it has lost its yellow hue. The biliary acids are not of necessity present in the urine of icterus.

The detection of the coloring matter of bile is effected by pouring a small quantity of urine on a white plate; a drop of nitric acid is then permitted to fall on the thin layer of fluid. Soon a play of color takes place, commencing with green and blue, passing to violet and red, and often finally to yellow or brown. According to Frerichs,[*] this reaction may fail in cases where the other symptoms of jaundice are undoubted, owing to the bile-pigment having already passed through stages of transformation. When this is the case, the urine is at one time of a brown or brownish-red color, and becomes red on the addition of nitric acid; at another time it is of a deep red, which is converted by nitric acid into a dark bluish-red. Dr. Murchison has made a similar

---

* Diseases of the Liver. Sydenham Soc. Trans., vol. i. p. 100.

observation* in rare cases where jaundice has resulted from a blood poison, and he has frequently found the urine to present those characters where there has been no jaundice, but obvious derangement of function, or alteration of structure of the liver.

Dr. Basham† speaks highly of the following test for bile-pigment as being very delicate. The urine is shaken up with a small quantity of chloroform, which dissolves out the bile coloring matter and retains it in solution. If this solution be then decanted and evaporated carefully, the pigment which is left gives, on the addition of a drop of nitric acid, a beautiful ruby-red color, after displaying the characteristic play of colors. This test is equally available for detecting bile-pigment in other fluids.

Dr. Carter tells us,‡ that urine containing an excess of indican, presents the same succession of colors, when treated with nitric acid, as urine holding bile-pigment in solution. To avoid this fallacy in a doubtful case, the urine should be treated with sulphuric acid, as described while discussing indican. If the mixture become black and opaque, depositing a deep blue or purple precipitate on being diluted with water, the play of colors may be attributed to the excess of indican.

The biliary acids are sought for by Pettenkofer's test. It consists in tincturing, with a few drops of a solution of sugar, a small portion of urine contained in a test-tube or in a china dish, placed in cold water. To this mixture an excess of concentrated sulphuric acid is added, drop by drop. The fluid assumes a yellowish-red color, which, if bile be present, passes into a crimson or violet. The test is not applicable to albuminous urine, unless the albumen be first coagulated and separated. And it is inconclusive; for urine containing an excess of indican when thus treated, may display a reaction exactly similar to that caused by the bile acids.§ Moreover,

---

* Clinical Lectures on Diseases of the Liver, p. 284.
† Renal Diseases, Am. ed., p. 280.
‡ Edinburgh Med. Journ., Aug 1859, p. 125.
§ On this point consult Murchison on the Liver, p. 425, and Neubauer and Vogel's Analysis of the Urine, Syd. Soc. Trans , p. 47.

Neubauer and Vogel state* that oleic acid and albumen give analogous reactions.

Sugar.—This substance is not a normal ingredient of urine, or exists only in traces too minute to be detected by the ordinary tests. When met with in healthy urine, it is probably due to the decomposition of the indican. Sugar may occasionally be found in the urine of those who live exclusively on a starchy diet, or who take large quantities of sugar; but the proportion even then is very small. The urine secreted while under the influence of ether, chloroform, or chloral hydrate, is found to respond to the copper tests for sugar. And Bordier† has grouped together many observations, which lead him to conclude that diabetes may be considered as an almost normal occurrence in the stage of recovery from acute diseases. Measles, pneumonia, erysipelas, in short, all inflammatory fevers are liable to its production during convalescence. At Guy's Hospital the urine of a large number of patients, laboring under various complaints, was found, in several instances, particularly in cases of phthisis, to give a more or less marked reaction of sugar.‡ But a large and persistent amount occurs only in diabetes.

Urine holding sugar in solution is light colored, of high specific gravity, and of very peculiar smell. It rarely deposits sediments, and, as is well known, the excess of water in it is enormous.

To detect the presence of sugar, several tests have been proposed, nearly all of which are easy of application.

Moore's test is the simplest. It consists in boiling the suspected fluid with an equal quantity of liquor potassæ. The mixture, if it contain sugar, becomes of a deep-brown color, which grows deeper the longer the boiling is continued. This method, although good, is not to be depended upon when the urine contains only traces of sugar; nor ought the change of hue, when slight, to be accepted as conclusive, for other things besides sugar alter it. Indeed, it is always better to corroborate the evidence thus obtained by other tests.

---

* Anleitung, etc , p 76, 5th ed. Wiesbaden, 1867.
† Archiv Gén. de Méd., 1868.
‡ Researches on Diabetes, by F. W. Pavy, M.D., 2d ed., p. 126.

Trommer's test is both more trustworthy and more delicate. A few drops of a solution of sulphate of copper are dropped into the test-tube holding the urine. Liquor potassæ is now added in excess. If the fluid be saccharine, the faint greenish tint is changed to a deep blue, the precipitate which is formed when the alkali is first added being soon redissolved. On heating the blue mixture it becomes brownish, then yellow, and finally a reddish-brown mass of suboxide of copper is thrown down, very different from the flocculent or greenish sediment noticed when no sugar exists. A very small quantity of sugar can be detected by this process: but, good as the test is, it has its drawbacks; for it has been proved that sugar is not the only substance which possesses the power of reducing the salts of copper. Chloroform, creatine, and to some extent uric acid, share with it this property. Furthermore, Beale has shown that the presence of ammoniacal salts will prevent the precipitation of the suboxide in urine containing but little sugar.

Fehling's test is a convenient modification test of the copper for ready use, and may be also employed for the quantitative determination of sugar. This is the direction for its preparation: dissolve 69 grains of crystallized sulphate of copper in five times its weight of distilled water, add a concentrated solution of 268 grains of tartrate of potassa, and then a solution of 80 grains of hydrate of soda in 1 ounce of distilled water; enough water is now poured into the vessel to make 1000 grains of the mixture—each 100 grains of which will be equivalent to 1 of grape sugar.* Pavy,† in his Researches on Diabetes, uses a liquid containing caustic potassa; of which 100 minims reduce exactly half a grain of grape sugar. It consists of sulphate of copper, 320 grains; tartrate of potassa (neutral), 640 grains; caustic potassa (fusa), 1280 grains; distilled water, 20 fluid ounces. This test will be found more delicate, as well as more striking, by boiling the test-liquid first, and then adding the urine drop by drop. If sugar be present it will produce a reddish or yellowish opaque

---

* Lehmann's Physiological Chemistry, vol. i. p. 255, Am. ed.
† Researches on Diabetes, 2d ed.

precipitate, the difference in color depending merely upon the deficiency or excess of the test-liquid. If no such reaction ensue, urine should be added until a bulk nearly equal to the test-liquid has been poured in, and the whole then boiled again; the characteristic change not yet occurring, the urine should be set aside to cool. If it contain less than half a grain per cent. of sugar, the precipitation will occur as the liquid cools. The mixture first loses its transparency, and passes from a clear olive-green to a light-greenish opacity, looking, as Roberts describes it, as if some drops of milk had fallen into the tube. This green, milky appearance is characteristic of a small amount of sugar. If no milkiness is produced, the urine can be confidently pronounced free from sugar.

For the quantitative analysis of sugar contained in diabetic urine, the test-liquid is used as follows: in an ordinary case of diabetes, the urine is diluted with four times its bulk of water, mixed in a narrow graduated glass divided into 100 measures. One hundred minims of the blue test-fluid are now placed in a small porcelain capsule with a fragment of solid caustic potassa about double the size of a pea, if Pavy's solution be employed. The contents of the capsule are made to boil over a spirit-lamp, and the diluted urine is dropped into it slowly from a graduated glass, until the blue color is entirely removed. The amount of diluted urine employed is read off from the graduated scale of the tube. Let us say it takes 30 minims to decolorize the 100 minims in the capsule, that would be $\frac{1}{2}$ gr. of sugar in each 30 minims, or 8 grains to the ounce of diluted urine, which, as it has been diluted to the extent of one-fifth, the 8 grains must be multiplied by 5 to get the amount of sugar really present in an ounce of the urine.

The oxides of other metals besides copper are reducible by grape sugar. In accordance with this well-ascertained fact, a test by *bismuth* has been proposed. Subnitrate of bismuth is boiled with urine, to which first some caustic potassa has been added. If sugar be present, a gray or black sediment announces the reduction of the oxide to metallic bismuth. I have used this test of late frequently, and have found it very satisfactory.

These copper solutions are liable, after having been kept for some time, especially if exposed to the light, to allow a slight reduction to occur on boiling without any sugar being present. The test-liquid itself, if not fresh, should be tested by boiling, and if any change occur, a fragment of caustic soda if Fehling's, or caustic potassa if Pavy's solution be used, will render it as fit as ever for use.

The *fermentation* test by yeast is another method in use to determine both the existence and the quantity of sugar; but for qualitative analysis it is too tedious. As a quantitative test, however, it is easy of application and trustworthy. It was suggested by Dr. Roberts, and its accuracy has been recently indorsed by Prof. Doremus, of New York.* It is known as the differential density method, and depends upon the fact that by fermentation of saccharine urine all the sugar is converted into carbonic acid, water, and alcohol, and consequently the urine is diminished in density, and each degree of density lost indicates one grain of sugar to the fluid ounce of saccharine urine. The method of procedure is as follows: about four ounces of the urine are put into a twelve-ounce bottle, and a lump of German yeast about the size of a small walnut, or if this cannot be had, ordinary brewer's yeast, is added. The bottle is then covered with a nicked cork (which allows the escape of carbonic acid), and is kept in a warm place to ferment. Beside it should be placed a closely-corked four-ounce vial containing some of the same urine without any yeast. The object of this is to obviate any error which might occur were the specific gravity of the urine, before and after fermentation, taken at different temperatures. In about twenty-two hours the fermentation will have ceased. The two vials should be removed to a cool place, so that the urine may acquire the temperature of the surrounding air. The specific gravity of the two specimens of urine should then be taken, and their difference of density, as determined by the urinometer, indicates the number of grains of sugar contained in each fluid ounce of the saccharine urine.

---

* Flint's Manual of Urine, p. 42.

The peculiar fungus which forms in saccharine urine has also been studied to confirm the diagnosis of the unnatural ingredient.

To estimate the quantity of sugar, various ingenious instruments have been employed. Of these, the polarizing apparatus proposed by Clerget and made by Soleil, or the color-tube of Garrod, would seem to be the best.

Inosite.—This is a substance belonging to the group of sugars, and occasionally found in the urine. It is not detected in health, and is, according to Cloetta, the observer who first discovered it in urine, associated either with glucose or albumen. It does not appear to be derived from the food, nor from the metamorphosis of glucose, and inosuria is a symptom rather than a disease.* The characteristic reaction of inosite is exhibited when a solution of the substance is evaporated with nitric acid nearly to dryness on platina, and the residue, moistened with a little ammonia and a solution of chloride of calcium, is again evaporated to dryness; a marked rose-color appears, which does not happen when true sugars are treated in the manner described.

Extractive matters, in certain diseased conditions, drain off from the blood, and, sometimes, in large quantity. Dr. Owen Rees, some years since, pointed out their value in diagnosis and suggested the tincture of galls as their test.† Healthy urine is scarcely affected by tincture of galls; the blood extractives are immediately precipitated by it. This precipitate must not be confounded with that of the earthy and potassa salts which is thrown down from all kinds of urine after the lapse of five or ten minutes, by the spirit contained in the tincture. Should albumen be present in the urine, it must be separated by boiling and filtration before applying the test.

The presence in the urine of the blood extractives indicates merely the escape of blood material, and proves the existence of congestion or inflammation of some part of the urinary surfaces. In a recent contribution to medical litera-

---

* Gallois, De l'Inosurie. 1864.

† See London Medical Gazette, 1851, N. S., vol. xiii. p. 136.

ture Dr. Rees has pointed out* that in Bright's disease the extractives can be found in the urine before albumen is met with, and also that they exist after the albumen has disappeared: thus, on the one hand, warning us of the approach of albuminuria, and, on the other, against too early a belief in convalescence; for, as Dr. Rees justly observes, so long as the blood is losing its extractives so long is our patient in peril. The presence of the extractives also enables us to diagnosticate nephritic irritation from renal calculus, before albumen, blood, or pus has appeared. It is highly probable that extractives will be found preceding albumen in urine in most cases.

Albumen.—Urine may be albuminous from an admixture with blood or pus, or from a transudation of the albumen of the serum of the blood through the walls of the vessels of the kidneys. Sometimes the albumen appears for but a short time in the urine; at other times it is permanent; and in accordance with the length of its stay its significance varies. But this important clinical point will further on engage our attention more fully. Let us here rather examine the tests announcing the presence of the foreign substance.

There are several methods enabling us to ascertain the occurrence of albumen. Of these, the chief are:

Heat, which coagulates the albumen;

Nitric acid, or *carbolic acid*, which causes a white precipitate;

Corrosive sublimate, which also occasions a precipitate.

The first and second of these tests are the most convenient and the most in use; but they must be employed with certain precautions, and care must be taken not to rush to a conclusion that albumen is present until several sources of fallacy have been guarded against. For instance, the application of *heat* may render the fluid thick by throwing down the phosphates instead of the suspected albumen. We can, however, easily avoid being led into error by adding nitric acid, which causes the turbidity to disappear, if it be owing to the phosphates.

Again, if the urine be alkaline and the quantity of albu-

---

* Guy's Hosp. Rep., 3d Series, vol. xiv. p. 431.

men small, heat will not produce coagulation.   Hence care must be taken to render the urine slightly acid before heat is applied.   Acetic acid, which does not precipitate albumen, may be added for the purpose of neutralizing the alkalescence.   A highly acid urine behaves like an alkaline urine; in it, too, albumen may fail to be exhibited by heat.

The addition of *nitric acid* may give rise to a precipitate, which is not albumen.   It may deposit the urates, or even uric acid.   But heat here supplies the touchstone.   The boiling urine clears quickly, if the opacity be not caused by coagulated albumen.

Now, as both the heat and the nitric acid test may lead to wrong conclusions, if trusted to exclusively, but as they are so manifestly complementary to each other, we must, to obviate all sources of error, in every case employ both.   The best method of proceeding is to boil the urine, after having ascertained it to be of acid reaction, in a test-tube, by the flame of a spirit-lamp, and then to add the acid.   Or a second specimen may be tested according to a plan proposed by Heller: a small, conical glass, filled about one-third full, is held in an inclined position in the left hand; twenty drops of nitric acid are then allowed to flow gradually down the side of the vessel; the acid collects at the bottom, and above it may be seen an accurately-defined layer of coagulated albumen.

The quantity of nitric acid used is always a matter of importance; it must be neither too much nor too little.   A large amount redissolves the albumen; merely a drop, on the other hand, may retard instead of favoring coagulation, which then does not take place even when the urine is boiled.   In testing for albumen by means of heat and nitric acid, there may be no immediate response; yet after a few hours a flocculent precipitate may form and fall to the bottom of the tube.*

Sometimes urine is encountered on which neither the heat nor the acid test yields the customary result.   This is owing to its containing a modified form of albumen.   Such a case

* Andrew Clark, Lond. Hosp. Reports, vol. i. p. 226.

was published by Dr. Bence Jones.* No coagulation was produced by heat, and none by nitric acid, unless the urine was subsequently heated and permitted to cool. The solid that formed on cooling, disappeared on heating. The substance which was precipitated by alcohol was the hydrated deutoxide of albumen. The patient was laboring under mollities ossium. Dr. Basham recommends the tincture of galls as a test for this modified form of albumen. Scherer, too, has met with a form of albumen precipitable·from the solution containing it by alcohol, but not by heat; boiling causing a mere turbidity.

Recently Méhu has recommended† the following *carbolic acid* solution as a test for albumen :

Of crystallized carbolic acid, 1 part by weight ;

Commercial acetic acid, 1 part;

Alcohol, 90 p. c., 2 parts.

This solution undergoes no change by keeping. It is used as follows: to 100 grammes of urine add 2 c. c. of commercial nitric acid, and thoroughly mix. Upon the addition of 10 c. c. of the carbolic acid solution the albumen is precipitated in white flakes. In testing highly albuminous urine or albuminous solutions charged with salts, the addition of nitric acid is scarcely necessary. This method I have frequently used of late, and have found it a very delicate and satisfactory test.

It is often of service to determine the exact amount of albumen voided with the urine. This may be accomplished by adding a small quantity of acetic acid to a weighed quantity of urine, which is then to be boiled. The precipitate is collected on a filter, dried and weighed. An easier and ordinarily sufficiently accurate method consists in adding a small quantity of acetic acid to a specimen of urine, boiling and.allowing the flaky precipitate to settle in the test-tube ; the proportion of precipitate to the entire bulk is then expressed as one-fifth, one-eighth, etc., as the case may be.

Blood.—The passage of blood with the urine constitutes

---

* Philosophical Transactions for 1848.

† Archiv. Gén. de Méd., Mars, 1869, p. 268.

the phenomenon known as hæmaturia. The urine voided is of a red color, or of a more or less dingy or smoky hue, and deposits, on standing, a reddish-brown or a dark coffee-ground sediment. If much blood be present, small, irregular masses are seen at the bottom of the vessel.

The appearance of urine containing blood is therefore not uniform. But, whatever the look to the naked eye, the diagnosis is at once rendered certain by the use of the microscope. And only by this means can it be rendered certain; for urine may be red or black, from the admixture of various pigments derived from substances swallowed as food or medicine, or belonging to the economy. Thus, beet-root, some kinds of strawberries, logwood, and rhubarb impart a deep-red color, which may be the cause of groundless alarms; or urine deeply tinged with bile, or discolored by fever, may be thought to signify the occurrence of hemorrhage from the urinary passages.

The corpuscles are not always of uniform appearance, yet they are never seen collected in rouleaux. But, after having found blood corpuscles to indicate the true nature of the changed hue of the excretion, the question remains to be solved, at what point has the blood been poured out? Is it really from the urinary organs? and if it be from them, whence?—from the kidneys, from the bladder, or from some other portion of the tract? Again, what morbid state lies at the root of the hemorrhage?

Now, the first of these questions must always be answered at the onset. Blood may flow from the vagina or uterus and become mixed with the secretion from the kidneys, or it may have been added for purposes of deception. In the former case, a careful inquiry into the state of these organs, or, if necessary, a digital examination, will eliminate the source of error; in the latter, having the patient watched, and drawing his urine off by the catheter, detects the imposture. When we have fully satisfied ourselves that the blood is derived from the urinary organs, the next point to be ascertained—and clinically its importance cannot be overrated—is, whether it proceeds from the kidney or the bladder. To determine this, we have not only to study the character of the fluid excreted, but also closely to investigate all the conditions of the accident.

If the blood come from the bladder, it is not equally diffused through the urine; the fluid discharged is at first clear or nearly so, but at the end of the act of micturition is much more deeply colored, or pure blood, in a liquid form or in clots, is voided. Then, too, there is usually pain over the bladder, with a frequent desire to pass water, or a stoppage in doing so.

When the blood is derived from the kidney, we discover, on the other hand, pain in the lumbar region, and other symptoms pointing to the affected organ, such as dropsy, the existence of albumen in considerable quantities in the urine, or the passage of gravel. Clots are not encountered in renal hemorrhage, excepting when the blood coagulates in the infundibulum or the ureter, and is gradually forced downward. Such clots are of a whitish color, and generally of cylindrical shape. In their transit toward the bladder, they become often the source of distressing pain. They are very significant, yet they are not absolutely pathognomonic of renal hemorrhage; for coagula formed in the bladder may be retained there for some time, and lose their color before they are expelled.

But aid in diagnosis may be derived from the study of the shape of the clots, which for this purpose should be floated out in water. According to Mr. John Hilton,* they will oftentimes be found to be exact moulds or casts of the cavity in which the blood was effused. Thus, for instance, coagula formed within the bladder are found to have a somewhat irregular, circular outline, and to be flattened in shape, with bevelled and serrated edges. In their passage through the ureters and urethra, clots are often the source of distressing pain.

The use of the microscope, furthermore, affords most valuable aid in the differential diagnosis. The epithelium which is mixed with the blood is not flat and in scales, like that from the bladder, but small and more or less round. Some-

---

* Guy's Hosp. Rep., 3d Series, vol. xiii. p. 19 et seq.

times the blood globules are seen to be collected on casts that have been moulded within the renal tubes. These blood-casts warrant an absolute conclusion as to the source of the hemorrhage. But they do not always occur; and their absence, therefore, is not so complete and valuable a proof as their presence.

On the whole, then, although there is no one constant and unequivocal sign of either renal or vesical hemorrhage, we may generally arrive, by care, at a correct knowledge of the source whence the blood proceeds. In perplexing cases we should obtain specimens of urine for examination in the manner recommended in the early pages of this chapter.

But let us suppose that the origin of the flow has been satisfactorily settled; it still remains to determine what is the probable cause of the bleeding. Here, too, trustworthy knowledge is not to be obtained, save by careful analysis of the group of symptoms before us. Let us glance at some of the chief causes of hæmaturia.

When of *renal* origin, it is often due to an irritation or inflammation of the kidneys produced by some poison escaping out of the system through this channel, as is observed in scarlatina and other acute idiopathic diseases in which the phenomena of acute desquamative nephritis show themselves. Here we have the history of the malady, and the presence of tube-casts and of a considerable amount of albumen in the urine, to explain the meaning of the hemorrhage. The blood, it has been demonstrated, is derived from the engorged and ruptured Malpighian corpuscles.

A congestion of the kidneys of very analogous nature, and leading to the same consequences, is occasionally encountered in typhus fever, in small-pox, in malignant measles, and in acute rheumatism. Irritant medicines, too, such as turpentine and cantharides, cause congestion and bloody urine. In all these varied circumstances, a knowledge of the history of the case and a careful survey of its symptoms render the diagnosis positive.

Renal hæmaturia of a more chronic character is generally due to cancer of the kidney; to ulceration within the pelvis of the organ; or to irritation, with or without ulceration, set up by a calculus. In the first of these affections there is nothing peculiar in the sensible qualities of the urine to point out the source of the hæmaturia until the disease is far advanced, when pus, and sometimes disorganized cancerous tissue, may be detected in the sediment. The signs of a non-calculous pyelitis are not sufficiently definite to enable us to distinguish this rare malady with anything like accuracy. The existence of a calculus—one of the most common, if not the most common of the agents producing hæmaturia—is indicated as the source of the hemorrhage by the bleeding having followed active exertion, or a jar of the body from a fall, and by its recurring from time to time under circumstances like those just mentioned, favorable to the disturbance of a calculus lodged in the kidney. The presumption of this being the reason of the repeated bleeding is converted almost into certainty if there be localized pain, and if on any occasion one of the stony concretions should have been expelled.

There has been described, under the name of paroxysmal or *intermittent hæmaturia*, a disease which differs from ordinary renal hemorrhage in that in the latter the urine is not only coagulable by heat and nitric acid, but contains blood corpuscles; while in the former, although coagulable by heat and nitric acid, it exhibits very few or no blood corpuscles, and the coloring matter is not deposited on standing. Besides, the urine shows an increased proportion of urea. According to Greenhow,* crystals of oxalate of lime are constantly passed during a paroxysm and are absent at other times. This affection is unattended by any permanent lesion of the kidneys. It is paroxysmal in form, and is not of malarious origin.† The disease is ushered in by rigor, which is followed by only an imperfect hot stage, and more rarely by sweating. The urine voided is of a deep-blood color, and within an hour or two, perhaps, changes suddenly to a pale-straw color. The etiology of the disease is unknown.

There is also a form of hæmaturia which is endemic, and depends upon the presence of a parasite (Bilharzia hæmato-

---

* Trans. of Clinical Society, 1868, vol. i.

† Vide Greenhow, loc. cit.; also Pavy, Trans. of Path. Soc. of Lond., xviii.

bia). It prevails in the Mauritius, certain parts of the Cape of Good Hope, Natal, Egypt, and Brazil. The parasite inhabits chiefly the small vessels of the mucous membrane of the urinary passages and the kidneys, and it gains access to these parts chiefly during the act of bathing in the rivers. Persons affected with the Bilharzia hæmatobia are often observed to pass small renal calculi of oxalate of lime, which have for their nuclei the ova of this parasite.*

Besides these causes, renal hemorrhage may result from an altered state of the blood. Hæmaturia of this kind is encountered in purpura and scurvy.

To consider now *vesical* hæmaturia. One source to which it may be owing is a congestion of the bladder, as witnessed in fevers of a low type. Another is inflammation, whether acute or chronic, and whether of traumatic origin or brought on by a stone. In all these contingencies, the history of the case and the local symptoms establish the diagnostic distinctions; in arriving at which we are often materially aided by the introduction of a sound into the bladder. It has been claimed for the *endoscope* that it also assists greatly in the diagnosis.†

Another form of hemorrhage from the bladder is dependent upon malignant growths on its mucous coat. Generally these are attended with pain, with a constant desire to empty the viscus, and with considerable emaciation and a general cachectic condition. The fluid which is passed frequently contains pus, and, as the malady advances, from time to time large quantities of blood. Yet it is not a little singular that the appearance of the blood in the excretion may be the first sign of disturbance of the urinary apparatus.‡

Vesical hæmaturia, more frequently than renal, occurs as a vicarious discharge. Persons who are subject to bleeding piles, lose blood occasionally from the bladder, instead of

---

* For a full description of endemic hæmaturia, see Dr. Geo. Harley, in the Medico-Chirurgical Transactions, vol. xlvii. p. 55, and vol. lii. p. 379.

† See Desormeaux, De l'Endoscope, Paris, 1865; and Cruise, Dublin Quart. Journ., May, 1865.

‡ An interesting case in point is reported by Dr. Todd, Case XI. Lectures on Urinary Diseases.

from the rectum. But in obscure cases of this kind, before arriving at a definite conclusion, it is necessary to bear in mind that some writers, Thudichum prominently among them, believe that true vesical hæmorrhoids are not uncommon.

Blood may be discharged from other parts of the urinary apparatus as well as from the bladder or the kidneys. It may come from the *prostate gland* or the *urethra*. Now, in either case the bleeding is usually very profuse, and large quantities of blood are passed pure, or at first unmixed with urine. Besides, there are local signs of diseases of these parts, furnishing important points of discrimination. But this subject cannot be here pursued; it belongs rather to the domain of surgery than to that of medicine.

Such, then, are the various conditions under which hæmaturia may be noticed. As regards its prognosis, it is evident that this depends less upon the hemorrhage itself than upon the disorder of which the hemorrhage is a symptom. The flow of blood in itself is very rarely fatal. One of the worst consequences it may entail is the retention of a clot which serves as a nucleus for the formation of a calculus. The treatment, too, varies of necessity with the cause of the affection. Without entering into particulars, I will merely say, that for the arrest of the hemorrhage rest is indispensable; and where we desire speedily to check the discharge, gallic acid is very valuable.

Pus.—Urine containing pus, deposits an opaque creamy sediment, or a glairy mass, is generally alkaline, and always slightly albuminous. If the deposit be agitated with an equal quantity of liquor potassæ, a dense gelatinous mass results. This is the chemical test for pus; but it is a clumsy one, compared with the rapid and absolute diagnosis of the pus corpuscles by means of the microscope.

Sometimes a large amount of mucus is mixed with the purulent sediment, or a deposit due wholly to the former ingredient is so considerable that it is mistaken for pus. Yet the mucous deposit shows distinct points of difference: it is less dense, and collects more in clouds at the bottom of the vessel. And here again there is no means of discrimination as certain as that afforded by the microscope. Quantities of epithelium are always seen to be entangled in the transparent mucus, and the action of acetic acid develops the filaments of mucin. Sometimes, also, there are thin flakes or cylindrical bodies, unlike any appearance exhibited by pus.

FIG. 40.

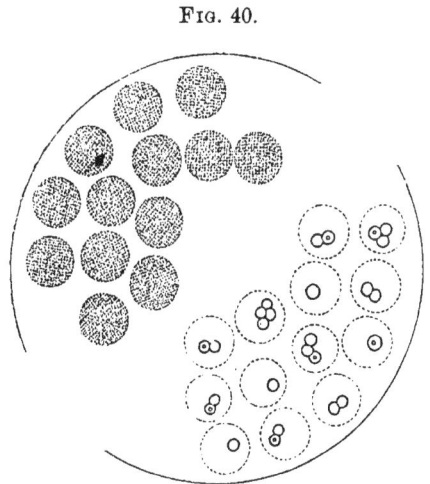

Pus corpuscles; those at the lower part of the field exhibit the action of acetic acid on the corpuscles.

Yet when the urine is strongly ammoniacal, even the microscope does not furnish a certain test; for the salts of ammonia obliterate the distinctive pus globules and convert pus into a slimy mass.

The occurrence of pus in the urine is a sign of suppuration somewhere in the genito-urinary system, or a proof that an abscess has opened into, and is being discharged through this channel. But as to the exact seat of the formation of the abnormal product, its existence in the urine affords no clue. To some extent, however, we can judge of this by the microscopical appearance of the corpuscles. When these are round and well developed, with their characteristic nuclei readily brought out by acetic acid, they generally have their origin in a catarrhal inflammation of the mucous membrane, especially of the bladder. On the other hand, as Vogel points out, pus corpuscles of irregular contour, exhibiting irregular nuclei when treated with acetic acid, or an ill-defined granular mass, consisting of irregularly-shaped pus corpuscles and partially-destroyed cells, indicate the probable existence of deep-seated suppuration, ulceration, or tubercular disease.

Fat.—Fatty matter may occur in the urine in various forms and in different conditions. It may be found in the shape of globules, when oil or milk has been added to the urine for purposes of deception, or when the former article has been swallowed for some time in considerable quantities, as for instance during the administration of cod-liver oil. It is also encountered in globules of varying size, either free, in cells, or in tube-casts, as in fatty degeneration of the kidneys.

In some cases it is met with in a molecular state, imparting to the urine a milky appearance, to which the name chylous urine has been given. The cause of this milky urine is not positively known. Dr. Beale considers* that the condition does not depend upon any permanent morbid change in the secreting structure of the kidney, and that the chylous character of the urine is intimately connected with the absorption of chyle, but precisely how the urine acquires that character is uncertain. It may continue for years without impairment of the general health, being always perceptibly increased by exercise. The disorder is best checked by the use of astringents.†

The tests for fat are its solubility in ether, and its microscopical characters. Lea and Atlee have recently pointed out‡ an error which is apt to occur in analysis of urine, viz., an illusory detection of fat. They found, in testing a specimen of urine, that the ether rose to the top so charged with matter as to resemble a half-liquid pomade. Separated by a pipette and spontaneously evaporated, it left a dirty-whitish greasy mass. A careful examination of this residue showed that instead of consisting of fatty acids, it contained nothing but the normal constituents of the urine, for it was soluble

---

* Kidney Dis. and Urin. Deposits, 3d ed., p. 309.

† See the cases of the disorder in the papers of Bence Jones, Medico-Chirurg. Transact., 1850-53; of Gubler, Gazette Médicale de Paris, 1858; and of Isaacs, Transact. of New York Acad. of Medic., vol. ii.; also Beale, Kidney Dis. and Urinary Deposits, 3d ed., p. 299.

‡ Am. Journ. Med. Sciences, April, 1869, p. 357.

in water, reappearing as normal urine. It was then ascertained that almost any specimen of urine will form an emulsion when violently agitated with ether, especially if the ether contain a small amount of alcohol, but this condition is not essential. When, therefore, ether appears to dissolve out fatty matter from urine, the ethereal solution should be separated, allowed to evaporate spontaneously, and, if the residue be soluble in water, it cannot be held to contain fat.

When passed in large amounts, fat may be evident to the unassisted eye. But there is no certainty of its presence unless the sediment be examined chemically and microscopically. Much error has indeed been occasioned by trusting solely to the look of the fluid. Thus the opalescence of urine caused by a sediment of urates has been mistaken for that from oily matter, and so also has been the pellicle which often forms on urine, and which consists not of fat, but of vibriones, fungi, and crystals of the triple phosphates. The "kyestein" pellicle observed in the pregnant state is of similar kind, though some oily matter may enter into its composition.

Sediments.—In connection with the different ingredients of the urine, the nature of the various urinary sediments has been discussed, and it has been insisted upon that they cannot be accurately determined, save by a careful microscopical examination. I will therefore here only group together their general characteristics:

1. A light and flocculent cloudy deposit is commonly mucus, entangling epithelial cells, or spermatozoids.

2. A dense, abundant, white deposit is generally composed of urates or phosphates; but it may be pus or extraneous matter.

3. A yellow or pink deposit is almost always due to urates.

4. A granular or crystalline deposit, of reddish color and small in quantity, is uric acid.

5. A dark, sooty or dingy-red deposit, is blood.

So much for the sediments. The following table may serve a useful purpose, in showing how both they and the soluble urinary ingredients are affected by the reagents commonly employed:

TABLE EXHIBITING THE ACTION OF THE MAIN REAGENTS EMPLOYED IN THE
EXAMINATION OF THE URINE.

SPECIFIC GRA-
VITY ....

High................ { Urine high colored............... { Increase of urea,
uric acid, etc.
Urine pale......... Diabetes.

Low................ { Urine high col-
ored or normal. { Certain forms of
Bright's disease.
Urine pale......... Excess of water.

HEAT ....

Throws down de-
posit .... { Soluble in acid.... Phosphates.
Insoluble in acid.. Albumen.

Dissolves deposit. { Urates.

Does not dissolve
deposit .... { Uric acid.
Phosphates.

NITRIC ACID......

Precipitates........ { Quickly ....{ Albumen.

More gradually...{ Uric acid.
Crystals of nitrate
of urea.

Dissolves .... { Earthy phosphates.
Alkaline phos-
phates.
Oxalates.

Causes decompo-
sitiou under ef-
fervescence..... { With heat.......... { Urea decomposed
into carbonate
of ammonia.

Without heat...... { Carbonate of lime
Uric acid.

HYDROCHLORIC
ACID..............

Precipitates........ { Uric Acid.

Transforms......... { Urates into uric
acid.

Detects, by violet
change of color. { Uroxanthine or
Indican.

SULPHURIC
ACID...............

Changes color of
urine............. { Brown. ....{ Urohæmatin.

Crimson or violet
(if sugar have
been added.) { Biliary acids.

Violet ....{ Indican.

ACETIC ACID .....

Precipitates de-
posit (not solu-
ble in excess of
the acid.) { Mucus.

TABLE EXHIBITING THE ACTION OF THE MAIN REAGENTS EMPLOYED IN THE EXAMINATION OF THE URINE—(Continued).

LIQUOR POTASSÆ.	Precipitates.........	Earthy phosphates.
	On boiling, turns urine brown....	Sugar.
	Dissolves............	Uric acid. Deposits of urates.
	Forms gelatinous mass.............	Pus.
LIQUOR AMMONIÆ	Precipitates.........	Earthy phosphates.
	Dissolves............	Cystine.
SOLUT. OF CHLOR. OF BARIUM.....	Precipitates.........	Deposit soluble in free acid. — Phosphates. Deposit insoluble in acids. — Sulphates.
NITRATE OF SILVER...........	Precipitates.........	Yellow deposit, soluble in nitric acid and ammonia. — Alkaline phosphates. White deposit, insoluble in nitric acid, but soluble in ammonia. — Chloride of sodium.
ALCOHOL, OR ETHER.	Precipitates.........	Albumen.
	Dissolves............	Hippuric acid.
	Does not dissolve..	Uric acid.
ETHER...............	Dissolves............	Fat.

URINARY ORGANS.

Diseases of the Kidney of which Pain is a Prominent System.

This group embraces acute inflammation of the kidney, and those painful affections classed under the term nephralgia.

Nephritis.—Acute inflammation of the kidney is chiefly observed in old persons and in damp climates. It may be

occasioned by an attack of acute rheumatism, by direct violence to the organ, or by the irritation of a calculus; but
probably its most frequent cause is exposure.

It commences with a chill, soon followed by fever. The
pulse is small and hard, the skin is frequently dry. There
are nausea and vomiting, and at times diarrhœa with tenesmus. The urine is voided drop by drop; it is red, and may
contain blood. The patient complains of a pain in the renal
region, sometimes dull, at others sharp and lancinating, and
augmented by pressure and by moving. The pain is not
limited to the kidney, but radiates to the diaphragm and to
the bladder. With it are often associated a numbness of the
thigh on the affected side, and a retraction of the testicle.

The disease may occur in both kidneys; yet it rarely affects
more than one. It lasts from one to three weeks, and generally terminates in resolution. But it may lead to suppuration and disorganization of the organ.

The disorder is recognized by the pain, the fever, the retraction of the testicle, and the appearance of the urine. It
differs from an attack of colic by the signs of disturbance
of the urinary organs, by the seat of the pain and the fever;
from rheumatic pains in the back, by the former of these
symptoms. Then, in lumbago we rarely find much febrile
excitement, nor are there nausea and vomiting, nor numbness along the course of the anterior crural nerve; but, on
the other hand, the pain is much more influenced by movements, especially by stooping and such other motions as call
the muscles of the back into play. Congestion of the kidneys is distinguished from inflammation by its affecting both
sides, by the absence of protracted or severe pain, and the
comparatively slight derangement of the urinary functions.
Further, the congestion is not idiopathic, and we can generally trace it to the swallowing of some irritating substance,
or to the poison of a febrile malady, such as small-pox or
typhus.

Chronic nephritis, if such a disease really exists irrespective of the forms of it associated with albuminous urine, and
belonging therefore to Bright's disease, is so ill defined and
uncertain a malady, that it has no signs which positively announce its presence.

Nephralgia.—Severe pain in the kidney, unconnected with inflammation of the organ, is ordinarily caused by the passage of a calculus. In such cases we have all the symptoms of acute inflammation, save the fever; the pain, too, is generally much more violent, and ends as suddenly as it commenced. With reference to the diagnosis, the complaint may be confounded with the same maladies as nephritis, and the differences are identical as between nephritis and the ailments resembling it, excepting, of course, that we must leave any indications afforded by febrile signs out of consideration. The greatest similarity nephralgia exhibits is to colic; but elsewhere this has already been discussed at some length; and in particular cases we are often much aided by the knowledge that our patient has on a former occasion passed renal concretions.

The amount of pain varies according to the magnitude of the stone and its character. As a rule, those composed of oxalate of lime give rise to most pain. We may distinguish them by their roughness and irregularity; those of urates and uric acid are much softer and not jagged, and, unlike calculi consisting of the salts of lime, are combustible on platina foil.

As already stated, we have in the severity of the pain a sign indicative of the probable nature of the case. Still, there are states in which paroxysms of pain referred to the neighborhood of the kidney are attributable to far other causes than the passage of a calculus. Leaving that obscure and doubtful disease, a pure neuralgia of the kidney, out of consideration, we find a few affections, very rare, it is true, which closely simulate the passage of a renal calculus.

The first of these is the pain occasioned by an inflamed and ulcerated ureter. Dr. Todd relates a case of the kind.* The patient had severe attacks of lancinating pain, referred to the right loin, lasting for weeks, and accompanied by constant and intractable vomiting. The urine contained pus in varying quantity, but neither blood nor calculous matter could be detected. At one time he continued free from any

---

* Lecture Second, on Diseases of Urinary Organs.

paroxysm for four years. After death the most careful search was made for a calculus, but no sign of one could be discovered. The ureter of the right side was thickened throughout the greater part of its course, and deposits of lymph adhered to its mucous membrane. A somewhat similar train of phenomena may occur from an irritation or inflammation of the ureter, caused by the poison of rheumatism or gout, although the paroxysms of pain are apt to be neither so severe nor of so long duration.

Another morbid condition closely resembling the passage of a renal calculus may result from the presence of the malarial poison in the system. How close this resemblance may be, the following case will show :

A soldier, twenty-four years of age, of fair complexion, and evidently of strong constitution, was seized rather suddenly with pain over the left kidney. The loin was sensitive to the touch, and appeared somewhat red and swollen. The skin was hot; the pulse 100. The urine was not found to be abnormal, though containing a reddish coloring matter. The pain continued for several days, becoming more severe, notwithstanding that by Dr. Hilborne West's direction, under whose charge the man was, and with whom I saw him, six ounces of blood were drawn from near the affected part. On the fourth day of the disorder the patient was assailed with excruciating pain along the course of the ureter, attended with the voiding, at short intervals, of a high-colored urine. The attack lasted from six o'clock in the evening until five o'clock the next morning, leaving the patient much exhausted; the only relief throughout its duration being obtained from the inhalation of chloroform. At six o'clock in the evening another seizure of equal violence set in; and, after the lapse of twenty-four hours, again another. Seeing the recurrence of the paroxysms at about the same time of each day, and learning from the patient that a few months before he had had a remittent fever, which had left behind an irregular intermittent, we resolved upon the administration of large doses of sulphate of quinia in the interval between the paroxysms. The seizure did not take place that night; but the remedy being a day or two afterward suspended, the fourth night was again a night of anguish. The antiperiodic was resumed, and continued, in lessened doses, for three weeks. The patient remained, for about six weeks after the last attack, under Dr. West's observation, gradually recovering his health and spirits. When he was lost sight of, there was still a dull pain in the left lumbar region, with inability to stand erect; but no return of the excruciating intermittent neuralgic pains.

In a case of this kind, it is evident that nothing but a knowledge of the history of the patient, and noting the regularly recurring onsets of the pain, could have led to a correct appreciation of its cause. We sometimes meet with a so-called neuralgia of the bladder, of similar origin, and having much the same symptoms, excepting that the distressing pain is distinctly referred to the bladder. As in the case just detailed, the attacks occur at night.

These remarks are all based on the assumption that the renal pain is very severe and paroxysmal in its character. Let us now briefly inquire into the significance of a steady and less acute pain, premising that we have excluded from consideration abdominal aneurism, affections of the muscles of the back, of the spine, and of the tissues surrounding the kidney, in which diagnosis, of course, we are materially assisted by an examination of the urine.

We meet with persistent pain referable to the kidney itself, in inflammation of the organ, especially in that variety of inflammation affecting the infundibula and pelvis, termed pyelitis. We also encounter it in malignant disease of the kidney; sometimes, although it is not then of long duration, from the irritation of concentrated and highly acid urine; much more generally from the presence of a stone lodged in the kidney. The pain in the latter complaint often extends along the course of the ureter to the testicle, which is retracted and swollen. Not unfrequently there is also tenderness on pressure over the affected kidney, and the pain is greatly increased by active exercise; and it is not uncommon to find, associated with these exacerbations of pain, nausea and vomiting, and the appearance of blood in the urine.

But there is yet another point in the diagnosis of the passage of calculi which we must not overlook, namely, that the pain may be referred to other parts than to the region of the kidney. It may be felt near or at the sacrum, and not merely on one side; or it may be referred to the right hypochondrium and extend downward, but not be perceived in the loin. Under the latter circumstances, there may be, with pain of great intensity, coexisting distention of the colon, vomiting, and constipated bowels, and the symptoms so closely resemble those of the passage of a biliary calculus, that, as we learn from a case recorded by Owen Rees,* nothing but the detection of blood in the urine prevents error. Again, as happened in two cases which came under my notice, the pain may be referred to the left hypochondrium or along the course of the colon, be associated with soreness to the touch and digestive disorders, and closely simulate an organic lesion of these structures. Nothing but careful and repeated examinations of the urine, and observing the irregular and whimsical course the supposed intestinal malady pursues, will enable us to arrive at a knowledge of the truth.

Nor must we be unmindful that a calculus may be months in passing, and that as it changes its position the seat of the pain changes. I had a case of the kind under my charge in a lady of about fifty years of age. She suffered for weeks at a time from excruciating pains, commencing in the left kidney; then felt somewhat below it; and finally localized in the neighborhood of the left ovary. She was occasionally free from pain for five or six days. But it was only after fully nine months of recurring suffering that the passage of a stone the size of a plum-stone, and followed by a discharge of large amounts of a gritty substance and a soapy-looking urine, removed her distress. The stone consisted of urates.

The symptoms of renal calculus may, after having existed for a longer or shorter time, entirely cease, owing either to the calculus becoming encysted and thus remaining innocuous, or to its obstructing the ureter, causing retention of the urine, and, by pressure, producing gradual atrophy of the cortical and tubular structures, the kidney being finally converted into a mere bag.

---

* Guy's Hospital Reports, 3d Series, vol. x.

In concluding the consideration of this subject, it may be useful to group together the symptoms by which we may infer the existence of a *calculus in the kidney*. They are: frequent micturition, often attended with pain at the end of the penis, pain in the loin, with or without accompanying soreness, occasionally passing suddenly into a violent paroxysm, with a tendency to shoot along the course of the ureter to the testicle and hip of the aching side; and in some cases the discharge of pus due to coincident pyelitis. These symptoms become very positive evidence if the blood extractives are present in the patient's urine, or if this, when examined microscopically, is found to contain blood corpuscles; or if we know that attacks of hæmaturia have previously happened, and that small urinary concretions have at any time been discharged. But all of these indications are far from being always present. Any one of them, or several of them, may be absent.

Diseases marked by an Albuminous Condition of the Urine, associated with more or less Dropsy.

Since the great discovery of Bright, that dropsy was frequently dependent on a disease of the kidney, revealing its existence by the occurrence of albumen in the urine, a host of laborers have endeavored to enlarge the edifice he had both planned and erected; but thus far the results of their work are not so extensive as to have materially changed the original fabric. Certain it is that, beyond the researches on the minute character of the urine,—researches which, by detecting the tube-casts, have added to our knowledge in a way not to be overestimated,—little has been brought forward that, in a clinical point of view, can be said to have altered the structure reared by the celebrated physician. The work progressing aims mainly at denying the unity of the affection which Bright described, and at proving that the disease which bears his name consists of a group of maladies having the common feature of a more or less albuminous state of the urine. Now, it is not at all improbable that this view will ultimately be fully accepted;

41

but as yet the distinctions proposed are, for the most part, neither very definite nor so constant and undoubted as to warrant us in making them the groundwork of a practical separation. I shall, therefore, in this sketch, prefer to consider the disorder as it is seen separated by broadly-drawn lines into an acute and chronic one, merely indicating the disputed points of pathology as I proceed, and endeavoring to incorporate such recently acquired facts as have a readily discerned and valuable diagnostic bearing.

Acute Bright's Disease.—In this form of the affection the symptoms are of an acute character. Especially so is the dropsy, which is quickly developed, and soon becomes the most marked token of the malady.

The history of a large number of cases is as follows: after exposure to wet or cold, a fever sets in, accompanied by nausea, and by a dull pain in the region of both kidneys, extending along the course of the ureters. The eyelids and face become puffy and swollen, and soon a general edematous condition of the skin is observable, showing itself very plainly in the extremities, scrotum, and abdominal parietes. Subsequently dropsical effusions frequently take place into the interior cavities.

A similar group of symptoms is apt to be noticed in the acute Bright's disease which so constantly attends scarlatina, excepting that, following as it does an exhaustive disease, there are from the onset much greater pallor and general debility.

The urine in both these forms of the acute malady is of high specific gravity, and dingy from its admixture with blood. It contains a large amount of albumen; a minute examination brings to light casts, lined here and there with blood corpuscles. As the malady progresses, these " blood-casts" disappear, and we find the coagulable material which has been effused into the tubes coated with epithelium, which may be normal or slightly fatty, and with free nuclei, or slightly granular, or quite homogeneous; or we may discern pus globules taking the place of the epithelial cells. Furthermore, crystals of uric acid, of urates, even of oxalates, and a considerable amount of renal epithelium are objects often seen in the sediment.   The normal constituents of the urine are considerably changed.   The chlorine may have disappeared altogether; the uric acid and the pigments are increased.   The amount of urea fluctuates much: it may be either augmented or diminished.   There is a frequent desire to void the urine, although the whole quantity passed is rather below the natural average.

FIG. 41.

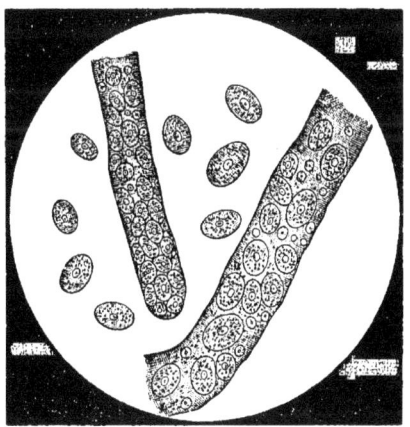

Epithelial casts and epithelial cells from the kidneys found in a case of acute Bright's disease (*acute desquamative nephritis*); magnified about 460 diameters

The constitutional disturbance is not, as a rule, extreme; the pulse, however, may be very quick, tense, and full.   The skin is generally harsh and dry; nausea and vomiting are of common occurrence.

The urgent symptoms last ordinarily for several weeks.   When recovery is about to take place, they abate; the skin becomes moist, the pulse is no longer accelerated, and hand in hand with a diminution of the dropsy, the quality of the urine largely increases.   But this, although fortunately the most common, is not the invariable issue.   The disease may gradually lapse into a chronic form, or, as sometimes happens, the patient's condition decidedly ameliorates: he leaves his room, as he thinks, well, yet with a certain amount of albumen in his urine; and often then he remains to all appearances in good health, until after a fresh exposure the albumen increases in the urine, and the dropsy and most of the acute symptoms return.

And whatever the attending circumstances when an attack has been at all prolonged, the risk to life is greatly increased by the supervention of local inflammations—as of the pleura, lungs, peritoneum, or pericardium; or by the sudden effusion of fluid into the pulmonary structure; or by the retention of urea in the blood and consequent uræmic intoxication. If from any of these complications death take place, the kidneys are found to be enlarged and somewhat irregularly congested. The medullary cones are of dark color, their bodies are compressed, while their bases expand into the swollen cortical substance. The surface of the organ is smooth, and the investing capsule is easily detached.

The recognition of the disease is readily effected The puffy, pale face; the general dropsy; the albumen in the urine, associated with tube-casts, form a combination of signs so remarkable, that it is difficult to mistake their meaning. The same phenomena are encountered, although not always to the same degree, in the chronic form of the malady. What is therefore about to be said of the differential diagnosis of the acute complaint, applies with almost equal correctness to both varieties of the ailment.

The main disorders with which acute Bright's disease is apt to be confounded are:

ACUTE NEPHRITIS;

SUPPURATIVE NEPHRITIS;

HÆMATURIA AND PURULENT URINE;

SIMPLE ALBUMINURIA;

PULMONARY ŒDEMA;

PLEURISY AND PERICARDITIS;

DROPSY;

COMA; CONVULSIONS.

Acute Nephritis.—This differs from acute Bright's disease, by its affecting generally only one kidney, by the much greater pain and tenderness in the lumbar region, by the retraction of the testicle, and the higher degree of febrile excitement. Then, too, the deeply-colored urine which is voided contains little or no albumen.

Suppurative Nephritis.—There is testimony proving that in rare cases the suppurative process may coexist with Bright's disease. But, on the whole, the two disorders are totally distinct, and may, as a general rule, be readily discriminated. Suppurative nephritis occurs from external· violence, from exposure to cold and wet, from a morbid condition of the blood, or the impaction of a renal calculus, and may lead, like Bright's disease, to uræmic symptoms. But it usually attacks only one kidney, occasions much local pain, is frequently attended with a fever more or less remittent or intermittent in its character, and at times with a well-defined swelling, which may be felt in the lumbar region, and extending far downward. Now, all this is very different from Bright's disease, which always affects both kidneys, and in which no enlargement of the organs can be perceived through the abdominal walls. Then, we detect blood and pus in the urine of cases of suppurative nephritis, and any casts that are found are seen to be covered with pus corpuscles.

Hæmaturia and Purulent Urine.—In both these complaints, if we can speak of them as such, and otherwise than as symptoms, there is albumen in the urine; and, on the other hand, traces of blood and pus may be present in the urine of Bright's disease. But the quantity of albumen met with in hæmaturia or in purulent urine is small; in fact, it is in exact proportion to the amount of· pus or blood the excreted fluid contains; whereas, on the contrary, if the secretion from a Bright's kidney be mixed with pus or blood, the amount of albumen is very large.

Simple Albuminuria.—By this is meant an albuminous urine unconnected with any marked structural lesion, such an albuminuria as is sometimes observed as a transient phenomenon in the course of several diseases; as, for instance, in the exanthemata, in typhus, in cholera, in hectic fever, or as a consequence of surgical diseases and operations.* An albuminuria of similar kind is also met with when the kidneys become congested from interference with the circula-

* Henry Lee, Lectures on Practical Path. and Surgery, 3d ed., Lond., 1870, vol. ii. page 380.

tion, as in disease of the heart, or from the pressure of a gravid womb. Albumen in the urine may also be encountered in diphtheria, in pneumonia, in acute rheumatism and gout,* consecutively to a blister, or after partaking plentifully and exclusively of albuminous food.† But in all these conditions the quantity found is small and transitory, very unlike what it is in the persistent albuminuria of Bright's disease. Then the constitutional symptoms in the morbid states referred to are so dissimilar to those of Bright's disease, that they become a safeguard against error. But the most valuable aid in forming a judgment is derived from a microscopical investigation of the urinary sediment. In simple albuminuria there is no exudation; hence no tube-casts can be detected in the urine. This, at least, represents the general truth. But we must admit that repeated and searching examinations may detect occasionally a few. Yet their inconstancy, their character, the small amount of albumen they are commonly associated with, are of significance; and the general nature of the symptoms again helps to explain their meaning. Then, too, the kidney may really be, in several of the morbid states under discussion, in the same condition as in the earlier stages of acute Bright's disease, but it is unlike the fully developed malady with its marked clinical features which we have above described.

Pulmonary Œdema.—Bright's disease is one of the most frequent causes of pulmonary congestion and dropsical effusion into the air-cells; oppression in breathing, inability to lie in the recumbent position, cough, frothy expectoration, are therefore common among the symptoms attending the renal affection. And, to distinguish this œdema from that produced by other morbid states, we have only to examine the urine carefully,—a matter, indeed, which ought not to be neglected in any case of œdema of the lungs.

Pericarditis and Pleuritis.—The tendency to internal inflammations, especially to those of the serous membranes, is a remarkable peculiarity of Bright's disease. We may dis-

---

* Thudichum, *op. cit.*
† Hammond's Physiological Memoirs; Simon's Animal Chemistry.

criminate pericarditis, or pleuritis complicating the malady, from either of these affections of other origin, by noting the far greater amount of dropsy than is ordinarily found in these disorders, and by detecting albumen and tube-casts in the urine.

Dropsy.—By an examination of the urine, too, may be distinguished the dropsy of the complaint under consideration from that produced by other causes. And independently of the physical properties of the urine, we see very often the evidences of the true nature of the dropsy in its commencing with swelling of the face, and then becoming universal, and in the striking and characteristic physiognomy which it has a share in developing. But more will be said hereafter on these points.

Coma ; Convulsions.—A common and very dangerous complication of Bright's disease manifests itself by signs of great derangement of the nervous system, prominent among which are drowsiness and convulsions. Now, it is evident that it is very important to distinguish the cases produced by uræmic poisoning from epileptiform convulsions and kindred states in which there is no appreciable change of structure in the kidneys. Let us see how they differ.

Uræmia, or uræmic intoxication, is most commonly preceded by a diminution in the urinary secretion. There is headache, with indistinct vision, great drowsiness, and vertiginous sensations; the pupils are sluggish and usually dilated; the hearing is impaired; the countenance is dusky; the skin cool, with short exacerbations of heat, and the patient suffers from constipation and nausea and vomiting. Paralysis of sensation may be observed in the extremities. The dulness of mind is apt to deepen into stupor or coma, or convulsions set in as precursors of the coma, which terminates in death, unless the urinary secretion be freely re-established. The coma may at one time be so profound that it is impossible to arouse the patient, whilst at another time he rouses himself, and acts with considerable intelligence.

In some cases the marked phenomena set in with a chill, by which the eliminating function of the skin is suppressed; in other cases, however, there is no such obvious beginning.

And as regards the decided lessening, or even suppression of the urinary secretion, though this is the rule, it is not constant. I wish here particularly to call attention to this point; for I have known many an error in diagnosis committed, and the symptoms of uræmia many a time receive an erroneous interpretation, by supposing that this state could not exist, as the quantity of urine passed was about normal. We must test for urea and the other urinary ingredients, which may be profoundly changed in amount, notwithstanding the seemingly healthy aspect of the secretion, and notwithstanding, too, that it may be found free from albumen.

Cases of uræmic coma differ from ordinary comatose conditions, as witnessed in apoplexy, in fevers of a low type, or following narcotic poisoning, by the dissimilar symptoms ushering them in. The coma is much more suddenly developed than that in fevers; far less suddenly than that of apoplexy or narcotic poisoning.* Then, the stertorous respiration, to adopt the observation of Addison,† is peculiar — the loud sounds of the expired air are of much higher key, not like the low, guttural tones of apoplexy. Furthermore, we have in the general dropsy a clue to the nature of the case; but of course the most certain light is thrown on it by the analysis of the urine. And often, indeed, until this has been effected, no positive judgment can be given; for the dropsy may be so very slight as to escape observation, and the other signs be ill defined.

The same remarks apply to the delirium or to the epileptic convulsions of uræmia. And here the difficulty in diagnosis is increased by the first seizure oftentimes happening unexpectedly; so much, in truth, increased, that, unless we are aware of the history of our patient and have previously examined his urine, the true explanation of the symptoms is not to be reached. Cases of uræmic convulsions may occur in pregnant women; in them, however, the tendency to dis-

---

* There may, however, be exceptions to this rule, as in a curious instance reported by Moore in the London Medical Gazette, 1845, in which a person became comatose after taking laudanum; yet his death was found to have been caused by contracted kidneys.

† Guy's Hosp. Reports, 1859.

order of the kidney is so great, that we are rarely in error in concluding the convulsions to be of uræmic origin. Uræmic delirium is rare, but I have met with it under circumstances in which nothing preceded it to indicate its nature, and in which it was very marked.*

The fact that the grave phenomena are thought by some to be due to the urea, by others, to its decomposition into carbonate of ammonia, has been already alluded to. A distinguished physician, Prof. See, has recently suggested that they may, in different cases, be owing to either, and has indicated the features by which *uræmia* may be distinguished from *ammoniæmia*. In the former there is no fever; a clean tongue; a smooth, elastic skin; a disordered respiration, but not a disordered circulation; convulsions and coma. In the latter, we always find mucus or pus in the urine, and an affection in consequence of which the urine is retained somewhere in the urinary passages; there are chills, followed by burning heat of surface; a dry, grayish skin, exhaling, like the breath, an ammoniacal odor; a dry tongue; emaciation; rarely vomiting; the respiration is free, the circulation deranged; headache occurs, but the intelligence remains good.

Chronic Bright's Disease.—An acute attack of Bright's disease may become very prolonged, and gradually pass into a confirmed malady, or the complaint may come on insidiously from the onset, and develop itself very slowly. In either case we have a dangerous chronic affection established.

The transition from the acute to the chronic disease is indicated by the disappearance of blood from the urine, by its lessened specific gravity, and the smaller amount of albumen it contains; and not uncommonly by a temporary diminution of the anasarca and an increase in the quantity of urine voided.† When the disease runs a more or less chronic course from the commencement, its initiatory steps are very

---

* Case at the Penn. Hosp., April, 1865.

† Dr. Ringer (Lancet, Nov. 1865) states that a sign more trustworthy than any of those mentioned is afforded by the temperature of the body. When the acute stage ceases, the thermometer indicates a normal temperature, and not a temperature ranging from 100° to 105° Fahr.

obscure. We generally find such cases in persons who are poorly fed and half clad, who live in damp, ill-ventilated houses, are intemperate, or whose constitutions are ruined by syphilis or scrofula. The first symptoms they notice may be a frequent desire to urinate; a swelling of the extremities or of the face; an increasing pallor and general debility. They seek medical advice, and an examination of the urine reveals at once the cause of their protracted indisposition. Yet the renal disease may lead suddenly to a fatal termination without the patient having previously experienced any manifest or urgent signs of ill health. And even after the malady has been fully recognized, it is very difficult to predict its course. In truth, different cases present very different symptoms. We meet in many with the same phenomena as those encountered in the acute variety, and life is threatened by the same dangerous complications; but in others the signs are dissimilar—the dropsy, for instance, is very slight or wholly wanting, or the amount of albumen is small. The only constant and characteristic manifestations are the profound and increasing anæmia, and the presence of albumen and tube-casts in the urine. Generally, too, the fluid is of low specific gravity.

Now, the altered specific gravity can only be dependent upon a diminution of the urinary solids. The urea is lessened, and so are, as a rule, the uric acid, the pigment, and the salts. Commonly, also, the urine is not so abundant as in health, and its reaction is less acid.

The albumen is very variable in amount; its quantity may, indeed, fluctuate much in the same patient, and even change from day to day. It is persistent; yet the observations of Christison and Rayer forbid us to doubt that it may, in some cases, disappear for a short time.

The tube-casts, too, are not uniform—not nearly as much so as in the acute variety of the affection. We meet with casts almost or quite homogeneous, and small or large; with casts besprinkled with shrivelled degenerating epithelium; with casts covered with granules or with oil-drops. In the progress of a particular case, nearly all of these forms may be encountered, although, as we shall hereafter see, the preponderance of any one of them affords an indication as to the exact state of the kidneys. There is only one kind we do not find in the chronic disorder: the one covered with well-developed epithelial cells or blood corpuscles. The apparent absence of casts from albuminous urine is not absolute proof of non-existence of renal degeneration. In some cases their absence is only temporary, while in others, they are small and few in number and easily escape detection, even after most careful search.

Other minute features, too, it has been sought to turn to advantage. Thus it is suggested by Dr. J. G. Richardson* that we may derive additional aid in diagnosticating the form and stage of the renal affection by a careful study of the white elements of the blood, found in varying proportion in the urine.

From these remarks, it is obvious that a great diversity of phenomena is witnessed in chronic Bright's disease; so great, in truth, is this diversity, that the opinion is fast gaining ground that there are several distinct pathological affections embraced under the one term, and attempts have of late years been made to define the train of symptoms significant of each. But, notwithstanding that a means of separation is also afforded by the very varied aspect of the organ,—enlarged or fatty in some instances, diminished or waxy in others,—it is not clearly enough proved, certainly not proved as regards all, that the dissimilar appearances may not be different stages of the same malady to make it incumbent to arrange the symptoms with reference solely to the morbid anatomy of the kidney. I shall, therefore, consider the differential diagnosis of chronic Bright's disease continuously, and point out, after having done so, the clinical features which are supposed to be indicative of the various forms of the malady.

Leaving out of consideration those affections for which both the acute and the chronic disease may be mistaken, and which have been already discussed, chronic Bright's disease may be confounded with—

---

* Am. Journ. of Med. Sciences, Jan. 1870.

Anæmia;
Neuralgia;
Chronic Rheumatism;
Chronic Bronchitis;
Cardiac Dropsy;
Gastro-intestinal Disorders;
Cancer; Tuberculosis; Cysts of Kidney.

Anæmia.—There are few diseases which alter the blood so completely as does chronic Bright's disease. The blood corpuscles go on steadily diminishing, while the fibrin holds its own, and the quantity of albumen fluctuates considerably, being ordinarily much reduced. Besides these changes, the blood often retains its effete ingredients, since the kidneys are incapable of performing their function. The alteration and gradual impoverishment of the blood make themselves manifest by the increasing debility, and by the pallor and waxy look of the countenance.

We may discriminate this anemic or chlorotic condition from that unconnected with renal disease by the existence of albumen and tube-casts in the urine, and often also by the prominence of the dropsical symptoms. But it is essential to know that some of the phenomena—certainly albuminous urine and dropsy—may attend the anæmia following profuse or frequently-repeated hemorrhages, without the structure of the kidneys having been impaired. It is difficult to distinguish these cases from true Bright's disease, except by taking into account the diminution of the albumen as the hemorrhagic tendency is lost, and the absence of the fibrinous moulds of the tubules. The dropsy, unless it be considerable, can hardly be looked upon as a valuable differential index, for a slight or moderate amount of dropsy, or even none at all, may be encountered in either morbid state.

The ophthalmoscopic appearances presented by the retina, and described in a previous part of this work, afford help in distinguishing between the anæmia of Bright's disease and that produced by any other cause. The white patch upon the retina, opposite to and around the optic entrance, with hemorrhagic effusions, is quite characteristic, and, according to

Dr. Dickinson,* it especially belongs to that state of the kidney known as granular degeneration.

Neuralgia.—As this is not at all infrequent in the chronic form of Bright's disease, we must always, in obstinate cases, examine the urine, so as to see whether or not a renal affection lie at the root of the painful malady. The neuralgia may affect the fifth, or other nerves; sometimes it takes more the form of hemicrania, and it is often associated with disordered vision, or impairment of other special senses; or it may coexist with strange and anomalous nervous symptoms.

Chronic Rheumatism.—Very frequently patients affected with chronic Bright's disease complain of muscular pains. The pain is dull, not increased on pressure ; sometimes shooting, more like that ordinarily called neuralgic, and to which we just called attention. The pain is oftenest met with in those instances in which the dropsy is slight or wholly wanting, and an examination of the urine is then the only means of determining its real significance.

Chronic Bronchitis.—This is one of the most common complications of Bright's disease ; so common, indeed, that Rayer observed it in seven-eighths of his patients, and Wilks† states it, from an extensive analysis of cases, to have been more universal than any other single symptom, albuminous urine alone excepted. It is hardly necessary to add that the last-mentioned sign is the one that distinguishes this secondary pulmonary trouble from all other forms of bronchial disease.

Cardiac Dropsy.—A chronic disorder of the kidney is often connected with disease of the heart; and knowing the frequent combination of an organic cardiac malady with Bright's disease, it becomes our duty, in every instance of dropsy associated with a cardiac affection, to examine the urinary secretion, for both the prognosis and treatment are influenced by the result of a search of this character.

Let us suppose that in cases of so-called cardiac dropsy we find albumen in the urine; is this a proof of coexisting Bright's disease ? No; not unless the amount of the abnormal ingredient be considerable, or tube-casts accompany the

---

* Pathology and Treatment of Albuminuria, p. 134.
† Guy's Hospital Reports, 2d Series, vol. viii.

albuminuria. Mere congestion of the kidneys, resulting as it does from an obstruction to the flow of the venous blood along the vena cava, may occasion albuminuria; but the presence of albumen is temporary, and its quantity small. A large amount, persistent and conjoined with tube-casts, shows that changes have begun in the renal textures.

Gastro-intestinal Disorders.—These, it is well known, are among the most common consequences of the renal malady. They manifest themselves in various ways. Some patients suffer from flatulency and indigestion; others from diarrhœa; others, again, from nausea and vomiting. The latter symptoms are very apt to occur when urea accumulates in the blood, and the phenomena of uræmic intoxication are clearly developed. They may be, however, also met with at any period of the disease without the concurrence of other urgent symptoms; and become so prominent as to throw into the background most of the other signs of the renal affection.

To cite a case in point: an assistant nurse in the medical ward of the Philadelphia Hospital was attacked suddenly with nausea and vomiting, which persisted, in spite of the remedies employed, and became so troublesome that the man had to desist from his occupation. There was no febrile disturbance; the tongue was clean; the epigastric region not tender to the touch. Excepting a slight bronchitis, there were no apparent signs of disease in any organ in the body, and nothing to account for the gastric irritability. A close inquiry into the history of the patient revealed that he had had an attack of dropsy some time previously, from which he had recovered. But of late he had again noticed a swelling of the feet; and, on examination, a slight edematous condition was indeed found to exist. From the combination of these signs, I drew the conclusion that a chronic renal disease lay at the bottom of the gastric disturbance; and the detection of albumen and of casts in the urine proved the opinion to be correct.

Cancer; Tubercle; Cysts of Kidney.—These morbid products affect the kidneys but rarely—at all events but rarely in a form so marked as to give rise to conspicuous clinical phenomena. In all of them there may be albumen present in the urine, but it is generally in very small amount, and mixed with some ingredient having a more specific meaning. Thus in *cancer* of the kidney we may find blood with the albumen, and in some instances cells like those observed in any cancerous growth; sometimes the hemorrhages are profuse and frequently recurring, and we may detect a palpable tumor in the flank. In cases of melanotic cancer, whether it have its seat in the urinary apparatus or elsewhere, Eiselt and Bolze* have noticed that the urine on standing assumes the color of porter, and that on the addition of concentrated nitric acid it instantly presents the same dark color; facts which they regard as highly diagnostic.

In *tubercle*, little yellow, cheesy masses of degenerated tubercular matter collect as a sediment, as in the cases referred to by Frerichs in his work on Bright's disease. The constant presence of this sign is, however, doubtful. The tubercular matter is derived from the ureters or pelvis of the kidneys. The deposit it forms in the urine is insoluble in acetic acid; and Vogel describes the microscopical characters of the deposit, as irregular corpuscles not exhibiting, when treated with acetic acid, normal nuclei, or only showing small, irregular nucleoli, and an ill-defined detritus, with fragments of cells and an indistinct and finely granular mass, with which crystals of cholesterine are sometimes mingled. The signs of chronic pyelitis are also present. and there is no other assignable cause for its existence than tubercle. We may be assisted in the diagnosis by finding tubercles in other organs. Rayer tells us that scrofulous disease of the vertebræ has repeatedly been observed to be associated with tubercular kidneys.

In *cysts* of the kidney—those at least inclosing echinococci —small vesicles containing the characteristic structures of the parasites may perhaps be detected. Ordinary cysts are not to be recognized with any certainty during life; nor can they be distinguished from Bright's disease, since they are very frequently developed in the chronic varieties of this disorder.

Having now treated of chronic Bright's disease as *one* affection, I shall here briefly refer to the distinctions that have been made between its forms. In so doing, I shall

---

* Prager Vierteljahr., vols. lix. and lxvi.

follow the classification proposed by the English physicians, which is chiefly based on the diversified anatomical aspect of the kidneys.

There is first the chronic *enlargement* of the organ, of which several kinds exist:

1. The fatty kidney, pre-eminently Bright's disease. The kidney is very large and fatty. The deposit may occasion yellow scattered granulations, or the enlarged organ is pale,

FIG. 42.

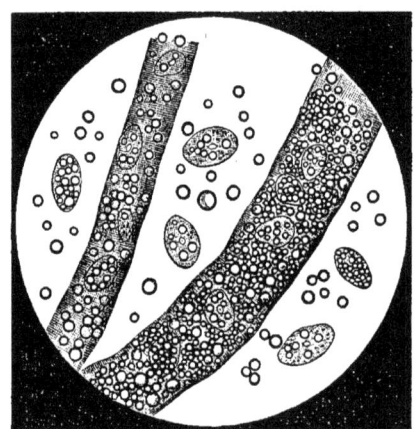

Fatty casts and epithelial cells filled with fat, as seen in the discharge coming from a highly fatty kidney.

and mottled by red vascular patches. The convoluted tubes are filled with oil, accumulated in their epithelial cells. The fatty disease is recognized by the numerous oily casts, fatty cells and free oil cells which appear in the highly albuminous urine. It is a very dangerous complaint,—perhaps the most fatal of all the forms of the malady,—is generally very chronic in its course, and attended with persistent dropsy. This morbid condition must not be confounded with a simply fatty kidney, such as is sometimes found in phthisis, or oftener in drunkards, and which is not associated with albuminous urine.

It is thought by several, by Dr. Dickinson especially, that the fatty kidney may follow a high degree of inflammation in the acute form of Bright's disease, particularly in that form brought on by exposure to cold. The acute form attending scarlet fever is more apt to pass into the large white kidney.

2. The enlarged, chronically inflamed kidney. I allude to the chief form of the large white kidney so frequently mentioned by English physicians. This is probably the chronic non-desquamative nephritis of Johnson;* it is the kidney represented by the third, fourth, and fifth form of Rayer's albuminous nephritis;† it is the chronic form of the tubal nephritis of Dickinson. The organ is white, enlarged, dense; its tubes are filled with exudation matter, their walls thickened. The cortical portion of the kidney is pale, and increased in breadth, evidently full of an inflammatory deposit; the medullary cones retain their vascularity. This variety of the malady often follows acute Bright's disease. It may last for a few years, but generally terminates before that time unfavorably. The dropsy it occasions is very extensive and persistent, and there is usually little difficulty in tracing it to an acute attack. This large kidney is not supposed ever to contract.

3. The waxy kidney, an affection in which the enlarged organ is smooth, of firm look, and of pale-yellow color, and is the result of a general disease involving the kidneys in common with other organs. It originates in the exudation from the minute arteries of a waxy material which infiltrates the tissues. This disease, as Dickinson ably enforces,‡ very generally follows upon protracted suppuration from whatever cause, either wound or disease, as dysentery or phthisis. The urine is increased in quantity in the earlier stages and contains much albumen, but not many casts. Those which are seen are pale, and, for the most part, transparent, structureless moulds of the tubules, generally of large diameter. Blood is but rarely present in the urine, and the urea is but slightly diminished in quantity. Diarrhœa frequently coexists, and the liver and spleen are apt to be enlarged. The dropsy is very trifling in amount, yet its persistence while the urine is increased in quantity is peculiar to this form of renal dis-

---

* Diseases of the Kidney.

† Traité des Maladies des Reins, tome ii. and Atlas.

‡ Med.-Chir. Trans., vol. l. p. 39; also Pathology and Treatment of Albuminuria.

ease; the patient is sallow looking and emaciated; his disease may last for years.

FIG. 43.

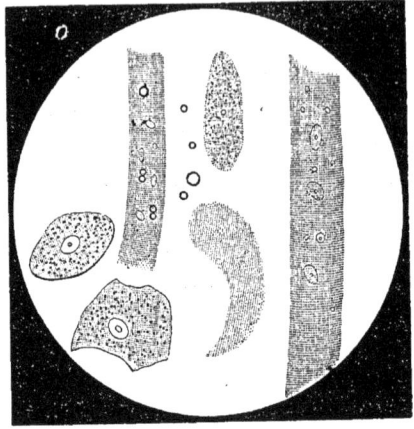

Hyaline or waxy casts, magnified about 460 diameters, taken from the urine.
On some of them are scattered a few shrivelled epithelial cells and oil drops; the
large cells to the left are epithelial cells from the bladder.

The kind of casts here depicted may be found in any form of Bright's disease,
acute as well as chronic. In the waxy kidney, however, they vastly preponderate, and are of large size—many much larger than those in this figure.

Then we have the small *contracted* kidney, which is viewed
as the last stage of Bright's disease by those who believe in

FIG. 44.

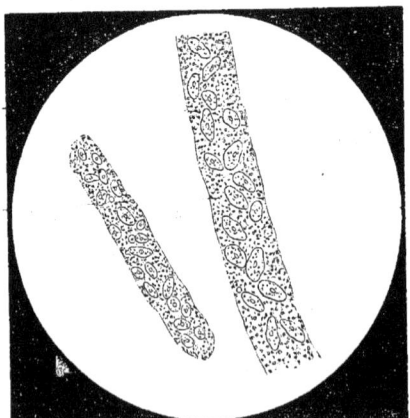

Granular casts, or casts covered with disintegrating epithelium and granules.
Casts of this character are chiefly found in the disease which leads to the contracted kidney. They are never seen in the acute complaint, excepting at its
close, when it is assuming a chronic form.

the varying appearance being only successive stages of the
same morbid process. This form of disease is frequently

found in gouty persons.   The urine contains but an incon-
siderable amount of albumen; the tube-casts are granular,
or simple fibrinous moulds, generally small, sometimes large;
here and there a little oil is observed.   Dropsy is absent in a
certain proportion of cases, and when present is generally
slight.   It often disappears for awhile and returns.   The
urine is increased in quantity, although toward the termination it becomes scanty or even suppressed.   The disease runs
a very chronic course.   It is chiefly characterized anatomically by an affection of the fibrous tissue lying between the
tubes, a slow increase, followed by a slow contraction of the
intertubular fibrous tissue.   The disease is often described as
the granular kidney, or as granular degeneration of the organ.

In the following table, part of the framework of which is
taken from one contained in Dr. Todd's Lectures on the
Urinary Organs, the clinical differences between the different
forms of Bright's disease are set forth:

TABLE EXHIBITING THE CLINICAL DIFFERENCES BETWEEN THE PRIN-
CIPAL FORMS OF BRIGHT'S DISEASE.

Cases in which Dropsy is Urgent and Acute.

Acute desqua-mative, or tu-bal nephritis; or acute drop-sy from expo-sure, or after scarlet fever..	Dropsy extensive; usually febrile symptoms. Recoveries fre-quent; but dis-ease may termi-nate in the large white kidney.	Urine deep color-ed, of high spec. grav., contain-ing much albu-men, often blood; also casts covered with epithelium.	Kidneys enlarged and vascular, shedding their epithelium.

Cases in which Dropsy is very Variable in Amount, Chronic, and may be Absent.

Fatty kidney....	Persistent and ob-stinate dropsy, coming on grad-ually; face pale and puffed. Always fatal.	Urine contains much albumen, fatty casts, fat cells, free oil. Spec. grav. rather high, usually from 1015 to 1030; rarely 1010. Quantity mode-rate or dimin-ished.	Kidneys in a state of enlargement, and fatty; some-times have a mottled appear-ance.

Cases in which Dropsy is very Variable, etc.—(Continued.)

Waxy kidney...	Dropsy trifling, or entirely absent; great emaciation; striking sallowness of face; liver and spleen enlarged. Unfavorable prognosis.	Urine increased in quantity, contains much albumen, but comparatively few casts, which are pale and transparent. Spec. grav. varying, usually above 1010.	Kidneys enlarged, smooth, and waxy looking.
Chronic contraction of the Kidney.........	Dropsy moderate, less than in fatty kidney; face sallow, yet not so much so as in the waxy disease; often retention of urea, tendency to coma, and to convulsions; impoverished blood; epistaxis; liver may be cirrhosed. May exist for years without being suspected; is a very chronic disease.	Urine more copious than in health, yet extremely small amount of albumen; hyaline and large granular casts, altered epithelium, a little oil. Spec. grav. very low: rarely above 1010, much oftener below.	Kidneys waste slowly, are full of a deposit, become small, dense, and contracted; the capsule very adherent; the thickness of the cortical substance diminished.

The indications for treatment are, to keep up the action of the skin; not to allow the kidneys to become clogged,—however much we ought, as a rule, to avoid stimulating diuretics; to prevent the dropsy from gaining; and to check the drain of albumen from the system, or counteract the bad effects of this drain.

The food taken should be very easy of digestion. Exercise in the open air is permissible, if the dropsy allow of it, excepting in the acute form of the malady, in which rest in the horizontal position should be rigidly enforced.

Diseases associated with Purulent Urine.

There is a group of affections in which pus is found in the urine, and in which the presence of this abnormal ingredient becomes of great value in diagnosis; yet to distinguish the individual members of the group from each other, and to ascertain the source of the purulent urine, we have to look, for the most part, to the other symptoms. In every case in which pus in any quantity is detected in the urine, it becomes of great importance to ascertain primarily that it is not derived from the urethra, from the vagina, or from an abscess that has opened into the urinary passages. The first point we may decide by examining into the history of the case, and, if necessary, by an exploration of the parts, as well as by an examination of the urine procured in the manner recommended in the first part of this chapter; the second, by the same means, and by determining that a discharge takes place equally when no urine is voided; the third is more difficult to make out, but there is generally something in the symptoms and in the history of the case furnishing a clue to its interpretation,—such, for instance, as the sudden appearance of a large quantity of pus in the urine. Having excluded each of these morbid states as the source of the purulent urine, we next turn to see which of the maladies that are its most common cause is before us. They are:

Acute Cystitis. — Acute inflammation most frequently affects the mucous membrane at or near the neck of the bladder. The inflammation may spread from the mucous membrane to the muscular coat; but it very rarely reaches the peritoneal covering. In some cases it is propagated along the ureters, and even to the kidneys. The morbid action is not often of idiopathic origin—much more usually is it due to the extension of an attack of gonorrhœa, to disease of the prostate, to traumatic causes, to protracted retention of urine, or to the irritation produced by medicines or stimulating drinks. Sometimes it is owing to the poison of rheumatism or gout.

Acute cystitis is much more frequently encountered in men than in women, and in adults than in children. Its main symptoms are a feeling of weight and pain in the hypogastric region, augmented by movement and by pressure. The pain does not, however, remain confined to the region about the bladder, but is also felt in the iliac and sacro-lumbar regions. It is attended with considerable febrile disturbance and an extreme irritability of the affected viscus. The urine is voided drop by drop, and its passage is usually accompanied by straining and a scalding sensation at the neck of the bladder; it is high colored, cloudy from increased vesical mucus, and contains blood and pus. The acute disease generally terminates within a week, leaving often an irritable bladder or a chronic inflammation.

The symptoms of acute cystitis are similar to those of acute nephritis, and the exciting causes too are much the same. But acute inflammation of the bladder differs from acute inflammation of the kidney by the greater severity of the pain, its much lower position, and the distress occasioned in voiding the urine. Neuralgia, or spasm, of the bladder may be distinguished from acute inflammation by the absence of fever, and the sharp, lancinating, but paroxysmal pain of the former malady, each onset of which lasts hardly longer than from two to six hours, and is attended with difficulty in making water, which, however, disappears as the pain subsides.

Metritis exhibits several of the traits of cystitis: we find the same hypogastric pain shooting downward to the thighs or toward the anus and loins, the same feeling of weight in the perineum, and the same signs of irritation of the bladder and of fever. As it, however, generally occurs in the puerperal state, we have the history, and, moreover, the character of the discharges from the vagina, to guide us; and should doubt still exist, the knowledge to be gained by a digital and a specular examination.

Chronic Cystitis.—This affection, often called catarrh of the bladder, is very common in advanced age. It generally comes on in an insidious manner, and is excited by some obstacle to the evacuation of urine, such as a stricture, or by the presence of a stone in the bladder, or by an enlargement of the prostate gland. A paralysis of the viscus leading to retention of its contents, or a serious structural disease of its coats, whether malignant or non-malignant, may, however, also establish the morbid process.

The symptoms are partly those of constitutional debility, partly those of local disease.   The most usual of the latter, and indeed in every way the most characteristic of the malady, are the dull pain, a frequent desire to make water, and the passage of a large quantity of pus with each act of micturition.   The urine, on standing, deposits a thick, glairy, viscid sediment, in which, under the microscope, triple phosphates and large pus corpuscles, extremely regular both in contents and in shape, may be detected.

The diagnosis of the disease in males is easy.   The only affection with which it is liable to be confounded is abscess of the kidney.   In females, uterine disorders may so closely simulate it that we cannot be certain of the existence of a disease of the bladder until, by careful inquiry into the history of the case, and, if need be, by aid of the speculum, we have ascertained with accuracy the state of the organs of generation.

But having decided the case to be one of chronic cystitis, it is always more difficult to discover its exciting cause.   We have to depend, to a great extent, upon the history of the malady; its association with a stone can only be determined by the use of the sound.

Abscess of the Kidney.—This dangerous condition is the result of suppurative inflammation of the kidney, or of abscesses forming in connection with a poisoned blood, as in pyæmia, or of embolism.   The suppurative inflammation is sometimes traceable to an acute attack of nephritis brought on by exposure or external violence, to retention of urine, or to the impaction of a renal calculus; but at other times it originates without any assignable cause, and in a very insidious way.

When the disorganizing process has continued for some time, and the abscesses are fairly formed, we encounter these signs: a fulness on one side of the spine in the lumbar region, associated with some tenderness on deep pressure and with more or less constant pain; occasional rigors and feverishness; and the presence of blood and pus in the urine. In some cases a marked tumor is found in the loin, extending toward the iliac fossa. If the abscess burst into the calices there occurs, simultaneously with a subsidence of the tumor, a sudden and copious discharge of pus with the urine, or if into the intestine, with the fecal evacuation.

The disease almost never affects more than one kidney; hence so-called uræmic symptoms are very rarely met with, as the healthy kidney enlarges and becomes capable of performing a double amount of work. The disorder gradually leads in most cases to a fatal issue, from the irritation, the wasting discharge, and the protracted hectic. There is, however, a possibility of recovery if the patient have strength enough to withstand the purulent drain until the abscess empties itself. It may do this through the urinary passages, through the colon, through the lumbar muscles, through the diaphragm, and be evacuated by coughing, and the cavity of the abscess then cicatrizes; or the abscess may burst into the peritoneal cavity and cause rapid death.

The diseases for which the malady is most apt to be mistaken are chronic cystitis, perinephritis, and pyelitis. From cystitis it may be distinguished by the dissimilar local signs and the different appearances of the urine. Thus, in the affection of the bladder the quantity of pus constantly discharged is far greater—for in abscess of the kidney there are times when but little or no pus is voided; on the other hand, the urine of the vesical disorder is less albuminous. Yet this is not a certain guide, for we may have a Bright's kidney associated with a catarrh of the bladder, and thus both a highly purulent and a highly albuminous urine be produced. In this case, however, a diligent search with the microscope will detect casts and other renal products in the sediment.

Perinephritis unconnected with inflammation of the kidney is a very rare disease. I have seen but one instance of it, which occurred in a young gentleman, who, returning home from a long walk, strained his back in jumping a fence. An abscess very gradually formed, giving rise to a slight fulness in the left lumbar region, and severe pain, which disappeared as matter was discharged through the integuments. The function of the kidney was not affected : proving that the disorder was in the neighborhood, and not in the structure of the organ.*

But an external opening may be established when the process of inflammation and suppuration has commenced in the kidney and thence spread to the loose tissues surrounding it. Under these circumstances, the appearance in the urine of pus prior to its discharge through the muscles of the back, would be the only certain means by which we could judge where the suppuration had primarily taken place.

The prominent symptom in perinephritis is pain, which at times is so severe as to confine the patient to bed with knees flexed, with a sense of fulness and dragging weight in the region of the kidney, and with lameness owing to the interference with the play of the psoas muscles. The urine is generally unaltered; the bowels may be constipated, owing to the pressure of the tumor on the intestine. A rounded, doughy, and generally indolent tumor is usually found in the renal region. In Dr. Bowditch's three cases the abscess extended up into the right pleura, without apparently affecting the liver, after having probably forced its way behind that organ and along the psoas muscles under the right crus of the diaphragm, and caused pulmonary or pleuritic complications, but not jaundice. As the disease advances, severe chills, with fever and copious night-sweats, occur, and emaciation and marked debility.

As regards the treatment in these cases, when the diagnosis is established, an external incision, permitting the escape of pus, is demanded.

Pyelitis.—This is the name given by Rayer to inflammation of the mucous membrane of the pelvis of the kidney —an affection very rarely, in fact almost never, idiopathic, being commonly caused by a calculus that has been arrested at the commencement of the ureter, or by a retention of urine from an obstacle in the ureter, bladder, or urethra, or

---

* Trousseau, in the second edition of his Clinique Médicale, Lect. XCIV., cites several instances of perinephritic abscesses, and Bowditch narrates three cases in the Boston Med. and Surg. Journ., 1868, N. S., vol i. p. 357.

by an extension upward from the bladder of an inflammation.
Bright's disease and diabetes are usually, and, according to
Roberts, typhus and the eruptive fevers, pyæmia, scurvy,
diphtheria and carbuncle, are occasionally, complicated
with some degree of pyelitis. The urine is commonly acid.

The symptoms of the malady are, therefore, in part those
produced by the morbid states exciting it, especially those
denoting a calculus lodged in the kidney or arrested in its
transit toward the bladder; partly those directly traceable to
the inflammation of the pelvis and infundibula. The manifestations of the latter disorder are, a constant pain in the
loin, felt also in the course of the ureter, and the passage of
pus and occasionally of blood with the urine.

The most difficult point connected with the recognition of
pyelitis is to be certain that the purulent discharge does not
proceed from the bladder. And there is no positive sign to
guide us excepting the existence in the urine of epithelium
from the pelvis of the kidney, distinguishable by the frequent
occurrence, in a cell, of clearly-defined, dark-colored, round
granules, and of two nuclei. But this epithelium may not
always be found, and we have then to fall back upon the
history of the case, upon the attacks of renal pain, upon the
hæmaturia caused by a calculus, and the combination of
signs as pointing more to one disease than the other. In
some cases there is a perceptible swelling in the loin, which
assists us materially in coming to a conclusion ; at times,
too, owing to coexisting congestion or degeneration of the
kidney, the amount of albumen is wholly disproportionate
to that contained in pus, and this becomes a valuable indication of the affection not being vesical. But if there be a
coincident disease of the bladder, the differential distinction,
on Rayer's own showing, becomes impossible.

Supposing, however, the point settled, and the vesical
origin of the pus disproved, the diagnosis is limited to an
inflammation of the ureter, an abscess in the substance of
the kidney, and to pyelitis. Here again the history of the
case comes into play. Furthermore, in the former of these
affections—a very rare one, unless associated with pyelitis—
the amount of pus in the urine is very trifling; in the second,

too, it is less than in pyelitis, excepting when the abscess empties itself. The pus is also, as already indicated, not constant, alternately appearing in and disappearing from the urine, and the disease is attended with much greater constitutional disturbance. Yet here again we must admit that the disorders are sometimes very obscure, and very difficult to distinguish, and it may be impossible to discriminate between them should any of the morbid states coexist.

In those cases of pyelitis in which there is a decided obstruction to the flow of urine through the ureter, caused by a calculus, clot of blood or viscid pus, or other débris, the discharge of pus is suddenly arrested and the cavity of the pelvis dilates very much; gradually the gland tissue is compressed, and a large pus-containing sac is formed, giving rise to a condition known as *pyonephrosis*, and to a distinctly limited swelling in the side. These kind of tumors are ordinarily not painful to the touch, are sometimes very indolent, and, as a rule, do not materially affect the general health. They not unfrequently subside gradually by very free discharges of pus, and the patient recovers.* They have been known to occur in both kidneys, but this is of great rarity.

When the changes resulting from an impediment to the flow of urine are unassociated with suppuration of the mucous membrane of the pelvis of the kidney, we have the condition designated by Rayer as *hydronephrosis*. It is often due to congenital malformation of the ureter, and sometimes is double. The swelling to which it gives rise may subside simultaneously with a sudden and copious discharge of urine. When this symptom is absent, the diagnosis must be based on the existence of a fluctuating renal tumor and the absence of signs of suppuration.

Hydatid tumor of the kidney is of comparatively rare occurrence and is very apt to be confounded with hydronephrosis. When the urine contains no hydatid vesicles or their débris and the hydatid fremitus is absent, the diagnosis is extremely difficult and must rest chiefly on the history of the case.

---

* See, for instance, Cases XLVIII. and L. in Dr. Todd's Clinical Lectures on the Urinary Organs.

Disorders in which a very large Amount of Urine is discharged.

Diabetes.—An excessive flow of urine was formerly called diabetes; it is now customary to restrict the term to the excessive flow accompanying the excretion of sugar, the diabetes mellitus, or glucosuria, of many authors.

Diabetic urine is of pale color and of high specific gravity, ranging generally from 1030 to 1050. The quantity passed is enormous; seventy pints and upwards have been known to be discharged daily.

The symptoms attending this drain of fluid from the system are, as may be supposed, great thirst, constipation, and generally a dry, harsh skin, and a feeling of constant emptiness and of hunger. To these are added a steadily progressing waste of the body, debility, chills, a somewhat hurried breathing, peevishness of temper, and a tendency to boils and carbuncles. Cataract and other kinds of defective vision are not infrequent; and M. Galezowski* has described a form of retinitis which has been observed, in some rare cases, to accompany diabetes.

The disease is a very fatal one; yet it is impossible to foretell its exact mode of termination. Some are cut off rather suddenly; others drag out a long existence, and die worn out and dropsical, or of superadded phthisis. For some days, or even for weeks before death, the sugar may disappear from the urine.†

Whence comes the sugar? Is it from the food, the blood, the kidneys, the stomach, the liver? These are questions that cannot be satisfactorily answered. Since Bernard's discovery of the sugar-forming properties of the liver, saccharine urine is thought to proceed from an inordinate formation in this viscus of sugar, which is not fully destroyed in the lungs, and is excreted by the kidneys. But the experiments

---

* Compte Rendu du Congrès Ophth. de Paris, 1862.

† In a case for a long time under my charge, in which the diabetes lasted for several years, sugar entirely disappeared from the urine as the signs of phthisis became fully developed, and for several months before death.

of Pavy seem to throw some doubt on this simple and ingenious theory. That the sugar is not derived from the food,
is very certain; for patients kept even on the most rigorous
meat diet still pass sugar. In some cases diabetes has been
found associated with paralysis of the tongue, palate, and
vocal cord, and other signs of disease in the floor of the fourth
ventricle.

Starchy and saccharine substances increase the quantity of
diabetic sugar. Nay, they may be the cause of a little sugar
appearing in the urine of healthy persons. Yet those in
whom a saccharine state of the urine is readily induced are
in great danger of becoming diabetic.

In the aged, sugar may be present in the urine without
being attended with distressing symptoms. It is in such
cases that we are most apt to meet with the intermitting diabetes to which attention has been called by Bence Jones.*
When the abnormal ingredient thus disappears from the
urine, it is replaced by uric acid and by oxalates.

There is still another form of intermitting diabetes. Sugar
is sometimes—Dr. Burdel† says uniformly—found in the
urine during the paroxysms of intermittent fever; but it
vanishes entirely during the intervals.

Chronic Diuresis.—This disease is otherwise known as
hydruria, or diabetes insipidus. It is characterized by the
habitual discharge of a very large quantity of urine containing an excess of water, but no sugar. The general symptoms are much the same as those of diabetes; the thirst is
generally extreme, and, if some of the recorded observations
can be fully relied on, more water is passed than is drunk.

The cause of this singular malady is obscure. It would
seem to be connected with some abnormal state of the nervous system. It certainly was in the following marked instance of the affection:

A young man, twenty-four years of age, was admitted
into my ward at the Philadelphia Hospital. He was thin,
greatly troubled with thirst, and discharged daily from

* Med.-Chir. Transact., vol. xxxviii.
† L'Union Médicale, No. 139, 1859.

thirty-six to forty pints of limpid urine of a very low specific gravity, in which, by several tests repeatedly employed, not a trace of sugar could be detected. He stated that he had been in good health until about five months previously, when he had a sunstroke while laboring on a building. He was for awhile insensible, and from that time had had constant pain in the head, and had been unable to work. He lost flesh rapidly, and was much annoyed by frequent and excessive emission of urine. Beyond the symptoms mentioned, little was found in the case. All the internal viscera appeared to be healthy; the bowels were constipated.

The patient drank an enormous amount of water, though, unless he obtained the coveted liquid by stealth, not so much as he habitually passed. For upwards of a week he improved on tonics, especially on the ignatia amara, voiding once only seventeen pints in the twenty-four hours. But he then relapsed, discharging as much water as before, and growing daily weaker and weaker. Suddenly he was seized with very great irritability of the stomach and a complete suppression of urine, repeated catheterizations proving the bladder to be empty. He was cupped over the kidneys, placed in a warm bath, and active diuretics were administered, with the result of re-establishing the function of the kidneys. But the diuresis did not return; the man passed about a pint of high-colored fluid daily until his death, which took place on the fifth day after the suppression of urine, and about six months after the sunstroke. Toward the last, he was much troubled with uncontrollable vomiting and obstinate constipatiou, became very dull and stupid, and his features and skin assumed the appearance of the stage of collapse in cholera. Unfortunately, permission to examine the body could not be obtained.

We meet with cases of polyuria also under other circumstances. Lanceraux tells us that it is not uncommon in syphilitic affections of the nervous centres.*

We must take care not to confound cases of chronic hydruria with true diabetes. They differ by the low specific

---

* Sydenh. Society's Transl., p. 76.

gravity of the urine and the utter absence of a saccharine ingredient.* Sometimes a state of diuresis is found to exist temporarily during the removal of dropsical effusions, or when the action of the skin is insufficient. We also meet with apparent cases of diuresis in hysterical women and in persons who suffer from incontinence of urine, whether due to an external injury, or dependent upon simple irritability, or upon inflammation or paralysis of the bladder. In all such, however, we can establish the diagnosis by laying stress on the history of the patient, and by measuring, as accurately as possible, the amount of urine passed in the twenty-four hours—which amount may be large, but is not inordinate.

Disorders in which little or no Urine is discharged.

Suppression of Urine.—Suppression of urine, unconnected with already existing degeneration of the kidney, is a rare disorder. Yet it may occur in previously healthy persons, or in the course of fevers of a low type, and probably associated with no other morbid state than congestion of the kidneys. It is occasionally met with as one of the freaks of hysteria, or is caused seemingly by the irritation reflected to a healthy kidney from a diseased bladder.

The symptoms it occasions, independently of the absence of the discharge of urine, are drowsiness, nausea, vomiting, coma, sometimes convulsions; in one word, the symptoms of uræmic poisoning. Irrespective of these, the formidable complaint may give rise to marked urinous smell of the perspiration and breath, and to exceeding and very general cutaneous hyperæsthesia.†

Concerning the exact cause of the suppression, we are often kept in the dark until the termination of the malady;

---

* See, on the examination of the urine in instances of the disorder, the cases collected by Parkes, On the Composition of the Urine. London, 1860.

† This was, next to the suppression of the discharge, the most obvious symptom in a case under my care in 1864 at the Philadelphia Hospital, in which no urine was secreted for many days, the catheter being repeatedly introduced into the bladder. The patient recovered. She had, previous to the attack, and had still, when last seen, vesical catarrh.

for, unless we are familiar with the patient's antecedent symptoms, we are unable to determine, in the absence of the urinary secretion, whether or not a disease of the kidney lies at the origin of the mischief. If not speedily relieved, the affection generally ends in death.

Retention of Urine.—Unlike what happens in suppression of urine, the kidneys, when the urine is simply retained, perform their secretory function; but the fluid collects in the bladder and is not voided. The distended viscus forms a swelling in the hypogastrium, discoverable both by palpation and by percussion. The urine is generally not wholly kept back, for a slight discharge every now and then takes place, or there is a constant dribbling—a matter which in itself should always suggest the introduction of a catheter.

Retention of urine, if soon recognized, is not in itself a dangerous complaint, as it can be ordinarily at once relieved by the passage of a catheter; but if the ailment escape observation, or be inefficiently dealt with, the bladder is very apt to burst, or the patient dies from the absorption of the noxious urinary ingredients.

The causes which lead to retention are various; prominent among them, at least in a medical point of view, is paralysis of the bladder, especially that form of paralysis which occurs in low fevers; it is also one of the symptoms of paraplegia; then inflammatory swelling of the neck of the bladder, organic stricture, or enlarged prostate may give rise to it; again retention or incontinence may be due to hysteria.

The disorder is readily detected. It may be discriminated from suppression of urine by the existence of the hypogastric tumor, and by the introduction of a catheter—a means which, in cases of doubt, ought never to be neglected. Sometimes the abdominal swelling is so great as to lead to the belief of the existence of dropsy; and the error is fostered by learning that the patient has been passing his water and has a constant desire to discharge it, or by seeing that it dribbles from him.* But I have already discussed these points in con-

---

* In a case reported by Schneider, and quoted in Br. and For. Med.-Chir. Rev., April, 1864, urine was passed: yet when a catheter was introduced,

nection with abdominal swellings, and need only here again draw attention to the errors in diagnosis which are likely to arise.

The retention from paralysis is distinguished from that due to other causes, as to obstruction, by observing that the catheter enters readily, and that the urine flows out in a continuous stream, increasing and lessening with the respiratory movements, but does not come out in jets.

---

because the peculiar shape of the tumefaction seemed to indicate that the swelling was produced by a distended bladder, 14 pints of urine, and subsequently 8 more, were removed.

43

CHAPTER VIII.

AN abnormal collection of watery fluid in the areolar tissue or in the serous cavities of the body, constitutes dropsy. Now, dropsy is but a symptom, and as such we have already examined into it as associated with various disorders of which it forms a striking manifestation; but, though only a symptom, it is one so obvious and prominent, and comprises so often apparently the whole complaint, that it will serve a useful purpose to investigate connectedly the clinical meaning of its typical forms.

Dropsy, according to its Seat and Extent.

Dropsies may be external, or confined to internal parts. To the latter variety belong hydrothorax, hydrocephalus, and ascites—affections elsewhere described, and which we shall only consider here so far as they may form part of a general dropsy.

External dropsies are illustrated by *anasarca* and *œdema:* the first, a universal accumulation of serous fluid in the areolar textures; the second, a more localized collection in the same structures, and differing, therefore, in nothing but extent. Both, as ordinarily met with, exhibit painless swelling of the surface, devoid of redness; a skin often stretched and shining, pitting upon pressure, and retaining for some time the mark of the finger; and in both, the tumid part, if punctured, allows a watery fluid to run out. Œdema is most commonly perceived around the ankles; the tumefaction of anasarca is found generally not only in the lower extremities, but also in the arms and in the face.

(674)

Anasarca is usually dependent upon disease of the kidneys, or of the heart; hence an extensive infiltration of the areolar tissues must always lead us to examine these viscera with care. The swelling rarely shows itself at all parts of the body at once: it ordinarily begins at the feet and ankles, and extends, more or less rapidly, upward; but it may commence in the face. It becomes greatest where the areolar tissue is loosest.

Œdema may be due to the same causes. Yet a limited collection of fluid is very often the consequence of a purely local trouble unconnected with a visceral disease, but of a character interfering with the venous circulation. Thus, the compression or obliteration of a large vein occasions œdema below the point of the disorder. We see œdema happening if a bandage be applied too tightly, or if swollen glands press upon the main vein of a limb. We also meet with it in the adhesive form of venous inflammation, and in milk-leg, or *phlegmasia dolens*—a condition observed in puerperal women, or as a sequel of typhoid fever, in which the whole of one lower extremity becomes edematous, in consequence of inflammation, or, to adopt the view which is much more probably the correct one, of blocking up of the femoral vein by a coagulum. In all of these forms the œdema is one-sided; and the cause being external to the thoracic or abdominal cavities, there is usually little difficulty in its recognition. A circumscribed œdema also accompanies erysipelatous inflammations of the skin or subjacent tissues; so, too, do we find œdema confined to a limb the general nutrition of which has been lowered by the occurrence of paralysis.

When the dropsical effusion is dependent upon some tumor seated in an internal cavity and interfering with the passage of the blood, it may possibly be very local and one-sided; but it is most apt to be found on both sides of a portion of the body, although more particularly marked on one side. The extremities which are edematous or anasarcous exhibit usually also a marked enlargement of the veins.

Another source of a double-sided œdema is a watery condition of the blood. This form of dropsy is often seen in chlorotic girls without there being any disease of an internal organ. The state of their blood is highly favorable to the transudation of the serum, and this collects, first about the ankles, and subsequently, perhaps, in other parts of the body. The absence of any discoverable organic affection, the pallid countenance, and the venous murmurs in the neck furnish the key to the recognition of the origin of the dropsy.

A dropsical effusion in part of similar origin, but much more often connected with internal dropsy, especially with ascites, is the dropsy we observe in those broken down by malarial poisoning. The state of the liver and spleen added to the condition of the blood determines the greater extent of the effusion. One of the most extraordinary forms of dropsy connected with debility and altered blood is furnished by the disease known as *beriberi* to the physicians in India, and in which the anæmia culminates in acute œdema associated with stiffness of the limbs, numbness, extreme prostration, anxiety, and dyspnœa. General anasarca, too, and, in some instances, paralysis of the extremities, happen.*

Dropsy, according to its Causation.

Having viewed anasarca and œdema as in the main uncombined with internal dropsies, and as forming the sole signs of the dropsical complaint, let us now look at them when associated with effusions of serum elsewhere. The same remarks will also apply to hydrothorax and ascites, the meaning of which, when occurring alone, we have inquired into already, but which we shall here consider in their relations to *general* dropsy, or that form of the disorder in which anasarca or œdema coexists with dropsy of one or several of the large serous cavities.

And first, let us examine into the causes of general dropsy. The most common are a disease of the heart, of the kidneys, of the liver; so common, in truth, that in every case of dropsy we must examine these organs carefully. Accord-

---

* For a full account of this curious malady, see Aitken's Pract. of Medic., vol. ii.

ing as the dropsical accumulation originates in a morbid state of these viscera, it is called cardiac, or renal, or hepatic.

Cardiac dropsy arises in consequence of the deranged or enfeebled circulation, produced by a disease of the walls and cavities of the heart, associated or not with a valvular lesion. The dropsy begins in the feet and ankles, being very much influenced by position, and gradually extends upward; but it is rarely very obvious in the face or upper extremities. The thighs and scrotum are sometimes greatly swollen, and there is a watery effusion into the pleural cavities or into the pulmonary parenchyma.

Renal dropsy is usually much more general than cardiac dropsy. It does not, like this, begin in the most dependent parts, but is often first noticed in the face and eyelids. There is hardly a space in the body where, as the complaint progresses, fluid may not accumulate. The proof that the dropsy is renal is furnished by the presence of albumen in the urine, and by the other signs of a diseased kidney.

Occasionally the dropsy is owing to an affection of both the kidney and the heart; when the question may occur, which of the organs was primarily disturbed and gave rise originally to the dropsy? But this is a matter we cannot more than indicate, since it would otherwise involve the discussion of a much-vexed question in pathology, namely, whether, when Bright's disease coexists with a disease of the heart, the renal affection has produced the cardiac malady, or the cardiac malady the renal affection. And should it be of importance, in an individual case, to determine the point alluded to, we may be enabled to arrive at a conclusion by a close examination of the history of the case : did the patient suffer from palpitation and shortness of breath prior to or coincident with the anasarcous condition, and has he ever had rheumatic fever; or did he have an attack of acute dropsy before the persistent swelling of the feet or of the face occurred? It is scarcely necessary to add, that if this have happened, there is a very strong probability of the renal disease having been antecedent to the cardiac disorder.

Hepatic dropsy may, like the preceding forms, be more or less general; but it is, on the whole, very rarely so, unless of long standing, or unless there be coexisting disease of the heart or kidneys. The most usual kind of dropsy depending upon an affection of the liver is abdominal dropsy, and this is so well understood that ascites is very frequently looked upon as constituting a proof of hepatic disorder. But it is a mistake so to regard it; for ascites, as we found when examining into the causes of abdominal swelling, may also be produced by peritoneal tumors or inflammation, by enlargement of the spleen or pancreas, or by the pressure of diseased glands,—in fact, by any lesion which occasions a decided impediment to the portal circulation.

Besides these sources of general dropsy, we may find deterioration of the blood, with, perhaps, a simply enfeebled condition of the heart, giving rise to it. But such a state is much more likely to occasion œdema, or, in some instances, anasarca, than general dropsical effusions; and it is thus that while the former phenomena are not uncommon in exhausting diseases or in marked impoverishment of the blood, the latter are rarely met with unless there be at the same time some cardiac or renal complaint.

Dropsy, according to the Rapidity of its Development.

Dropsy may come on suddenly, or be gradually developed. The first is called *acute* or *active* dropsy; the second, *chronic* dropsy. To the latter class belong the majority of instances of the forms of dropsy we have just been discussing, in which the watery accumulation is thought to arise from defective action of the absorbent vessels, or in which, in other words, the dropsy is passive. Acute dropsy has active symptoms much like those of an inflammatory fever. The effusion takes place suddenly, and in consequence of exposure to cold and wet, or of a checked perspiration. In the vast majority of examples it is accompanied by albumen in the urine, and is, in truth, due to a disturbance of the kidneys. Yet there are cases of acute dropsy which are not of renal origin, and in which the rapid occurrence of universal anasarca is not susceptible of being traced directly to a definite lesion.

The *prognosis* of dropsy depends upon the cause of the

effusion. The least dangerous variety of the complaint is that happening in connection with changes in the blood. The acute dropsies are, as a rule, much more curable than the chronic or passive forms of the disorder; but their prognosis is very much influenced by the extent of the effusion and the seat it may occupy. An accumulation of liquid in most of the serous cavities of the body is, of course, vastly more perilous than one which occupies only the loose subcutaneous tissues. Local dropsies are influenced by treatment in proportion to the readiness with which the obstruction producing them is susceptible of being removed.

In the *treatment* of dropsy, we find constantly two indications recurring: the first, to remedy the cause of the accumulation; the second, to remove the latter from the system. The former of the indications is the most direct way of getting rid of the watery collection, and of preventing its return; but it is not always possible to accomplish the object. For example, we cannot do so if the dropsy be caused by an incurable organic disease of the heart, liver, or kidneys. The second of these indications is fulfilled by attempting to carry off the water by the skin, by the intestines, or by the kidneys, selecting, in individual instances, the channel which the circumstances of the case indicate as being the best suited, or making use of all, if there be nothing which forbids us from so doing. When we cannot get rid of the fluid in this way, we may let it out by an operation—by tapping the internal cavities, or, as in anasarca, by puncturing the skin.

CHAPTER IX.

IN the following sketch I shall attempt to describe only those disorders of the blood which constitute the essential or principal forms of blood disease, which are seemingly, for the most part, idiopathic, and may be recognized by well-marked clinical traits. Prominent among these, and to a certain extent characteristic of all blood disorders, are general debility, a changed aspect of the mucous membranes and of the skin, especially in color, and alterations of nutrition.

Anæmia.—This is the name given by Andral to poverty of blood. The morbid state is met with as a consequence of profuse or frequently recurring hemorrhages, of insufficient nourishment, of affections which prevent the nutriment taken from being properly absorbed or assimilated, thus impoverishing the blood by depriving it of its most needed constituents, and of profuse chronic discharges, which drain the blood of many of its important elements, and especially of its albumen. Besides these causes of anæmia, we find it occasioned by particular poisons, as by malaria, or by the retention of noxious ingredients in the blood, or by diseases of certain glands. Again, it is sometimes encountered without our being able to trace it to any obvious source. But under all these circumstances, we have to deal with a watery blood deficient in red corpuscles; in other words, with an anemic condition.

Now, whatever may have given rise to the anæmia, the manifestations of the disorder are much the same. The patient is weak and pale; his lips and tongue have lost their red color; his pulse is feeble, but generally accelerated; the appetite is deficient or depraved; the bowels are apt to be costive. Exercise induces great fatigue, shortness of breath, and palpitations; and the disturbance of the heart may be associated with cardiac murmurs or with blowing sounds in the cervical veins, and is sometimes so persistent as to lead, as will be found elsewhere described, to structural changes in the heart. In some cases, further, we meet, among the symptoms of the affection, with obstinate headache and dropsy, and in very many with a persistent pain in the left side in the region of the spleen.

Chlorosis.—As a marked form of anæmia, we may consider chlorosis. Here the pallid, waxlike countenance, the very pale lips, and the pearly eye afford unmistakable evidence of the deterioration of the blood. The complaint is especially encountered in young females, and is, as a rule, associated with amenorrhœa. Indeed, many restrict the term to the obvious anæmia combined with suppression of the menses, so often affecting girls about the age of puberty.

Addison's Disease.—There is another form of anæmia which requires to be specially mentioned, namely, that connected with disease of the *supra-renal capsules.* Dr. Addison, whose name the complaint now bears, met with a form of general anæmia which had no perceptible cause whatever; in which there had been neither loss of blood, nor mental shock or anxiety, nor exhausting diarrhœa; which was concomitant with neither malignant nor scrofulous disease, nor with any affection of the spleen, kidneys, or lymphatic glands, nor, in fact, with any lesion that the most careful examination could detect.

While seeking for the explanation of these puzzling cases, he discovered that the peculiar anæmia always occurs in connection with a diseased condition of the supra-renal capsules, and is characterized by distressing languor and very great general prostration, remarkable feebleness of the heart's action, irritability of the stomach, and a singular alteration in the hue of the skin. This consists in a dingy or smoky appearance of the surface; or the color may be of a deep amber or chestnut brown, or the altered skin has a bronzed tinge. The discoloration may occur in patches, which are usually most obvious on the face or superior extremities, or it may extend over the whole body. The patient may seem, at first sight, to be jaundiced; but the pearly whiteness of the conjunctiva soon dispels such an idea. The nails are pale and bluish; the body and breath of the sick person at times exhale an offensive odor; and the blood has been found to contain an excess of white globules.

The disorder is a chronic one, generally lasting for years; but it almost invariably destroys life. Yet cases have been recorded in which most of the symptoms of Addison's disease were present and which nevertheless recovered. In these cases, the diagnosis is not, however, beyond doubt, for we now know well that several of the most striking features of the malady may occur without disease of the supra-renal capsules. Thus, the discoloration of the skin may happen in other affections, as in pregnancies attended with much constitutional disturbance—as occurred for instance in a case that I recently had under my observation; or during exhausting lactation; and again, particularly in those examples of the disorder which progress rapidly, the bronzing may be absent. As regards the character of the altered color of the skin when present, by far the most significant change is a gradual and uniform discoloration approaching to the hue of skin of a mulatto, and dependent upon a layer of pigment in the rete mucosum. The discoloration in patches is both less constant and less significant. And under any circumstances, before we attach full weight to the bronzed look of the skin, we must be very certain that it is not the effect of the sun. In Addison's disease the discoloration is most evident on the face, neck, superior extremities, penis and scrotum, and in the flexures of the axillæ and around the umbilicus.

With reference to the other symptoms, the most conclusive of them are remarkable prostration, generally without any marked waste of the body, feebleness of pulse and obvious anæmia. These symptoms precede in most, but far from in all cases, the discoloration of the skin; and they are not unfrequently associated with pain in the back and gastro-intestinal irritation, with breathlessness upon exertion, and dimness of sight. A peculiar odor of the body, like that perceived in the colored race, was observed in two cases placed on record by Mr. Hutchinson.

Death may take place gradually from the constantly growing asthenia; or it may occur suddenly, and where the amount of prostration does not appear so excessive as to foreshadow it. The post-mortem examination shows generally the organs totally destroyed, and, if we may adopt the researches of the observer who, next to Addison, has done most to elucidate the subject—Dr. Wilks, that destruction is dependent upon a peculiar scrofulous degeneration. Should this prove to be the correct view of the case; should, in other words, the nature of the disease of the capsules influence its symptoms more than the mere fact of their being diseased, it would explain why in some cases of absence of the gland, or of its cancerous degeneration or suppuration, no signs of Addison's disease existed. Many of the symptoms of the fully developed malady may be due to the implication of the nervous branches, derived from the sympathetic and pneumogastric, which go to the gland. And as regards all the symptoms, it must, in a diagnostic point of view, be borne in mind that it is their combination rather than the presence of any one which gives them their value, and that this combination consists chiefly in the association of a peculiar discoloration of the skin with a pearly eye, well-marked anæmia, and prostration, and without the existence of any other disease than of the supra-renal capsules to account for the train of abnormal phenomena.*

Leucocythæmia or Leukæmia.—This morbid state consists in a decided increase of the white corpuscles and a decrease of the red. Under the microscope, which furnishes indeed the surest means of recognizing the disease, the white globules of the blood, instead of bearing the normal propor-

---

* See the cases collected by Addison, in his work on Diseases of the Supra-renal Capsules; by Wilks, Guy's Hospital Reports, vol. viii. and vol. xi., 3d Series; by Harley, Brit. and Foreign Medico-Chirurg. Review, 1858; by Laycock, ih. Jan. 1861; by Habershon, Guy's Hosp. Rep , 3d Series, vol. x ; by Copland, in Dictionary of Pract. Medicine; by Greenhow, quoted in Amer. Journal of Med. Sciences, Oct. 1866; and the very complete report in the Transact. of Path. Society of London, 1866.

tion of about 1 to 50 of the red, are found in the proportion
of 1 to 6, or even of 1 to 2; and after death, grayish coagula,
consisting almost entirely of colorless blood-cells, are met
with in the heart or large veins.

The abnormal condition exists in connection with hypertrophy of the spleen or of the liver, with other diseases of
these viscera, and with various malignant or non-malignant
affections of the lymphatic glands or of the thyroid body.
But none of the blood glands is as constantly and as markedly affected as the spleen.

The disorder may occur at all ages, and in both sexes; but
it is more common in men than in women. Besides the obvious pallor and cachectic appearance, it often occasions diarrhœa, hurried breathing, hemorrhages from various parts,
especially from the nose, fleeting abdominal pains, and dropsy
attendant upon the enlargement of the spleen or liver, which
is so usually present.* In some cases a swelling of the
glands on both sides of the throat, attended with inflammation of the mucous membrane of the mouth and pharnyx,
and followed by swelling of the axillary and inguinal glands,
precedes the enlargement of the liver and spleen.†

As regards the symptoms, the closest similarity to leukæmia
is presented by the affection described as pseudo-leukæmia,
or, more frequently, as *Hodgkin's disease*. It consists in an
enlargement of the lymphatic glands of the body, which
soon becomes complicated with extreme anæmia and signs
of cachexia, with dropsy, with attacks of suffocation, and
leads usually, in the course of not many months, to death.
A few superficial lymphatics are first affected, others follow; the disorder then extends more decidedly, the spleen
and the liver increase in size, other organs, too, may become
involved; but the spleen is the one most constantly disturbed. The chief anatomical lesion is found to be an
augmented formation of the structure of the glands. But

---

* Compare the cases of Bennett, in his work on Leucocythæmia, 1852, and
of Virchow, in his collected Essays (Gesammelte Abhandlungen), etc.

† Mosler, in Virchow's Archiv, xliii., quoted in Amer. Journal of Med.
Sciences, July, 1868.

although we might expect decided alteration in the blood, the distinguishing mark from leukæmia is that there is not an increase of the white corpuscles.*

Pyæmia.—Purulent contamination of the blood is an affection much more apt to be met with by the surgeon than by the practitioner of medicine; yet it is one sufficiently often encountered by him to require that he should be familiar with its symptoms. These are, great depression of the vital powers, profuse sweats, rapid pulse, and the formation of purulent deposits in different portions of the body. The symptoms may be of gradual development; but often they set in suddenly with a chill, to which a fever of low type soon succeeds; or the shivering is followed even from the first by copious sweating, and the febrile phenomena subsequently appear.

The pyæmic fever rarely lasts longer than a week, and during its continuance it usually presents the most marked variations in temperature. Yet the disease is not always alike in this respect; for we find, as Heubner has proved, not only cases in which the most decided increase of animal heat is constantly followed by an equally decided decrease, but also cases in which there are febrile attacks, followed by striking intervals, during which the temperature is almost normal; and cases in which continuous fever exists with intercurrent decided rises in temperature.† Still, in all the maximum of the temperature is apt to be very high, ranging from 106° to 108°.

The disorder may arise after injuries and operations; or where sinuses or abscesses exist that have no free vent for the pus; or in consequence of the contamination of the blood which happens in phlebitis or arteritis; or results from the breaking down of coagula which have formed in the blood-vessels; or it may supervene upon diffuse cellular inflammations, or upon puerperal fever,—in fact, it will be found

---

* See the cases of Hodgkin, Med.-Chirurg. Transact., vol. xviii.; of Wilks, Guy's Hosp. Reports, vol. xi., 3d Series; of Black, Amer. Journ. of Med. Sciences, April, 1866; of Wunderlich, Archiv der Heilkunde, 1866; and a review by Spillman, Archiv. Géné., 1867, vol. ii.

† Archiv der Heilk., ix., 1868.

under many dissimilar circumstances. But without stopping to explain its varying sources of origin, let us look at its diagnostic traits.

Now, there are several complaints with which pyæmia is likely to be confounded, the chief of which are typhoid fever, rheumatism, acute glanders and farcy, and acute affections of the liver.

It is liable to be mistaken for *typhoid fever*, on account of the adynamic character of the fever, and, it may be, the occurrence of diarrhœa and of cerebral symptoms. But the history of the case is very dissimilar; there is no eruption, or if there be an eruption, it consists, as Bristowe so particularly points out, of sudamina surrounded by a zone of congestion, and is therefore not the eruption of the typh-fevers; and, on the other hand, we find in typhoid fever neither the profuse sweating nor secondary deposits of pus, and the thermometry of the disease is very different. We must not forget, however, that pyæmia may happen as a complication of the febrile malady.

The pain in the joints and their swelling in succession, the fever, the perspirations resemble very much at times the symptoms of *rheumatic fever*. But the difference consists in the greater severity of the constitutional phenomena caused by the poisoned blood, in the marked exhaustion, in the rigors, and in the history not being that of rheumatic fever. Moreover, the frequent signs of formation of abscesses in internal organs or around the joints, the development of pustules on the skin, and the striking redness of the tumid joints assist materially in the diagnosis.

Acute glanders or *acute farcy* is a disease scarcely distinguishable from pyæmia, since it occasions, for the most part, the same manifestations. The knowledge that the patient who has apparently pyæmic symptoms has been working among horses, the ulceration of the mucous membrane of the nose, and the fetid discharge proceeding from it, which occurs in acute glanders, and which is apt to be associated with nasal hemorrhages, with an offensive breath, with enlargement of the lymphatic glands in the vicinity of the affected mucous membrane, and with hurried breathing, or sometimes with gangrene of various parts,—afford us the only means of discrimination. Then we find a peculiar tuberculated or pustular eruption which appears upon the skin, and in farcy the lymphatic glands and vessels specially suffer. But more significant than all, in point of diagnosis, is being able to trace the distinct history of the contagion; for the grave coryza and some of the other prominent symptoms mentioned do not happen in all forms of equinia,—certainly not, at least it is generally so stated, in farcy.

Acute affections of the liver resemble pyæmia on account of the jaundice which may attend the latter disorder; but the history of the case, the rigors, the sweats, and the purulent deposits distinguish it.

In conclusion, let us inquire where and how these secondary deposits are formed. They may take place in the parenchymatous organs, particularly in the lungs and liver; in the synovial sacs, in muscles, or in areolar tissue, especially in that under the skin. To account for their formation is not easy; and there is very great difference of opinion among pathologists concerning this point. The views now most generally received are, that they are owing to a suppurative form of capillary phlebitis, or—and this is becoming more and more the accredited opinion—that the vitiated blood coagulates either in the veins, heart, or arteries, usually in the former, and that the clots, becoming disintegrated, are washed into the smaller vessels or capillaries of individual tissues, and there give rise to inflammation and the development of pus.

It has just been indicated that the altered blood may coagulate in the arteries. Now when, from this cause, or from disintegration of fibrin in the arterial system, the fibrinous masses occasion deposits in solid organs, as in the liver or spleen, we may have, with the similar pathological states, similar symptoms arising to those of true pyæmia. Indeed, in the *arterial pyæmia*, as it has been called, rigors, febrile symptoms and sweating, and pains in the joints are observable. In connection with the obscure febrile condition, the liver and spleen are often observed to increase in size slowly.* The heart may or may not be affected.

The description of pyæmia given represents it as an acute affection, and so it almost always is. Yet there are cases much slower in their course, and extending over months. These *chronic* or *relapsing* instances of the disease have been described by Mr. Paget,† in his usual concise and happy manner. The symptoms presented are the same as in the acute malady; but the local evidences of the complaint are more often seated in different parts of the same tissues, and less frequently in internal organs. The malady is not nearly so perilous a one.

Septæmia.—This is a poisoned state of the blood, produced by mineral and vegetable, but especially by animal poisons, such as the bite of venomous serpents or the absorption of putrid matters which have been generated in the economy, or by their inoculation. The continued exposure to the breathing of foul air and of septic gases will also occasion septæmia. The symptoms of the blood poisoning vary somewhat with the individual poison that has occasioned it. They are, in the main, the symptoms of pyæmia,—which indeed may be viewed as a form of septæmia,—excepting that secondary pus formations belong to the former rather than to the latter, and the same of course may be said of embolism and its results. In many instances the altered condition of the blood leads to hemorrhages from internal organs, to petechiæ, to delirium and coma, to extreme rapidity of pulse, to burning heat of skin, to enlargement of the spleen, to cough and bronchial catarrh, and to gastric and intestinal disorders.

Thrombosis and Embolism.—While discussing endocarditis, the phenomena of embolism have already been alluded to, and they have also been mentioned in connection with several other subjects, as of obstruction of the cerebral arteries, and of some diseases of the kidney. Yet it may serve a useful purpose to view here connectedly, though

---

* Samuel Wilks, Guy's Hospital Reports, vol. xv., 3d Series.
† St. Bartholomew's Hospital Reports, vol. i.

chiefly in their diagnostic bearing, some of the results of the formation of the clots in large vessels or in the heart, and of their being carried along with the current of the blood and driven into remote vessels. The whole of the process of the formation of the clots is included under the term "thrombosis," while the projection onward of a thrombus, or of the fragments detached from it and the phenomena thus occasioned, are designated by the great pathologist to whom our knowledge of the subject is chiefly due—Virchow, as "embolia."

The subject of embolia, or embolism, is that which more particularly concerns the physician in its immediate practical bearing; but though thrombi do not as often produce symptoms which the medical practitioner is called upon to be acquainted with from a bedside point of view, he must have closely studied their cause and meaning to appreciate those of embolia.

The embolus may produce manifestations in the venous system, either in the peripheral veins; or in the venous trunks of the great internal cavities of the body; or portions of the thrombus may have been washed into the pulmonary artery from the right side of the heart; or it may have become impacted in the arteries of the general circulation, in the larger arteries, or in those of fine calibre; or it may have been washed into the very structure of organs through these arteries, as into the liver structure through the hepatic artery, into the splenic parenchyma through the splenic artery. Let us examine some of the symptoms thus occasioned a little more closely, premising that arterial embolism is of much more frequent occurrence than the other forms.

In the *veins* thrombi may form, which, so long as they do not produce an obstruction of the canal, give rise to no marked signs. A slight hardening and pain on pressure if the coagulum be in the more superficial veins, their enlargement if the clot be in the deeper veins, are apt to be the only evidences of the disordered condition. But when the occlusion is considerable, and especially when the collateral circulation is insufficient, œdema is developed, which may be attended with very great tenderness of the swollen part, and, if the impediment be of long duration, with changes

44

in the nutrition of the structures sufficient to produce phlegmonous inflammation. These phenomena are all encountered
to a greater or less degree in milk-leg or phlegmasia alba
dolens, which in all likelihood depends upon an obstruction
by a coagulum of the venous circulation in the affected limb.
In some cases profuse hemorrhages occur as a consequence
of the stoppage in the vein—as cerebral hemorrhages produced by thrombosis of the sinus, or, as in a case referred to
by Virchow,* enormous hemorrhagic infiltration of the sub-
peritoneal and subcutaneous tissues, as well as of portions
of the muscles of the abdominal walls, as the result of a
coagulum in the external iliac vein, the epigastric, and the
crural vein.

Now, portions of the clot, situated in any part of the venous
system, whether peripheral or not, and however remote from
the heart, may become, by being broken off and driven onward with the circulation, sources of great danger. Thus, in
cases of milk-leg they may be propelled from the veins of the
extremity to the heart; or the same may happen when a clot
has formed in the pelvic veins, subsequent to the ligation
of internal piles. Again, when the blood clogs in veins connected with the portal system, the detached fragments may be
washed into the liver, and these lead to secondary abscesses.
This, for instance, is the most likely causation of the so-called
metastatic abscesses of the liver in dysentery. But when
coagula occur in the venous system and are wholly or in part
carried away with the circulating blood (if we exclude those
which, from their situation, could only reach the liver), we
generally find the manifestations of disturbance arising in
the heart or lungs. Arriving at the right side of the heart,
the concretion, if at all large, or if it become so by serving
as a nucleus for a larger clot, occasions symptoms of exhaustion and collapse; an intermitting, feeble pulse; irregular
and confused beating of the heart, and cardiac sounds, enfeebled or lost over the right side of the organ; rapidly developed
distress in breathing, referred, by the sufferer, to the heart,†

---

* Pathologie und Therapie, p. 172.
† B. W. Richardson, Medical Times and Gazette, Nov. 1868.

and signs of asphyxia, though all the time the patient is taking deep inspirations; great agitation; and a swollen state of
the veins of the body. Death may then take place suddenly
if a portion of the clot separate and obstruct the pulmonary
artery.*

But the mode of death, and the symptoms preceding it in
embolism of the *pulmonary artery*, are not always the same,
and depend very much upon the size of the embolus and
where it is arrested. A large-sized clot, whether it be merely
part of one occupying the right heart, or be washed at once
into the pulmonary artery, will occasion much the same
signs as those alluded to as indicative of a large clot in
the right side of the heart; the craving for air is particularly
intense, and this craving is increased by every movement of
the body; the muscular debility, the lowered temperature,
the cyanosed look, the turgid veins of the neck and their
undulations, the increased, irregular cardiac impulse, though
the heart's action is not sufficiently disturbed to account for
the disturbed respiration and disordered general circulation,
are also noticed: and in some cases a systolic blowing sound,
and where the case is at all protracted, vertigo, albuminuria,
and œdema of the limbs may be observable. The intellect is
always apt to remain clear. As regards the pulmonary phenomena proper, collapse of the lung, hemorrhagic effusions,
œdema, or capillary bronchitis are likely to happen, excepting in those instances in which the principal trunks of the
pulmonary artery are blocked up, and almost instantaneous
asphyxia ensues. If the fragments be very small, the amount
of dyspnœa is not of necessity great, nor are the symptoms of
asphyxia marked; and inflammations of the parenchyma of
the lungs may take place, occasioning often secondary obstructions and metastatic abscesses in the lungs, from which
recovery even may possibly take place. These kind of metastatic abscesses are observed in pyæmia, and are not unusual in puerperal fever.

Blood clots in the *arteries* as a consequence chiefly of gangrene and of ulceration. The vessels for instance passing

* As in a case recorded by Druit, Med. Times and Gaz., July, 1862.

from a gangrenous part contain coagula forming in a direction from the periphery to the centre. We may find the clots in gangrene of internal organs, as of the pulmonary tissue. Again, atheromatous disease of the coats of the arteries may lead to the development of thrombi. But the most important phenomena connected with obstruction of arteries are those not of coagula forming in them, as of their being washed into them; the phenomena of embolism therefore rather than those of thrombosis. Now, the phenomena of embolism are distinguished from those of the mere formation of clots by what is always the most significant sign of either arterial or venous embolism—the suddenness of the manifestation of the abnormal state. And in point of fact the symptoms arise not so much as the result of any of the conditions alluded to that occasion coagulation, but very much more often as the consequence of deposits, fibrinous concretions, and excrescences which are seated on the valves on the left side of the heart, and portions of which are carried away by the circulating blood into remote parts. When these bodies become impacted in a vessel the calibre of which is such that it does not permit them to pass on, we find rapid changes taking place in the portions of the body supplied by the obstructed artery; coldness, pallor of the parts, a diminished functional activity, a shrinking; and if, as often does happen, the first obstruction is followed by others, and the collateral circulation cannot be established, local death and gangrene ensue.

All these changes are of course only discernible in external parts, especially in the extremities; the disturbances of function are the most, or indeed are the only, obvious signs where the internal organs are the sufferers. If the emboli be driven to the brain, we have, as has been already elsewhere alluded to, softening as the result, and this may be preceded by disorder of intellect, without motor disturbances, and by severe attacks of vertigo, in cases in which merely the smaller arteries supplying the surface of the cerebral hemispheres are obstructed. But where, as is indeed the most common seat of emboli, the arteries of the fissure of Sylvius are clogged, the phenomena are those of apoplec-

tic hemiplegia; and the palsy affects the whole of one side
of the body, even the face, and, though ushered in by only
very passing or imperfect unconsciousness, is apt to be permanent. The brain may also suffer from the seat of the obstruction being in the carotids; and indeed of all organs the effects
of embolism are most plainly perceptible in the brain. The
presence of emboli in the splenic, renal, and mesenteric
arteries is generally rather to be inferred from the history of
the case, and does not occasion any obvious discernible signs.
But tenderness, enlargement of the spleen, and pain in the
splenic region in splenic embolism, or disordered secretion
of urine and pain in the loins in embolism of the renal
artery, may be very marked.

The occurrence of pain in these cases of internal embolism
must not be overlooked; and in embolism of the arteries of
the extremities pain is a symptom of as great or still greater
prominence. It may be like a violent neuralgia, or so constant that it is mistaken for rheumatism; and, as happened in
a case of embolism of the right iliac artery, under the charge
of Dr. Hutchinson,* and which I saw, it may recur in paroxysms of intense severity, and be referred to the foot, though
this be already in a condition of sphacelus. Besides the
pain, we are apt to find extreme hyperæsthesia in some parts
of the affected limb; and pricking sensations, formication,
and loss of tactile sense, followed by complete anæsthesia in
others. Then painful spasms of the muscles, and a more or
less perfect paralysis of motion may occur. If we join to
these symptoms an absence of pulsation in the arteries below
the seclusion until the collateral circulation is decidedly established, a strong beat of the vessel on the cardiac side of
the obstruction, the coldness of the limb below this obstruction, and the signs of defective supply of blood, we have a
group of phenomena which, taken in connection with the
history of the case, render the diagnosis a positive one. And
in reviewing the history of the case, the state of the heart and
the cardiac symptoms must be always carefully examined

---

* Published Proceed. of Path. Society of Phila., Am. Journ. of Med. Sciences, Oct. 1863.

into. It is there in truth where the mischief generally begins; and a close inquiry may show that the sudden manifestations of arterial obstruction were preceded by an attack of palpitation and irregular action. A change in the physical signs of the diseased organ, as of its murmurs, may not be evident; but should it be evident, it is a sign of the utmost moment. Indeed any change in what may be viewed as the centre from which the embolus may be detached, is of great significance. And this holds good quite as much for venous as for arterial emboli. Thus, in a case of coagulum in a vein, a sudden disappearing of swelling and œdema of the affected limb, with the supervention of signs of embarrassed circulation and respiration, would at once tell what had taken place.

In regard also to the diagnosis of embolism we must always bear in mind the causes which are likely to give rise to it. Several of the causes of arterial embolism have already been mentioned; those of venous embolism are the same as of venous thrombosis, or, to speak more explicitly, the breaking up of the clots and their transportation may occur in any of the conditions which have occasioned them. Now, these conditions, too, will produce arterial clots, and indeed some are more apt to lead to coagulation in the arteries than in the veins. Prominent among them are a narrowing of the calibre of the vessel, as by pressure; dilatation of the vessels and of the heart; failure or great diminution of cardiac power, with consequent retardation of the blood stream—a state which is more likely to occasion venous than arterial thrombosis; a breakage in the continuity of the vessel, as when it is torn or cut; changes which take place in the coats of the vessels, especially inflammatory changes; and contact of the blood within the vessels with foreign bodies. Then it is very likely that special states of the blood, by altering the cohesion of the globules, predispose to, if they do not absolutely cause, the clotting, which, if one of the other elements alluded to then favor, is readily accomplished.

Another cause of embolism is that due to accumulations of pigment in the blood, the result of malarial fever. The pigment may obstruct the capillaries in the brain and thus occasion capillary apoplexies; or be driven to the liver and there produce signs of disturbance of its circulation, and abscesses. As in all forms of capillary embolia, the symptoms are very obscure: the suddenness of their development, generally so characteristic of the other forms of embolism, is wanting; and the diagnosis, as throughout in capillary embolia, is always nothing more than a matter of conjecture, based on a close study of the general phenomena and history of the case.

In conclusion, the subsequent changes of the thrombus must be alluded to. It may organize and be converted into connective tissue and yield an impaired passage to the blood; and perhaps the collateral circulation be freely established; or, what is not so favorable a result, it may soften and undergo fatty metamorphosis. But even when large portions are not detached and occasion the marked symptoms of embolism, small ones may be wafted into capillaries and there lay the foundation of abscesses. It is thus that in a case of thrombus or embolus we may have the secondary results of pyæmia to deal with—metastatic abscesses caused in the manner described, and attended with a blood profoundly altered and vitiated by the decomposing products circulating in it. It is almost needless to add that under such unfavorable circumstances the therapeutic means at our command in the treatment of embolism too generally prove wholly nugatory.

Scurvy.—This disease is not often met with in civil practice; but it is one very familiar to the military and naval surgeon. It consists in a deterioration of the blood, produced by living for a long period upon the same kind of food, and especially upon salted meats, without the requisite supply of fresh vegetables being taken. Indeed, the privation of the latter for a length of time is by far the most constant and most potent cause of scurvy; so constant and potent, in fact, that it is by many regarded as the sole determining source of the disease. Now, this influence of vegetables is attributed to the large quantity of potassa they contain; and as it has been found that there is a deficiency of the salts of potassa in scorbutic blood, it was concluded that this deficiency is the cause of scurvy, and has only to be remedied in order to cure the scorbutic taint. But this theory has not been so positively proved that it may be definitely adopted. Another cause of scurvy is the want of proper assimilation of food, as has been noticed in prison scurvy.*

Scurvy is usually slow in its development. The patient becomes low spirited, easily fatigued, is loth to exert himself, and complains much of general debility. The appetite is impaired; there is a craving for acids and for vegetable food; the tongue is large and flabby; the breath fetid; the pulse feeble; the skin dry. The bowels are usually constipated; but a tendency to diarrhœa may exist, and indeed is apt to occur as the disease advances. Neuralgic pains, referred to any part of the body, but chiefly to the lower extremities, to the bones, and to the back or thorax, are common. The face is pale, or has a yellowish tinge; the eyes are surrounded by a dark ring. During the progress of the ailment, or in severe cases almost from the onset, we find swollen, spongy gums, which bleed on the slightest touch; hurried breathing; a rapid pulse; weakened eyesight, sometimes night-blindness; epistaxis; painful swelling and hardness about the joints of the extremities and in the calves of the legs; and purple spots and bruiselike stains on the skin. Should the malady remain unchecked, the symptoms described heighten in severity, ulcers form which have a fungoid look and a great tendency to bleed, hemorrhages take place from internal organs, old sores and wounds reopen, well-knit fractures become disunited, there is a constant tendency to swoon, and the patient perishes miserably exhausted, and with his blood in a complete state of dissolution. In some cases death takes place from diarrhœa or dropsy, which may be suddenly developed. Even under the most favorable circumstances, recovery from scurvy is slow.

Purpura.—Scurvy is not a disease difficult to recognize; only one affection resembles it at all closely, and that is *purpura*. In this disorder also red or purple spots or livid blotches, uninfluenced by pressure, and passive hemorrhages from the mucous membranes happen. But there is this

---

* See Med. Memoirs of the U. S. Sanitary Commission, p. 278.

difference between the two complaints: purpura is common in fruit seasons, and often attacks persons who have not been in any way deprived of vegetable food. The gums are not soft and spongy, as in scurvy, nor do we find the same weakness of mind and body. Then, the stain of the skin in purpura is apt to be more generally diffused, and the purple blotches are smaller, or, at all events, the large patches of discoloration consist clearly of an aggregation of very many small spots. Moreover, although, like scurvy, the disorder may be benefited by iron, by bark, and the mineral acids, it is not controlled, like scurvy, by fresh vegetables, by lemon-juice,—in fact, by agents which are most decided antiscorbuties.

From a clinical point of view we find several forms of purpura. In the mildest, the purpurous spots are apt only to appear on the legs. They come in crops, which fade, and there are no constitutional symptoms excepting a little lassitude, and perhaps aching of the limbs and pain in the back. In the graver cases, "purpura hæmorrhagica," we find, in addition to the cutaneous hemorrhage, epistaxis, hæmatemesis, hæmaturia, or other internal hemorrhages, and extravasations of blood may happen into the substance of the muscles. The amount of pain attending the malady is very different. There may be none, or it may be trifling; or deep-seated pains in the cavities of the body, or extended neuralgic pains may accompany the purpurous complaint. In some instances the pains are chiefly felt in and around the joints, and the apparently rheumatic aches subside in a few days, and spots of extravasated blood become visible. This "purpura rheumatica," a variety particuarly described by Schönlein, is usually met with in the strong and healthy. It is, indeed, one of the peculiarities of any kind of purpura, that it may come on in the midst of seemingly excellent health. This is a matter to be borne in mind; for while it is true that the disorder may be preceded for some time by signs of general debility, or occur in the course of disease of the liver, of Bright's disease, or as a sequel to the exanthemata and rheumatic fever, it also happens where, from previous looks, we should least expect it. Its production, as the result of a sudden shock to the nervous system, such as fright, and its occasional intermittent character, have been noticed by various observers.

The duration of the malady is very variable,—only a week or several months may elapse before the spots disappear. Its pathology is unknown. It is clearly, however, not merely a disease of the blood; the capillaries lose their retentiveness, either, as has been actually demonstrated, in consequence of degenerative change, or as the result of impaired power, from the morbid action affecting directly or indirectly the part of the nervous system that controls them — the vaso-motor system.

In some cases purpura presents an *acute* form. It is ushered in by a chill, and by intense pains in the back and limbs, but is generally unattended with fever or severe constitutional disturbance. The purple spots usually first appear on the legs, and are wholly uninfluenced by pressure. They last five or six days, or somewhat longer, then gradually change their color and fade. The patient feels languid, but unless from loss of blood his strength is not materially impaired. The effusion of blood happens in some cases into the loose connective tissues of the body, or blood is lost from the lungs, and still more frequently from the bowels or urinary organs. Under these circumstances the pulse, which other-wise is apt to preserve its normal frequency, becomes very rapid; but until exhaustion begins to tell on the nervous system—not as a rule long before dissolution—the mind remains clear, and cerebral or spinal symptoms are absent. It is thus that we are able to distinguish severe cases of acute purpura, which may indeed prove fatal in forty-eight hours,* from spotted fever.

---

* As in a remarkable case reported by Dr. Harrison Allen, Proc. of Path. Soc. of Phila., Am. Journ. Med. Sci , Jan. 1865.

CHAPTER X.

RHEUMATISM AND GOUT are affections having a strong tendency to change their seat, and are dependent upon the presence in the blood of some poisonous material which probably accumulates there in consequence of malassimilation. The poison which is supposed to occasion the most frequent of these disorders—rheumatism—is lactic acid; and it is during an effort at its elimination that the phenomena of rheumatism, or at least the phenomena of acute rheumatism, are best studied.

The rheumatic poison has a singular predilection for the fibrous, serous, and muscular textures. Hence we find it attacking principally such structures as the joints, the fasciæ, the endocardium and pericardium, and the muscles in various parts of the body. According to its main forms, it is sometimes divided into articular and muscular; but the more usual division into acute and chronic is simpler, and will answer our purpose best.

Acute Rheumatism.—Here the rheumatic poison gives rise to the symptoms of an acute, active disease, and attacks especially the larger joints. These swell, become hot, red, tense, tender, and the seat of pain aggravated by the slightest movement; an effusion also takes place into the surrounding structures, or into them and the synovial membranes of the joint itself. The rheumatic inflammation may either remain confined to the joints first affected until the disease is over, or, what is more common, it shifts from joint to joint, implicating most of the large ones in succession, yet often invading fresh joints before the swelling has subsided in the parts first attacked. The articular disorder is ushered in and aecom-

(699)

panied by high fever, soon attended with a full, bounding pulse, with profuse, sour perspirations, with a deeply-coated tongue, a scanty, turbid, highly acid urine, and a countenance singularly expressive of suffering.

Now, there is ordinarily little difficulty in recognizing the complaint. The pains in the joints, their tumefaction and tenderness, the shifting character of the disorder, and the peculiar constitutional symptoms form a group of phenomena eminently characteristic. Then the absence of the symptoms so usual in continued fevers, such as dulness of intellect or delirium, gastric and intestinal disturbance, and sordes on the teeth and gums, enables us at once to separate the rheumatic disorder from these febrile states, and renders its distinction still easier. In truth, excluding acute gout, the only affections at all likely to be confounded with acute articular rheumatism are pyæmia and glanders, acute synovitis, and milk-leg. The diagnosis of the former has already been discussed in connection with diseases of the blood; it only remains, therefore, to point out the marks of similitude and contrast between acute articular rheumatism and the other maladies just mentioned.

Acute synovitis resulting from an injury, or from cold, occasions, like articular rheumatism, pain and heat in the joint, with distention. But the disorder, excepting, perhaps, if it happen in a rheumatic constitution, does not affect more than one joint; and as there is scarcely any or no effusion into the surrounding tissues, the outline of the joint can be distinctly discerned, and fluctuation is very readily detected. Often, too, the accumulation of fluid reaches an extent far greater than in rheumatic inflammation; moreover, the febrile and constitutional derangement is not so severe as in acute rheumatism, and the affection has no tendency to change its seat. Still, we must not forget that acute synovitis may be rheumatic.*

Milk-leg, or phlegmasia dolens, occurs most usually in women after delivery, or as a sequel of continued fevers. Generally only one leg swells, and this becomes throughout,

---

* See Adams, Med. Times and Gazette, Feb. 1869.

or sometimes only around the calf, preternaturally white, firm, hot, and shining. The tumefaction is uniform, and very painful, especially so when touched. It does not pit, or pits but very slightly, upon pressure, unless at the lower part. There is in some cases tenderness with a sense of hardness in the course of the femoral vein, though this is by no means, constant; and we are apt to find signs of much debility and of altered blood and febrile symptoms. But these are unlike the peculiar constitutional disturbance of rheumatism, and equally dissimilar are the history of the case and the local signs. Among these, two giving rise to striking differences may be mentioned: the almost entire loss of power in the affected limb in phlegmasia alba dolens, and the much higher temperature it shows by the thermometer than the other members. And while alluding to its heat, we may remark that an increase of general temperature corresponds to an increase of pain and swelling in the limb, and of constitutional distress.*

Rheumatism may be modified in its manifestations by happening in connection with, or consequent upon other disorders. For instance, the febrile phenomena may be of an adynamic type when the disease occurs consecutively to typhoid or typhus fever; or we may find the local signs of acute rheumatism strangely mixed with the symptoms of puerperal fever, and in some of these cases pus may fill the tumid joints; or the presence of the syphilitic poison or of gonorrhœa may imprint peculiar features upon the rheumatic complaint. Thus, in the latter instance there is usually less febrile distress, the articular pain is not so severe nor acute; the integument covering the affected joint is apt to retain its normal color; there may be but one joint—and there are not generally many—implicated; the inflammation is confined to the synovial membrane; the joint affection resembles rather an acute or subacute rheumatoid arthritis than acute rheumatism; and the eye, too, unlike what happens in ordinary acute rheumatic fever, is often attacked. But the

---

* See case at the Pennsylvania Hospital, described in vol. ii. of its Reports, by Dr. Elliott Richardson.

most significant of all signs is finding a running from the urethra, which diminishes when the gonorrhœal rheumatism sets in, but which does not cease.

The traits of an attack of acute rheumatism are, however, still more frequently altered by certain complications in internal organs which the contaminated blood is apt to occasion. Prominent among them are the cardiac troubles, which are in fact so common that they may be looked upon as forming part of the rheumatic manifestation rather than as being one of its complications. The affection of the membranes of the heart disturbs the pulse and renders it irregular, hurries the breathing, and, unless carefully managed, is very prone to leave some lasting mischief. It is, as a rule, not difficult of diagnosis; but this is a matter we have investigated already, while examining the signs of endocarditis and pericarditis.

Other complications are inflammation of the lung, particularly of the bronchial tubes and of the pleura, or cerebrospinal disturbances, exhibiting themselves by headache, violent delirium, convulsions, and coma, and occurring either in connection with a thoracic disorder, or solely in consequence of the action of the vitiated blood on the nervous centres, or again, as has been recently suggested, in consequence of multiple capillary embolism, or the sudden exhaustion of the nervous centres.* This explanation has been more particularly applied to the cases in which an excessive temperature attends the rapidly-developed signs of cerebral disturbance, a temperature of 107° or more. But speaking from a bedside point of view, we must remember that such cases are comparatively rare, and that rheumatic delirium is far from always of the same nature. It may be of the kind just mentioned. It may develop itself with or without the signs of cardiac trouble. It may come on early in the disorder during the violence of the fever; or late, and clearly from debility and impoverished blood, yielding to nourishment and stimulants. It is very rarely the result of meningitis. When this happens, the swelling of the joints usually lessens; the delirium is marked by great talkativeness, or, on the

* Weber, Clinical Society's Transactions of London, vol. i.

other hand, the patient is extremely taciturn. Headache is rarely, and vomiting is not at all among the symptoms.

In a few instances of rheumatism we find arteritis arising, and especially inflammation of the fibrous structures of the aorta. This condition may be suspected should we observe intense general uneasiness and distress, with pain, increased pulsation, a distinct murmur in the course of the vessel, and tumultuous action of the heart without there being obvious signs of disease of that organ present. Still, the diagnosis is never a positive one.

Acute rheumatism is not a disease either of children or of persons advanced in years. Its duration is very variable. By judicious treatment it may be conquered in about two weeks; but often convalescence does not set in for three, four, or five weeks. It rarely ends fatally; its cardiac consequences are more to be feared than the acute attack.

Cases occur not unfrequently in which the inflammation in the joints is somewhat lingering, and in which the febrile symptoms are not intense. These cases form an intermediate grade between acute and chronic rheumatism, and are generally spoken of as *subacute*. The disorder is more apt than the acute variety to affect the muscles as well as the joints; nay, the former may be alone attacked. It may be witnessed in the joints of one extremity, or in one joint, and might then be mistaken for synovitis. But the dissimilar history of the complaint will guard against error: no accident has happened to account for the swelling of the joint, and often the patient will tell us that he has had previously an attack of rheumatism. This subacute form of rheumatism is very apt to be confounded with rheumatic arthritis; we shall presently refer to their distinction.

Chronic Rheumatism.—This may be either a sequel of the acute disease, or the disorder from the onset assumes a lingering form, the constitutional symptoms being very slight. The affection may show itself in the joints, giving rise to stiffness, a dull aching, and pain produced by motion, but without heat or very obvious swelling, tenderness, febrile excitement, or marked sweating; or it may implicate the muscles in various parts of the body, occasioning stiffness, as well as pain when they are moved; or it attacks both joints and muscles; or is seated chiefly in the sheaths of nerves, leading to what is called neuralgic rheumatism, of which, for instance, sciatica often affords a striking example. In any case, the occurrence of the pain furnishes the starting-point in diagnosis, and we must ascertain, by careful examination, whether it be augmented by motion, whether it be more or less shifting, whether it be not combined with stiffness either of the muscles or joints, whether it be influenced by changes of temperature, whether it be not neuralgic, or associated with a disturbance of some viscus, such as of the liver or kidneys,—before we conclude that the complaint is really rheumatic.

This is especially necessary in the most common form of chronic rheumatism—*muscular rheumatism*. All kinds of pains in the muscles or their surroundings, the cause of which is not at once apparent, are apt to be pronounced rheumatic. And indeed it is not always easy to say whether they are or are not of that character. We may distinguish them from the anguish of neuralgia by the pain in the latter complaint being ordinarily confined to the distribution of one nerve, and not being increased by movement or by pressure; nor is it so steady, or attended with soreness, excepting over a few spots at some distance from each other in the course of the affected nerve. As regards the pains caused by organic structural disease, we can generally discriminate them from those of rheumatism by close attention to the history of the case, and by a careful exploration of the internal organs. Thus, for instance, we shall find pain radiating from the right hypochondrium to the shoulder to be dependent upon hepatic disease; or pain shooting down to the groin, thigh, and testicle, to be caused by a disturbance of the kidney; or a bearing down and an aching near the sacrum, to be probably due to uterine disorder.

Muscular rheumatism may affect the neck, the scalp, the muscles of the face, and the parietes of the chest or of the abdomen. It may be not only chronic in any of these situations, but also acute; or, what is more frequent, when it occurs with fever and is transient, it is a sudden acute exacerbation in persons who are rheumatic and suffer more or less persistently from rheumatism, though perhaps in a different part of the body, from the one in which the acute affection has happened.

One of the most common seats of muscular rheumatism is in the loins. It then constitutes the disease known as *lumbago*. The patient is unable to stand erect, and finds it nearly impossible to stoop forward, on account of the severe pain occasioned when the muscles of the back are called into action. Unless the attack be very severe or acute, there is no constitutional disturbance; but the disorder is very often obstinate. It is easy of recognition. We distinguish it from pain in the loins due to disease of the kidneys, chiefly by an examination of the urine, and by the different way in which movement affects the rheumatic pain; from lumbo-abdominal neuralgia, by the two or three sore spots in the course of the affected nerve; from rheumatism of the vertebral articulations, by the absence of tenderness and swelling around the spinous processes; from lumbar abscess, by the want of a local bulging or fulness, of fluctuation, and of fever. Then, we must be careful not to consider as lumbago the pain in the back caused by disease of the spine, or disorder of the uterus, or by the passage of abnormal urinary constituents, such as oxalate of lime, or consequent upon strains, or blows, or scurvy, or malaria, or anæmia, or a general or local muscular debility.

Thus there are many causes of pain in the loins, and where the case is of any duration or of any doubt, we must not rest satisfied until we have excluded these causes from consideration before we assume the disease to be really rheumatism of the muscles and fasciæ of the back. This caution is very necessary in investigating the cases of "weak back," so prevalent among soldiers, and which, though commonly spoken of as rheumatic, are really, for the most part, due to strains or injuries which have, perhaps, produced a weakness of the muscle and a persistent cutaneous hyperæsthesia; or to an impoverished blood, to neuralgia, to scurvy; or to digestive disorders attended with the passage from the kidneys of large amounts of urates or oxalate of lime.

45

The remarks made with reference to this form of muscular rheumatism, and the states which simulate it, are also applicable to pains apparently muscular, affecting other portions of the body. We may have pain and soreness of the muscles developed by overwork and attended both with muscular and cutaneous hyperæsthesia,—a condition very different from rheumatism, and designated by Dr. Inman* as "myalgia." This soreness of the muscles is thought by him to be always in direct proportion to the debility of the muscular system, and is chiefly caused by long-continued exertion beyond the power of the muscle, or by a very ordinary amount of action when the muscle itself or the individual is extremely dehilitated. The morbid state is most marked during the convalescence from scarlet fever, where it may be looked upon as due to overexertion of the weakened muscles. The soreness of the muscle is almost constantly accompanied by heightened sensibility of the skin over it; and this coexisting cutaneous tenderness may be in any case regarded as a very important diagnostic sign.

Another form of muscular rheumatism which we may here allude to is the wry-neck, or *torticollis*. This depends chiefly upon contraction of the sterno-cleido-mastoid muscle of one side, and occasions the ungainly appearance with which most persons are familiar. But we must be careful not to consider every case as of rheumatic origin. The disorder may be spastic, or depend upon nervous injury, and when chronic may lead to alteration in the muscular structure. Injections of atropia, hypodermically, may generally be used, not only for their good therapeutic effect, but because, in chronic cases even, they may show us, by the difficulty or impossibility of relaxing it, how much of the muscle is really changed.

A form of chronic rheumatism which also may be briefly mentioned is that affecting chiefly the fibrous membranes, such as the *periosteum*. This becomes thick, and tender on pressure; its thickening may even be very perceptible, to the touch as well as to the eye. This kind of rheumatism happens in those who have syphilis; but it also occurs where no

---

* Spinal Irritation explained, or a treatise on Myalgia.

such taint exists. The pains are generally much more severe at night; and this is sometimes assumed to be a proof of the syphilitic character of the disease. But incorrectly so; for many varieties of chronic rheumatism are aggravated by the warmth of the bed. Indeed, the only really diagnostic signs of syphilitic rheumatism are the obvious evidences of constitutional syphilis, or the history of the infection. Still to cases in which several nodes exist, and in which the pains more particularly affect the long and flat bones, and in which iodide of potassium speedily modifies them, we shall be rarely wrong to attribute a syphilitic origin.

Chronic rheumatism is often feigned, especially by malingerers in the army and navy, and the deception may be very difficult of detection. They pretend to be scarcely able to walk, or hobble around with a cane, and complain much of the pain and stiffness in their joints. Yet there is not the least sign of deformity or real stiffness; the pain is always stated to be the same; and their general health is excellent. Their way of using the stick, too, is characteristic: they move it each time they move the seemingly crippled leg, but, as a rule, not immediately, thus not employing it as a support. Anæsthetics are of great value in enabling us to decide as to the real amount of immovability of the limb.

Gout.—This disease, so closely allied to rheumatism, may be, like the latter, either acute or chronic. Instead of describing its phenomena, I shall at once point out the marks of difference between the two maladies. In gout, the small joints are chiefly or alone affected; in rheumatism, the large. The gouty inflammation is accompanied by more local pain and redness than the rheumatic, and by œdema, by enlargement of the veins, and desquamation of the cuticle, and implicates, at least at first, only one or a few joints, especially the joint of the great toe; while rheumatism attacks the joints of the upper as well as of the lower extremities. In gout there is a tendency to disease of the kidneys, but we meet with no cardiac complication, as so constantly happens in rheumatism, with a moderate febrile disturbance, and no profuse sweats. Gout is much more decidedly hereditary than rheumatism; its early attacks are apt to recur with a certain amount of periodicity, and last about a week—therefore a much shorter time than those of rheumatic fever.

Gout occurs generally in those who live high or drink large quantities of malt liquor, and especially in men about middle age; while rheumatism is usually seen in the weak, is excited by cold and damp, is as common in females as in males, and is oftener found ·in the young and before middle age. Gout is frequently combined with a deposition of chalk-stones in the joints; rheumatism never. Then, if we accept the observations of Dr. Garrod* as conclusive, we possess an absolute means of diagnosis in the examination of the blood. Uric acid is always present in large excess in gout, and absent in rheumatism. This, should further researches prove it to be an invariable rule, will be a positive and invaluable diagnostic test, and will render easy of discrimination even those cases which, with the usually employed means now at our command, are very perplexing to distinguish. Nor is the method of detecting the uric acid difficult, if we make use of Dr. Garrod's ingenious plan. It consists in obtaining the crystals of uric acid on a thread placed in a mixture of the serum of the blood or of the fluid from a blister, with acetic acid, in the proportion of six minims of the acid to each fluid drachm of the serum.

Nearly all the remarks just made apply more especially to the distinction between acute gout and acute rheumatism. The chronic disorders are more difficult to separate. Indeed, unless there be external deposits or chalk-stones, their discrimination may be impossible. In these obscure cases, however, the history and an examination of the blood may throw considerable light on the diagnosis. In many subjects, too, Dr. Garrod informs us, the exploration of the external ear will assist us in arriving at a correct diagnosis: we find one or several spots of deposit of urate of soda on the helix.

Gouty persons are subject to indigestion, flatulency, pains and cramps, or palpitation of the heart,—phenomena which

---

* Gout and Rheumatic Gout, 2d edit. London, 1863.

are due to the gouty poison, and which are generally ameliorated by a fit of gout. Sometimes the gouty inflammation
of the joints retrocedes during an attack, and severe epigastric pain, nausea, vomiting, flatulence and acidity, faintness
and a feeling of sinking, and a quick, feeble pulse, show that
the morbid action is transferred to the stomach; or it flies to
the head, and apoplexy or maniacal symptoms occur; or to
the heart, and there is violent palpitation, with difficulty of
breathing, and intense anxiety.

Rheumatic Arthritis or Rheumatic Gout.—The painful
malady last discussed is, fortunately, comparatively rare in
this country. But the same cannot be said of that distressing disorder known as *rheumatic gout*, and which is generally
viewed as a blending of the two diseases, though there are
many who believe that it is neither rheumatism nor gout,
but a distinct affection. The disorder may be acute or
chronic. It is not very often the former; many of the acute
cases indeed being rather subacute than acute. Even in
those belonging to the *acute* form there is comparatively little
febrile disturbance; and though we observe pain and aching
in the joints and some discoloration, we find less redness than
in acute rheumatism, and certainly the tongue less furred,
the pulse not so bounding, much less profuse perspiration, no
such heavy deposits in the urine, and an utter freedom from
cardiac complication. The acute arthritic disease has rather
inflammation of the pleura and of the eye as its attendants, and
is often accompanied by a sallow skin, yellowish conjunctiva,
and discolored, costive stools. It implicates the large and small
joints equally, thus differing from gout, and causes very great
swelling, due to an effusion, not around the joint, but into its
capsule. It fastens upon several joints, and though it may
pass from joint to joint, it shows but little migratory tendency; the joints first attacked remain the seat of disease.
Unlike gout, it is apt to affect the smaller joints of the hands
without a previous affection of the toes, and exhibits no
periodic paroxysms or exacerbations. Moreover, an acute
attack is of very much longer duration. Unlike subacute
rheumatism, it does not affect the muscles, and is, both in

the suffering at the time and in its ultimate results, a very much graver malady.

The great danger in rheumatic arthritis is from the effects of the inflammation on the joints. The changes there produced are very obvious in the *chronic* form, for each joint attacked is apt to be permanently damaged. The chronic complaint may follow the acute, or it may commence, without any febrile symptoms, with pain and stiffness in the joints. These soon become much distended with fluid, which is gradually absorbed, and the structure of the joint alters, the cartilages become, sooner or later, implicated, and gradually waste, and there are often chronic changes and permanent deformity produced, as Dr. Adams* has so well described. The alterations may go on getting worse and worse in consequence of repeated attacks, until complete immobility ensues, and the joints becoming permanently affected, the ends of the bones are dislocated and enlarged. But although there is much swelling of the joints, no deposits of urate of soda are found in them.

Rheumatic arthritis is more common in females than in males; may be, like rheumatism, excited by cold and damp, and is very apt to occur in the weak and unhealthy. It often, even in cases that recover, persists for months. Nor will it yield to the remedies usually administered in acute rheumatism; nor to colchicum and the alkalies, so beneficial in gout. Guaiacum, cod-liver oil, arsenic, quinine, and other tonics are much more serviceable agents; and often, too, we may use in addition, with advantage, the medicine so valuable in most of the forms of chronic rheumatism—the iodide of potassium.

---

* Treatise on Rheumatic Gout, or Chronic Rheumatic Arthritis, etc. London, 1857.

CHAPTER XI.

THE lassitude, the heat of skin, the excited circulation, and the altered secretions—in one word, the group of morbid actions recognized as fever, is often consequent upon some strictly local malady. But here the fever is a symptom, and does not constitute the only obvious affection present. It is only in the latter case that the disorder merits the name of essential fever. The first step, therefore, when fever has been recognized, is to determine whether it is symptomatic or idiopathic; whether, in other words, it is but a complement to a disease, or, so far as can be ascertained, the disease itself. This is not generally a difficult matter. The history of the case, the absence or presence of the marked peculiarities of serious local disturbances soon determine the scale of evidence to rise on the one side or sink on the other. And it is astonishing, with the progress of medicine, how many affections have been passed over from the domain of fevers to the narrower circle of inflammation of individual organs; how many a case of gastric fever, for instance, turns out to be subacute inflammation of the stomach; and with what a different eye the brain and lung fevers of the olden times are regarded. While thus the group of idiopathic fevers has been considerably winnowed, some of their broad traits have been very prominently brought forward. It is now well understood that, with few exceptions, they are characterized by the want of definite and invariable anatomical lesions. That in all constant changes occur in parts of the nervous system, or in the blood, is highly probable; but these changes are not of a nature to be recognized by our present means of research. Certainly there is no invariable injury perceptible in the organs of the body: sometimes one, sometimes another suffers; sometimes nearly all; at times, none.   When we contrast this with symptomatic fever, the difference is striking.

The visceral lesions, then, of an idiopathic fever are not the starting-point of the fever; but rather secondary and uncertain complications influenced by and subordinate to the profound disturbance of the whole system.   In idiopathic fever, the fever controls the lesions; in symptomatic fever, the lesions control the fever.

Most fevers run a definite course, showing a strong tendency to a spontaneous termination at a given time.   At their commencement, too, they are for the most part very similar. There is a prodromic state, marked generally by unsound sleep, pain in the back, and lassitude.   This is followed by chills, which are succeeded by heat of skin, arrested secretions, quick pulse, and evident fatigue upon the least exertion.   The fever has now reached its full development.   Its precise character becomes evident; the symptoms caused by disorders of individual organs stand forth.   After awhile the disturbance declines, or speedily ceases under the influence of critical discharges.   The functions are re-established, and a convalescence, more or less rapid, sets in.   An unfavorable termination, on the other hand, may take place at any period after the system has been fairly invaded.

Such is a brief outline of the general phenomena of a fever.   But varied causes and secondary changes of course modify these phenomena, and occasion signs serving to distinguish one febrile disorder from the other.   In some, the fever is continued; in others, it exhibits a distinct periodicity.   Again, some fevers are attended with symptoms of extremely high action; others with the signs of most profound prostration and blood-poisoning.

The marked features impressed upon the fever, either by the course it runs or by the specific nature of the symptoms, go to form what is called its *type*, and may be made the basis of the classification of all febrile disorders.   But as opinions have been and are still singularly diversified as to what really constitute the most palpable characteristics, so the classification of fevers is as yet, to a great extent, a matter of speculation. Nor has the difficulty been lessened by the disposition to assign a separate place to each fever presenting any, however minute, points of dissimilarity. Certain it is that very many divisions are uncalled for; for Nature herself, by the readiness with which she permits even essential traits to be interchanged or to become blended in the same attack, proves that even groups are not widely distinct, and that minor differences are, therefore, wholly unworthy of forming the touchstone of systematic arrangement. In the following table no attempt is made at an exhaustive or strictly scientific classification. Some disorders, such as cholera and puerperal fever, considered by many eminent pathologists to belong to idiopathic fevers, have no place assigned to them; while others, such as influenza and yellow fever, the claims of which to be here mentioned are undoubted, might have their positions fairly impugned. But in a diagnostic point of view, the arrangement adopted is convenient, and is sufficiently accurate to be free from grave objections.

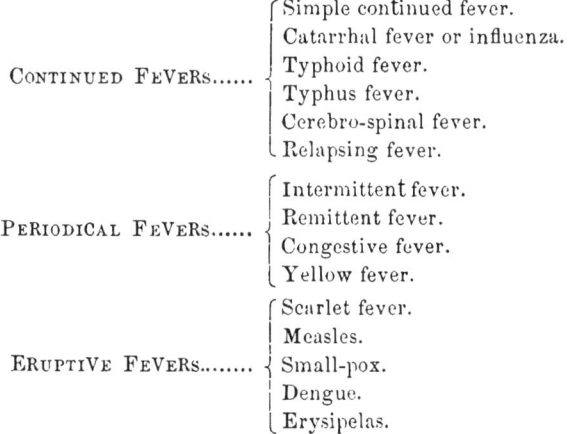

FEVERS.

CONTINUED FEVERS......
- Simple continued fever.
- Catarrhal fever or influenza.
- Typhoid fever.
- Typhus fever.
- Cerebro-spinal fever.
- Relapsing fever.

PERIODICAL FEVERS......
- Intermittent fever.
- Remittent fever.
- Congestive fever.
- Yellow fever.

ERUPTIVE FEVERS........
- Scarlet fever.
- Measles.
- Small-pox.
- Dengue.
- Erysipelas.

Continued Fevers.

All continued fevers are characterized by a steady progress of the febrile movement without either decided exacerbation or relaxation, the rise and fall observable being too slight to modify the impression of a sustained action.

Simple Continued Fever.—In simple fever we find all the phenomena which constitute a fever. It sets in with feelings of lassitude and chilliness; to these succeed hot skin, excited pulse, thirst, headache, pain in the limbs. The bowels are generally confined, the urine high colored. The fever is soon at its height; it then either gradually declines, or is more suddenly relieved by copious perspiration or by a critical discharge from the bowels. Generally it runs through all these stages in a few days; but it may be protracted for several weeks. On the other hand, a day may witness both its commencement and termination. The convalescence is almost always rapid.

The exciting causes of this form of fever are fatigue, errors in diet, change in mode of life, exposure to cold and moisture, or to the sun. When brought on by mental overwork or by grief, it is not uncommonly attended with considerable prostration, simulating typhoid fever, but differing from it by the absence of the peculiar abdominal symptoms and of the eruption. More frequently the fever has the appearance of one of high action. At times, indeed, it is so intense, and the vascular system so wrought up, that the distemper assumes what is called an inflammatory type. It now exhibits the characteristics of the fever described by the physicians of the last century as synocha. Burning heat of the surface, throbbing of the temporal arteries, severe headache and delirium are among its symptoms. This variety of the fever is not, however, a disease at present encountered, save in tropical latitudes. In point of diagnosis, it is most apt to be confounded with internal inflammations, especially with inflammation of the brain. On the history of the case, and on the full consideration of all the symptoms before us, alone can a trustworthy opinion be based. In truth, in all the grades of what appears to be at first sight simple continued fever, we ought, before assuming the febrile state to be the disease and sufficient to explain the abnormal phenomena, to examine carefully all the organs, and see whether the symptoms may not be wholly accounted for by some visceral disturbance. And often then, under what seems to be a very active or "ardent" fever, will, on closer scrutiny, be found lurking the traits of an inflammatory lesion.

Catarrhal Fever.—It is not common to class this epidemic malady with the idiopathic fevers; it is oftener described as a mere variety of bronchitis, because inflammation of the bronchial mucous membrane constitutes one of its most prominent symptoms. But this is not a just view. With as much reason might typhoid fever be omitted from the list of febrile maladies, and described as a variety of enteritis or diarrhœa.

Catarrhal fever is essentially an epidemic disease, and one which has visited the human race from remote antiquity. Its history is thus not confined to any particular time, nor to any particular nation; yet, in spite of its frequency and wide prevalence, its cause is still unascertained. We know nothing further of it than that it is an atmospheric poison traversing continents with extreme rapidity, just as cholera does, affecting animals as well as man, and leaving behind it an influence which shows itself long after the epidemic visitation. But what this peculiar state of the atmosphere is, which produces such potent results, is not understood. It is certainly neither heat, nor cold, nor damp, nor any recognizable physical changes in the surrounding air; for the disease has occurred at all times of the year, and with every kind of weather.

Each epidemic does not furnish precisely the same train of symptoms; but they all agree in this: the disorder always sets in suddenly, and always attacks pre-eminently the mucous membranes. Generally it is the mucous membrane of the nose, eyes, and bronchial tubes which suffers most, and we find the signs of coryza and bronchial inflammation—a watery eye, sneezing, uneasiness about the throat, and cough. But associated with these are usually an extraordinary amount of lassitude and impairment of strength; much more than the cold in the head or the bronchitis will account for. The skin is hot, the pulse only of moderate volume, or weak, the tongue white and coated; the patient complains of his debility, and of the aching pains in his back and limbs. Often there is disturbance of the alimentary tract, evinced by loss of appetite, nausea and vomiting, or by diarrhœa. Commonly after three or four days these symptoms begin to subside, the cough and debility outlasting the other morbid signs.

But all epidemics do not run precisely this course. In some, the prostration is not so evident, and the febrile signs are more active and of an inflammatory type; in others, the pain and soreness of the limbs and in the joints constitute the most prominent symptoms, or we may find hemicrania, or capillary bronchitis, or pneumonia, as distressing complications.

Influenza is not ordinarily in itself a fatal disease. It is only so in the very young or the very old, in both of whom it is apt to become combined with inflammation of the smaller bronchial tubes or of the lung.

Catarrhal fever is easily discriminated from other maladies. Its peculiar epidemic character prevents us from mistaking an ordinary cold or bronchitis for it. Occasionally the attending debility makes it look like the onset of a low continued fever. But brain symptoms are only present in rare instances in influenza; and, on the other hand, decided catarrhal symptoms are not common in typhoid or typhus fever. Before long, too, the occurrence of the eruption of these diseases clears up whatever doubt may have existed. The all but constant absence of an eruption in influenza comes also elsewhere into play; it serves to distinguish this disorder from measles or small-pox.

When influenza is prevailing on a large scale, it is often found peering out from under the garb of other diseases, and it may be difficult then to separate its manifestations from those of the malady it accompanies.

Typhoid Fever.—In this country and on the Continent of Europe a form of continued fever largely prevails, marked by great prostration and disturbance of the nervous system, and, unlike most essential fevers, by constant and appreciable anatomical lesions. To this disease the various designations of typhoid fever, enteric fever, entero-mesenteric fever, nervous fever, and abdominal typhus have been applied.

The disorder either attacks single individuals, or shows itself as an epidemic. It occurs at all seasons of the year;

but in this country, at least, is most frequent in autumn. In some localities it is thoroughly at home; in others it is only occasionally seen. It avoids both extremes of age, seizing mainly on young adults for its victims. It is not commonly regarded as contagious; yet there is no lack of trustworthy evidence to prove that it has been communicated by contact.

The distemper may set in suddenly, but more generally it has an insidious beginning. For some days preceding the access of the fever the patient feels weak and out of spirits. He is listless and without animation, and his countenance fully expresses his languor. He complains of soreness and fatigue, of dull pain in the head, of loss of appetite. His sleep is unsound; all exertion is wearisome. He is sick; something is evidently weakening his nervous energies. A fever now appears, preceded mostly by a chill, or, at all events, by chilly sensations, which alternate with flushes of heat. The muscular prostration accompanying the febrile movement is so great that the patient is obliged to seek his bed. His appetite is entirely gone, the tongue coated, the bowels loose, the abdomen somewhat swollen and tender to the touch. On close inspection, a few reddish spots, resembling flea-bites, are found on its surface.

The malady has now completed its first week. It enters the second week with fever unabated, and with the signs of disturbance of the alimentary tract and of the nervous system more and more unmistakable. There is sometimes nausea or epigastric distress, often pain in the right iliac fossa, increased by pressure, and tympanites. The tongue dries and becomes reddish or brownish; the gums and teeth are covered with dark crusts. The mind is dull and wandering; cough and great restlessness exist; the debility is extreme.

The disease now begins to draw to its close. It has reached the third week, and a change, for better or for worse, may be looked for. Slowly recovery sets in, marked by a brightening of the countenance and a gradual increase in consciousness and strength; or deepening insensibility, jerking of the tendons, feeble pulse, and cold, clammy sweats indicate that dissolution is fast approaching.

Thus, in one way or the other, the fever itself is apt to terminate by the twenty-first day. Yet such is not always the case. Death may take place at an earlier period; or, on the other hand, the malady, by troublesome complications, may be lengthened beyond the second month. Under any circumstances, convalescence is protracted. The nervous system rallies but gradually from the shock it has received.

Among the symptoms enumerated, some are so striking, and tend so clearly to characterize the disease, that, in examining them more closely, we become at once familiar with the features distinguishing typhoid fever from a host of other maladies. And first, of the more purely *febrile* symptoms. The skin is hotter than natural; this is especially perceptible in the evening exacerbations of the fever. Frequently the surface is covered with an acid perspiration, very manifest during the whole course of the disorder, and also encountered long after convalescence has set in. The pulse is accelerated, and remains so after the heat of skin has left; but it is rarely tense, and even in intercurrent acute inflammations it seldom loses its compressibility. A jerking, irregular beat, or very great rapidity, is an unfavorable sign.

When we investigate the febrile symptoms by the thermometer, we find them striking, and, in many respects, peculiar. Wunderlich's* observations on very many cases show that the temperature on the first day of the fever, in the morning, may be stated at 98·5°; in the evening, at 100·5° Fahr.; on the second day, in the morning, it is apt to be about 99·5°, in the evening 101·5°; on the third day, in the morning, 100·5°, in the evening 102·5°; on the fourth day, in the morning, 101·5°, in the evening 104°. From that time on the evening temperature ranges between 103° to 104°, the morning temperature being about 1 degree lower, until the middle of the second week, when, certainly in the milder cases, although the evening temperature may remain quite or nearly so high, there is an abatement of heat of 1° to 2° in the morning. These changes between morning and evening become very

---

* Archiv der Heilkunde, vol. ii., or Edinb. Med. Journ., Nov. 1862; also Die Eigenwärme in der Krankheiten.

evident toward the end of the week, and are still more evident in the third week, when the morning and evening temperatures may vary between 4° to 6°. During this week, too, the evening temperature gradually decreases; but in severe cases it remains high, and there are no decided remissions, either in the second or third week. The morning temperature is high, 104° or more, and there may be still greater heat of skin in the evening, or else it differs but little from that of the morning.

Among the abdominal symptoms, *diarrhœa* is the most prominent. It is never absent, excepting when the disease is unusually mild. Generally, and especially in grave cases, it is a very early symptom. The clue to its cause is found in the state of the abdominal glands; in the enlargement and ulceration of the glands of Peyer, of the solitary glands, and in the tumefaction of the mesenteric glands. And in these morbid alterations, which are so constant in typhoid fever as to constitute its anatomical characteristics, we find not only an explanation of the occurrence of the diarrhœa, but also of its frequency. The stools are thin, of a yellow or dark-brown color, and of offensive smell. When the affection is at its height, from three to four evacuations occur during the twenty-four hours; but the passages may become much more numerous, and with their number the danger rises. If they take place without the knowledge of the patient, his situation is precarious.. Sometimes the stools contain blood. Should this be present in considerable quantity, it is a very unfavorable circumstance. Yet intestinal hemorrhage is by no means necessarily fatal.

Enlargement of the spleen is a very constant attendant upon the fever. In fact, whenever we can be certain that the evident increase in size is not due to some previous malady, the extended percussion dulness in the splenic region becomes an element of importance in our diagnosis.

Another abdominal symptom of significance is *pain*. It varies much in its severity and character; and is, indeed, not always present. It is rarely acute; oftener a heavy, aching feeling. In some patients it is of a griping kind, preceding the loose discharges; in others, it only seems to be called into existence by pressure. Its most common seat is in the iliac fossæ; yet the testimony of the sick man himself as to its exact situation must be received very cautiously. He is too ill to answer intelligently, is apt to reply in the affirmative to any leading question, and thus may be made to say that almost any part hurts him which is touched. Still the expression of suffering on his face, when pressed on either side at the lower part of the abdomen, is strongly indicative of the pain corresponding, for the most part, to the seat of the irritation. And often while the hand is exploring this region, a movement of the fluid and gas in the distended bowel, attended with a gurgling noise, becomes perfectly appreciable. This sign is best elicited near the ilio-cæcal valve, and is full of meaning.

During convalescence, griping pains are not unfrequently complained of. They are colicky pains, produced generally by errors in diet, and may be followed by a return of the diarrhœa or by a relapse of all the other symptoms of the malady. Occasionally—fortunately not often—during such a relapse, or even during the latter period of the fever, a sudden pain sets in, of great intensity, unremitting, and attended by spreading tenderness. Such a pain forebodes evil. It shows that peritoneal inflammation has been lighted up in consequence of the intestine having been perforated.

Hardly inferior to the abdominal symptoms in import—in many respects of even greater significance—are the signs of disturbance of the nervous system. The fever is, as its old name implies, pre-eminently a " nervous" fever: the nervous symptoms are, in truth, never absent; but, though always present, they are less extensive in some cases than in others, and not the same throughout all the stages of the disease. Thus, early in the disorder, dull headache, mental languor, and a perverted state of the senses, such as ringing in the ears and dulness of hearing, are encountered; while later, great restlessness, delirium or coma, and jerking of the tendons are phenomena more likely to be met with. The *delirium* especially requires to be noted. It sets in generally during the second week, for the most part at night, and terminates with convalescence or else ends in coma. It is not a wild delirium, but a confusion of mind associated with rambling thoughts. If the patient's attention be strongly engaged, he may almost always be roused, and does for a time as he is told; but, after a short interval, his muttering lips indicate that some curious fancy has again taken possession of him. In some cases, not in many, the delirium is attended with great restlessness and much agitation, and the sick man, if not prevented, attempts to walk about the room. This kind of frenzy is of bad augury, and often ends in fatal coma. Equally unpromising is early or unremitting delirium.

When contrasted with the mental wandering in other acute disorders, the delirium of typhoid fever exhibits peculiar traits. It is ordinarily more active than that of typhus; far less demonstrative or talkative than the mania of drunkards; as aimless as, but less continued than, the ravings of inflammation of the brain.

In some cases of typhoid fever appear, however, symptoms not only of cerebral, but also of spinal origin; and they may indeed assume a high degree of intensity. We find cutaneous hyperæsthesia, extending over a large portion of the body, spinal pain and tenderness, with a sense of pricking along the vertebral column, and, in some instances, cutaneous and muscular anæsthesia, numbness of the extremities, partial paralysis or convulsive contractions of the respiratory muscles, convulsive cough, paralysis of the sphincters, contractions of the extremities, and even rigidity of the muscles of the neck.* These spinal symptoms are more common when the disease is epidemic than when sporadic, and are always indicative of a very serious form of the disorder. They sometimes persist after the fever has left, or indeed, and this is especially true of paralysis, may not appear until convalescence. The palsy may or may not be linked to an organic lesion. It may be preceded by trembling movements, suggesting the idea of sclerosis of the cord; but the tremor is rather the result of general debility, and, unlike sclerosis, it

---

* Fritz, Etude clinique sur divers Symptomes spinaux observés dans la Fièvre typhoide, referred to in Arch. Génér. de Méd., June, 1864.

occurs before, and does not follow, the complete loss of muscular power in the limbs.

Two other prominent symptoms of the malady must still be inquired into: one is epistaxis; the other, the cutaneous eruption. *Epistaxis* is not often absent in grave cases. It may happen at any period of the complaint; but it is most apt to take place before the disorder is far advanced. The quantity of blood lost is rarely considerable; and for this reason the occurrence of the hemorrhage is frequently overlooked.

The *eruption* which is peculiar to the disease is commonly spoken of as the rose-colored rash. It appears about or shortly after the seventh day; but occasionally not until the end of the second week. It can hardly be called a papular eruption, as it consists rather of small, red spots, only very slightly elevated above the skin, somewhat similar to flea-bites, yet differing from them in lacking the central mark and in their finer, paler color and less obvious outline. The spots are seen upon the abdomen and chest, almost never upon the extremities or upon the face. They disappear totally on strong pressure, yet return immediately when the pressure ceases. They are generally few in number, and not persistent. Each spot does not last for more than three or four days; then it fades, and a fresh one near by replaces it, and runs the same course. Spots thus appear and pass away for more than a week, after which, in most cases, they entirely vanish. During convalescence not a trace of them can be found; but should the patient get up too soon, or be imprudent in his diet, and a relapse take place, they again show themselves with the other symptoms of the malady.

This eruption, although very common, is not invariably present; at all events, it is not invariably found. Beyond doubt, too, it is in some epidemics more constant and marked than in others.

Late in the disease another eruption appears, consisting of very minute transparent vesicles, scattered plentifully over the body. These sudamina are not so frequently encountered as the rose rash, and are certainly not so characteristic; yet they are seen often enough to be regarded as a feature of the affection.

After this analysis of the symptoms of typhoid fever, it would be useless repetition to discuss at length how the disease differs from all other idiopathic fevers. The attempt will rather be made to explain its diagnosis from those maladies, whether essentially febrile or not, to which it bears the closest resemblance. And here we find that the disorders with which typhoid fever may be confounded are, owing to its varying aspect, not the same at all the stages of the complaint. Early in the affection it is most likely to be mistaken for simple continued fever, or for one of the exanthemata. But diarrhœa is not present in these, nor are there marked prodromes; and whatever doubt may exist with reference to simple continued fever, is cleared up in a few days, as the symptoms come to an end at a time at which in typhoid fever they begin to be more and more developed. Still the exanthematous fevers cannot, before their eruptions appear, be distinguished with absolute certainty; though we may suspect measles by the attending coryza, scarlatina by the sore throat, and small-pox by the lumbar pains and high fever.

At a more advanced period, typhoid fever may be confounded with typhus, and with these morbid states:

GENERAL DEBILITY;

TYPHOID CONDITIONS;

ENTERITIS;

PERITONITIS;

MENINGITIS:

ACUTE PULMONARY AFFECTIONS.

General Debility.—It does not at first sight seem very likely that so acute and dangerous a disease as typhoid fever could be mistaken for mere debility; yet such an error may occur where the disease is latent, or so very light as hardly to confine the patient to his bed. In these so-called "walking cases" of the fever, the debility, however, sets in suddenly, and not gradually, as in weakness from general constitutional causes. Moreover, the abdominal symptoms are rarely wanting; and there is always more or less confusion of mind. Due attention to these circumstances will prevent mistake; but the greatest safeguard against error is to be aware that the disease assumes at times a latent form, and to examine every case of great and sudden debility, to see if under its mask are hidden the features of typhoid fever.

Typhoid Conditions.—No blunder is more common than to misconstrue into typhoid fever a typhoid condition of the system. We may find this condition in many different complaints, both acute and chronic; but more especially are purulent infection, some forms of pneumonia, dysentery, and erysipelas attended with delirium, drowsiness, dry, brown tongue, and extreme prostration,—in one word, with a typhoid state.

Yet a typhoid state is not typhoid fever; it is simply a low condition of the system which may be present in very many dissimilar maladies, and which is present in its most perfect form in typhoid fever. But in this malign complaint we have other signs than those of vital depression : we find joined to it diarrhœa, tympanites, epistaxis, an eruption, and special manifestations of disturbance of the nervous system, —all symptoms bearing no direct relation to the adynamia, and thus serving as valuable distinctive marks. An examination, too, of the urine is often of signal service. There are, indeed, cases of Bright's disease and of abscess of the kidney, in which the poisoning of the blood which happens occasions a very deceptive likeness to typhoid fever—so deceptive that only a minute examination of the urine can fully explain the true meaning of the symptoms. The following case well illustrates this :

A man, about forty-five years of age, was admitted into the Philadelphia Hospital in January, 1863. He was very prostrate, and hardly able to give an account of himself. It was, however, ascertained that he was not a person of intemperate habits, and that he had been attending to his work until within two weeks. He was evidently stupid, and, when questioned about himself, seemed to have great difficulty in remembering, and in collecting his thoughts. He had fever; a pulse above 100; a dry brown tongue. The heart sounds were feeble, the heart increased in size. The urine was at times turbid, and contained a slight whitish sediment, which was not, however, examined with the microscope. His mind wandered at night; the abdomen was distended and in parts slightly tender; several doubtful red spots were detected on its surface. In fact, he appeared to have almost every one of the more constant symptoms of typhoid fever, excepting the diarrhœa. A few days after his admission he became comatose, and sank. The intestinal glands were found in a healthy condition; but both kidneys were thoroughly disorganized and filled with pus.

Enteritis.—The great difference between enteritis and typhoid fever consists in this: in enteritis the inflammation of the intestine constitutes the disease; in typhoid fever the irritation of the intestine and morbid alteration of its glands are merely elements of the disease. In enteritis, therefore, there are no further symptoms than those referable to the inflamed intestine. We find no great prostration; no mental wandering; no enlargement of the spleen; no rose spots and sudamina; no signs of abnormal processes due to a typhoid dyscrasia. The disorder, too, gives rise to much more abdominal pain, and is of shorter duration.

Peritonitis.—The same remarks apply to peritoneal inflammation. Here, moreover, the expression of the face, the constipation and the very great abdominal tenderness serve as marks of discrimination. But we must not forget that acute inflammation of the peritoneum may appear in the course of typhoid fever. Generally this untoward event happens at a late period of the disease, and after the patient has been under observation for some time; we are then at no loss to understand the meaning of the spreading tenderness, the rapid, small pulse, the marked tympanitic distention, the sweats, the nausea and vomiting, the collapse, and the pinched features. But the accident may occur in cases which we have not previously seen, or in which the affection has run so latent a course as hardly to have attracted even the patient's attention. The cause of the peritonitis is then commonly first revealed by the autopsy, which shows actual perforation of the intestinal walls, in consequence of ulceration of a solitary or aggregate gland. Whenever, indeed, in typhoid fever the signs of peritonitis can be clearly traced, the exciting cause of the inflammation may be announced to be perforation; for the evidence on which it has been assumed

that peritoneal inflammation may take place without the
giving way of the intestine is not so positive as to cause us
to abandon this diagnostic rule.

Meningitis.—Typhoid fever has some symptoms in common
with inflammation of the brain; but the signs of difference
have been fully discussed in connection with acute and with
crebro-spinal meningitis, and need not here be re-examined.

Acute Pulmonary Affections.—In a large number of cases
of typhoid fever—in fact in the majority—we find cough, dependent upon an affection of the bronchial tubes. The bronchial inflammation, if it really can be called an inflammation, gives rise to the peculiar signs of extreme loudness of
the rales, with a cough disproportionately slight; sometimes,
too, owing to the blood gravitating to the most dependent
portions of the lungs, the resonance over the posterior part
of the chest is impaired. From these phenomena, added to
the abdominal and cerebral symptoms of the fever, there is
no difficulty in discriminating between idiopathic bronchitis
and typhoid fever. Nay, even before the symptoms of the
febrile malady are clearly defined, we may suspect the true
explanation of the rales from the coexisting extreme vital
depression.

Not unfrequently we find pleurisy combined with the
bronchitis, and in some cases, not in very many, the cough
is associated with exudation into the pulmonary structure.
Now, it may be extremely difficult to distinguish a pulmonic
lesion of this kind from inflammation of the lung setting in
amid signs of prostration, until the appearance of the eruption and of the marked abdominal symptoms solves the difficulty. Generally, however, it is not a matter of much doubt,
as the condensation of the lung in typhoid fever does not
occur early in the disease—not, in fact, until the symptoms
of the fever are clearly developed. Occasionally a cough
remains after the febrile symptoms have begun to decline
and the mind is regaining its clearness. The cough increases
in severity, and the patient soon loses the strength he may
have acquired. On listening to the chest, we find scattered
over both lungs many fine, dry and moist sounds. The
percussion note is here and there dull; the expectoration is

profuse; there are dyspnœa and excessive sweating. Here is a group of signs which, if not absolutely, are at least almost invariably, associated with the occurrence of acute phthisis. The further progress of the disease reveals its nature more and more distinctly, and many of the symptoms of the typhoid state reappear. But there is no difficulty in establishing the fact that the formidable complication followed, or was at least fanned into life by, the attack of fever. Sometimes, however, we observe acute phthisis with most of the symptoms of typhoid fever without that affection being really before us: even the delirium, the stupor, and the enlargement of the spleen may be present; but the eruption never is, and the diarrhœa very rarely.

Typhus Fever.—The term typhus is not very definite in its signification. The German, Swedish, Irish, and most of the British physicians comprise under it all low forms of fever, including typhoid. In this country and in France it is applied solely to that low continued fever prevailing in jails and camps, among crowded populations, or in badly-ventilated localities, and which is not characterized by any constant structural lesion. Without entering into the discussion whether or not it ought to be separated from typhoid fever; whether it be, as so many still affirm, nothing but a cerebral form of that same typhous disorder of which typhoid is regarded as the abdominal form, having the same cause, obeying the same laws,—without entering into this vexed question, we cannot but recognize in it many phenomena so different from those of typhoid or enteric fever that, on clinical grounds alone, if on no others, a separate recognition is called for.

Typhus fever very rarely occurs sporadically. It is a highly contagious malady, almost always met with in an epidemic form, and generally among those whose systems are depressed or blood impoverished. It is either preceded by a brief stage of lassitude and dejection, or is ushered in with a chill and pain in the head and back. The skin soon becomes dry and of pungent heat; the pulse rises very much in frequency, and is at first full, sometimes even tense. The patient lies in a state of half consciousness; very dull, very drowsy, very weak, with evident signs of his nervous and muscular system being overwhelmed by the influence of some fearfully depressing poison. The face is flushed; the eye injected; the odor from the body extremely unpleasant.

By the fifth day all these symptoms are plainly marked, and about this time a coarse, red, cutaneous eruption makes its appearance. But it occasions no change in the gravity of the symptoms. On the contrary, the confusion of mind and stupor increase, the patient wanders, picks at his bed-clothes, and ceases to complain of the pain in the head or limbs. The pulse is frequent and feeble; the tongue dry and dark; sordes collect on the gums and teeth. The bowels remain as they were at the onset—constipated. The urine often comes away drop by drop; or, as the bladder loses the power of contracting, is retained. The case has now reached its height; the signs of a prostrated nervous system, of dete-riorated blood, and of utter loss of muscular strength either commence to pass away or deepen from hour to hour, and clearly show the doom that awaits the fever-stricken patient. From the beginning of the distemper until the unfortunate issue, is rarely over thirteen days. If the sick man can with-stand the poison until the third week, he is apt to throw it off and recover; but it may be so virulent as to overpower him almost at the onset.

Let us examine some of the symptoms of this pestilential disease in detail.

The *physiognomy* of typhus is very peculiar. The expres-sion is stupid, and coarser than in health. The face wears a deep flush, of a dusky-red hue. The eye is much injected, the pupil often contracted. The skin is very hot and dry, and covered with a characteristic *eruption*, from which the disease takes its name of "spotted" or "maculated" typhus. The rash is well defined, at first slightly elevated and usually much like that of measles. It is of a dark tint, and fades but does not vanish on pressure. It makes its appearance from the fifth to the seventh day, and is permanent; not consisting of successive eruptions, but of the same spots, which deepen or lighten with the changes in the disease, and do not pass away before the fourteenth day. Each spot thus lasts until recovery or until death, and no new ones show themselves after the second or third day of the rash. They are generally very numerous on the trunk and extremities, but are rarely observed upon the face. Some are much lighter than others, and thus a mottled aspect of the skin is produced, on which Dr. Jenner*—who has described the typhus fever eruption, or, as he calls it, the "mulberry rash," with much fidelity—lays great stress. Sometimes the spots are of purple color and uninfluenced by pressure. These petechiæ are the attendants of the worst forms of the malady.

The different forms of eruption, however, are different in degree rather than in kind. The poison leads to local interference in the capillary circulation, and then to transudation from and rupture of the distended vessels; and it may do this partly in consequence of the vitiation of the blood, partly by its action on the sympathetic nervous system. This is likely the cause of the eruption, and the extent and consequences of the paralysis of the capillaries explain the more or less obvious effect of pressure on the rash in many idiopathic fevers.

The skin of a typhus fever patient is often very sensitive, and, as already stated, generally very hot. In some cases the thermometer indicates a *temperature* of 107°, or more; and most commonly it ranges above 104°. The heat is very sustained: it does not show the marked differences between morning and evening which are observed in typhoid fever: the daily variations to the middle of the second week being rarely 1° Fahr.; and from that time onward the morning abatement does not amount to more than about 1·5°, until the defervescence is reached. The passing away of the high temperature—"the defervescence"—occurs, however, not as in the enteric fever by gradual though more and more evident remissions, but suddenly. Early in, or toward the middle of, the third week, the temperature falls quickly, and for the most part in twenty-four or thirty-six hours a normal standard is reached.

The *cerebral* symptoms of typhus fever are never absent,

---

* Identity or Non-Identity of Typhoid and Typhus Fevers, London, 1850; and Medico-Chirurg. Transacts., vol. xxxiii.

although they vary much both in intensity and character. In some epidemics they constitute the prominent feature of many cases, and dangerous and fatal these cases are apt to be. One of the most striking and frequent proofs of the disturbance of the brain is seen in stupor. The patient's mind seems gone: he lies in a heavy slumber, occasionally muttering some incoherent words; or he is sleepless, his eyes remain wide open, yet he cares nothing for, and takes no notice of, anything going on around him. Either of these states may deepen into coma.

In other cases delirium is the most conspicuous symptom. Now, this delirium rarely sets in before the end of the first week, though it may precede the eruption. In type it is low and muttering, and unaccompanied by great restlessness; or it may be associated with constant movements and trembling of the limbs, or jerking of the tendons,—in fact, with symptoms resembling those designated as hysterical. Sometimes the mental wandering is active and very persistent. The patient tosses about, is constantly talking, and can hardly be restrained from getting out of bed. He has illusions of hearing and of sight; his eyes are injected, the pupils often contracted; there is great headache with intolerance of light. Here we have the true brain typhus, with its formidable cerebral symptoms simulating closely those of idiopathic inflammation of the brain, and differing from them only by their union with a cutaneous eruption, by the dissimilar aspect of the tongue, and the beat of the pulse, which is rarely very full, and never so tense as that of meningitis. Then, the nervous excitement is accompanied, or, at all events, soon succeeded, by greater and more rapid prostration of strength, and is often exchanged far more suddenly for coma than is observed in the meningeal disorder.

The cause of this violent disturbance of the brain is either due to the direct effect of the poison on the nervous centre, or to the impure blood which circulates through it; and however strange it may seem that phenomena so vehement and so like those of true inflammation should not be really owing to this morbid process, yet it is beyond doubt that the signs of the severest nervous derangement in these fevers may coincide with a mere congestion — nay, even with a brain and spinal marrow presenting, to all appearances, a perfectly healthy structure.

These head symptoms of typhus are, as those of enteric fever, sometimes connected with a very noisy, shallow, and irregular respiration. This kind of breathing can be clearly traced to the abnormal state of the nervous system, as no signs of alteration in the lungs coexist. Often, as Dr. Flint* has lucidly pointed out, it is a forerunner of fatal coma. In one case I found the strange phenomenon associated with great distention of the bladder, and subsiding very materially after the introduction of a catheter.

The remarks made with reference to the cerebral phenomena of typhus apply to those cases in which there is no inflammatory disorder within the cranium. But we must not overlook the fact that this may ensue. Such cases are very difficult of recognition. The pulse, as a rule, is slow and irregular, the pupils contracted, there is a frown on the forehead and intense headache, sometimes screaming. Vomiting is not always encountered. We may find with these symptoms acute hydrocephalus, and the morbid appearances may be confined chiefly to the base of the brain.†

The *circulation* in typhus exhibits some peculiarities worthy of note. The pulse, after the disease is fully developed, is generally rapid, and either of moderate volume or feeble. As the disorder advances, and the strength becomes more and more impaired, it rises in frequency, while it diminishes in force. As convalescence is established, it falls; if it remain frequent, this is generally indicative of some concealed visceral disorder, often of a disease of the lungs. It does not always correspond closely with the condition of the heart, so far, at least, as this is revealed by the impulse. The beat may be excited and violent, while the pulse is very weak. At times the cardiac impulse undergoes a singular diminution, and with its change the first sound becomes enfeebled; in fact, it is sometimes almost lost, and only very gradually re-

---

* Clinical Reports on Continued Fever.
† Kennedy, Dublin Quarterly Journal, Feb. 1867.

gains its natural tone. Occasionally, at the height of the disease, it is replaced by a soft, systolic murmur; not here a sign of inflammation, but dependent upon the depraved state of the blood. The sphygmograph may show an improvement in the pulse by demonstrating a slight return of its dicrotism before any improvement can be ascertained by the finger.*

The *urine* is generally high colored at first, but may become very pale as convalescence sets in, depositing an abundance of urates and phosphates. There is an absence of the chlorides, or they are reduced to a trace. The urea, as ascertained by an analysis of Dr. Parkes† in a case in which no medicine was given, is increased, and its augmented excretion is remarkably regular during the height of the malady. Indeed, the increased amount of urea is, as determined by repeated examinations of the urine of typhus fever, very constant, and is a proof of the more active metamorphosis of tissue. During convalescence the urea sinks below the physiological standard, and then gradually rises to it. These observations, however, must be compared with those of Rosenstein,‡ which we have referred to when discussing the chemistry of urea.

Notwithstanding the amount of water drunk, the water passed is lessened, and it would appear to be retained in the system. The urine is apt to contain a large amount of uric acid, and, as a rule, preserves its acidity. In 8 out of 21 cases that I examined during a late epidemic,§ it contained albumen, and this ingredient was only present in the severer cases. In some instances the microscope exhibits in the deposit, besides the salts of the urine, renal as well as vesical epithelium, and tube-casts, either finely granular or hyaline, or epithelial. Very much the same condition of urine as regards most of the constituents is also found in typhoid fever. But the pigment which in typhus fever was detected by Parkes throughout only in small amounts, has in typhoid fever been found to be immensely increased.

The complications encountered during the course of the

---

* Dublin Quarterly Journal, Feb. 1867.
† The Urine in Disease, p. 258
‡ Med. Times and Gazette, 1869.
§ See Am. Journ. of Med. Sci., Jan. 1866.

fever, or during convalescence, are much the same as those of typhoid fever, although they do not in the two diseases occur with equal frequency. We meet with abscesses, with large sloughs on the trunk and extremities, with milk-leg, with erysipelas, with inflammation of the parotid gland, with œdema of the glottis, and with pulmonary troubles. The latter are very common, and mostly very alarming. Sometimes they consist merely in affections of the larger bronchial tubes; but very often we have to deal with a dangerous capillary form of bronchitis, commencing very insidiously, not attended with much cough, and very easily overlooked. A coarse crepitation or fine bubbling sounds are heard over the whole chest, and the respiration is hurried. At times, instead of these signs, or associated with them, may be noticed dulness on percussion and bronchial respiration over the lower lobes of the lungs, depending upon congestion, with consolidation more or less perfect, of the pulmonary tissue. Here is one of the worst of all the complications—a low form of pneumonia. During the last stages of the fever, or after convalescence has set in, acute tubercular deposits occasionally develop themselves in the lungs with the same symptoms as during or subsequent to typhoid fever. One of the most significant signs of this untoward event is the utter want of response of the system to stimulants and tonics.

To discuss now the differential diagnosis of typhus fever. We find various maladies resembling it, but none so closely as typhoid fever. The subjoined table shows both their similarities and their differences:

TYPHOID.	TYPHUS.
Age generally from 18 to 35.	At all ages; often in persons beyond middle life.
Not contagious, or but feebly so; often sporadic.	Highly contagious; generally epidemic.
Attack generally insidious.	Attack generally sudden; no lengthened prodromes.
Duration fully three weeks; very frequently much longer.	Duration somewhat shorter; often not prolonged beyond second week.
Death hardly ever before end of second week; more generally in, or after third week.	Death not unfrequently at end of first week, and often before conclusion of second.

TYPHOID.	TYPHUS.
Cerebral symptoms come on gradually; last longer.	Delirium or decided stupor comes on soon, sometimes almost from the onset; headache has appeared and disappeared by about the tenth day.
Great emaciation.	Less emaciation; greater prostration.
Face pale, or flush confined to cheeks.	Face deeply flushed, of dusky hue; eye dejected.
Skin hot, sometimes covered with acid perspiration.	Skin of pungent heat; sometimes emitting an ammoniacal odor.
Abdominal symptoms, such as diarrhœa, tympanites; intestinal hemorrhage not unusual.	No abdominal symptoms; bowels constipated; meteorism rare; intestinal hemorrhage extremely rare, if it ever occurs; sometimes acute dysentery during convalescence, or as a sequel.
Epistaxis common.	No epistaxis.
Bronchitis and pleurisy.	Pneumonia, or, at all events, more marked intense congestion of the lungs, and bronchitis of finer tubes.
Eruption light red, and not on extremities.	Eruption darker color, and all over body.
Post-mortem appearances are: morbid state of Peyer's patches; enlargement of mesenteric glands; ulceration of mucous coat of intestine; enlargement and softening of spleen; ulceration of pharynx.	No constant post-mortem appearances; the most frequent are the dark-colored, liquid state of the blood, and enlargement of the spleen. Softening of the heart is more common in typhus than in typhoid. There are no intestinal lesions.

The points of contrast between the two affections are here so manifest that it would seem impossible ever to confound them. Yet it must be remembered that all the signs are not present in every case. Nor does this table go to prove anything beyond the clinical distinction between the kindred maladies; certainly not a different cause of production, nor a dissimilar nature. Neither can it be denied that occasionally the symptoms of the two diseases are strangely blended or interchanged. Thus we may have constipation in typhoid, and diarrhœa in typhus, or the eruption may be curiously mixed. For instance:

A boy, sixteen years of age, was received into the Philadelphia Hospital, with evident signs of a commencing fever of a low type. A day or two after his admission, and corresponding, as nearly as could be ascertained, to the fifth day of the disease, an eruption showed itself all over the body. It was dark colored, petechial in its aspect, and did not disappear on pressure. Associated with it were drowsiness and constipation. In a few days more, however, the symptoms changed. The dark eruption faded, and rose-colored spots were perceptible on the chest and abdomen; diarrhœa set in, and the fever ran its course to a favorable termination with the character of typhoid, just as at the onset it had assumed the character of typhus.

Besides typhoid fever, typhus may be confounded with meningitis, with inflammation of the lungs, with measles, with small-pox, and with the plague. The distinctive marks between the first two and typhus fever have been rendered apparent while discussing the cerebral and pulmonary complications of the latter malady. I shall here only dwell again upon the great value of the eruption in a diagnostic point of view. The symptoms which approximate measles, small-pox, and yellow fever to typhus, will be analyzed in connection with these affections. One word here as to its difference from the *plague*.

This pestilent disease, which during several centuries left almost annually its deep indent upon the human race, is hardly known to us at present, save by description. And the descriptions leave on the mind the impression of an exposition of a familiar malady; for the authors who have most carefully delineated its traits have produced a picture which, with very slight changes, may be suited to a representation of epidemics of typhus fever. Thus, we read of a highly contagious fever setting in suddenly, attended with constipation, with a rapid, feeble pulse, with delirium, with a dry tongue, with noises in the ears and deafness, with starting of the tendons, with watchfulness or stupor, and with red patches and purple spots scattered over the whole surface of the body. The features which typhus does not share with the plague are nausea and vomiting, an alarmed, despairing look of the countenance, hæmoptysis, and, above all, the buboes and carbuncles in different parts of the body.

In concluding this description of typhus fever, let us inquire what are its relations to that extraordinary affection which has but comparatively lately been committing such ravages in some of the New England States, in parts of New York, and in Pennsylvania, and with which we have had to contend in this city and its environs—the so-called *spotted fever*.

This malignant complaint is not a new disease; it has prevailed before in this country, and has been sketched by Miner, Hale, Gallup, North, and others, who witnessed it in the New England States, and by Ames, of Montgomery, Alabama. It assumes different forms, according to the organs which bear the brunt of the disturbance. The form which we have had to encounter was the cerebro-spinal: in truth, the phenomena were those of the disease usually called cerebro-spinal meningitis, and the symptoms of which have been described in a previous chapter. Prominent among these symptoms were: intense headache; pains in the back and extremities; restlessness; great prostration of strength; increased cutaneous sensibility; stupor, delirium; irregular pulse; dilated pupils; dimness of sight; nausea and vomiting; hurried, shallow breathing; a feeling of spasmodic constriction of the chest; and throwing back of the head. The urine was high colored, containing large quantities of urates, and often a small amount of albumen; the skin was seldom more than slightly heated, sometimes even cold, and frequently but not invariably the seat of a petechial eruption, usually of purplish color, wholly unchanged by pressure, and appearing ordinarily on the first day of the disease. The affection ran generally a very rapid course. Many died on the third day; some perished in a few hours; occasionally it was protracted for several weeks. Those who survived the fifth or sixth day were apt to recover, and entered on a tedious convalescence.

Now this strange complaint, which, on account of the soreness of the throat which may attend it, was by some believed to be malignant scarlet fever, was by others regarded as modified typhus, and by others again as cerebro-spinal inflammation. That it is the disease described as cerebro-spinal meningitis, or cerebro-spinal typhus, admits now of no doubt. But whether it be a separate disorder, or a mere variety of typhus fever, is a question still at issue. Let us contrast its phenomena with those of this affection, which in many respects it so closely resembles. Both diseases are apt to prevail at the same time ; both attack all classes and ages; both are evidently attended with dissolution of the blood,— but this alteration in the blood occurs much more rapidly and is much more marked in spotted fever than in ordinary cases of typhus;* the eruption is different from that of the common form of typhus; there is less delirium; a less intense fever; the affection is of much shorter duration, and not nearly so contagious, if in truth we can regard as proved that it is contagious at all; the countenance is not of a dusky hue and stupid, but pale or of a sallow color, and dull or expressive of suffering. And certainly, whether or not spotted fever be a peculiar form of typhus, clinically its manifestations are very dissimilar to those of the usual varieties of this complaint. But they are not so dissimilar to those occurring in some epidemics of malignant cerebral typhus which have been described. Indeed, while fully admitting that we cannot, from the evidence in our possession, as yet decide with certainty on spotted fever being merely modified typhus, and developed by the same poison, a larger experience with the disease than I had when this work was first published, makes me adhere still more decidedly to the opinion that it is not an inflammation, but a fever of a typhous type, a cerebrospinal fever, kindred, to say the least, to typhus fever.†

---

* The deterioration of the blood occurs, indeed, very soon in spotted fever. In an autopsy of a child who died in twenty-four hours, I found the blood diffluent and black ; in an adult patient who had been sick but two days, I detected blowing sounds in the heart, evidently of blood origin. The poisoned blood unquestionably gives rise to many of the nervous symptoms, and it is on the blood and the nervous centres that the poison mainly acts. In this respect the malady is very like typhus fever. In fact, I think it may be designated as a fever of a typhous type, varying somewhat in its manifestations, according as the nervous centres, the intestinal tract, or the lungs are chiefly attacked.—*Note to first edition.*

† An extraordinary case, bearing on the relationship of the complaints under discussion, was under my charge in 1865 at the Pennsylvania Hospital : see case xii. of a series of typhus fever cases, published in Amer. Journ. of Med. Sci., Jan. 1866. For accounts of the late epidemic, consult the observations of Dr. Upham, in the Boston Med. and Surg. Journ., vol. lxviii.,

Relapsing Fever.—This is a form of fever characterized by its rapid course and its proneness to relapse. Epidemics of this disease—and it only occurs in epidemics—are frequently encountered in Ireland and in Scotland. In this country it was, until lately, almost unknown.

The disorder is decidedly acute. Its invasion is sudden, and marked by rigors, pain in the back and limbs, vertigo, severe headache, and nausea and vomiting. Fever is soon developed, and rises high; there are severe muscular pains, particularly in the muscles of the extremities; the pulse is very rapid; the temporal arteries throb; the tongue is covered with a thick, white fur. The bowels are, as a rule, constipated. In many cases there is engorgement of the liver with yellowness of skin; in nearly all epigastric tenderness and marked enlargement of the spleen. The matter ejected from the stomach is greenish, or sometimes black and like coffee-grounds. Minute points of extravasated blood are not uncommonly observable upon the integument. On the fifth or seventh, though sometimes not until the tenth day, the symptoms subside as speedily as they have set in, a profuse perspiration preceding their decided abatement. Convalescence is now apt to be rapid, and apparently complete, the patient being up and going about; but the intermission does not last long. Ordinarily after a week, therefore on the twelfth or fourteenth day from the first beginning, sometimes sooner, rarely later, the attack returns, presenting again the same signs, and again terminating by a critical sweat in convalescence. This second attack may be short and mild; but it may be both longer and of graver character than the first. It is, at times, followed by another, and yet another relapse.

1863; the communications of Drs. Gerhard, Jewell, and others, in the Transactions of the Phila. College of Physicians, Am. Journ. of Med Sci., 1864 and 1865; the Publications of the Massachusetts Medical Soc., vol. ii.; also Dr. Stillé's monograph on Epidemic Meningitis; Dr. Githens, Amer. Journ. Med. Sci., July, 1867, and various papers, by Dr. Liddell and others, published in the same journal. To contrast our epidemic with that in Great Britain and on the Continent, see discussions and papers by Murchison, Sanderson and others, in Med. Times and Gazette, London Lancet, and Med. Press and Circular, of the past few years; and Reports in Brit. and For. Med.-Chirurg. Rev., Oct. 1868, and in Dub. Quart. Journ., Aug. 1868; Ziemssen and Heis, in Archiv fur Klin. Med., Bd. i., and Klebs, Virchow's Archiv, 1865.

When the patient finally throws off the disease, he is very weak, and his blood is much impoverished. He shows a tendency to dropsy of the extremities; and blowing murmurs, evidently not organic, are perceptible while listening to the heart. These murmurs, however, may also be heard during the paroxysms. Is the patient really well during the intermission? He appears so, yet his spleen remains enlarged, the pulse is apt to be slow, the action of the heart weak, and the arthritic pains do not entirely disappear.

Relapsing fever has an intimate connection with destitution. It is contagious, but far from a very fatal disorder. In fatal cases death sometimes happens during the first paroxysm as the result of syncope, of hemorrhage into the brain, or from the lungs; or it may occur suddenly during the intermission from paralysis of the heart. But the most common termination of the cases having an unfavorable issue is in consequence of states which have been induced by the malady, such as lobular inflammation of the lung, abscess of the spleen or kidney, chronic diarrhœa, dropsy, parotitis, palsies. At times the patient perishes in a condition similar to the collapse of cholera, though the collapse is more protracted and the pulse can be felt, and discharges from the bowels are by no means a constant accompaniment. The extreme prostration, attended with great coldness of the skin, may last for days. It is more particularly met with in the "bilious" or "bilious typhoid" form of the malady—a very dangerous variety in which severe vomiting, jaundice, and delirium are encountered, and the paroxysm is not followed by a distinct intermission or remission, but often by the signs of collapse alluded to, and in which uræmic symptoms have been more particularly noticed.* The collapse, however, may happen not only at the close of the paroxysm, but in the remission, whether this be distinct or not, or in a subsequent paroxysm; and this may be the case no matter what variety of the disorder we have to deal with, and whether or not the grave symptoms are due to uræmia.

Yet it will be probably found that the state of the kidneys

---

* Hermann, Account of St. Petersburg Epidemic; Schmidt's Jahrb., No. 6, 1865; see also further observations in Meissner's article, ib., No. 2, 1870.

and of the urinary secretion has very commonly a great deal to do with the graver phenomena of the malady. Acute renal disease with albumen and tube-casts in the urine was discerned by Obermeier* in two-thirds of his cases; and as regards the urine, Riesenfeld† found that the urea during the first paroxysm was always increased, and that this increase continued beyond the crisis. The products of the heightened tissue metamorphosis may be retained, and thus grave symptoms arise.

There is no constant lesion in relapsing fever, unless it be the lesion in the spleen. This organ is enlarged, and presents numerous round or irregularly shaped bodies, of white or yellowish-white color.‡

The description of the malady has been chiefly taken from the epidemics which have been commented on by Jenner, Lyons, and Murchison. But we have lately had relapsing fever both in New York and Philadelphia; and I have encountered the disorder. Its features have appeared to me much the same as in the epidemics already described; and this, to judge from the interesting lectures of Dr. Alonzo Clark,§ is also the case with the fever as met with in New York.

The diagnosis of the malady cannot be made positively during the primary seizure. Yet the presence of the fever, while an epidemic prevails, may be suspected from the sudden fierce beginning of the attack; and the fact of the high fever heat of 104° to 107° C. showing itself in less than twenty-four hours, and exhibiting but little difference between morning and evening, until the rapid and great fall which takes place at the crisis; and the character of the gastric symptoms. Relapsing fever resembles yellow fever in its short duration and in some of its manifestations; but there is this evident difference; in yellow fever the remission constitutes part of the paroxysm, the symptoms do not subside nearly as completely, nor does the black vomit come on until the stage of collapse is reached.

---

* Virchow's Archiv, 1869., Bd. xlvii., quoted in Glasgow Med. Journal, Nov. 1869.

† Ib., quoted ib.   ‡ Pastau, ib., quoted ib.

§ Medical Record, March, 1870.

From typhoid and typhus fevers, relapsing fever may be distinguished by the shorter prodromes, the presence of jaundice, which hardly ever occurs in these maladies, and by the very brief period during which the symptoms last. Again, critical sweats with the rapid cessation of the fever are not likely to be seen in these disorders, certainly not in typhoid fever; and the intense continuous febrile heat, as indicated by the thermometer, the severe muscular and arthritic pains, and in some cases the early collapse without apparent cause are characteristic; and, on the other hand, delirium and stupor are very rarely encountered in relapsing fever. After the relapse has taken place, the diagnosis is easy, if the case have been watched during the first attack. But should it not have been under notice before, it may be at times very difficult, if not wholly impossible, to say whether we are dealing with relapsing fever or with that rare condition, a relapse of typhoid or typhus fever. And this difficulty is enhanced by the want of uniformity of the symptoms in the second onset of the strangely recurring malady, and the close similarity they occasionally show to those of typhoid or of typhus fever. Another difficulty, too, is presented by the fact that relapsing fever may exhaust itself in the first paroxysm. But this is a very unusual occurrence.

In looking at the different forms of continued fever which have just been passed in review, we cannot help being struck with the many features which they possess in common. They are nearly all apt to occur as epidemics or endemically. They are nearly all more prevalent in densely-populated parts of the country, or among masses of men, than in localities where the population is scattered. They all exhibit a strong disposition to run a certain well-defined course before terminating. In truth, it is very doubtful whether any medical means can cut short this course; for a specific treatment for any of the forms of continued fever, by which they may be controlled with the same readiness as the malarial fevers, has not yet been discovered. But we can accomplish much by seeking to remove all sources of irritation, and by close attention to the complications which arise. In simple fever we materially aid the system in throwing off the morbid matter by stimulating the secretions; in the low forms of fever we interpose, by art, to prevent the disease from undermining, step by step, the vital powers. The greatest peril in these fevers is generally from exhaustion. Usually, if that can be guarded against, the malady is nearly conquered. To use the forcible words of Stokes:* "In a disease which is under the control of the mysterious law of periodicity, every hour of compelled life is a clear gain."

Periodical Fevers.

These fevers are characterized by the distinct periodicity of their phenomena: they exhibit intervals during which the patient is wholly or nearly free from febrile disturbance. With the exception of one (and its place here is, indeed, doubtful), they are all owing to that poison, so prolific of disease, termed marsh miasm or malaria, of the intimate cause of which as yet we know, unfortunately, nothing more definite than that heat and moisture, and probably vegetable decomposition, are essential to its production. This noxious agent gives rise to a group of fevers, ever betraying their common origin by their strong family resemblance: alike in occurring in low, swampy localities; alike in most of their symptoms, and in the difficulty of eradication from the system; alike in the secondary lesions, in the enlargement of the spleen and of the liver, and in the altered condition of the blood, which they leave behind them; and also alike in being under the control, absolute and immediate, of cinchona in its various preparations.

Along with the forms of miasmatic fever, I shall describe yellow fever; not because I believe it to be of identical nature, but on account of the similarity of the prominent symptoms.

Intermittent Fever.—The phenomena presented by an attack of intermittent fever are so well understood, that a short general description of them will be sufficient.

The paroxysm comes on with a chill: the face becomes pale, the lips bluish; the teeth chatter; the skin is cold to

---

* Clinical Lectures on Fevers, London Med. Times and Gazette, 1854.

the touch; there is generally a feeling of uneasiness and fatigue. After a period varying commonly from half an hour to an hour, this cold stage passes off. Now we find decided heat of the surface, with restlessness, thirst, a full, rapid pulse, muscular pains, a scanty secretion of urine; in other words, active febrile symptoms. These continue for hours, for a period always much longer than the first stage: then a sweat breaks out all over the body; the pulse becomes softer and less frequent; the secretions are fully re-established; and this sweating stage terminates the paroxysm.

The patient is now for the time being well; but the disease soon recurs: in from twenty-four to seventy hours the paroxysm repeats itself. In the former case we call the fever a *quotidian;* in the latter, a *quartan.* The *tertian* type is before us when the paroxysm sets in again in about forty-eight hours; the *double tertian,* when we find a daily attack, but those of alternate days alone corresponding in time and severity. The period between the ending of one attack and the beginning of another is spoken of as the *intermission* or *apyrexia;* while the time between the beginning of the two paroxysms, including the first with its succeeding intermission, is called the *interval.*

The varied types of the fever present marked differences in the character and duration of the several stages. The tertian has generally the longest hot, the quartan the longest cold stage. In the quotidian there is a very short cold stage, followed by a hot stage which may last for upwards of fifteen hours. Occasionally the stages are very irregular and anomalous. Thus, the sweating stage may precede the cold stage, or it may be the only one which shows itself; or, again, the rigor may be altogether wanting. Sometimes there are no distinct stages; but the patient has a "dumb ague," which manifests itself at definite periods by a feeling of great depression, or a severe pain at some portion of the body, or by chilly sensations, or headache, or by nausea and vomiting, or, as I have seen in one instance, by excruciating pain over the kidneys, and almost entire suppression of urine.

Now, cases of this kind are difficult to distinguish from organic disease. We can only do so by laying stress on their strictly periodical nature; by noting that the curious manifestations cease entirely to recur with intensity. This does not happen where the symptoms are not caused by a lurking malarial poison: for idiopathic disorders exhibit the phenomena of structural change or of deranged function at all times; not merely on certain days or at certain hours. It is true that, among the inhabitants of miasmatic districts, some complaints, and particularly those of the nervous system, display a well-defined periodicity; but here, too, are found the significant traits of organic or functional disturbance between the decided exacerbations of the symptoms.

Then again we must remember that diseases may assume an apparently intermittent character, being worse every second day, and yet not be malarial at all. Even mania, as Schroeder van der Kolk tells us, may take this type. The whole aspect of the symptoms and a tentative treatment with quinine will help to inform us as to the true nature of the malady.

The temperature in intermittent fever shows a peculiar record, and one which, in doubtful cases, may be turned to great advantage. Notwithstanding the marked sense of chilliness, the thermometer rises suddenly and rapidly to a high degree. Even during the decided chill of the beginning of the paroxysm, it indicates 105° or more. But with the ending of the paroxysm, it is found that the fall has been equally rapid. In the interval it marks about a normal heat; rising quickly with each paroxysm. No other malady presents these variations.

The diagnosis of an ordinary and regular intermittent is easy. Leaving the other malarial fevers out of consideration, only two morbid states present recurring rigors and febrile excitement, and are, therefore, apt to be confounded with it: hectic fever and chills attending upon suppuration in deep-seated parts. Now, hectic fever differs in this from an intermittent: it is simply a fever of irritation, the cause of which a careful scrutiny will generally detect. We find it accompanying many chronic diseases in which destruction of tissue occurs, especially phthisis; and the chronic affection has its own signs, which exist at all times, whether the symptomatic fever be present or not. Then its outbreaks are irregular. Several often take place within the twenty-four hours; their intermissions are incomplete; the temperature does not fall as in intermittent fever, for there is not complete defervescence; and although the paroxysms may commence with chilliness, they are not ushered in by a well-defined rigor. Further, they are apt to be morning paroxysms, and are not modified by antiperiodics. Whenever, indeed, we find an intermitting fever not influenced by these agents, it ought to arouse suspicion, and all the internal organs, particularly the lungs, should be carefully explored. Thus, and thus only, can serious errors in diagnosis be positively guarded against.

When pus forms, and especially when it forms in internal cavities, it betrays its presence by rigors, followed by more or less fever. But these, unlike the chills of ague, do not repeat themselves at definite periods. Moreover, in the midst of the apparent intermission, febrile signs or other manifestations of a seriously disordered system may be discovered. The chills of ordinary pyæmia are distinguished by the same phenomena; then the rigors, unlike the malarial malady, are often characterized by the profuse sweating which immediately follows them rather than by an active development of the fever.

An affection which on account of the chill succeeded by fever might be mistaken for the malarial disorder is the curious so-called *urethral fever* which sometimes arises after the passage of a bougie, and which may even terminate in death.* Our knowledge of the introduction of the instrument and the non-recurrence at a fixed time of the rigor and febrile phenomena furnish the points of distinction.

Yet another affection liable to be mistaken for intermittent fever is *syphilitic fever*. The fever may occur in attacks consisting of a chill, followed by a hot stage and sweating, and be so similar to the malarial disorder as to lead to error.† The apparent ague fits happen, however, toward

---

* Roser, quoted in Brit. and For. Med.-Chirurg. Review, Oct. 1867.

† See cases of Bassereau, referred to by Bumstead in his Treatise on Venereal Diseases.

evening, and are succeeded or accompanied by severe headache and pains in the bones,—in fact, by the same symptoms
as the more ordinary form of syphilitic fever. In the form in
which the febrile symptoms are continuous, these generally
precede the eruption for a week or more, and may continue
after this appears.

Remittent Fever.—This is a fever pre-eminently of hot
climates and malarial districts. It is the fever of Hungary,
of the Pontine Marshes, and particularly of Africa and the
southern portion of the North American Continent. Occasionally, not often, we meet with it in winter and in early
spring; very generally, during the summer and autumn
months.

Remittent fever has no well-defined and constant prodromic
symptoms, excepting, perhaps, a singular sense of gastric
uneasiness. It is ushered in by a marked chill, soon succeeded by violent fever, which, after a varying period, decreases, and then breaks out again. By this time the symptoms of the disease are very apparent. The patient complains
of pain, of fulness and throbbing in his head. He is restless
and distressed; his limbs ache; his tongue has become coated;
he suffers from thirst, and rejects the contents of the stomach.
After continuing at their height from six to eighteen hours,
these symptoms again subside: a sweat breaks out all over
the body; the irritability of the stomach lessens; the patient
is composed, even cheerful; his headache has nearly ceased;
and he falls into a quiet slumber. But this lull is not of long
duration. Soon the fever is rekindled: the skin is as hot and
dry as before; the pulse as full, frequent, and hard; and the
other symptoms return with increased intensity, again to
abate, again to recur, until either the exacerbations are
effaced and the fever assumes a continued type, or else the
remissions become better and better defined,—more, indeed,
like intermissions than remissions.

The average duration of the fever, unless protracted by
complications, is about nine days. Its most common type
is the double tertian; the exacerbations of alternate days
corresponding in severity, duration, and even in the nature
of the symptoms.

The urine in remittent fever presents much the same changes, though in a different degree, as those occurring in intermittent fever. Its color is much deeper and its acidity greater, but during convalescence the urine passed rapidly becomes alkaline, throwing down the most abundant deposit of phosphates. During the active stages of the fever, there is an increase of urea, not simply above the standard of health, but even above that in intermittent fever; and this increase of urea during the fever is attended with a diminution of uric acid—unlike what happens during the paroxysm of ague—and of the coloring and extractive matters; while, as convalescence sets in, the urea decreases in amount, and the other ingredients mentioned increase.* A copious deposit of urates, forming with the phosphates as it were a critical discharge, is noticed as the fever subsides, and is analogous to what takes place after the paroxysm in intermittent fever. At no stage does the urine contain albumen, as it often does in typhus, and so very generally in yellow fever.

Remittent fever is readily recognized: the rise and fall of its febrile signs are too striking to escape observation. Its characteristic traits are more closely allied to those of intermittent fever than to those of any other disorder. But there are these points of contrast: in intermittent fever, each paroxysm begins with a chill, which is not the case in remittent fever; for after the first paroxysm there is rarely a marked chill, and even the chill ushering in the disease is usually not violent. After each febrile exacerbation comes an abatement,—not an intermission, for the fever does not wholly leave; the tongue remains coated, and the gastric derangement does not entirely cease; the patient is not well, as after a fit of ague. The symptoms grow and decline; they do not appear and disappear.

Owing to the presence of jaundice in many cases of bilious remittent fever, the disease is often mistaken for acute congestion of the liver. Here, again, the exacerbations and remissions serve as distinguishing marks; and so, too, in

---

* Joseph Jones, Observations on Malarial Fever. Extr. from the Transact. of the Am. Med. Association.

separating the gastric complications of bilious remitting fever from acute gastric inflammation. The severe headache is also a distinctive feature of value.

Under ordinary circumstances, there is very little likelihood of confounding with each other typhoid and remittent fevers. The lines between the two diseases are too strongly drawn : no marked periodicity exists in typhoid fever, and, on the other hand, we find no diarrhœa, no eruption, no thoracic symptoms, no deafness, and no very great prostration in remittent fever. But instances are met with in which the diagnosis is not easy, because the symptoms of the two mala-. dies are blended. Thus, in a typhoid fever occurring in a malarious region there are often distinct exacerbations and remissions obscuring the real ailment. The malarial influence has set its stamp on the disease, and may for several days completely veil it; but soon its real nature becomes manifest. The great weakness; the low delirium; the tympanitic abdomen; the thin passages, so unlike the dark, hard stools of remittent fever,—all unfold to the careful physician the true character of the disease before him. Sometimes a certain periodicity is witnessed in typhoid fever as it is approaching a favorable termination. The skin becomes hot every afternoon or evening, while it is cool during the night or in the morning. Here a knowledge of the previous history of the case guards against error.

Not unfrequently, after an attack of remittent fever has lasted for ten or twelve days, these symptoms are noticed: great muscular debility, jerking of the tendons, picking at the bedclothes, dark, dry tongue, and weak pulse. The fever becomes of a continued type, and the whole aspect of the malady is now that of a typhoid disease. It is these cases which have given rise to the opinion that bilious fever often changes into typhoid fever. But in reality it is not so much the peculiar specific typhoid fever, with its enteric lesions, as a typhoid condition, that is ordinarily developed. The abdominal signs are not encountered, nor do we find an eruption, and there is very rarely persistent diarrhœa.

During the exacerbations of remittent fever, the cerebral symptoms are sometimes almost identical with those of idio-

pathic inflammation of the brain. There is severe headache, with violent beating of the arteries of the neck and
face, a wild eye, intolerance of light, and even delirium.
Were the patient now seen for the first time, he would be at
once pronounced to be laboring under acute meningitis, and
probably be bled and freely purged,—a treatment which, fortunately, is of advantage to him. Suddenly the pulse loses
its throbbing character, a perspiration covers the surface,
and, as if by magic, the cerebral disturbance ceases until the
next paroxysm redevelops it.

Cases of this kind are readily enough recognized, if we
know something of their history. If we are not familiar
with it, we have to await the remission for their explanation;
and after the sudden withdrawal of the signs of disorder of
the brain, it is hardly possible to have doubts as to the meaning of the acute nervous symptoms, should they recur. It
cannot be a meningitis we are dealing with,—a steady, progressing disease, and one never exhibiting such strange
freaks of intermission. But occasionally the symptoms show
themselves under circumstances where a malarial poison is
not suspected to be at work.

A young gentleman, of studious habits, while diligently
preparing for a college examination, was seized with violent
headache and fever. The sense of fulness in the head was
unbearable, the fever was high, there was nausea with great
gastric irritability. These symptoms lasted for nearly twenty-
four hours, and then subsided in the forenoon, to become
aggravated in the evening. Delirium followed by great
drowsiness was perceived at an early hour of the third day
of the disease. The case now assumed a very alarming
aspect. Local blood-letting was resorted to with some relief,
and in a few hours the symptoms were, fortunately, favorably
modified: the headache was much less, the mind was again
quite clear. Although the patient had never suffered from a
malarial fever, he had spent part of his summer vacation in
the marshy neighborhood of Washington; but several
months had elapsed, and winter was setting in. The time
of the year, therefore, and his immediate occupations rather
favored the view of an inflammation of the brain. But the

evident remission in the cerebral symptoms, the coated state of the tongue, and that indescribable malarial look of the countenance, which became daily more apparent, decided me upon administering quinine,—a course which, under other conditions, would have been very injudicious. The evening exacerabation came, but was far less severe. The nature of the case was now evident; the quinine treatment was vigorously pursued, and the patient soon recovered.

The violent headache and delirium were in this case observed to be in connection with well-defined febrile signs. Occasionally one or both of the symptoms mentioned last during the remission, while the fever abates. I have even met with them occurring in paroxysms without fever being present, as in the following case:

A young lady of delicate constitution was attacked, in September, with remittent fever. The disease ran its course without any unusual symptoms; a violent headache, but little if any wandering of the mind, being observed during the daily exacerbations. After the tenth day, the fever lessened, and the disease assumed a continued type; but very soon afterward, every evening for three days, between five and six o'clock, a boisterous delirium set in, lasting for three or four hours, and once nearly all night. It was followed by a profound sleep, from which she woke up with a clear mind. Strange to say, during these fits the pulse was not accelerated, and there was no heat of skin. The third attack was not so very severe, as the patient was already in part under the influence of decided doses of quinine; the fourth was, I am sure, prevented by this drug.

In both these cases the symptoms approached those of the congestive type of the disease, and the issue appeared at one time doubtful. Generally speaking, remittent fever, unless it be of the congestive variety, has a favorable prognosis. It is difficult for us, living in a century in which the remarkable effects of bark are so well understood, to believe that the complaint was once so fatal, and that so many deaths should have taken place from a disorder over which we now exercise so undoubted a control. But the long list of distinguished names that have fallen victims to it, and among them we find Cromwell, James I., and the Emperor Charles V.,* proves the medical skill of former times to have been iusufficient for its cure. In our day, the consequences of remittent fever are more to be dreaded than the disease itself. We often find, as its sequelæ, most obstinate intermittents, enlargement of the liver and spleen, dropsy, protracted auæmia, headache, and impaired activity of mind.

And it is in this malarial cachexia that, on pricking the finger and examining a drop of the blood thus obtained, we are apt to detect a large number of those particles and masses of black or dark color and irregular shape to which Frerichs has so particularly called attention. Not that the pigment matter is merely found in the cachexia following remittent fever. We observe it in the blood in the severer forms of any malarial disease; and it is very probable that the spleen is the principal seat of its formation, and that it is chiefly derived from a destruction of the red globules. The pigment is in great part carried from the spleen to the liver, where it remains; or it passes through this viscus to the lungs, brain, and kidneys. The clogging of the coarser fragments in the capillaries of the liver may, as Frerichs suggests, by interference with the portal circulation, explain the intestinal hemorrhage and diarrhœa which attend some severe cases of remittent fever; while the cerebral phenomena or albuminuria, hæmaturia, or suppression of urine may also be caused by retention of pigment, in the one case in the capillaries of the brain, in the other of the Malpighian bodies. Thus, then, would be solved some of the anomalous symptoms of malarial fevers. But the abundance of pigment does not occur in all; and whether a peculiar quality or an unusual intensity of the miasm produces it, is undetermined. In a diagnostic point of view, though from the very evident grayish or ash-colored hue of the skin, and the singular character of the symptoms, we may suspect that we have to deal with the

---

* From the record of the Emperor's sickness, as given by the historian Mignet (Charles V. au Monastère de Yuste), we may learn, what fortunately now we hardly have an opportunity of observing, the features of remittent fever when left to itself.

pathological state under discussion, yet we cannot be sure of it until we have examined the blood microscopically. And here, too, it seems to me that the question of the amount of pigmentary matter present must not be overlooked. For pigment may be found in the blood of those who never, to their knowledge, have had intermittent fever, and who certainly present no signs of malarial poisoning.*

FIG. 45.

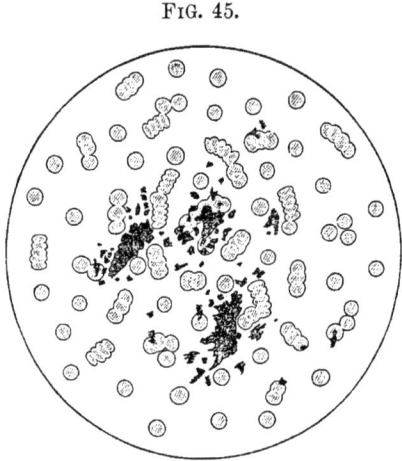

A drop of blood taken from the finger of a man the subject of malarial cachexia. The granules of pigment, as well as the larger fragments of irregular form, are seen among the blood globules. The pigment was for the most part black; some of the particles were reddish brown.

Another test of malaria has been recently proposed. Since the discovery of Bence Jones of the existence in animal textures of a substance resembling quinia, the diminution of this "animal quinoidine" has been thought to occur in malarial disease. The interesting experiments of Rhoads and Pepper† strongly favor, indeed, this view; though we cannot as yet regard the matter as settled, since it has been stated‡ that the fluorescent substance is introduced in the food taken, and is rapidly excreted. The more rigid diet of fever patients

---

* This whole subject has been recently most thoroughly investigated by my colleague Dr. J. F. Meigs. See Pennsylvania Hospital Reports, vol. i., 1868.
† Pennsylvania Hospital Reports, 1868.
‡ Chalvet, Gaz. Hebd., v. 1868.

might thus explain the apparently abnormal decrease of the animal quinoidine.

In children, a fever of remittent type is observed, the nature of which has been a subject of the gravest controversy. By some it is ascribed to the irritation of worms; by others it is regarded as only a variety of the ordinary malarial fever. Now, there can be little doubt that what is called *infantile remittent* is rarely a miasmatic disorder. It is often a gastro-enteritis connected with verminous irritation, or produced by errors in diet; or a typhoid fever,—an affection which now and then occurs, even in very young children. What has given rise to this confusion is, that all febrile diseases in children exhibit a much greater periodicity than in adults, and in all cerebral symptoms are apt to be present. To distinguish the two maladies alluded to from true remittent fever, we must study particularly their manner of commencement and probable origin, and note the peculiarities of the abdominal symptoms. Then we may lay stress on the irregular mode and unequal duration of the febrile exacerbations. Sometimes, also, by close scrutiny, the characteristic eruption of a low continued fever may be found in an apparent remittent.

But some of these cases of remittent fever are really of malarial origin; even in very young children this may be their source. I saw, for instance, some years ago, a little girl, three years of age, who had a distinctly malarial remittent fever, which was checked by antiperiodics. During the violent exacerbations she was very delirious; her face had a most anxious, frightened look; her screams could be heard all over the house. In the remissions she was perfectly sensible, but there was gastric irritability, and the bowels were very constipated.

Congestive Fever.—This is a malignant, destructive, malarial fever, which may be either of the intermittent or remittent form. The pernicious attacks are of the tertian or quotidian type. While they are at their height, there is intense congestion of one or several internal organs, and with the abnormal condition of the circulation a dangerous perversion of the function of innervation is associated. From

48

this state the patient may rally, but only to fall a victim to another paroxysm, unless art intervenes to shield him from his doom.

The symptoms of this violent malady vary according to the organ more specially disturbed, and to the extent of the derangement of the nervous system. We have, thus, several distinct varieties, of which I shall describe the most prominent.

The *gastro-enteric* form is very common in our Southwestern States. Its distinctive features are nausea and vomiting, purging of thin discharges mixed with blood, intense thirst, and an equally intense desire for air. There is little abdominal pain or tenderness, but a weak, frequent pulse and very great restlessness. The patient complains of a sense of sinking and of weight, and of burning heat in the stomach. His breathing is deep drawn; to each expiration succeed two short inspirations. The face, hands, and feet are pale and cold; the features shrunken. Sometimes these symptoms continue for several days, and gradually increase in intensity, in spite of nature making several efforts at reaction. More frequently reaction does take place; the skin becomes hot, the pulse feeble, and the stormy symptoms subside or wholly yield until another outbreak, which is very apt to be deadly, occurs. The usual length of the fatal paroxysm is stated by Dr. Parry,* in his short but interesting sketch of the disease, to be from three to six hours.

The *thoracic* variety of the malady is often combined with the one just described. Its most characteristic trait is violent dyspnœa, caused by overwhelming congestion of the lungs. It is, perhaps, the most rapidly destructive of all the forms of the disastrous affection.

In the *cerebral* variety there is intense congestion of the brain; and sometimes effusion of serum into the ventricles takes place, or even rupture of the blood-vessels. The abnormal state of the brain manifests itself either by coma or by delirium. In the former case, there is usually preceding stupor with occasional delirium; the pulse is slow and full;

---

* Amer. Journ. of the Med. Sciences, July, 1843.

the face dull, and either flushed or livid; indeed, some of the symptoms which are observed in apoplexy show themselves. When, on the other hand, delirium is marked, we have much the same morbid phenomena as in acute meningitis: the patient is wild; he sings, he cries. He may die in this state without coma supervening; but a comatose condition generally succeeds rapidly to the fierce excitement. Should recovery take place, the delirium gradually ceases.

Another variety much dwelt upon by authors is the so-called *algid* form. This is not often seen in this country; I abridge Maillot's* description of it as he noticed it in Corsica and Algeria. The disease is more than a mere continuation of the cold stage of a paroxysm; most commonly the characteristic symptoms manifest themselves during the period of reaction. The pulse slackens, and finally ceases; the extremities, face, and trunk become in succession rapidly cold. There is no thirst; the skin feels like marble; the breath is cold; the voice broken. The mind is clear; the expression of the countenance impassive, and like that of a dead man. There may be vomiting and choleraic discharges. These symptoms go on steadily toward death, unless decided reaction be brought about.

Now, in none of these forms of congestive fever is the first paroxysm apt to be of a pernicious character. In the majority of instances the disease begins as ordinary periodic fever; and it is only in the second or third paroxysm that the alarming symptoms appear. Nor is the first congestive paroxysm very likely to prove mortal; generally it is not until the second or third that a fatal issue is to be apprehended. But this is no excuse for neglecting to provide for the patient's safety by the promptest treatment. Indeed, whenever we are dealing with a periodical fever in districts where intermittents or remittents are known to assume a malignant form, we must be constantly on the lookout for the possibility of their becoming of the pernicious type. Proper watchfulness will sometimes detect, even at the onset of the attack, by the unusual prolongation

---

* Traité des Fièvres Intermittentes. Paris, 1836.

of the cold stage, or by irregularity of the pulse, by the great sensitiveness in the splenic region and by the pain pressure there may occasion all over the body, or by an imperfect hot stage, or by the feeling of internal heat while the surface is really cold, the danger that is approaching, and arrest its further steps by the bold use of antiperiodics.*

The cause of this desperate disease is evidently a highly active malarial poison; and once in the system, it remains for a long time. Thus, should the patient even weather the first attack completely, he is not wholly out of danger; for he has not entirely gotten rid of the morbific influence. He may have a second seizure quite as dangerous within the same season.

Before proceeding to the discussion of another subject, I shall here devote a few pages to the consideration of some of the irregular forms and modifications of malarial poisoning, and to its share in producing febrile disorders of blurred and uncertain type. Practically, this is of very great importance, and specially of importance to American physicians.

In the first place, I shall speak of the chronic malarial poisoning so often seen among inhabitants of malarial districts. It manifests itself by lassitude, debility, torpor of the liver, and enlargement of the spleen. The stools are often black, the digestion is impaired, the complexion sallow. Occasionally attacks of jaundice occur, which rather relieve than aggravate the unhealthy state of the system. Sometimes the noxious influence shows itself in another way: the patient is seized with nausea, and gastric irritability so great that almost everything he takes is instantly rejected. The tongue is coated, the skin dryish; but he has little if any fever. The bowels are confined, the urine is turbid. He is restless, and as weak as if he had typhoid fever; but he has neither an eruption nor diarrhœa. His

---

* For observations illustrative of the different forms of the disorder, see Louis, New Orleans Journal, vol. iv.; Ames, *ibid.;* Holmes, American Medical Intelligencer, vol. xxxix.; Ford, South. Medic. Journ., vol. iv. Also Bartlett on the Fevers of the United States; Dickson, Elements of Medicine; Semenas, De la Fièvre Pernicieuse chez les Enfants, Paris, 1848.

sleep is disturbed, and he often suffers with hyperæsthesia of the scalp, and neuralgic pain shooting over the forehead and causing twitching of the eyelids. After remaining from six to seven days in this condition, his nails, perhaps at a certain hour every day, are noticed to become bluish; or he feels chilly, and a slight fever immediately afterward sets in. The return of these febrile symptoms is checked by quinine, and the patient enters upon a slow convalesence, remaining for a long time enfeeblèd.

Cases of this stamp were, during the late war, frequently noticed among those who had been poisoned by malaria in the Southwestern States or in the vicinity of Washington, and who had returned from the army to their homes in the condition set forth. The poison was often very obscure in its manifestations; at times it became the occasion, remote if not immediate, of a state resembling typhoid fever, although by no means identical with it. Probably for the most part of similar origin, and in several respects of kindred nature, was that curious fever which so many soldiers brought with them from the swamps of the Chickahominy. Without attempting to describe it in full, I shall give a sketch of the phenomena I noticed among those who had been with the army during the Peninsular campaign and were sent to the city for medical treatment.

The fever, I was informed, generally commenced with a decided chill, to which febrile excitement soon succeeded. This chill was sometimes, but not always, repeated. Many cases of the disorder showed at first distinct remissions; but if the fever lasted for more than a week, it became continued. Diarrhœa was a prominent symptom from the first; sometimes it preceded the disease by several weeks. In the cases that I saw in Philadelphia, nausea, and vomiting of bile, and great thirst were often present; the stools were very frequent and offensive; the eye was injected. There was generally mental confusion, and not unusually wild delirium; but no eruption—certainly no rose-colored spots. The tongue was sometimes coated, but often smooth, clean, and moist. The debility, after the affection had reached the middle or the end of the second week, was extreme. The face was pale, dull in its expression, and became, from day to day, like the rest of the body, more and more emaciated. It was mostly of a very sallow hue, seldom really jaundiced; at least the conjunctivæ, although injected, were not discolored. The skin was dry, and not very hot. The heart sounds were feeble, as was also the pulse. The lungs generally remained healthy. In the third week of the disease, the patient was apt to enter upon convalescence, or he died utterly exhausted, the freest stimulation exerting but little effect.

The post-mortem examinations were only to a certain extent satisfactory, as regards the light they threw upon the symptoms. In a large number of instances, perhaps the majority, neither the solitary nor Peyer's glands were ulcerated. They were frequently, however, found to be swollen, and sometimes of very dark color. The mucous membrane of the lower portion of the ilium and of the colon was often seen to be congested, even inflamed. The heart was several times noted as flabby. None of the other organs presented any constant lesions.

The convalescence from the fever was very slow; and during this protracted recovery symptoms occurred quite as striking as those of the fever proper. Those who got well did so with a broken constitution, and showed for months, by their wan face and their great debility, the hold the disease had had upon them. Sometimes, after gaining strength slowly for some time, they lost ground again, and relapsed into a typhoid condition very similar to that of the first attack, excepting in exhibiting an almost undisturbed state of the mind and a more continued character of the fever.

The blood was left very much impoverished. This fact manifested itself by the pallid face, the blood murmurs heard over the heart or the irritability of that organ, and the dark-purple spots, unchanged by pressure, which showed themselves at times all over the body, and often did not appear until long after the fever had left.

As other sequelæ of the fever, for in a certain sense they were sequelæ, I noticed milk-leg, enlargement of the liver, tympanites, parotitis, and diarrhœa, which ceased at times, but only to break out again. The looseness of the bowels was not generally associated with ulceration or thickening of the intestinal mucous membrane; the solitary and agminated glands were prominent, and contained blackish pigment. This diarrhœa was very obstinate, is still met with, and will probably be encountered long after all other signs of the "Chickahominy fever" have vanished from view.*

Yellow Fever.—This formidable malady is known under more than one name. It is the disease of Siam, the malignant pestilential fever, the Mediterranean fever, the malignant bilious fever of America, the sailor's fever, typhus icterodes. It takes its familiar appellation of yellow fever from the yellow tinge assumed during its course by the skin.

Yellow fever is a distemper met with in hot climates in low and level localities on the sea-coast. It is a virulent disorder, presenting many valid claims to be recognized as a separate member of the family of fevers. Its source is unknown: and though in many respects like malaria, it is so unlike it in others that we cannot call the complaint a miasmatic one. All we know of its cause is, that it does not exist without a high temperature, and that frost is its greatest enemy.

Yellow fever is an affection of very short duration: it rarely lasts a week; many die on the third or fifth day of the disease. It has but one paroxysm, which is never repeated. This paroxysm may be divided into three stages, which are well marked in some epidemics, far less so in others.

The first stage, called that of reaction, is pre-eminently

---

* According to Dr. Woodward (Outlines of the Chief Camp Diseases), this fever is one of those belonging to a group named by him "typho-malarial," which was the most frequent form of camp fever during the late war. It consists of mixed cases, in which the malarial and typhoid elements are variously combined with each other and with the scorbutic taint, now one, now the other of these elements preponderating. Prominent among the peculiarities of the malady are stated to be a decided tendency to periodicity, hepatic tenderness, with an icteroid hue of the countenance, gastric disturbance, excessive enlargement of the spleen, a very protracted convalescence, and the appearance throughout of the signs of a scorbutic affection. The rose-colored rash and the tympanites of typhoid fever are generally absent. Diarrhœa is ordinarily very marked, and is apt to be persistent. A plate, representing very artistically the intestine in the so-called typho-malarial fever, may be found in Circular No. 6, War Department, Surgeon-General's Office, Washington, 1865.

the febrile stage. Its average duration is from thirty-six to forty-eight hours. It generally commences suddenly, and is very frequently ushered in by a chill. Soon, however, the febrile excitement becomes established. The skin is harsh and hot; the pulse quick and tense, although sometimes it is both easily compressible and not very accelerated. The face is flushed; the eye brilliantly injected, yet watery. The patient is conscious, restless, anxious, and complains much of the torturing pains in his forehead, loins, and legs. The breathing is hurried; the stomach irritable, the epigastrium painful on pressure; there is great thirst. The bowels are constipated; the stools very dark colored. The tongue is more or less coated and moist; sometimes it is red, while at others it remains natural throughout the disease. The febrile signs increase toward evening, and lessen toward morning; but do not distinctly remit until after from thirty-six to forty-eight hours, when a remission does occur, or . when, to speak more correctly, the whole aspect of the case changes.

The disorder now appears in its second stage: the fever subsides; the pulse falls and becomes easily compressible; the headache is relieved; the breathing is no longer oppressed. But the gastric irritability does not wholly disappear, and a deep-yellow or orange hue gradually tinges the eye and the whole surface of the body. The patient is cheerful, and wishes to get out of bed. And indeed his sufferings may be over, his convalescence may have set in: after a few dark-colored, biliary stools, the yellowness of the skin fades, and he is well.

But it is not often that the disease relaxes its hold so easily; more generally the deceptive improvement does not last a day, and after the brief lull the struggle for life begins. The patient grows again very uncomfortable and anxious. In truth, the symptoms of the first stage reappear with increased intensity. In addition, new signs of the gravest import show themselves: the pulse sinks, and becomes slow and extremely irregular; the skin is cool, dry, very dark, and in some cases of a bronze hue, and spots may occasionally be seen on its surface. The stomach is as irritable as before, but the act of vomiting is easier; and, without much retching, large quantities of altered blood, or "black vomit," are ejected. Blood oozes from the mouth, from the gums; sometimes from the eyes and nostrils, from the bowels, and from the vagina;* or hemorrhage takes place into internal cavities, and the blood is retained.†

The phenomena of collapse become now more and more unmistakable: the black vomit often ceases, because the contractile power of the stomach has ceased; a low, muttering delirium sets in, and the patient dies prostrated. Yet the mind may remain clear almost to the last, and the strength be but little impaired. Should reaction take place, recovery is only very gradual.

But yellow fever does not at all times and in all localities present precisely the same degree of intensity, or the same group of symptoms. Sometimes it exhibits frank, active febrile phenomena; at other times there is little febrile excitement, but a disposition to internal congestions and to early prostration. This congestive form is far more dangerous than the inflammatory; yet both are highly destructive. From 10 up to 75 per cent. are the figures representing the mortality of this fearful malady. Omitting the instances of an exceptionably mild type, the average is calculated, in the elaborate work of Dr. La Roche,‡ to be 1 in 2·32. The more rapidly the stages succeed each other, the more dangerous the case. The occurrence of black vomit, of very great epigastric tenderness, of hiccough, of suppression of urine, of delirium, of early jaundice, of oppression in breathing, of convulsions, of a fiery, glistening eye, and of petechiæ,— warrant an unfavorable prognosis. "Walking cases," or those in which the patients walk about until they suddenly eject black vomit, always terminate fatally.

The recognition of yellow fever is, generally speaking,

---

* Cases in the epidemic of 1856–57 at Lisbon, reported upon by Lyons, London, 1858; also by Da Costa Alvarengo, Fièvre jaune à Lisbonne, Paris, 1861.

† In a case at the Pennsylvania Hospital, in 1853, the pericardium was filled with blood resembling black vomit.

‡ Yellow Fever. Philadelphia, 1855.

easy. The intense pain in the back, limbs, and forehead; the appearance of the eye, the color of the skin; the short duration of the febrile symptoms; the nausea; the epigastric tenderness; the black vomit,—constitute a group of symptoms which unmistakably mark the disease.

But let us look at the points of contrast which yellow fever presents to other affections. It differs from *plague* by the absence of buboes and of carbuncles, and the much more frequent occurrence, on the other hand, of jaundice and black vomit. Then, too, the red, suffused eye and the single paroxysm are not witnessed in plague. The febrile malady may run on to a state of collapse as complete as in *Asiatic cholera;* but, unlike this destructive disease, the symptoms of entire prostration are preceded by fever, and not by vomiting or purging of rice-water.

The lines of demarcation between the ordinary forms of continued fever and yellow fever are very broadly drawn. It is distinguished from *relapsing* fever by the different countenance, by the supra-orbital pain, and, above all, by the extreme rarity of a relapse and the infinitely greater mortality. To *typhoid fever* it bears so slight a resemblance that it is scarcely possible to confound the two affections: one, a short, severe disease, with its peculiar physiognomy and gastric symptoms; the other, a long-continued malady, of low type, with its characteristic eruption and enteric signs. It is only when yellow fever is protracted beyond the ninth day that the diagnosis is rendered doubtful; and then we have generally the history to guide to a correct understanding of the case. The likeness between yellow fever and *typhus* is much closer. But one is a short fever, with distinct stages; the other is a longer, much more continued fever. One has no marked cerebral symptoms; in the other, the cerebral symptoms are the most prominent feature. One has but rarely an eruption, but often hemorrhages; the other has always an eruption, and hardly ever hemorrhages.

The disease most likely to be confounded with yellow fever is *bilious remittent.* In truth, the symptoms are very similar, and many of them differ only in intensity. The diagnosis of the milder forms of yellow fever from remittent fever is indeed extremely difficult, unless the epidemic influences prevailing be taken into account. Then, as is well known, the affections may be blended, and yellow fever become obviously periodical in its febrile phenomena. The occurrence of black vomit is not in itself a distinctive sign between the two diseases; for black vomit may be absent in yellow fever, and, on the other hand, it may, although it rarely does, occur in remittent fever, just as it has been known to occur in child-bed fever, in the plague, and even in typhus fever.*

The least doubtful sign, a recent writer tells us, is derived from an examination of the urine. Unlike what happens in bilious fever, albumen appears in from twelve to fourteen hours after the fever sets in, as becomes manifest by the cloud which nitric acid causes; then the albumen increases, and the traces of urea and the uric acid diminish and gradually disappear, so does the bile pigment.†

When yellow fever is well marked, it differs in this way from remittent:

YELLOW FEVER.	BILIOUS REMITTENT.
Of short duration, ending commonly in from three to seven days.	Lasts nine days or upwards.
Period of incubation from five to nine days.	Period of incubation very variable; may extend to months.
A disease of one paroxysm, terminating in recovery or collapse..	A disease of several paroxysms, with intervening remissions.
Very severe nausea and vomiting throughout; early and decided epigastric tenderness; black vomit.	Nausea and vomiting not so severe, and rarely as marked at the onset; neither as early nor as constant and decided epigastric tenderness; vomiting of bile and of the contents of the stomach.
Hemorrhages from gums and various parts of the body.	No hemorrhagic tendency.

* This statement with reference to typhus fever is made on the authority of Dr. Stokes. The occasional occurrence of black vomit in remittent fever is admitted by many authors. Several winters ago, a physician of this city brought to me, for examination, a specimen of black vomit which had the same microscopical characters that I have been in the habit of finding in the black vomit of yellow fever. The patient undoubtedly had remittent fever, from which he recovered.

† Ballot, Archiv. Génér., Nov. 1869.

YELLOW FEVER.	BILIOUS REMITTENT.
Tongue clean, or but slightly coated; pulse very variable, becomes slow in last stages.	Tongue heavily coated; pulse varies less, is always quick until convalescence sets in.
Highly injected, humid eye; often fierce, or anxious expression of face.	Eye not peculiar; different physiognomy.
Supra-orbital pain, and pain in back and in calves of the legs.	Headache; sense of fulness in head; often no pain in loins or in legs.
Very rarely delirium; mind generally clear.	Delirium frequent; mind always dull.
Urine generally contains albumen; suppression of urine common.	No albumen in urine; suppression of urine rare.
Little muscular prostration; often rapid convalescence; no sequelæ.	Much greater muscular prostration; slow convalescence and tedious sequelæ.
Almost certain immunity after one attack.	One attack seems rather to predispose to others.
Very high mortality; disease is epidemic.	Slight mortality; disease more endemic in its nature.
Treatment unsatisfactory.	Very amenable to treatment.
Autopsy shows inflammation, or very great congestion of stomach, and sometimes ulceration or softening. Liver enlarged, of a yellowish color; its secreting cells filled with oil globules. Heart often exhibits disintegration of muscular fibres.	Autopsy shows congestion of stomach; more rarely a high degree of inflammation. Liver of an olive or bronze hue, not fatty.

Eruptive Fevers.

The eruptive or exanthematous fevers form a group having numerous features in common. They are all characterized by a period of incubation, during which the poison lies dormant in the system; by a fever of more or less intensity preceding the eruption; by an eruption which presents a distinct aspect in each disease, and which pursues a definite, clearly-defined course until it, and with it the febrile malady, disappears. Moreover, they are all very prone to occasion serious sequelæ; are all, in the main, disorders of childhood; rarely attack the same person twice; are contagious; and have not as yet been brought under the influence of specific treatment,—the most important part of our treatment relating to remedying the complications that arise while the febrile affection is held on its regular course. Their origin is as yet unknown, and their prevention, as a group, uncertain. One of them, however, has been checked in its ravages by a wonderful discovery, and it is not too much to hope that, one of these days, all will be brought similarly under the control of science.

These remarks apply particularly to the three chief exanthematous fevers: scarlet fever, measles, and small-pox. In great part, too, they hold good in regard to erysipelas, described here in connection with the eruptive fevers.

Scarlet Fever.—This disease, known also as scarlatina, is one of the gravest of the exanthemata, affecting both children and adults, and marked by great heat of skin, frequent pulse, sore throat, and an early scarlet eruption. These symptoms are often preceded by an uncertain period of incubation, but soon exhibit their striking features. The febrile excitement is characteristic; the skin very hot and generally dry, and the rapidity of the pulse so great that often by this sign alone we may, especially in the midst of an epidemic, predict the coming eruption. Vomiting, too, is a frequent symptom at the beginning of the illness.

The *rash* appears on the second day of the disease. It comes out almost simultaneously all over the body, although, on close scrutiny, it may be soonest perceived on the neck and breast. At first the surface exhibits an almost uniform red blush, which disappears momentarily on pressure, or rather pressure leaves a white stain on the skin, which quickly again reddens from the periphery to the centre. Soon, however, the eruption presents an unequal aspect: it is of more vivid scarlet hue in some parts of the body, as in and around the flexures of the joints, and is not everywhere smooth. Here and there are seen elevated rough points of darker tint edged by the red integument, and not unfrequently vesicles containing a thin fluid. The skin is very hot and itchy, and, especially on the hands and feet, tumefied. On the fourth or fifth day of the eruption, it declines; by the seventh, the cuticle begins to come away in large flakes. Sometimes the rash, when at its height, recedes, and then appears again. In malignant cases it comes out late, and is either pale and indistinct or dark and livid. In some instances it is wholly wanting. Some years ago, I saw a case of this "scarlatina sine exanthemate" in a lady, who, watching over the sick-bed of her daughter, contracted the disease and went regularly through it, even to its sequelæ of disorder of the kidneys and swelling of the salivary glands, but in whom not a trace of an eruption could be detected.

The *sore throat* of scarlatina is almost as constant and as characteristic as the scarlet rash. It shows itself very early, sometimes before the eruption, and rarely waits until the third day of the complaint. At first the throat trouble consists in a diffused redness extending over the tonsils, palate, and half-arches, and in a swelling of the tonsils: the patient complains of pain in his throat, augmented by pressure and by swallowing, and of stiffness of the muscles of the neck. After a few days, if the disorder be severe, irritating discharges occur from the inflamed surfaces, and patches of false membrane and superficial ulcerations are seen in the fauces. The glands at the angle of the jaw become much tumefied, and, by pressing on the cervical vessels, produce a tendency to drowsiness and stupor. These are grave symptoms; their occurrence, indeed, is indicative of one of the main dangers in these "anginose" cases of the disease.

The false membranes which are developed last about five or six days; they form as well as re-form in patches, and are very easily removed. Sometimes they extend to the larynx; but this does not often happen, and even when it does, the symptoms of croup, in the opinion of Barthez and Rilliet,* do not arise. The acrid discharges and the decomposing membranes often occasion a most fetid breath, and, by being swallowed, a persistent diarrhœa.

The *tongue* has a peculiar look. At first it is thickly coated, and its borders only are red; but soon the fur is cast off, and the whole organ becomes very red and its papillæ prominent. After it has presented this appearance for six or eight days, it returns to its normal condition. In bad cases it is extremely dry and of a brownish hue.

---

* Maladies des Enfants, tome iii.

In children, the disease frequently sets in, as the eruptive fevers are apt to do, with convulsions. In truth, cerebral symptoms of one kind or another are not uncommon at all stages of the malady; yet very great differences are observed, in this respect, in different epidemics. In some cases of malignant character, the vomiting, the screams, the grinding of the teeth, the occurrence of delirium and insomnia, make the attack look, at the onset, like one of acute meningitis; but the eruption soon sets all doubt at rest, and even before it is noticed, the great heat of the skin and the extreme rapidity of the pulse point to the source of the mischief. The nervous symptoms in these dangerous instances of the affection do not, however, cease with the eruption; they may last to the end of the malady. Sometimes they are not noticed until late in the disorder, and after the period of desquamation has fully begun; but the convulsions and stupor—for these are the morbid manifestations then more specially encountered—are owing rather to a diseased state of the kidneys that has been induced, than to the immediate effect of the fever poison.

Occasionally some of the larger joints swell up, and present the appearance of subacute rheumatism. The joints are not, however, very painful on pressure, and generally only two or three are enlarged. This form of rheumatism is evidently owing to the retention in the blood of some morbid material, and would seem to simulate ordinary acute articular rheumatism in presenting endocarditis and pericarditis as complications.*

Further complications of the disease are dropsies, passage of blood from the kidneys, pleurisy, tendency to gangrene, œdema of the glottis, diphtheria,† and a very low state of the system. These complications are not apt to arise until at or soon after the period of desquamation; sometimes they lead to long-continued trouble, and become thus the most hazardous of the sequelæ of the malady. Other consequences of the affection, lasting, it may be, for years after

---

* Scott Alison, Medical Gazette, 1845.
† Trousseau, Clinique Médicale, tome i.

the febrile attack, are a tendency to boils, swelling of the parotid and of the lymphatic glands of the neck, diarrhœa, chronic inflammation of the eyelids, and deafness from in-flammation extending up the Eustachian tube to the mem-brane of the tympanum, or from suppurative destruction of portions of the ear.

Of all these morbid states, *dropsy* is the most common. The effusion of fluid may be caused by the altered state of the blood; but much more generally it is owing to an ab-normal condition of the kidneys, produced by their efforts to eliminate the poison from the system. The organs take on the disease described as acute desquamative nephritis: their secreting function is impaired; albumen, tube-casts, epithelial cells, and sometimes blood are found in the urine; and we meet with severe headache, great restlessness, and œdema of the face and extremities, as the attending vital symptoms. Still, notwithstanding these grave phenomena, the majority of the cases recover, and the kidneys are rarely permanently injured.

The dropsy is apt to show itself between the tenth and twentieth day of the malady. The albuminous condition of the urine may precede it by several days; yet albumen in the urine is not always associated with dropsy. In most cases of scarlatina, it is found at some period of the disease for a short time and in small quantities; but this transitory albu-minuria is not, like the albuminuria coexisting with marked anasarca, connected with many tube-casts in the urine and numerous epithelial cells.

The *state of exhaustion* noticeable at the close of the fever and while desquamation is still going on, is at times very great,—so great that, in young persons especially, the case wears the look of typhoid fever. And the resemblance is heightened by the occurrence of diarrhœa associated with and perhaps dependent upon, a swelling of the solitary and agminated glands. But the signs of desquamation, the sore throat, the enlargement of the cervical glands, and the his-tory of the affection furnish distinctive marks of the utmost value.

The allusions that have just been made to the diverse

complications of the malady are mainly of interest, on account of their exhibiting the intricate diagnostic questions which may arise. Of the recognition of the disorder during the febrile stage it is not necessary to say much, as ordinarily it is not difficult. The distinction between it and the other exanthematous fevers may be seen by glancing at the table, to which a place is elsewhere assigned, showing their similitudes and their differences. I will only here mention, as bearing upon the distinction between scarlet fever and measles that cases are occasionally encountered in which the eruption alone is too ill defined to become the sole basis of an opinion, and that then we have to lay the greatest stress on the presence or absence of catarrhal symptoms and sore throat, and on the march of the symptoms. So, too, with reference to small-pox. The rash preceding the formation of the pustules may have so strong a resemblance to that of scarlet fever, that a scrutiny of all the attending circumstances, and a careful watching of the eruption for at least a day, are requisite to the detection of the true nature of the case.*

An erythematous rash, appearing in blotches everywhere except on the face, has been noticed in membranous croup and laryngeal diphtheria after the operation of tracheotomy.† But it is very irregular, runs a rapid course, and is not followed by desquamation.; a point, it may be here mentioned, distinguishing all the forms of irregular rashes, happening at times—though very rarely—in diphtheria, from the scarlet fever eruption.

Like measles, scarlatina may be mistaken for that curious form of eruptive fever called by the Germans *rubeola*, or "fire measles," and which is regarded by some as roseola, but is more generally looked upon as a hybrid of measles and scarlet fever. It displays a red eruption, ushered in by a chill, followed by fever, which is accompanied by coryza, cough, and sore throat. The fever prior to the eruption lasts for three or four days. The rash then comes out all

---

* The disorders may also be combined. See the cases of Marson, Medico-Chirurg. Trans., vol. xxx.

† Bericht des K. K. Krankenhauses Wieden, 1865.

over the body at once. It is most distinct on the trunk, neck, and face, being more scattered on the extremities. It first resembles measles, but the spots soon run together in irregular patches, unlike the well-defined crescentic eruption of measles. These patches are of variable size and surrounded by healthy skin. They are of deepest color in the centre, distinctly elevated, and very much influenced by pressure. The eruption lasts ordinarily four or five days, but in severe cases eight or ten. It gradually fades, and desquamation ensues, though the scales are small, and never in size like those of scarlet fever. During the continuance of the rash, the general symptoms are much aggravated; the sore throat may be very severe, and attended with inability to swallow and hoarseness. As the eruption fades, the constitutional symptoms subside. Swelling, and even suppuration of the cervical glands, are not uncommon sequelæ.

Another affection with several features corresponding to scarlatina is the breakbone fever, or *dengue*. The points of dissimilarity may be learned by referring to the description of the malady further on given.

Measles.—The symptoms precursory to the specific eruption of this affection are fever, watery eyes, frequent sneezing, flow from the nose, and cough; in fact, all the manifestations of an acute coryza or catarrh. To these diarrhœa is in many instances added, indicating a simultaneous irritation of the intestinal mucous membrane. On the fourth day after the commencement of the morbid signs, a rash is perceived on the face and neck; thence it continues to extend until, in the course of two or three days, the whole body is covered. The eruption does not alleviate the febrile symptoms; on the contrary, while it is spreading to the trunk and lower extremities, the constitutional disturbance increases. But as soon as it begins to fade, which it does on the fourth day of its appearance, the fever lessens; and by the ninth day of the disease, both fever and rash have left. Frequently then the cuticle comes away in fine scales, and this desquamation is attended with very annoying itching. The patient, now that he is convalescent, shows his sickness: he is pale and somewhat emaciated. Often he still coughs, and his eye is slightly inflamed. These signs are not unusually the last to disappear.

Of all the symptoms mentioned, two are, in a diagnostic sense, of pre-eminent importance: the catarrh and the eruption.

The *catarrh* is nearly constant. It is true that a variety of measles is recognized—" rubeola sine catarrho ;" but this is very rare. Generally speaking, the coryza and catarrh decline with the eruption; occasionally, however, they remain for some time after the rash has left. The feature which distinguishes these catarrhal symptoms from those of influenza consists in the eruption; before this happens, the diagnosis is uncertain, though we may often suspect measles by the look of the face, the greater intensity of the febrile signs, and a knowledge that the disease is prevailing in the community.

The *eruption* is very peculiar: it consists of slightly raised red spots, which coalesce and form blotches of an irregular, crescentic shape; between these blotches the skin is of natural color. The eruption disappears first from the face; in other words, it disappears in the same order in which it appeared. As it fades, it becomes brownish, and subsequently of a yellowish tint. In its earliest stages it is similar to the papulæ of small-pox; and this similarity may be heightened by its being mixed, as it sometimes is, with a few miliary vesicles. But after the first day of the rash there is little room for doubt. In the one case the spots remain as they were; in the other, they change into pustules.

A question may sometimes arise as to whether the eruption is that of typhus fever or of measles. Both are coarse, both often not unlike in color, and both may be developed about the same time. Generally speaking, however, the eruption of typhus fever shows itself several days later than the rash of measles; and although coarse, it is not crescentic, and is found on the trunk and extremities rather than upon the face. Moreover, the physiognomy, the excessive prostration of strength, and the marked cerebral symptoms of the low fever are such as to render a differential diagnosis seldom difficult.

Measles is usually met with in children; but it may be encountered in adults, especially among soldiers, and is, in adults, a much more severe complaint than in children. In the latter it is not an alarming disease. Only occasionally does it occur in epidemics which present a malignant character. Its greatest danger commonly consists in the eruption disappearing prematurely or appearing but partially, and in the severity of the thoracic complications.

These are either acute bronchitis or acute pneumonia. The former may occur at any period of the disorder, and involve the finer tubes. But it does not generally set in with severity until the eruption has reached its height or is beginning to fade. In young children, symptoms of inflammation of the larynx, or of croup, are at the same period apt to manifest themselves. Acute inflammation of the lung, too, is met with, at this stage of the malady, or sometimes even after convalescence has apparently commenced. We may suspect that mischief is going on within the chest, if the breathing be very oppressed and the pulse continue to be rapid; but so as to detect early the hazardous and insidious complication, and guard against it, the chest should be examined daily, both anteriorly and posteriorly. Occasionally the thoracic affection leaves a chronic bronchial disease; or a persistent cough and night-sweats make us fearful, and often but too justly, that tubercles have been awakened by the inflammation; and it may, in individual cases, be extremely difficult to decide with which of these morbid states we have to deal. Emaciation and a chronic cough are found in both chronic bronchitis and phthisis; and the physical signs of tubercular consumption are, in children, notoriously ill defined and untrustworthy. Then, the nummular sputum may occur in the bronchitis of measles. We may, therefore, be obliged to await the progress of the abnormal phenomena before coming to a definite conclusion.

At times we meet with anomalous forms of measles. The peculiar disease called "rubeola," which presents in its symptoms a mixture of scarlet fever and measles, has already been alluded to; irrespective of this, there is a kind of measles with a papular eruption like ordinary measles, but distinguished from it by the papulæ not being arranged in crescentic clusters, being less obvious and not appearing at all, or showing themselves but imperfectly on the limbs. The patches are of dusky hue, and there is no distinct sore throat, but considerable constitutional disturbance. This "rubeola notha" prevailed extensively in London a few years since.* A somewhat similar anomalous exanthem was common in Philadelphia during the winter of 1865–1866, occurring at the time when both measles and scarlatina were frequent, and particularly the former. The eruption, more partially papular than, but of dark hue like measles, was principally confined to the face. It appeared at the end of the first or on the second day of a slight malaise; though in some instances I saw there had been a marked chill at the beginning of the complaint, in others, the rash was the first sign of disease attracting attention. There was very little constitutional disturbance, a slight watery appearance of the eye, no sore throat, or a mere faucial reddening, and cough; yet this symptom was not constant. The eruption, which occurred chiefly in patches, not, however, distinct and crescentic, lasted from five to seven days, gradually fading and not being followed by desquamation. In only one instance did I observe a peeling of the cuticle, and this happened on the hands and feet. An almost invariable sequel was swelling of the cervical glands. The urine in the cases I examined contained no albumen, and convalescence was rapid. In one family I attended, the exanthem attacked three out of four children, all of whom had had measles two years previously.

Small-pox.—This fearful disease, which formerly ravaged all parts of the globe, is now, fortunately, much less seldom seen in civilized countries; at all events, we do not now encounter those frightful epidemics so dreaded and so disastrous to the human race.

Small-pox, or variola, attacks both children and adults. It is a highly contagious malady, spreading very rapidly among those unprotected by vaccination, and among masses of men; hence its presence on board ship or in camps is especially to be feared.

---

* Babington, London Lancet, May 7th, 1864.

The chief symptoms of the stage of *invasion* are chills, fever, and pain in the back. The fever runs very high, and exacerbates markedly toward evening. The pain in the back is very severe, and particularly severe in grave cases; there are also nausea, vomiting, headache, and great restlessness. All these symptoms subside at the end of the third or on the fourth day, when an eruption shows itself on the lips and forehead, but soon extends to the trunk, and from the trunk to the extremities.

At first the *eruption* has the appearance of papulæ; but on the second and third day the coarse spots undergo a decided change. At the top of each papule appears a vesicle, which gradually becomes larger and larger, and fills up with a milky, thick fluid; in short, becomes a pustule. By the fifth or sixth day this change has been fully accomplished, and the pustules are spheroidal and lose the umbilicated look which they had while forming. On the eighth day matter begins to ooze from their edges, and a secondary fever sets in, lasting for three or four days, until, indeed, all the pustules are broken. Now crusts form where previously there had been pustules; and as these crusts dry and fall off, the skin beneath is seen to be of a red color which only very gradually fades, and here and there are noticed those scars and pits which the patient carries during the remainder of his life.

When the pustules are in great abundance, they run together; such cases are very grave, and constitute the variety of the disease known as *confluent* small-pox. The eruption may be discovered a day earlier than in the discrete form, and the rough, red blotches are often so thickly clustered as to give a uniformly red aspect to the whole surface. When the pustules completely fill up, whole portions of the face or of the trunk seem to be covered by one extensive pustule, which gradually dries into a continuous brownish and most disfiguring crust. While the process of maturation is going on, the features are observed to be greatly swollen; the eyes may be hidden from view; the nose and lips are tumid. The patient complains of the tension of the skin, and not unfrequently of sore throat and of a steady flow of saliva from the mouth. The secondary fever is very violent, far more so than in discrete variola. It may not show itself until a day or two later, lasts longer, and is the period of danger, since it is at this time that death is most apt to happen.

A fatal issue is often preceded by dry tongue, by delirium and great restlessness; by what, in fact, are called typhoid symptoms. Sometimes it is brought about by attacks of dysentery or of diarrhœa, by passive hemorrhages, by affections of the larynx or trachea; by some complications, therefore, which the worn and irritated frame is unable to withstand. Now and then death takes place from supervening pneumonia or bronchitis; but an unfortunate termination from maladies of the respiratory organs does not occur only in the secondary fever, as these affections are, perhaps, oftener encountered during the period of eruption. Sometimes the patient sinks at the very onset of the disease. In these malignant cases, he dies from the virulence of the poison. He is stupid, delirious; the eruption seems, as it were, to struggle to reach the surface, is of a livid hue, and may fail to appear until after death.

Small-pox is occasionally met with, during the progress of other disorders, blending its symptoms with those of the complaint to which it becomes superadded. It is thus found as an intercurrent affection in typhoid fever, in typhus, in scarlet fever, and in measles; yet even then there is no difficulty in recognizing its peculiar traits—its lumbar pain and characteristic eruption. Ordinarily the detection of variola is extremely easy, excepting at its onset. But the points of similarity it may present, in its early stages, to typhus fever, to erysipelas, and to several other diseases, have been already discussed, and need not be repeated; elsewhere it has been noticed that we have often to await the course of the eruption before framing a positive diagnosis from the symptoms alone, and without taking the epidemic influences prevailing into account. When the disorder is fully developed, all difficulty in its diagnosis ceases. Let us here look at the marks of distinction between it and the other principal eruptive fevers, premising the statement that, in the period of invasion, the pain in the loins is the most significant differential sign:

TABLE EXHIBITING THE DIFFERENCES BETWEEN SCARLET FEVER, MEASLES, AND SMALL-POX.

SCARLET FEVER.	MEASLES.	SMALL-POX.
Period of incubation very uncertain; may be only a day, or may be weeks.	Period of incubation variable; generally seven to fourteen days.	Period of incubation from six to twenty days; generally about ten days.
Fever, with very great heat of skin and very frequent pulse; persists unabated during eruption.	Fever, with heat of skin and moderate frequency of pulse; not relieved, but rather increased by eruption.	Fever often very violent, with bounding pulse and pain in the loins; great relief from occurrence of eruption.
Eruption on second day, first on neck and chest; spreads rapidly.	Eruption on fourth day, first on face; spreads gradually, in the course of about forty-eight hours, to rest of body.	Eruption at end of third, or on fourth day; first on lips and forehead.
Eruption uniform or in very large patches of scarlet hue, with interspersed raised spots and some vesicles; rash, followed, after the seventh day from its appearance, by very complete desquamation.	Eruption in crescentic patches, with intervening portions of healthy skin; lasts about five days; followed by partial and very incomplete desquamation, and scales are, as a rule, very fine.	Eruption first papular; remains so about a day; then becomes vesicular, then pustular; on the eighth day of eruption, pustules maturate.
Sore throat; rarely coryza or bronchitis.	Coryza and bronchitis very constant; much more rarely sore throat.	Often sore throat and dry cough; bronchitis only as a complication.
Red "raspberry" tongue.	Tongue coated; may be red at edges; but does not lose its coat.	Tongue coated and swollen; may become red at edges.
Cerebral symptoms frequent and grave.	Cerebral symptoms neither frequent nor grave.	Cerebral symptoms, especially convulsions in children, frequent
Temperature very high; may range from 105° to 112°; no rapid fall soon after eruption, nor decided increase of heat preceding it; high temperature, though not so high as at first	Temperature during fever preceding the eruption high, 103° to 106°; rises rapidly toward breaking out of eruption. It may remain high for from twelve to twenty-four	Temperature during fever preceding the eruption, often 106°; then speedy defervescence taking place within thirty-six hours; subsequently thermometer indica-

SCARLET FEVER.	MEASLES.	SMALL-POX.
or at height of eruption, to the tenth day, when it begins to subside gradually. According to Ringer, a fall of temperature takes place on the 5th, 10th, and 15th day of the disease.	hours after appearance of rash; then sinks very speedily, a return to almost a normal temperature being arrived at on the second day from the beginning of its fall. Thus the defervescence is both rapid and complete; a protracted defervescence, or the maximum of temperature lasting for a considerable time after the coming out of the eruption, or a very high degree prior to it, indicates a severe case.	ting a temperature of about 100°, notwithstanding the progressing development of the pimples into pustules. Decided rise of temperature during secondary fever, and then gradual and protracted defervescence; slight rise during desiccation. (*Wunderlich.*)
No secondary fever.	No secondary fever; although sometimes a slight increase of fever just before eruption leaves.	Always secondary fever.
Pneumonia rare; pleurisy more frequent.	Pneumonia a very frequent complication.	Pneumonia not a very frequent complication.
Sequelæ: Bright's disease; dropsy; conjunctivitis; deafness; phthisis; chronic diarrhœa; glandular enlargements.	Sequelæ: chronic bronchitis; phthisis; conjunctivitis.	Sequelæ: chronic diarrhœa; glandular enlargements; various diseases of the eyeball and eyelids.

The contagion of small-pox does not always manifest itself by an attack of variola. Sometimes it is modified by happening in a person who is partially protected by vaccination. This *varioloid* disease is mild. It is distinguished from variola by the pustules passing more quickly through all their stages, and, above all, by an utter absence of secondary fever. Very soon after the eruption, within thirty-six hours, the thermometer shows entire freedom from fever, and unless serious complications happen, the heat of the body remains at very nearly the normal temperature.

Another modification of the affection, to express the current view, or a specific disorder very similar, to state in these words an opinion which has been the subject of many fierce disputes, is *chicken-pox*. Without entering into the controversy, it may be shown to differ, as regards its symptoms, from small-pox in the leniency of the introductory fever; in the eruption beginning generally first on the trunk, occurring often on the second day, though it may not appear until the end of the third, and continuing to appear and disappear in crops, the mass of the eruption, however, having appeared within twenty-four hours; in the vesicles being surrounded by little or no inflammatory redness; in their remaining vesicles, and not becoming pustules; in their attaining their height on the third or fourth day of the eruption, and then bursting and shrivelling without presenting depressions at their apices, and in the crust which falls off about five days subsequently being followed by a smooth, shining, round, and irregular pit. Then the eruption is rarely prominent on the face; and the disease does not protect, as mild forms of small-pox do, from a subsequent attack of variola. Sometimes the vesicles may be found, as are the pustules of small-pox, on the roof of the mouth and at the back of the throat. But, notwithstanding they may be everywhere very plentiful, the disorder is not a grave one. Yet I have known it to terminate fatally.

Dengue.—This is an arthritic fever with a cutaneous eruption. It has been prevalent in the form of epidemics chiefly in the West and East Indies, as well as in Virginia and South Carolina, and others of the Southern States.

It usually begins with pain, stiffness, and swelling of some of the smaller joints, or with severe muscular pains, aching in the back, and stiffness of the muscles of the neck. Fever follows, with suffusion of the eyes and headache; but, as a rule, without nausea and vomiting. On the third day the fever ceases altogether, or subsides very markedly, though the muscular and arthritic pains do not pass off entirely. The febrile paroxysm may last somewhat longer, or only six to twelve hours. In any case it is very apt to be succeeded by an interval of two to four days free from absolute suffering, though not from great debility and some pain. Then the pain returns, and with it the fever; nausea and vomiting and a thickly-coated tongue, too, are noticed. This new phase of the complaint is generally relieved by the appearance of an eruption, which shows itself on the fifth, sixth, or seventh day of the malady, and, therefore, very much later than the rash of scarlatina, which it resembles often in hue and aspect. But not invariably; for it may occur in patches and be papular, or even vesicular or like urticaria. The eruption is attended with a sense of burning and of itching, and disappears after two or three days' duration. Then convalescence sets in, marked by considerable muscular weakness and general depression, and frequently with the rheumatic stiffness or soreness persisting ·for some time. Swellings of the lymphatic glands of the neck, axilla, and groin occur in many cases, and may continue during couvalescence.

The cause of this singular malady—the breakbone fever of parts of our country—is unknown. It is a harmless disorder, clearly epidemic, and contagious. Such, at least, is the opinion of Dr. Dickson, to whom we owe one of the best descriptions of the disease, and from whose published statements, based on epidemics observed in Charleston, I have chiefly drawn this sketch.

Erysipelas.—This is an eruptive fever, accompanied by inflammation of the integument of some part of the body, generally of the head and face. This definition, of course, only refers to such cases as fall into the hands of the physieian, and to them alone the following remarks apply.

The disease begins with a chill and fever. Soon a portion of the face is noticed to be red and hot. The redness spreads, a clearly-defined edge marking its onward march; and generally it does not stop until it has occupied the whole of the face and a considerable portion of the scalp. The features are then so tumefied as to be hardly recognizable. The patient is very restless, has high fever, and not unfrequently enlargement of the glands at the angle of the jaw, and sore throat. By the seventh or eighth day the disease is over, and large patches of cuticle fall from the no longer swollen and disfigured countenance.

This is simple erysipelas; but we may have to contend with more dangerous forms and somewhat different symptoms. Thus the affection may extend—as is in truth always its tendency—from the true skin to the subcutaneous areolar tissue, and give rise there to collections of pus, which reveal their presence by chills and an obscure sense of fluctuation, and keep up an irritative fever until they are discharged. Irrespective of this, the tumefaction, while the complaint is at its height, is much greater in this phlegmonous variety of the malady, and there is more constitutional disturbance; but, on the other hand, not so much local irritation, for the morbid action travels less rapidly, and often remains more circumscribed. In some cases the inflammation extends to the brain, and, instead of the wandering at night, always a very common symptom, we have violent delirium, soon succeeded by coma and rapid sinking. In other cases, again, and they are generally very bad ones, we may find these active cerebral symptoms, and yet not be able to detect, after death, signs of inflammation in the brain or its membranes. Now and then the disorder passes to the throat, reaches 'the larynx and bronchial tubes, and places life in imminent peril from œdema of the glottis, or from a most hazardous form of capillary bronchitis. In some instances, a highly asthenic state becomes developed, and the patient dies exhausted.

The diagnosis of erysipelas is not beset with difficulties. Erythema resembles it most closely; but there is this manifest difference: in erythema there is scarcely any swelling, not much tendency to spread, and almost no constitutional disturbance. The ordinary exanthematous fevers may, at an early stage, be mistaken for erysipelas. But all of them, even scarlatina, have a longer period of febrile invasion; in all, too, although the eruption takes its origin at one spot, and generally on the face, it is not limited there. The thickly-clustered blotches of commencing confluent small-pox and the swelling attending them give at times to the face the look of erysipelas. But here, also, evidences can be found of a rash about to appear all over the body; and should doubt still exist, it is soon dispelled by the progress of the eruption. Sometimes vesicles and even irregular pustules form in erysipelas, and occasion some misgivings as to whether the malady be not a chronic disease of the skin, such as eczema, pemphigus, or impetigo; but these affections lack the constitutional symptoms and the history of a recent acute disease, and in reality the likeness is not a very striking one, if the inflamed surface be carefully examined.

Erysipelas may be confounded with *mumps*. This does not seem at first sight very likely, but I have known the error to have been committed. It was mainly caused by too much stress being laid on the redness which is frequently found beneath one or both ears in parotitis; but which, unlike erysipelas, is attended with much pain on moving the jaw, and with decided glandular tumefaction. The redness, moreover, shows no tendency to spread, and rarely continues for the four or five days during which mumps lasts. In very young children, however, there may be some difficulty in diagnosis. I have seen the glands at the angle of the jaw much swollen for one or two days prior to the slight discoloration over them taking on a deeper blush, and then spreading rapidly as marked erysipelas over the whole face and part of the scalp, reaching the other jaw, where subsequently the glands began to swell. In such cases great weight must be attached to the history of the case, to determine which disorder was primary, and whether the glandular complaint was or was not the complication. If the contagion of mumps can be traced, the matter is easily settled.

CHAPTER XII.

To facilitate the discrimination of diseases of the skin, they have been grouped into classes. These have been arranged by some authors in accordance with the obvious characters of the eruption, by others in accordance with its presupposed cause and attending structural alteration. The former classification is that of Willan and Bateman, and, with such modifications as the knowledge of the day has necessitated, is the one still generally followed. In compliance with its main features, cutaneous affections, omitting some of the less important ones, may be thus grouped:

DISEASES OF THE SKIN.

MACULÆ.................................	Ephelides. Vitiligo. Chloasmata. Nævi.
EXANTHEMATOUS DISEASES ...	Erythema. Roseola. Urticaria.
PAPULAR DISEASES	Lichen. Prurigo.
VESICULAR DISEASES	Eczema. Herpes. Pemphigus.
PUSTULAR DISEASES..............	Acne. Impetigo. Ecthyma. Rupia.
SQUAMOUS DISEASES..............	Lepra. Psoriasis. Pityriasis. Ichthyosis.

(782)

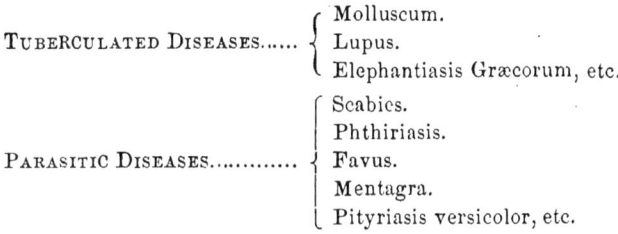

TUBERCULATED DISEASES......
{
Molluscum.
Lupus.
Elephantiasis Græcorum, etc.
}

PARASITIC DISEASES..............
{
Scabies.
Phthiriasis.
Favus.
Mentagra.
Pityriasis versicolor, etc.
}

Another system of classification which has much to recommend it, and which takes for its basis the anatomical seat and arrangement of the cutaneous malady, is that of Hebra. As developed by him, it is, however, not a purely anatomical, but a mixed system. All diseases of the skin are arranged in twelve classes: Hyperæmiæ; Anæmiæ; Morbid secretion of the cutaneous glands; Exudations; Hemorrhages; Hypertrophies; Atrophies; Neoplasms; Pseudoplasms; Ulcers; Nervous affections; Parasites.

The fourth class is the most comprehensive, and is divided into an acute and chronic; the acute being subdivided into a contagious class—the exanthemata, and a non-contagious—erythemata, dermatitis, phlyctænoses. The chronic exudations are the squamous affections—psoriasis, lichen, pityriasis rubra; the pruriginous affections—eczema, scabies, prurigo; the acneform affections—acne, sycosis; the pustular affections —impetigo, ecthyma; and the bullous affections—pemphigus.

But in this sketch of cutaneous affections, we shall adhere to the first classification; and in accordance with it, when a disease of the skin is presented for examination, we must first endeavor to ascertain the group it belongs to; for instance, is it vesicular, pustular, or erythematous? Having determined this, we next fix which one of the group it is. When this has been accomplished, we inquire into the history of the disorder and its duration, whether acute or chronic; take into account the presence or absence of fever and the general condition of the patient; search for the evidences of a cachexia or of some visceral disturbance; and trace, as far as possible, the cause of the affection and its exact seat. Having done all this, we have a groundwork upon which to institute a suitable treatment.

Most diseases of the skin are again subdivided into several varieties, based, for the most part, on their duration, situation, form, feel, and color. Thus we have constantly recurring the terms fugax, inveterata, capitis, facialis, palmaris ; or punctate, guttata or guttate, when like a drop on the skin ; nummular, when like a coin ; larvaris, like a mask, etc.; the qualifying words, læve, indurata ; and the adjectives of color, nigrum, rubrum, versicolor. But these divisions are all of secondary importance ; and I shall not, in this outline, regard them. Premising this statement, let us briefly examine the characteristics of the various cutaneous affections of more common form. The class of *maculæ* composed chiefly of the ephelides, comprising freckles, called also lentigo, and large patches of a yellowish-brown color, attended with slight desquamation ; and nævi or moles, spots of congenital origin, need not be further considered.

Exanthematous Diseases.—This group, regarded, too, as *rashes*, is often made to include rubeola, scarlatina, and erysipelas ; but these belong more strictly to idiopathic fevers than to diseases of the skin, and have been described already. There are only three affections which, strictly speaking, come under this division of cutaneous complaints : erythema, roseola, and urticaria. In all of these the skin is more or less red, and its surface unbroken.

Erythema is characterized by a uniform and continuous redness of the skin, occurring in irregular patches of some size, and attended with but slight swelling, if with any. The affection may or may not be associated with disturbance of the general health ; usually it is acute, and connected with some visceral disorder. There is only one variety apt to be combined with decided febrile symptoms—the hard, painful protuberances most commonly seen on the legs, and constituting the so-called " erythema nodosum." This form of the complaint is chiefly observed in those of rheumatic diathesis.

Roseola consists in circumscribed spots of a rose-red color, and of a more or less circular form. The spots are smaller than those of erythema. There is slight fever, and at times redness of the fauces. The affection is generally acute, and bears a certain resemblance to scarlatina and measles; but it is not contagious, its constitutional symptoms are much milder, and we find neither the marked sore throat of scarlet fever nor the catarrh of measles.

Urticaria, or nettle-rash, gives rise to prominent and perfectly smooth patches, the color of which is either redder or whiter than the surrounding skin. The wheal-like eruption is attended with more itching and tingling than the other exanthemata, and is much more evanescent, generally disappearing in two days at furthest. It may, however, exist in a chronic form. Its cause is irritation of the gastro-pulmonary or gastro-urinary mucous membrane. Certain kinds of fish, especially shell-fish, are particularly prone to produce it. Urticaria is thought generally to be an exudative disease of the skin; but there are those who believe that it is only a spasmodic contraction of the muscular tissue of the cutis;* and it seems to me most probable that it is wholly a reflex phenomenon caused chiefly by reflected irritation of the cutaneous vaso-motor nerves.

Papular Diseases.—A papula, or pimple, is a small elevation of the cuticle with an inflamed base; it does not contain any fluid, and usually terminates in desquamation.

Lichen furnishes the best-marked example of a papular eruption. It consists of minute conical papulæ, generally of reddish color, and occurring in clusters. It is most frequently encountered in the summer months and in adults, and often in persons of good health, but who have been exposed to much fatigue or anxiety. Sometimes it is evidently connected with disordered digestion. It is very commonly chronic. When assuming a circular form, it is designated as a species of ring-worm. The lichen of young children and infants is called "strophulus." There is often a mixture of papulæ with an eczematous eruption; indeed, there is a close relationship existing between the two disorders.

Prurigo is a papular affection of the skin attended with excessive itching. The pimples are generally torn by the finger-nails, and are surmounted by black scabs. They are

---

* Gull, Guy's Hosp. Rep., 3d Series, vol. v.

not red, as those of lichen so usually are, and are, as a rule, larger, and accompanied by much more pruritus and by thickening of the skin. The affection may or may not be attended with constitutional symptoms. It is very distressing and obstinate, especially when happening in old persons. It generally affects more particularly the arms and legs, very rarely the face and neck. The skin of the anterior and outer part of the leg is most changed; that over the flexors in the forearm is always healthy. The distressing disorder may be purely local, occurring around the anus, or on the scrotum and root of the penis, or on the pudenda. Some of these cases, however, though called prurigo, present no papulæ, and the disorder is really due to perverted sensibility of the cutaneous nerves alone.

Prurigo can often be traced to want of personal cleanliness. It is frequently found to be connected with deterioration of the health, and is indeed essentially an affection of the nerves. It may last a lifetime, beginning in childhood. Its local forms are associated with irritation of the bladder, rectum, or uterus.

Vesicular Diseases.—These are characterized by an effusion of a clear fluid beneath the epidermis, which is generally raised in small elevations. To the class of vesicular diseases belong especially eczema and herpes. Along with them pemphigus, usually grouped with the bullæ, will be described; for bullæ differ from vesicles only in size.

Eczema consists of minute vesicles collected together in irregular patches. The vesicles are often confluent, and it then appears as if the whole surface were secreting fluid. This may harden, from exposure to the air, into scabs of various thickness and color. The skin itself is often of a vividly red hue.

Eczema may affect the whole body, but is ordinarily limited to some portion of it. It is acute or chronic. The former is generally seen as the effect of local irritants, and may be met with in young and healthy persons. Chronic eczema is oftener the consequence of constitutional disturbance, and is very frequently found to be associated with some disorder of the digestive system. Dentition and unhealthy milk are common sources of the affection in very young children. In them the disease is extremely apt to attack the scalp and face, forming the complaint often described as "crusta lactea;" or, if the secretion be partly purulent, and dry into large, dark scabs, the malady is designated as "eczema impetiginodes."

In some of the forms of eczema, especially in its chronic varieties, the vesicles supposed to characterize the disorder can often not be found. This and other reasons have caused several recent dermatologists, especially Hebra* and Anderson,† to deny that eczema need be vesicular at all. Infiltration of the skin, exudation on its surface, the formation of crusts, and itching are held to be its distinctive signs, while the eruption is at its height; but the eruption may consist of clusters of papules, vesicles, or pustules, or there may not be a vestige of any of these, the skin being red and smooth and secreting a sticky discharge or covered with green or gummy crusts.

Eczema, particularly when it affects the scalp and face, must not be confounded with the morbid secretion from the sebaceous follicles giving rise to soft crusts. This disease, or "seborrhea," by preference attacks the parts mentioned, but its crusts, as Hardy has shown, are unlike those of eczema in the readiness with which they are detached, and susceptible of being moulded between the fingers. The surface beneath the crusts, too, is dissimilar. It has an oily, glistening look.

Herpes, like eczema, is classed as a vesicular affection, and differs from the obviously vesicular form of the latter disorder by the larger size of the vesicles. These are generally of globular form, and are arranged in clusters upon an inflamed patch of skin. Each vesicle is distinct, and remains so throughout its course. It lasts from about eight to twelve days, and often terminates by the formation of a thin incrustation.

Herpes has seldom a longer duration than three weeks. It happens usually in persons of delicate skin; is generally very local, having its seat on the lips, eyelids, prepuce, or pudenda; and is almost invariably associated with an internal disease, especially with irritation of some portion of the gas-

---

* Hautkrankheiten; or Translation by Sydenh. Soc.
† A Practical Treatise upon Eczema. London, 1863.

tro-pulmonary mucous membrane. It often appears at the termination of fevers. Its most distressing form is that extending around one-half of the trunk,—"herpes zoster," an acute disorder, which may show itself over the course of any of the superficial nerves. Indeed, herpetic or bullous eruptions often happen over the course of nerves, and a nerve lesion, the result of disease or of an injury, will produce them over the disordered nerve.

Herpes and eczema may both be confounded with scabies, which, like them, occasions a vesicular eruption which is apt to be found on the inner surface of the limbs and flexures of the joints. The distinction consists in the severe itching; in the small, conical vesicles, torn, as they so usually are, by scratching; and in the presence of the acarus, which may be removed from its burrow with the point of a needle or any sharp instrument.

Pemphigus is a disease not often met with. It appears in very large vesicles or bullæ, surrounded by a zone of erythematous redness. The blebs occur in crops, and look like small blisters filled with serum. The disorder may be acute or chronic. It is ordinarily chronic, and happens in persons of enfeebled constitutions. The chronic form is also called "pompholyx."

Pustular Diseases.—These are marked by circumscribed elevations of the cuticle which contain pus. Acne, impetigo, and ecthyma belong to the group. Rupia, too, although often classed among the vesicular or the bullous disorders, appertains more strictly to the pustular.

Acne is an eruption of hard, isolated, red elevations, due to chronic inflammation of the follicles of the skin. At the apices of many of these elevations pus forms, which is discharged, leaving a hardened base, which only gradually disappears. Acne is generally seen on the face and shoulders. Men of sedentary occupations and drunkards are very liable to it. In women it is frequently associated with uterine disturbances.

Impetigo presents small pustules occurring in successive crops and arranged in clusters. The pustules are but little raised above the surface, soon break, and a thick, yellowish or greenish crust is developed. When the disorder attacks the scalp and face, especially in infants and children, it gives rise to very extensive incrustations, and constitutes, particularly if conjoined with eczema, the affection designated as "porrigo larvalis."

Ecthyma differs from impetigo by the larger size and greater prominence of the pustules and their inflamed base. When the crust that forms on each pustule falls, a highly-congested surface or a superficial ulceration is seen, which leaves a cicatrix. The disorder is apt to be connected with a cacheetic state of the system. It bears a certain resemblance to sycosis; but the limitation to the hairy portions of the face, the yellow color of the pustules, their conical form and smaller size, and the brown crusts they occasion, distinguish this malady.

Rupia produces very large pustules, that desiccate into thick, brownish crusts, often of conical shape or resembling the shell of an oyster, and which, when thrown off, expose ulcerations of various depth that are slow to heal, and on which fresh crusts arise. The disease runs a chronic course. It occurs especially on the lower extremities, is almost always syphilitic, and coexists with a deteriorated constitution. It is very like ecthyma, and can be distinguished only by the history of the case, the persistent ulcerations, and the prominent, peculiarly-shaped crusts.

Squamous Diseases.—Here the predominant characteristic is the formation of small, whitish patches of unhealthy cuticle covering red papular elevations, or a deep-red surface. Lepra and psoriasis are the main disorders belonging to this group. Pityriasis is included by many authors, while others regard it as merely a variety of chronic erythema. It differs from lepra and psoriasis by the production of minute squamæ, which are constantly thrown off and re-formed, and which are seated on a reddened integument.

Lepra and *psoriasis* may be described together, since there is very little real difference between them. In both we find patches of red hue raised above the surrounding integument and covered by scales of dried epidermis. In lepra these patches have a circular or circumscribed shape, the scales are large and well defined. In psoriasis, on the other hand, while the scales more completely cover the morbid portion of skin, they are finer, and the patches are large or consist of very small ones which have coalesced into a single large one, are not of an annular form, and not separated by healthy skin.

Lepra and psoriasis occur most frequently among the poor and uncleanly, and are sometimes evidently hereditary. They are chronic affections, and often extremely obstinate. They are both liable to be mistaken for lichen, especially lepra. The latter is, however, distinguished by the distinct scales and by the smooth, red skin, which is at once perceived when the scales are detached. Psoriasis has a predilection for the vicinity of the joints. Sometimes it appears exclusively on the palm of the hand.

Ichthyosis, or fish-skin, is also a squamous disease; but it differs from the others of this class in being much more general, affecting as it does often the whole integument, and in the absence of reddening or any signs of inflammation of the surface. The skin is dry and rough, and covered with thickened and exfoliating cuticle. Ichthyosis is almost always of congenital origin.

Tuberculated Diseases.—These are hard, indolent, superficial, and generally permanent tumors of the skin. Molluscum, Lupus, and Elephantiasis of the Greeks illustrate this group.

Molluscum presents numerous globular or flattish tubercles, sometimes seated on a broad base or attached to a peduncle. They occur chiefly in groups on the face and neck, are filled with a peculiar atheromatous matter, vary in size from a pea to a pigeon's egg, show no tendency to inflame or ulcerate, and are not attended with increased sensibility of surface. They are of the color of the skin or of brownish hue. They may last during life and grow very slowly without affecting the general health. There is a variety met with specially in children, which has at the top or side of each tubercle a small orifice from which a creamy fatty fluid can be pressed. This variety is regarded as contagious; though there are many who still doubt the contagious nature of "molluscum contagiosum."

In *lupus*, the tubercles may or may not ulcerate. They are of a dull-red color, and, if they ulcerate, are apt to destroy the tissues in which they are situated. The ulcers also spread, and may occasion much devastation. When they heal, they leave a strongly-marked whitish cicatrix and an unhealthy-looking skin. The disorder occurs in syphilitic or scrofulous persons. There is a form of lupus occurring only in strumous subjects, and characterized by warty formations. This "lupus verrucosus" is without pain or itching, but cicatrices form, though there has been no previous ulceration.*

Elephantiasis of the Greeks is distinguished by tubercles, from the size of a pea to that of a walnut, of reddish, or whitish, or bronzelike hue, which may ulcerate, and which are preceded by erythematous patches. Often, too, there are symptoms of defective innervation, especially deficient sensation of the surface, and the blood is seriously affected. The face is frequently the seat of the malady, and becomes very much thickened and disfigured.

The Barbadoes leg, or elephantiasis of the Arabs, is an enormous increase in size of the limb, usually dependent upon an indurated swelling of the subcutaneous tissues, with some alteration of the skin proper. The tumefaction may be in swellings separated by deep furrows, giving somewhat of a tuberculated look to the part, or it may be uniform. It is similar in the structure it principally affects to the extraordinary induration of the cellular tissue, to which the name of *sclerema* or sclerodermia has been given. I had some years since a marked case of this strange affection under my charge at the Pennsylvania Hospital, in a woman, forty-two years of age, who, admitted with œdema of the feet, was at the same time noticed to have a swelling of both wrists and forearms as well as of the cheeks. The swelling was firm and resistant, and did not pit on pressure. The skin covering it was very smooth, and of redder hue than at other portions of the body; there was well preserved sensibility. The œdema disappeared from the feet, but the signs of the indurated cellular tissue did not leave the affected parts. On the con-

* McCall Anderson, Journal of Cutaneous Medicine, vol. i.

trary, the condition of these parts became worse, though the general health was excellent, all the internal viscera being in a normal state. Gradually the hands, particularly the fingers, were found to be more and more resisting and immovable, and she could scarcely bend them; occasionally they were the seat of pain. The skin lost all suppleness, and could not be raised up. At no time, while under observation, was albumen present in the urine. She left the hospital unimproved by the sulphur baths, the bichloride of mercury, and the various other alteratives she took; and I have since learned that she died of an acute pleurisy succeeding an attack of acute meningitis, from which she had not wholly recovered. Prior to her death, so great was the pressure exerted by the dense and contracting cellular tissue, that dry gangrene of a finger ensued, as well as of a toe, the disease having also been noticed in the lower extremities. In truth, the progress of the whole affection was in its effects on the adjacent muscles similar to that produced in cirrhosis by the increased and indurated cellular tissue. She died about one year from the beginning of the complaint. Examined after death, the skin over the diseased parts was firmly united by the dense and augmented areolar textures to the muscles beneath; thus, of necessity, their motions had been interfered with.

There is a form of enlargement of the leg which we may here briefly refer to—one in which the overgrowth of the affected limb is associated with *disease in the lymphatic system*. Vesicles form, which are connected together by ridgelike elevations, and which from time to time discharge a chylous fluid.* The subcutaneous lymphatics near the groin are usually found to be distended.

Parasitic Diseases.—These may be caused either by the presence of parasitic animals or of plants. To affections of the former origin, or to the epizoa, belongs especially scabies; though the various forms of lice producing the ailment, presenting for the most part, a pruriginous eruption —phthiriasis, must be alluded to. The other animal para-

---

* W. H. Day, Transactions of Clinical Society of London, vol ii., 1869.

site, the entozoon or demodex folliculorum, inhabits the sebaceous and hair follicles, but does not, so far as is known, cause disease.

The complaints associated with the vegetable parasites, the *epiphytes*, or as those on the skin are called, the dermatophytes, are chiefly favus, mentagra, pityriasis versicolor, and some of the forms of ring-worm, tinea circinatus, and tinea tonsurans. Pellagra, also supposed to be due to a vegetable parasitic growth, is not an affection met with in this country. Nor does the presumed parasitic fungus lodge in the skin. It is said to be found in diseased Indian corn or maize, which, when eaten, causes the general cachexia and cutaneous eruption which characterize the malady, of which the eruption moreover is determined by exposure to the sun.

Scabies, or the itch, is owing to the acarus scabiei. This burrows into the skin, particularly between the fingers and between the toes. The channels produced are generally somewhat curved, and may be traced as whitish or black streaks of several lines in length, in the situations just indicated. The disease is attended with excessive itching, and the eruption of conical vesicles, or even, in some cases, of pustules.

At the close of the late war we had a form of itch very prevalent in this country, and which was spread far and wide, as is presumed by contact with the troops—the so-called *Army itch*. It was a very chronic and very distressing affection, and no age or social state was exempt from it. Indeed, so prevalent was it that it almost appeared as an epidemic. The itching was intense, the eruption, as by far most frequently met with, was like prurigo, but vesicles, or even an eczematous condition of skin, or pustules attended the intolerable itching; and in cases of very long duration the appearance of the skin was altered, and all trace of a distinctive eruption was gone. The eruption was seen on the arm, forearm, chest, abdomen, and lower extremities, particularly on the ulnar side of the forearm and inner aspect of the thigh. It was sometimes found on the scalp, but very seldom in the groins, axillæ, on the hands or between the fingers. It was benefited by sulphur; for almost all the preparations recommended for it contain sulphur. Whether it was due to the same acarus, as ordinary scabies, or to a different species, I am unable to say.

Favus gives rise to bright-yellow umbilicated crusts, of circular shape and smooth surface, which often form yellow rings around the hair follicles and are not much elevated above the skin. There is no discharge. The disease very rarely affects any other part of the body than the scalp. In cases of doubt, the microscope furnishes us with a certain means of diagnosis, by exhibiting the cryptogamic plants.*

The vegetable origin of *mentagra*, or sycosis, is not so satisfactorily proved as that of favus. The distinctive marks are the development of yellowish pustules, having a bright-red base, around the roots of the hair of the beard. The tricophyton tonsurans is the parasite said to be found in sycosis, and it is also met with in *tinea circinatus*, the ring-worm of the body, and in *tinea tonsurans*, the ring-worm of the scalp.

Pityriasis versicolor occasions those yellow or yellowish-brown discolorations which may be not unfrequently seen on various parts of the body. The affection is common in women, especially in pregnant women. The microsporon furfur of Eichstädt is the parasite present in this disorder. In pityriasis affecting the scalp, we may also find parasitic growths of vegetable nature; and they are often the cause of baldness, as in porrigo decalvans.

The disorders of the skin which we have been considering do not always occur isolated; they may be combined. Again, they are altered by the existence of a special taint, as by the syphilitic. Now, without making any attempt to describe *syphilitic* diseases of the skin, I may briefly state that they differ chiefly by their copper-colored tint, and by the stained aspect they leave. Then, syphilitic lichen has more distinct pimples, and a well-defined scab on each. The ulcerations in the pustular affections are deeper; while in the squamous disorders the scabs are smaller and the papules larger than in the non-syphilitic eruptions.

As regards the *treatment* of cutaneous affections, we should

---

* For a good description of these, see Bennett's Clinical Lectures.

always recollect that many of them require both constitutional and local treatment. Constitutional treatment is carried out, to speak in general terms, by purgatives, diaphoretics, and diuretics, in the acute cases and where febrile excitement is present; by tonics, especially by arsenic, cod-liver oil, iodine, and iron, in the chronic disorders. Local remedies may be used for a twofold purpose: either to soothe the irritated surface and protect it from external injury, or to produce a stimulating and alterative action. The latter is effected by the application of mercurial ointments and lotions, of the preparations of tar, of sulphur, of carbolic acid, and of alkaline washes; but we must be careful not to employ such agents in the early stages of cutaneous disorders, as they only aggravate them. Simple cerate, glycerin in a diluted form, solutions of lead, and the oxide of zinc ointment,—in fact, remedies which are soothing or sedative rather than stimulating are far more appropriate, and may be often advantageously resorted to even in the chronic diseases of the skin.

CHAPTER XIII.

POISONS AND PARASITES.

In disorders due to poisons or parasites, the morbid phenomena are clearly occasioned by causes introduced into the system from without. Thus they agree in being affections of external origin; and as regards both the diagnosis and treatment, our chief aim is to ascertain precisely to what foreign substance the symptoms are owing.

POISONS.

Cases of poisoning are presented to the physician's notice under various circumstances. Sometimes they are the result of accident or carelessness; sometimes the life of the patient has been attempted by himself or by others. In either case it may be a matter of the greatest moment to make out a correct diagnosis as the starting-point for prompt and skilful treatment.

I cannot, of course, enter here at any length into the subject of poisons, but shall merely endeavor to set forth the main signs by which the consequences of the most common of them may be recognized and distinguished. And for this purpose, it will be convenient to consider cases of poisoning as divided into acute and chronic, subdividing these two classes again according to the character and effects of the different noxious substances. Now, as regards their character and effect, various arrangements of poisons have been made by toxicologists, as, for instance, into irritant, narcotic, narcotico-acrid, and septic; into metallic and non-metallic; into animal, vegetable, and mineral. In the following sketch, I shall not adhere closely to any of these arrangements, but shall be guided by them only to a certain degree in grouping the poisons to be discussed.

(796)

Acute Poisoning.

The attack comes on suddenly, the patient having been previously in perfect health, but having taken some food, drink, or medicine which has been followed by the urgent symptoms. And it is always, in a case of suspected poison-ing, of the utmost importance to be able to make out these points.

Irritant Poisons.—The chief articles which give rise to acute poisoning belong to the class of irritant poisons. The symptoms vary somewhat, but they are generally those of acute gastritis, attended often with more or less inflamma-tion of the mouth, fauces, and œsophagus. Sometimes the air-passages may be involved, either directly or by sympathy, and we find hoarseness and cough. Convulsions are occa-sionally observed, and collapse is apt to occur sooner or later.

The acute pain, the tenderness, and the vomiting come on shortly after a meal, or at least after something has been swal-lowed. This distinguishes the acute gastritis caused by pois-ons from idiopathic acute gastritis. And sometimes several persons are similarly affected, a circumstance always strongly in favor of the idea of poisoning. From perforation of the stomach or intestines, irritant poisoning is discriminated by noting that the acute signs in the former case follow upon the manifestations of some gastric or intestinal trouble; and the attending phenomena of collapse are not, as in poisoning, associated with cramps or convulsions. Cholera resembles poisoning in the suddenness and violence of the attack, but is distinguished by the rice-water discharges and by its epi-demic character. In strangulated hernia, the comparatively gradual onset, the pain, the tumor, and the absence of diar-rhœa will be significant. As regards the separation of those cases of poisoning in which blood is ejected, from ordinary hemorrhage from the stomach, we find that pain and purg-ing are both absent in the latter, while in irritant poisoning they are apt to be well-marked symptoms.

Let us now examine some special poisons. Strong acids are frequently used to destroy life. *Nitric* acid stains the lips and mouth orange yellow wherever it touches them; the matters vomited are very acid, and act upon copper or tin, with the disengagement of reddish fumes of nitrous acid. *Sulphuric* acid stains the skin or mucous membrane white or grayish; the pain is excessive, and if the vomited matter be mixed with a solution of nitrate of baryta, a dense white precipitate of sulphate of baryta is thrown down. *Muriatic* acid is less irritant and corrosive than sulphuric acid. It is recognized in the ejected substances by causing a white precipitate with nitrate of silver. *Oxalic* acid, when concentrated, is very rapidly fatal. If vomiting occur, the matter ejected may be tested with a solution of lime, when the oxalate of lime will form a white and insoluble deposit.

The strong *alkalies*, when taken into the stomach, cause inflammation of the organ. *Ammonia* may induce violent nervous symptoms, similar to those of tetanus; its vapor sometimes acts powerfully on the air-passages.

Iodide of potassium, iodine, bromine, and *chlorine* are all capable of destroying life by their intensely irritant effect. *Phosphorus,* which is not unfrequently taken as a poison, imparts to the breath, the feces, and even to the urine an alliaceous smell, and makes them luminous in the dark. It acts as an irritant, causing obstinate vomiting and purging, pain at the epigastrium, rapid and weak pulse, jaundice, and unquenchable thirst. The local pain and inflammation are usually extreme, and collapse, with or without convulsions, comes on early. In some cases painful cramps in the limbs occur and various disturbances of sensibility, and later, violent delirium and convulsions eventuating in coma and death. In other cases hemorrhage is a striking feature, the blood is very fluid, and it issues from all the passages, and petechiæ form beneath the skin.

Jaundice is a very constant symptom; it seldom, however, comes on before the third day and is never intense.* The spleen increases in size simultaneously with the liver. Albumen is occasionally present in the urine, and the biliary

---

* Schraube, Schmidt's Jahrb., quoted in New Syd. Society's Bien. Rep. for 1867–8, p. 449.

coloring matters usually. In cases of phosphorus poisoning, acute and extreme fatty degeneration of the tissues happens. It occurs with astonishing rapidity. It has been seen, in the bodies of persons poisoned by phosphorus, within so short a period as forty-eight hours, and has been found to affect the heart, liver, kidneys, glands of the stomach, and the voluntary muscles.*

Various salts of *potassa*, *copper*, *zinc*, *silver*, *lead*, and *iron* occasionally cause death. They act, for the most part, as irritants merely; but some of them are powerfully astringent, and even caustic, as, for instance, the chloride of zinc or the nitrate of silver. If the toxical phenomena are due to the nitrate of silver, the staining of the lips may afford a clue to the nature of the case. There are no really distinctive symptoms produced by large doses of *arsenic*, *antimony*, *mercury*, or their compounds, which are among the best known of irritant poisons; the peculiar effects of each of these substances, when insidiously introduced into the economy, will be presently alluded to.

Among animal substances, *cantharides* has sometimes been productive of poisonous effects; strangury, and in male subjects priapism, are the most marked symptoms in such cases; while the shining, green particles of the drug, if taken in substance, have been detected in the vomited matters.

The vegetable irritants are mainly articles commonly used as purgatives. Thus, *elaterium*, *aloes*, *colocynth*, and *colchicum* have all proved fatal when taken too freely. The symptoms do not differ materially from those caused by other poisons of this class. *Tobacco* and *lobelia* are very powerful local excitants, occasioning emesis and purging, with a speedy collapse of the system. *Savin* not only produces inflammation of the alimentary canal, but is apt also to give rise to strangury; it is most frequently resorted to with the view of bringing on abortion.

Narcotic Poisoning.—The symptoms of narcotic poisoning vary more, according to the special article taken, than those caused by irritants. Narcotic poisons affect chiefly the

---

* Tardieu, Étude Médico-Légale sur l'Empoisonnement, 1867, p. 445.

nervous system and the circulation. Many of them produce phenomena like apoplexy and intoxication, from which they need to be most carefully distinguished. Narcotic poisoning is, for the most part, of the acute form.

Opium is by far the most important of narcotic poisons. It induces giddiness, stupor, and lethargic sleep, from which, however, the patient can at first be roused, if sharply spoken to. Subsequently this sleep deepens into coma, and cannot be broken; the skin is relaxed and perspiring; the face is usually pale; the pupils are contracted and insensible to light. A more or less evident odor of opium may often be perceived about the person or on the breath. No distinction can be drawn between the effects of different forms of this poison; the stronger the preparation, however, the more marked and the more rapid will be the progress of the case. Morphia, narcotina, and the other alkaloids give rise to similar symptoms; but the smell of opium is, of course, absent, and it is said that convulsions are more likely to occur as the result of their operation.

The diagnosis of opium poisoning from apoplexy and from the coma of uræmia has been discussed in a former chapter. We may merely recall that the contracted pupil caused by opium is of very great significance, and does not, with the exceptions there referred to, exist in the other states. Moreover, the coma of apoplexy is at once developed; while in narcotic poisoning it is not sudden, but is preceded by drowsiness or stupor, which gradually passes into coma. These phenomena occur also in the same sequence in uræmia; but they are even slower in their progress, and are frequently associated with convulsions and with dropsy.

Alcohol, if taken in large quantities and not much diluted, produces symptoms very much like those caused by opium. The effect would not always seem to be due to the absorption of the poison, since the breath may be quite free from spirituous odor. This absence of odor of the breath may give rise to a confusion between alcoholic poisoning and apoplexy, and the discrimination of these conditions must then depend in some measure upon evidence furnished by the history of the occurrence of the insensibility, and the presence or absence of the signs of palsy.

Belladonna and *hyoscyamus* produce a more marked excitement of the brain than opium does, often causing delirium of an active kind, with convulsions. The pupil is dilated and vision is singularly deranged; there is intense thirst, with spasm and burning in the throat. *Conium* occasions stupor, or paralyzes the muscular system. *Aconite* has a powerfully sedative influence upon the action of the heart, brain, and spinal cord, as well as an irritant action upon the alimentary canal; slow pulse, giddiness, delirium, numbness, and tingling of the skin, loss of power in the legs, with vomiting and purging, are followed by syncope and death.

Digitalis causes great dilatation of the pupil, sometimes vomiting and purging, and suppression of urine; its chief effect, however, is upon the pulse, which is strikingly lessened both in frequency and force. *Veratrum viride*, or *American hellebore*, now so extensively used in this country, closely resembles digitalis in its action.

Hydrocyanic or *prussic acid* is a well-known poison; it usually leads to convulsive contractions of the muscles of the limbs and trunk, and destroys life by stopping the circulation and respiration. Sometimes the odor of the acid, resembling that of bitter almonds, is perceptible in the patient's breath; but too much reliance must not be placed upon this point. Unfortunately, the diagnosis of this poison has generally to be made after death, for medico-legal purposes.

The gases arising from burning *coal*, and the fumes of *charcoal*, may lead to death by asphyxia; and a knowledge of this fact has, particularly in France, led to many suicides. In those cases in which the asphyxia has not a fatal termination, yet has been decided, disorders in the peripheral nerves may show themselves, manifest either by the signs of neuritis, or by pain and swelling simulating a phlegmon, or by vesicular eruptions in the course of an affected vaso-motor nerve. The peripheral disturbances may appear immediately, or not until after some days. The signs of disorder of the vaso-motor nerves do not last long; those of the motor or sensitive nerves have a longer duration; may be incurable, extending from the centre to the periphery, or in the reverse direction; or lastly, cause an ascending acute paralysis.*

Calabar bean acts as a direct sedative to the spinal marrow, and produces muscular debility or relaxation or even paralysis, extending to the heart and respiratory muscles. The mental faculties remain unaffected, and in this it differs from the action of the cerebral sedatives. It is, however, irritant to the alimentary canal, causing vomiting or purging, and a peculiar epigastric sensation is generally experienced. Calabar bean contracts the pupil and also the ciliary muscle, thus making the eye myopic.†

Strychnia and *brucia*, the active principles of nux vomica, and of several allied plants, give rise to phenomena strongly resembling those of tetanus. A very short time, however,—from a few minutes to an hour or two,—will determine the issue of a case of poisoning; while tetanus may run a course of several weeks. The first symptoms of strychnia poisoning are apt to be a sense of suffocation and dyspnœa, followed by starting and twitching and rigidity of the arms and legs, but not by lock-jaw; tetanus, on the other hand, comes on with setting or locking of the jaws, and the limbs are not at first affected with spasms, indeed, the arms remain throughout nearly free from them. Again, idiopathic tetanus is extremely rare; almost always there has been some wound or injury as a proximate cause of the malady. But we need not pursue these points of diagnosis further; they have been already mentioned in connection with tetanus.

Chronic Poisoning.

When the patient has been subjected to the continuous action of a noxious substance, the case is said to be one of chronic or slow poisoning. Any of the irritant poisons, given in small and repeated doses, will keep up a morbid condition of the stomach and bowels much like ordinary chronic inflammation.

The narcotics, taken in the same manner, act primarily

---

* Leudet, Archiv. Génér. de Méd., May, 1865.

† T. A. Robertson, Edinb. Med. Journ., March, 1868.

upon the cerebro-spinal system, and through this upon the alimentary canal, so deranging digestion and nutrition as even indirectly to cause death. *Opium* is the most important of the articles thus used; it is often administered to infants, for the purpose of quieting their cries, and the frequent repetition of the dose induces a series of phenomena closely allied to those observed in the adult. With the effects, on the mind, of opium taken persistently for the sake of intoxication, the reading world is familiar through the published experiences of De Quincey and Coleridge.

The habit is here and in Europe generally acquired only by persons who have begun the practice for the relief of some painful affection; in the East, opium is used much more commonly, and in many Oriental countries, to smoke it is a favorite amusement. Those who employ it constantly are pale, or have a sallow, haggard countenance and a dull eye. They are troubled by loss of appetite, sleeplessness, and low spirits, which they remove by resorting to the opiate. Though, in spite of the pernicious custom, their general health may remain for many years good, yet sooner or later it gives way, and the opium-eater dies worn out; or death may be the consequence of disease of the liver, palsy, or inveterate diarrhœa, produced by long addiction to the vice. Persons who consume large quantities of opium are very apt to have, from time to time, attacks of extreme nervous prostration, attended, perhaps, with violent headache, and requiring free stimulation for their relief.

Ether and *chlordform*, habitually made use of, also cause serious disturbance of the nervous system; and so does *alcohol*. The abuse of spirituous liquors gives rise to a disorder of the mental, motor, and sensory functions, producing sleeplessness, headache, giddiness, hallucinations; as well as to a sensation of choking, a diminished vitality, a tendency to fatty degeneration, especially of the liver and kidneys; in short, to the symptoms often met with in drunkards, and constituting the state so graphically described by Huss[*] and Marcet[†] as chronic alcoholism.

---

[*] Alcoholismus Chronicus, or Chronic Alcohol Disease.
[†] On Chronic Alcoholic Intoxication. London, 1860.

Tobacco used in excess gives rise to tremors, impaired digestion, intermittence in the pulse, with irregular cardiac action and palpitations, which may become very annoying, and originate the belief of an organic disease of the heart. Like the persistent abuse of alcoholic drinks, tobacco may occasion amaurosis;* and it is also affirmed that an insidious, obstinate form of otitis is developed in inveterate smokers, and is attended with very minute granulations of the pharynx, nasal fossæ, tubes, and middle ear.† When employed in large quantities by those previously unaccustomed to it, tobacco produces emaciation, weakness, sleeplessness, dull hearing, cold sweats, feeble action of the heart, and will even cause death.

Let us now examine some of the features of slow poisoning by the metals.

Mercury in any of its preparations, may lead to chronic poisoning. The mouth is inflamed, the gums sore and swollen, the salivary glands act inordinately, and the breath is very offensive. Colicky pains, and sometimes diarrhœa occur. Tremors of the limbs, when any motion is attempted, evince disorder of the nervous centres: they are particularly frequent in cases where the poison has been inhaled in the form of vapor, and come on by degrees, and are associated with loss of power of locomotion and with digestive disturbances. The tremors may be incessant and the movements involuntary, like those of chorea, and so rapid as to prevent the patient from obtaining rest at night.‡ In some cases, an eczematous affection is observed.

Poisoning by mercury is generally the result of the exposure to its action incidental to certain occupations, such as glass-plating, gilding, and working in quicksilver mines.

---

* Sichel, Annales d'Oculistique, Mars, 1865, quoted in Brit. and For. Med.-Chirurg. Rev., July, 1865.

† Triquet, quoted ib. Le Briert, Gazette des Hôpitaux, quoted in Ed. Med. Journ., Aug. 1864.

‡ As in a case reported by Dr. Taylor, in which the patient died from the effects of the poison, without, however, having presented salivation or mercurial fetor of the breath, or a blue line on the gums. Guy's Hosp. Rep., 3d Series, vol. x.

Lead poisoning is by no means uncommon among painters, plumbers, and other workers in lead. Sometimes it may be caused by accidental circumstances, as when the patient has drunk water passed through leaden pipes, or taken snuff which has been impregnated with lead for the purpose of coloring it; poisonous properties are said also to be acquired by snuff wrapped in lead-foil, and lead poisoning has been observed among those engaged in the manufacture of lucifer matches or working in glass powder.*

In such cases, the physician may have to depend entirely upon a correct appreciation of the symptoms for the diagnosis. Pain and uneasiness in the course of the colon, constipation, loss of appetite, and emaciation are the earlier signs. A metallic taste is sometimes perceived; the breath is fetid, and the tongue pale and furred; the gums are almost always edged with a blue line. Colicky pains are felt from time to time, and a severe and long-continued attack of colic may form the culmination of the disease. Occasionally wrist-drop, or paralysis of the extensor muscles of the forearm, so well known as a phenomenon of lead poisoning, occurs among the first symptoms; but it is more generally preceded by one or more attacks of colic. We also find at times lesions of the tendons in saturnine palsy.† Yet as regards this palsy we must bear in mind that paralysis of the extensors may occur which is not due to lead.‡

Sometimes there is evidence, in cases of saturnine poisoning, of very grave cerebral disorder; epileptiform convulsions, attacks resembling apoplexy, or general tremors and extended paralysis of the muscles, with amaurosis and other signs of nervous disturbance, are noticed. Of course the diagnosis, under these circumstances, will be materially assisted by an accurate knowledge of the previous history of the patient as regards exposure to the action of the poison. The tremors are, like those caused by mercury, mostly peculiar in ceasing when the limbs are supported or at rest.

---

* Lacharrière, Archiv. Génér., December, 1859.
† Med Times and Gazette, May, 1868
‡ St. George's Hospital Reports, 1868, p. 86.

Another result of lead poisoning is that it leads to the form of Bright's disease known as granular degeneration of the kidneys. This is very apt again to coexist with a gouty condition, which, as Garrod has shown, is one of the results of the absorption of lead. But the kidney trouble may be found, whether or not the joints are markedly affected. The intertubular or fibrous tissue of the organs becomes thickened by a sort of chronic inflammation, and depositions of urate of soda between the tubes are not uncommon.

Arsenic, administered in small doses for a lengthened period, produces a state of chronic inflammation of the alimentary canal. Œdema of the face and limbs, in some instances associated with albuminous urine, irritability of the stomach, diarrhœa, and increasing nervous derangement mark the progress of these cases; the hair and nails occasionally fall out, and there is much frontal headache. Similar effects are noticed to follow the pernicious habit of arsenic-eating; and will be also encountered among persons employed in making artificial flowers and toys, in dyeing cloths, in manufacturing and hanging green papers, or engaged in the sublimation of arsenical ores. Besides the phenomena of internal poisoning, cutaneous eruptions occur.

The inhalation of the fumes of *zinc* gives rise to a peculiar form of poisoning, characterized by a sense of weariness, a feeling of tightness in the chest, and by attacks of shivering, followed by heat of skin and a profuse sweating stage. This irregular form of ague is common among brass-founders.*

Sulphuret of carbon produces toxical effects of a singular character, conspicuous among which are gastric disturbances, a cachectic condition, impotence, and, in severe cases, amaurosis, hallucinations, and complete perversion of the intellect.† These phenomena are met with among workers in India-rubber.

---

* Greenhow, Medico-Chir. Trans., 1862.

† Delpech, Mém. de l'Académ. de Médecine. 1856; and Heurtaux, Recueil de la Société Médicale d'Observation, 1860.

Phosphorus is often seen, particularly among those who work in lucifer match factories, to produce very serious lesions. It may occasion, as acute phosphorus poisoning does, alteration of the composition of the blood and a hemorrhagic diathesis, and a fatty degeneration of several organs, as well as of the voluntary muscles.* It also produces necrosis of the jaw, for which the whole lower jaw has been removed.† It leads, when taken internally in doses that gradually exert a poisonous effect, to chronic inflammation and thickening of the stomach, to colicky pains, to diarrhœa, hectic fever, general emaciation, falling out of the hair, and palsies, which are generally the precursors of a fatal termination.

Animal poisons may give rise to chronic as well as to acute poisoning. We find, for instance, syphilis, and gonorrhœa, hydrophobia, dissecting wounds, snake-bites, and acute glanders and farcy,—all disorders exhibiting the effect of an animal virus. But we have already discussed some of these, so far as is admissible in a work of this kind; and of the others, it need only be said that the antecedent circumstances generally place the diagnosis beyond a doubt.

Yet there are a few illustrations of animal poisons and their effects, which must here, however briefly, be mentioned.

One of these is the *malignant pustule*, a terrible malady, which is the cause of many deaths on the continent of Europe, and which is identical with the *charbon* of animals. The disorder is also prevalent in New Mexico.‡ It is communicated to man by direct inoculation; or by means of the skin or hair of the diseased beast, or by eating its flesh; or by insects which, sucking the poison from the sick animal, implant it on the skin of man. The poison produces a red speck, which develops into a vesicle, under and around which an extremely hard spot forms that becomes gangrenous. The surrounding skin inflames, new vesicles or pus-

---

* Lanceraux, l'Union Médicale, 1863, quoted in Br. and For. Med.-Chir. Rev., April, 1864.

† Cases of Hunt and Boker, Amer. Med. Journ., April, 1865; Wells, New York Med. Journ , Jan. 1866.

‡ A. H. Smith, Amer. Journ. Med. Sciences, April, 1867.

tules spring up, and the gangrene spreads rapidly, the patient speedily sinking, or the death of the parts is arrested, and separation takes place between the living and gangrenous textures. It is remarkable how little local pain attends the grave constitutional disturbance, and signs of low, irritative fever. The disease is found on the exposed portions of the body, as on the neck and hands. Though due to a poisonous influence communicated from a diseased animal to man, it has been affirmed to have been traced to the presence of the filiform infusoria, called bacteridia, which have also been found in the charbon.*

There is another form of animal poisoning which may be in this connection briefly considered, namely, *milk-sickness*. Now, its phenomena are so variously described by writers, that its characteristic signs are difficult to define. It prevails only in the southern and southwestern portions of North America, and is brought on by drinking the milk or eating the flesh of cattle which have been exposed to certain influences, the nature of which is as yet unknown. Gastritis and enteritis seem to be more or less blended in the early stage of this disorder, which, at a later period, is said strongly to resemble typhus fever. The symptoms more especially dwelt upon are lassitude, nausea and vomiting, with a sense of burning at the epigastrium, great oppression, intense thirst, hot, dry skin, obstinate constipation, and obvious abdominal pulsation. If at all, recovery takes place very tardily, the tone of the stomach being often left impaired for life.

The treatment of this affection consists in overcoming the very obstinate constipation apt to exist, in remedying the local irritant action of the poison, and supporting the powers of the system. Mercurials pushed to salivation would seem to have proved beneficial in some cases.

Besides these forms of animal poisoning, which are produced by the direct contact with the virus, or at all events by its introduction into the system through the stomach, we find morbid states occasioned by animal poisons which arise

---

* Davaine, Gazette Médicale, July, 1865.

from decomposing bodies or excretions, or from the crowding of many together, particularly of those of uncleanly habits, or of wounded. These poisons reach the blood for the most part by the lungs, in the shape of *poisonous exhalations.* They are very depressing in their action, may lead to low fevers, or to septicæmia, and in the case of the wounded to pyæmia and hospital gangrene. Persistent nausea, too, and a lowering of all vital energy are not uncommonly observed in those who breathe continuously the foul air under the circumstances alluded to—as in hospitals and in prisons, in which thorough cleanliness is not enforced, and due regard is not paid to ventilation.

In some persons deleterious emanations from the human body give rise to a form of toxæmia, one of the chief features of which is the marked anorexia which attends the great debility.*

The exposure to animal effluvia may also excite violent diarrhœa, or even symptoms like those of cholera, certainly like those of severe attacks of cholera morbus. Of the occurrence of the former we have an illustration in the dissecting-room diarrhœa, which is usually attended with very fetid discharges, and may be accompanied by colicky pains, by nausea and vomiting, and headache. The same kind of diarrhœa also happens in those who clean privies, or who are exposed to the emanations arising from sewers; or dysentery or choleraic attacks may follow the exposure. Nay, as in instances recorded by Becquerel, the instant disengagement of large quantities of putrid gases, arising from bodies far advanced in decomposition, where coffins have been opened, has caused sudden deaths, or resulted in so serious a state of poisoning as to have given rise to very grave illnesses, having mostly a fatal termination.† In individuals who, in consequence of their vocation, are habitually brought in contact with animal effluvia and liable to inhale noxious gases, besides the attacks of diarrhœa referrrd to, chronic disturb-

---

* See Dr. Hunt's case described by himself in Pennsylvania Hospital Reports, vol. i.

† Traité d'Hygiène, third edition, p. 218.

ances of the stomach and liver, with marked impairment of the general health, may happen.

PARASITES.

Parasites, properly speaking, are organisms which become secondarily implanted within or upon the body. There is much room for doubt concerning several of them, as to whether they cause disease or are merely its concomitants. Some parasites give rise to no symptoms at all; many occasion phenomena closely resembling those of other irritations. In any case, however, the only absolutely convincing evidence of the presence of a parasite is obtained by seeing it.

Vegetable Parasites.—The chief vegetable parasites have been mentioned in connection with diseases of the skin; the oidium albicans, present in thrush, and stated to have been met with in diphtheria, as well as the sarcinæ ventriculi, have also been alluded to. All these vegetable growths can only be detected by the microscope; and, particularly in those involving the skin or hair, it is of the utmost use to employ the liquor potassæ, under the action of which the structures become transparent.

One, and so far as is known only one, fungus penetrates the internal tissues—the chionyphe Carteri. This gives rise to that terrible disease known as podelcoma, or the *fungus foot* of India,—a complaint confined to the natives of India who go about with naked feet. The fungus, introduced either through a scratch or passing through the pores of the skin, soon spreads, eating its way into the bones of the tarsus, metatarsus, and into the lower end of the tibia and fibula, producing a species of caries, or rather a breaking up and absorption of the osseous tissues. The fungus particles or masses are generally of deep black color, firm and globular, and in size varying from a pea to a pistol bullet; or the fungus presents the appearance of sloughing tissue, and exhibits chiefly white granules; or it consists of particles of pinkish color. In any case the foot is enlarged about the ankle and over the instep; and on either side of the ankle-joint, and on the dorsum as well as on the sole of the foot are small, soft swellings, having pouting openings that lead to fistulous canals communicating with the bones, which they perforate in every direction. The fungus mass is for the most part situated in the cavities in the bones, and from the canals passing to them transudes a discolored, glairy, or purulent and fetid fluid. The toes are distorted, and the muscles of the leg atrophied; but the fungus does not spread up the leg. The tendency of the disease is to cause death by exhaustion; the only remedy is amputation.*

Animal Parasites.—When speaking of the affections of particular structures, I have already alluded to some of these intruders,—those found in the skin or liver, for instance. I have now to consider chiefly such as inhabit the hollow viscera and certain solid organs or the muscles, noticing the phenomena caused by them and the main points by which they may be distinguished from one another. But in so doing I shall only mention those of greatest import, for, as there are at least thirty-one distinct animals which in some phase or other of their existence infect man, and as a number of these reside in the structures just alluded to, it would not be possible to describe them all in detail.†

Intestinal worms are, perhaps, the most common of all parasites. The general symptoms induced by them are those of intestinal irritation with disordered digestion. The appetite is capricious; the bowels are very irregular, sometimes constipated, sometimes relaxed; the abdomen is frequently swollen and hard, and the seat of distressing uneasiness or of colicky pains; the tongue is furred; the breath fetid; and there is constant itching about the nostrils and anus. The patient, furthermore, grits his teeth during sleep, and is very often annoyed by nightmare. Phenomena indicative of a greater or less degree of nervous disturbance are also met

---

* See Carter, in the Transactions of the Bombay Medical and Physical Society; and Aitken, Practice of Medicine, vol. i.

† See, for their full description, the excellent works of Joseph Leidy, A Flora and Fauna within Living Animals, Smithsonian Publications, vol. v.; of Davaine, Traité des Entozoaires et des Maladies Vermineuses; of Cobbold, Entozoa; of Leuckhart, Die Menschlichen Parasiten, Leipzig; and Küchenmeister, Manual of Parasites, Sydenham Society's Translation.

with; they may range from mere fretfulness up to delirium, convulsions, chorea, epilepsy, or even insanity.

There are many kinds of worms known to infest the alimentary canal of man, and they belong to the orders of *nematoda*, or round worms, or to those of *cestoidea*, or tape-worms.

The round worms are parasites of an attenuated and cylindrical form, and present these varieties:

1. The *ascaris lumbricoïdes*, or *round worm*, bears a considerable resemblance to the common earth-worm, from which it is, however, anatomically different. It inhabits the small intestine, sometimes finding its way into the stomach, or ' even into the œsophagus, or being discharged through the abdominal parietes.* When it ascends to the stomach and œsophagus, it causes, before it is expelled by the mouth, sudden attacks of fever and gastric derangement, with nausea and vomiting; and even at times marked delirium.† The worms have been known to be so numerous as to obstruct the intestine. Calomel, pink-root, chenopodium, and other purgatives, given singly or variously combined, will dislodge or destroy the parasite.

2. The *oxyuris vermicularis*, *thread*, or *seat-worm*, is very small, the male being about two lines, the female about five lines in length. The parasite is white, slender, and extremely active; is found in the anus, and causes intense itching of this part. The annoyance is sometimes such as to excite a suspicion of the existence of piles. It may creep into the vagina, giving rise there to profuse discharges; or into the urethra. It affects children frequently, but is not uncommon in adults. Enemata containing vinegar or turpentine generally afford relief.

3. The *ascaris mystax*, a parasite which inhabits the cat, may also, as Bellingham and Cobbold have proved, infest the human body. It is a moderate-sized nematode, from two to three inches long, though the female may reach about four inches. Its head end is spear-shaped.

4. The *trichocephalus dispar*, or *long thread-worm*, is detected

---

* Garnier, l'Union Médicale, Oct. 1861.

† Schmidt's Jahrb., No. 10, 1868.

in very large numbers in the ilium near its termination, or in the colon, particularly at its head. It has been found in persons laboring under typhus or typhoid fever, or dying from cholera or diarrhœa. It is from an inch and a half to two inches in length, and is characterized by the hairlike appearance of the head, which is generally buried in the mucous membrane of the intestine. It is not a very common parasite, and it is doubtful whether its presence gives rise to any marked derangement. The *trichina spiralis*, belonging also to the round worms, was formerly stated to be the immature brood of the thread-worm; but this is now known to be incorrect.

The *tape-worms*, or cestoidea, are jointed entozoa, of a ribbon-like form. They embrace the true tape-worms, or tæniadæ, and the bothriocephali. Of the former there are eight varieties, all of which have been found in man, though only two—the solium and the mediocanellata—are at all common. The bothriocephalus latus is the usual species of bothriocephalus met with in the human intestine.

The *tænia solium*, or *common tape-worm*, consists of an immense number of joints in connection with a single head. It may attain an enormous length, and inhabits chiefly the small intestines. The researches of Küchenmeister,[*] Von Siebold,[†] and others have shown that its eggs become developed into the *cysticercus cellulosæ* discerned in the muscles of the pig, rabbit, and other animals whose flesh is used as food. Cysticerci have also been detected in the muscles, cellular tissue, brain, and even in the eye of man; being once introduced into the alimentary canal, they find there a nidus in which to undergo development into the tape-worm.

The parasite is nourished from its head, the newly-created segments pushing those already formed before them, so that the caudal extremity is the oldest portion of the animal. Each segment is flat and rectangular, and contains both a male and female organ, the orifices of which are joined at

---

[*] See Manual of Animal and Vegetable Parasites. Translation published by Sydenham Society, 1857.

[†] Origin of Intestinal Worms, ibid. 1857.

the apex of a lateral papilla. In the *tænia solium*, the papillæ are arranged alternately at one side and the other. The

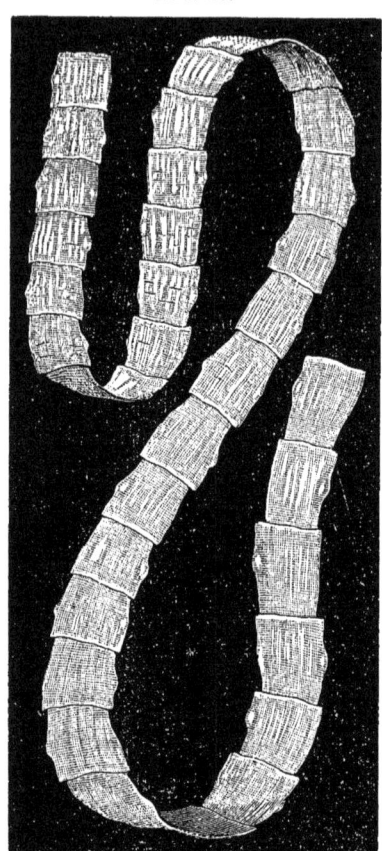

FIG. 46.

size of the segments increases gradually toward the caudal extremity, the largest being three or four lines in breadth. There may be upwards of eight hundred segments, and the worm may measure above ten feet; nay, it has been stated even to be above thirty. Upon the head, which is about as large as that of a pin, is a double circle of hooks contained in sacs, and around this circle are arranged four sucking-cups or mouths. The sleuder neck exhibits no segmentation. The sucking-disks in the *tænia mediocanellata* are much larger than those of the tænia solium, but the head, which is large, of blackish appearance, and obtuse, has no hooks.

Tænia solium. Drawn from a specimen.

Tænia occasions disordered digestion, colic, cramps, a feeling of uneasiness in the abdomen, irritation of the mouth, nose, and anus, anæmia, headache, dizziness, disturbed sleep, mental depression, cough, fainting fits, and various cerebro-spinal affections, such as convulsions and epilepsy; yet there are no absolute data for the diagnosis of this parasite, except its appearance in the discharges. In order that relief be permanent, the head must be expelled. Many remedies have been recommended for effecting this, among which may be mentioned pomegranate bark, extract or oil of male fern, kousso, powdered zinc or tin, and pumpkin seeds.

The *bothriocephalus latus, tænia lata,* or *broad tape-worm,* differs from the common tape-worm in having no lateral papillæ alternately arranged, but a single one at the centre of each segment; the segments themselves are much broader, and with the breadth greatly preponderating over their length; the head is of elongated form, has no hooks upon it, and only a pair of fissures instead of the four mouths of the tænia solium, and we find no traces of joints until about three inches from the head. The parasite is of yellow or grayish-white color.

Echinococci belong also to the family of the tæniadæ. They may take up their abode in the substance of almost any organ in the body, and are the immature brood of a species of tænia. They consist of a vesicle having at one portion of its wall a head, upon which are six hooklets circularly arranged. The whole animal is surrounded by an investing membrane, which may burst and allow it to escape; the term hydatid designates the enveloping cyst. It forms when the tænia embryo has bored its way to its resting-place in the liver, or has been carried with the circulation to other organs. The echinococcus, unlike other larval tæniæ, retains a more or less globular figure, in place of exhibiting a head, neck, and body. When the echinococci are arrested in their normal development and barren, not attaining to the production of scolices, they give rise to cysts with walls consisting of very distinctly developed, concentric layers, and having a peculiar gelatinous trembling — the so-called *acephalocysts;* and the same may be said of abortive cysticerci, embryonic forms of tæniæ, which, some suppose, may also occasion the hydatid cysts; though others maintain that the hydatids proceed from only one form of tænia—the tænia echinococcus.

The family of the *distomidæ,* belonging to the order of fluke-like parasites, is not at all uncommon in man.

A species of distoma, measuring from eight to fourteen lines in length, called the *distoma hepaticum,* very usual in the liver and gall-bladder of the sheep, has been seen in the human liver and gall-duct, and also, it is said, in abscesses of the scalp. Other species of distoma have been found in the portal vein, ureters, kidneys, and bladder, and upon the intestinal mucous membrane; yet in the portal vein and its larger branches—a common seat of the distoma—the parasite produces little or no appreciable derangement; but when in the intestine, it may give rise to congestion of the membrane, extravasation of blood, and the symptoms of dysentery. This has been specially noticed of the distoma hæmatobium, or Bilharzia hæmatobia, a worm very common in Egypt, and which has also been found to be the cause of the hæmaturia so prevalent at the Cape of Good Hope* and at the Mauritius.

A worm called the *strongylus gigas* has, in one or two instances, been observed in the kidneys; it need not, however, be more than alluded to.

The parasites which chiefly occupy the areolar tissues or the muscles still remain to be described. Of these there are two of special importance.

One is the *filaria medinensis*, or *Guinea-worm*. This is a very slender, flat, finely-ringed worm, which introduces itself into the subcutaneous cellular tissue: here it grows rapidly, and gives rise to swelling, with more or less inflammation; and severe constitutional disturbance is sometimes manifested. After a time the swelling points, breaks, and the worm may be laid hold of and carefully twisted around a little piece of stick or a quill until it is extracted entire; if broken off, the eggs with which it is filled, getting into the wound, will become the agents of fresh mischief. Very many of these worms may be found in the same patient, occasioning great annoyance and distress, even fatal exhaustion; but it is stated that there is often only one present. The number may vary between this and fifty. Some worms are twelve, others forty inches long, or even more. According to Busk, the parasite grows in the human areolar tissue at the rate of about an inch a week. Though it is most frequently found in the lower extremities, it has been observed to appear in the socket of the eye, the mouth, the cheeks, in the ears, and under the tongue and the scalp. It migrates rapidly from one part of the body to another. Where it exists, a pricking or an itching heat is felt; a vesicle forms

---

* John Harley, Medico-Chirurg. Transact., vol. xlvii.

when the worm is about coming to the surface, and this vesicle opens, leaving an angry-looking ulcer, in the centre of which the parasite shows itself. The period of incubation is about twelve months; thus a year elapses before the Guinea-worm makes itself manifest in the human body.* The disorder, common in Asia and Africa, is fortunately one with which we are unacquainted.

Trichina spiralis.—This parasite, which is now known to be of not unfrequent occurrence in the muscles of man, and to give rise to a very grave disorder, occasioning much pain and very often death, was formerly supposed to be perfectly harmless. It was discovered by Owen in 1835 in human muscles taken from the dissecting-room, and was named by him, as it was as fine as a hair and always coiled up in a more or less spiral line, trichina spiralis. The same parasite was subsequently found in animals, as by Leidy in the animal which it most infests,—the pig. But in the observations made, certainly in those made on man, the trachinæ were only detected in their cysts, and as these cysts become, after a certain period, filled with a calcareous deposit, which leads to the extinction of the worms, the whole subject of their presence in the human body was scarcely looked upon as other than one of curiosity, until in 1860 Zenker—the same pathologist who discerned the altered and granular condition of the muscular fibres in low fevers—proved, by a series of splendid observations, that trichinæ may exist free in the muscles of man, that they are encapsuled only after some time, and are the cause of what may be a very fatal disease. The first case was that of a servant-girl, who died in the hospital at Dresden with symptoms like those of typhoid fever. She, together with several members of the family in which she lived, and the butcher who had killed the pigs, had swallowed their meat uncooked, and had soon afterward been taken sick. At the autopsy, her muscles were found to be full of trichinæ, which were not yet encapsuled. One of the hams and some of the sausages, portions of which she had eaten, contained numerous encysted trichinæ. Thus the

---

* Aitken's Practice of Med., vol. i.

52

connection between the symptoms and their originating cause was clearly traced. It was soon verified by other observations; and it has since been well understood that the cases previously examined were cured cases, which had falsely given rise to the belief of the supposed innocuous character of the parasite, and that in the trichina disease, or *trichiniasis*, we find one of the most dangerous maladies to which the human frame is liable; so dangerous that whole families have perished from its effects amid great suffering, and that in the small village of Hedersleben, of 2000 inhabitants, 300 were affected, of whom 80 died.*

The parasite is always introduced into the body by eating ham, pork, or sausages made from the flesh of pigs containing trichinæ. It is very probable that the hogs themselves obtain them from rats, in which they are extremely common. It has also been stated that trichinæ may exist in beef,† but this is not generally admitted.

The trichina spiralis is the juvenile condition of a small nematode worm. It is incapable of generation, and becomes fruitful only, whether encapsuled or not, when introduced into the intestine. After being swallowed, if it be encysted, the capsule is dissolved, and the parasite remains in the intestine, where it rapidly grows to three or four times its former size, and, within two days, attains its full sexual maturity.‡ By the sixth day the female trichina contains an abundance of living young, and begins to throw off minute embryos, which are born without any covering from the egg, and at once begin to migrate to the muscular structures. When they reach these, they grow there, but do not generate others. A single female trichina may remain in the intestine for three or four weeks, or even longer, and may give birth, it is estimated, to from two hundred to two thousand embryos, which find their way to the muscles; while the trichinæ that have been swallowed never pass beyond the intestine. In six or eight weeks at furthest the

---

* Virchow, Die Lehre von den Trichinen, p. 33.
† New York Med. Journal, July, 1866.
‡ Leuckhart, Untersuchungen über Trichina Spiralis.   Leipzig, 1866.

intestinal trichinæ have, as a rule, died and left the intestinal canal; four to five weeks may be stated to be their average life.*

When the young trichina arrives in the muscles,—which it does, according to the current view, by piercing the intestinal walls and passing directly to the muscles, or, according to one of our own observers, Dr. Dalton,† by being conveyed

FIG. 47.

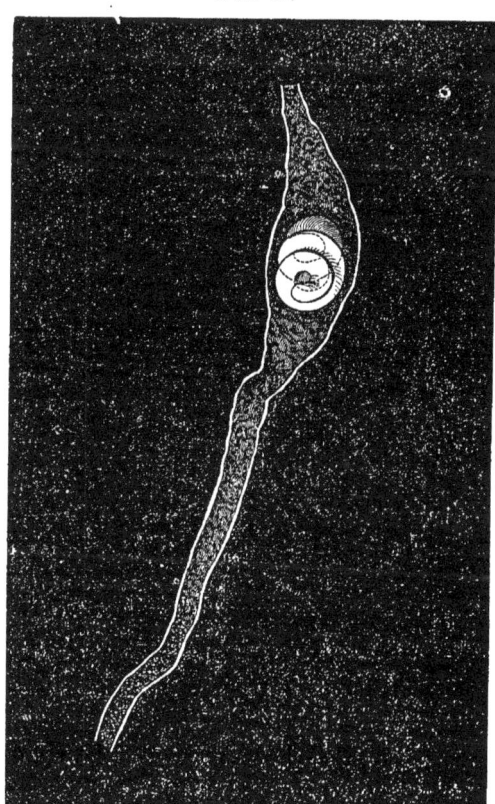

Trichina in recent human muscle, taken the thirteenth day of illness. (After DALTON.)

there by the circulating current,—it begins to destroy the muscular texture. It penetrates the sarcolemma, feeds on the fibre, particularly on the primitive fibrilles, and on the

* Leuckhart, op. cit.
† Transactions of the New York Academy of Medicine, 1864.

granules and disks of the contractile matter, or syntonine; and irritates the sarcolemma, leading to its gradual thickening, also to an increased development and multiplication of the nuclear elements, and to an exudation which finally fixes the worm to a particular spot. Thus is formed the cyst, which encapsules the worm, and which plays such an important part in the subsequent destruction of the parasite. This cyst in the human subject is oval, or, more generally still, spindle-shaped, the prolongations having a rounded end, and in its centre the worm lies coiled up. It takes a month or months for the cyst to form completely, though at the end of the third week after migration, the inflammatory irritation has reached its highest point, and the trichina is by that time—Leuckhart says in less, in fourteen days—nearly or entirely full grown. Several trichinæ may wander in the same track, and ultimately be inclosed in the same mass of exuded matter. Two are not unfrequently seen intimately coiled up, and the number may rise to five.*

After the perfect formation of the cyst, further changes take place in it. The masses of nuclei in the spaces at both extremities of the capsule become of greenish hue; dark or black particles of carbonate of lime and magnesia are deposited. The calcareous mass extends, and gradually covers the whole parasite, while around the prolongations of the cyst fat cells are deposited. The whole process is very destructive to the flesh-worm, and it is thus that the disorder is cured. But it is apt to be months before this result is accomplished. Nay, as we know from two cases recorded by Virchow, neither the encapsuling nor the calcareous transformation kills the worms, of necessity, at all speedily; for in the one case they had remained alive for eight, in the other for thirteen and a half years after the infection.†

FIG. 48.

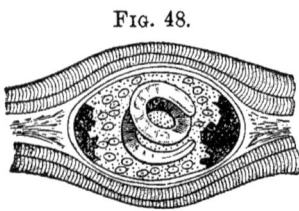

Trichina capsule with shell-like calcareous deposits. (After LEUCKHART.)

---

* Thudichum, Blue Book. Seventh Report of the Medical Officer of the Privy Council, p. 367.

† Virchow, op. cit., p. 40.

The appearances described are not to be recognized by the naked eye. Indeed, the cysts can scarcely be said to be visible excepting after the calcareous matter has been deposited in them, when they appear as very small gritty substances scattered over a piece of muscle. For the study of the cyst a low magnifying power only is requisite. To investigate the structure of the worm requires, however, one of at least 300 diameters. The parasite, which is truly a microscopical animal, being only $\frac{1}{3}$ to $\frac{1}{2}$ line in length, and about $\frac{1}{32}$ of a line in thickness, will be seen with this power to have an anterior extremity that is narrow and pointed, and where an alimentary canal commences by a mouth, followed by an œsophagus surrounded by cells. The cellular body extends through a very considerable portion of the animal, and passes into the less complex intestinal canal, which terminates with an anus at the rounded and comparatively thick posterior extremity of the worm. In the posterior third of the trichina lies the generative apparatus, which in part presents a dark, granular mass, but nothing else very marked, since in the trichinæ found in the muscles there are no developed sexual organs. The internal structures are protected by a thin but strong and elastic integument with minute grooves. The male intestinal trichina is only about two-thirds the length of the female, and the body is more transparent.

The number of trichinæ in the muscles may be from several hundreds to as many millions. Now, in accordance with their number in the muscles, with the character of the changes which there take place, and the quantity in the intestines, will vary the extent of constitutional derangement and the signs of local irritation. Thus the symptoms and the dangers of tri-

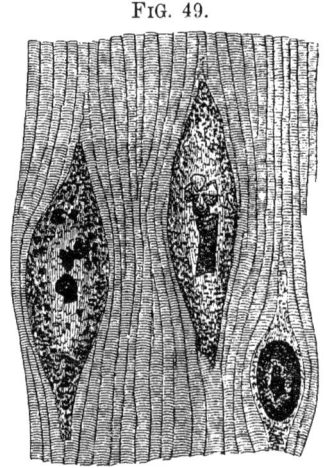

FIG. 49.

Encapsuled chalky concretions in muscle, due to dead trichinæ. Magnified about thirty times (After Leuckhart)

chiniasis are not always the same : we find indeed all degrees
of the malady. When merely a few thousand trichinæ occupy
the muscles, there is chiefly muscular pains with stiffness and
general debility; signs which gradually cease as the worms
become fully encapsuled, and cretaceous alterations occur.

Fig. 50.

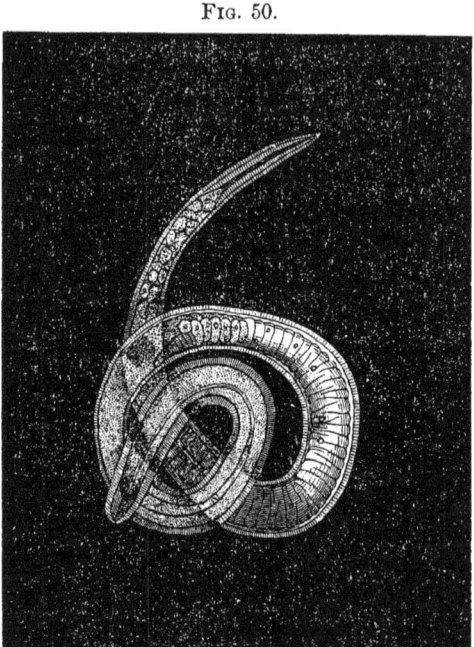

Trichina spiralis.   Magnified 300 times.   (Alter Virchow.)

When the muscles are occupied by millions of the flesh-
worms, the local phenomena are much more severe; there
may be almost complete immobility of the whole body, the
muscles of respiration and deglutition are implicated, irritative fever and the general cachexia are very marked, and the
patient is apt to perish by gradual exhaustion, or in consequence of the disordered respiratory function, or some pulmonary complication. The presence of large numbers of
trichinæ in the intestine produces diarrhœa, vomiting, abdominal pain and tenderness; or the worms may shortly
after being swallowed give rise to a kind of cholera morbus.
Speaking generally, we may recognize in trichiniasis three
stages : the first, lasting about a week, during which the

trichinæ are being generated in the intestines; the second, the passage of the brood through the intestinal walls into the muscular textures and the disturbances it there occasions; the third, the retrogressive formation which fairly sets in about three or four weeks after the beginning of the second. Now, it is this stage which yields the most striking manifestations of the malady:—loss of appetite; nausea; dry, somewhat coated tongue; diarrhœa; abdominal pain and meteorism; prostration; fever, with a quick pulse and copious sweating; edematous swelling of the face, followed in grave cases by almost general anasarca; sensitiveness of the muscles to the touch, or painfulness when moved, and their contraction or difficult motion; dyspnœa; sleepless nights; and emaciation.

Let us examine some of these phenomena more in detail:

The *fever* is a very marked symptom. It sets in early, owing to the intestinal irritation, though it is not until the end of, or after the first week, after therefore the migration of the young trichinæ has fairly begun, that it is strikingly developed. It is then, excepting in those cases in which fresh importations of trichinæ from the intestine in considerable numbers produce exacerbations, a continuous fever, with a pulse ranging from 100 to 130, with scanty urine and profuse perspirations having a very unpleasant odor, and which may continue in certain parts of the body after the general sweating has entirely ceased. The temperature is increased to about 101° Fahr., though it may pass beyond this; but it does not reach the high heat which is observable in other continuous fevers, particularly in grave cases. In this comparatively low temperature, joined to the profuse perspirations, the absence of enlargement of the spleen and of an eruption, the swelling of the face, the muscular symptoms, and a very red color of the visible mucous membranes, lie the points of difference between the febrile excitement of trichiniasis and typhoid fever,—a malady which, on account of the continuous fever, the prostration and diarrhœa and the sudamina, it resembles.

The *œdema* marks the distinct beginning of the second stage of the affection. It manifests itself first in the eyelids, and is very apt to be attended with a catarrhal state of the conjunctiva, dilated pupils, great susceptibility to light, diminished power of accommodation, and pain in moving the eye. The swelling may extend over the whole face. It is uninfluenced either by the sweats or the diarrhœa; but lessens generally very much, after lasting eight or nine days, or even disappears; at the same time, too, the diarrhœa is apt to diminish, or even gradually to cease. But instead of the œdema subsiding, it may extend to the chin, arms and legs, and the back; or it may show itself in the extremities subsequently to the disappearance from the face, and shortly afterward become perceptible over the trunk. In some cases an anasarcous condition, commencing at the ankles and extending upward, occurs during convalescence, and is of long duration. It is then probably connected with the state of the blood; whereas the œdema happening earlier in the malady is thought to be due to the pressure upon the arteries, exerted by the parasites and the exudation of plastic material they produce, or, in accordance with the observations of Thudichum, their presence within the lymphatic spaces, vessels and glands, and blood-currents.* It is a very striking fact connected with the dropsical swelling of trichiniasis that it is not associated with albumen in the urine, for, excepting an increased quantity of uric acid, the urinary secretion contains no abnormal ingredient. Boils, acne, and ecthyma are often noticed after the œdema has passed away.†

The *muscular symptoms* begin in the second stage with pain and stiffness in the limbs. Soon at all parts of the body the muscles give the impression of being swollen; they are extremely painful when touched or moved; and the patient lies in consequence as quiet as possible, or, in very severe instances of the affection, like a paralyzed person. The immobility is partially also due to the retracted state of the muscles which occurs in bad cases, and which produces a condition similar to a true spasm, manifest for instance in the semiflexed position of the extremities, and in the occasion-

---

* Thudichum, loc. cit., pp. 362 and 386.
† Meissner, Schmidt's Jahrb., No. 4, 1868.

ally present rigid, trismus-like setting of the jaws. The disturbance of function of certain muscles becomes particularly evident. The disorder of the muscles of the eye has already been alluded to; we encounter besides, impaired hearing and difficulty of deglutition and loss of voice, from the muscles of the ear, of the pharynx, and the larynx being filled with trichinæ. The respiratory muscles are commonly very much affected, and we find hurried and shallow breathing, and at times considerable distress in respiration. The muscles of the heart very usually, and the unstriped muscles of organic life constantly, escape infection; and as the trichinæ wander to the front of the body rather than to the back, the muscles anteriorly are more infested than those posteriorly.

The marked muscular pain, the stiffness, the fever, the profuse sweats, the acid urine, simulate the signs of acute rheumatism; but we find in trichiniasis diarrhœa, no articular swelling, and no heart complications. It is only as regards cases of acute muscular rheumatism—which is by no means frequent as a general state or associated ordinarily with obvious febrile phenomena—that error is likely to arise. The signs of prostration are, however, here wholly wanting.

The condition of the respiratory muscles gives rise, as already stated, to the embarrassed respiration, but it is not the only cause of the *pulmonary symptoms*. Yet whether it alone leads to congestion of the lung and to bronchitis or pleuritis, or other causes concur in producing them, it is certain that these states are very usual. They are also not uncommouly combined with pneumonia, which appears suddenly, and selects the lower portion of the left lung by preference, occurs about the twenty-sixth day of the disease, and is very apt to prove fatal. The sputa consist of dark unmixed blood; and the pneumonia is thought to be due to a trichinous embolism, the clots being derived from thrombi, which, forming in the venous system, are sent through the heart into the lungs.*

If the patient escape a serious pulmonary complication, if

---

* Rupprecht, Die Trichinen Krankheit im Spiegel der Hettstädter Endemie betrachtet, 1864.

he has strength enough to withstand the weeks of irritative fever and exhaustion, he enters at the end of a month of suffering upon a gradual convalescence. The fever declines; the respiration is less accelerated; the perspirations are far less copious; the urine increases in quantity; the pains decrease; and by about the sixth week of the malady, the patient is sufficiently free from pain to lie on his side, and is thus able to sleep. The pallor of his countenance gives way to a healthier hue; his appetite becomes insatiable; and he moves his limbs with more and more freedom. But it is a long time before he regains his full strength or his muscular power. Indeed, the latter may be always somewhat impaired; though we have the authority of Rupprecht for the statement that it may entirely return, and perfect health be recovered. In some cases the convalescence is greatly retarded by boils, inflammation of the lymphatic glands, and the very gradually yielding dropsy. The reduction of the power of accommodation of the eye to distances may also alter but slowly. Children are apt to convalesce more quickly than adults. They suffer, in truth, less from the disease, and are not so subject to it.

Now the diagnosis of the strange malady has been made evident while discussing the symptoms. It need be but further pointed out that its early manifestations might be mistaken for *irritant poisoning*, and that we can only tell their meaning prior to the development of the phenomena in the muscles by the detection of trichinæ in the stools. Again, it must be borne in mind that in some cases the first manifestations of the complaint do not happen for two or three weeks after the infected meat has been eaten; and that others show a very chronic course, and the whole disease is very protracted. The so-called "*sausage poisoning*," not dependent on trichinæ, differs from trichiniasis in its rapid course and the quick appearance of the symptoms after the spoiled sausages have been partaken of.* There is a peculiar disease of the arteries, *periarteriitis nodosa*, which, with the signs of acute desquamative nephritis and fever, gives rise to small swell-

---

* See Falck, in Virchow's Handbuch der Path. und Therap., vol. ii. p. 328.

ings under the skin, to rapid loss of muscular power with deficient electro-muscular contractility, and to such severe muscular pains that they are readily mistaken for those of the
trichinous affection.* But the history of the ailment, the
signs of the thickening of the vessels, and, if necessary, an examination of the muscles, will throw light on the cause of the
muscular distress. Indeed, in any instance, no matter what
be the complaint trichiniasis may simulate, there is but one
means of determining the presence of the flesh-worms positively—to examine a piece of muscle. This may be effected
by cutting down upon a muscle and removing sufficient of
its structure for a microscopical examination, or by using
Middeldorpff's harpoon or Duchenne's trocar to accomplish
the same purpose,—modes of diagnosis, it must be confessed,
of an aggressive kind, not likely to be readily submitted
to: though where they become necessary, I would suggest
anæsthesia, general or local, as a preliminary measure.

The chief epidemics of trichiniasis have occurred in Germany; but we have not escaped in this country.† Nor can
we claim that our hogs are not infected. On the contrary,
the report of the Chicago Academy shows that about 1 in 50
contains trichinæ in the muscles.‡ Our comparative immu-
nity from the affection is due to the pork being much more
generally cooked thoroughly before it is eaten; for the only
prophylactic is thorough cooking, prolonged exposure to high
temperature killing the trichinæ. Salting and smoking are
preventive means of some value, but do not insure safety.
Pickling has little if any effect.

In the treatment of trichiniasis we have, unfortunately, no
agents in our possession which kill the worms or prevent
their rapid development. The ordinary vermifuges, creasote, picrate of potassa, turpentine, arsenic, and benzine, have

---

* Kussmaul and Maier, quoted in Schmidt's Jahrb., No. 8, 1868.

† See, for instance, Dalton, op. cit., and Medical Record, vol. iv. p. 82;
Krombein, Buffalo Med. and Surg. Journal, June, 1864; also epidemic in
Iowa Med. and Surg. Rep., July 14, 1866; and Ristini, Med. Record, 1866,
vol. i. p. 249; Buck, ib. 1869, vol. iv.; Hun, Transact. of New York State
Med. Society. 1869.

‡ Chicago Medical Examiner, May, 1866; quoted in Med. and Surg. Reporter, June 2, 1866.

been employed in vain to destroy the dangerous parasites; nor is it certain that carbolic acid has any more effect. The most useful treatment at present known consists in removing as many of the intestinal trichinæ as possible by purgatives, particularly by scruple doses of calomel, to be repeated two or three times in as many days, unless the first dose produce mucous evacuations. Besides this treatment by large doses of calomel, we must support our patient's strength, relieve his more prominent symptoms, so far as they can be relieved by medicinal means, and be careful not to check the diar- rhœa by opiates. When the intestinal irritation subsides, which it generally does at the beginning of the third week; quinine, and in convalescence, iron, should be administered. Iron has been found of essential service in relieving the œdema dependent upon anæmia, which comes on at a late stage of the malady or during recovery.

INDEX.

Lightning Source UK Ltd.
Milton Keynes UK
UKHW012016220219
337761UK00009B/343/P